BRITANNICA

Medical and Health Annual

98

Encyclopædia Britannica, Inc.
Chicago • London • Paris • Rome
Seoul • Sydney • Tokyo

1998 Medical and Health Annual

Library of Congress Catalog Card Number: 77-649875
International Standard Book Number: 0-85229-659-2
International Standard Serial Number: 0363-0366

A few words from the Editor…

Even though anatomists have been dissecting cadavers for centuries, it seems they had missed some small but significant body parts. Not yet gracing the pages of *Gray's Anatomy* or any other standard text—but described in detail in this volume ("The Anatomist's New Tools," pages 16–29)—are several heretofore unappreciated structures of the head and jaw. The authors, trailblazing dental researchers from Baltimore, Md., attribute their discoveries largely to the use of some wondrous new technological "tools," including the National Library of Medicine's amazing $1.4 million Visible Human Project.

What contemporary American physician's name is known by anyone who has ever worked in a restaurant or institutional kitchen—and is probably on the tip of most people's tongues? (It is also in the dictionary.) The answer: Henry Heimlich. In "Rebel with a Cause: Saving Lives" (pages 60–77), this celebrated surgeon-inventor-humanitarian, who is credited with having saved more lives than anyone else in the world, holds forth on the cause that, at age 76, continues to drive him.

In "The Body Synchronic" (pages 78–91), British and Swedish scientists, both pioneers in the fascinating field of chronobiology, shed light on the role that circadian rhythms play in human health and disease. Among other things, they explain the role of the "body clock" in determining when and how much humans (and other animals) sleep.

In pondering body clocks, the editors of the *Annual* became curious about the sleep needs of people with frantic schedules and international itineraries. So they did their own (not entirely scientific) survey of some well-known achievers from many walks of life. In "A Good Night's Sleep: Celebrities' Strategies" (pages 92–109), a former surgeon general, an actress who plays a TV doctor, a Nobel laureate, the "father" of hatha yoga, a former first lady and U.S. president, and 21 others disclose their personal approaches to R and R—ranging from avoiding naps "like the plague" to discreet dozing during lectures.

In last year's *Annual* we introduced "The Bookshelf," which got rave reviews from readers. So we have expanded the section; on pages 124–144 are reviews of 26 new books in the very broad medicine-health-psychology fields—from a comprehensive child-care guide (Dr. Spock for the 21st century?) to a novel by a practicing psychiatrist to a collection of essays about the brains of celebrated athletes.

The Tuskegee Study of Untreated Syphilis in the Negro Male (1932–72)—the longest-running nontherapeutic experiment on humans in the history of public health—came to an *official* close only this year, with a presidential apology (***NewsCap,*** pages 280–281). The legacy of the Tuskegee study persists, however, in the form of a deep-seated distrust of the medical establishment by African-Americans. These attitudes and, in particular, their impact on AIDS awareness in the black community are examined in "Spreading the Gospel of AIDS Prevention" (pages 150–155). The authors propose some highly innovative ways that churches and gospel radio—sources that are trusted in ways that health professionals and government officials are not—can mobilize this community to confront the HIV/AIDS epidemic, by which it has been so hard hit.

Since the first HIV/AIDS cases were identified in the early 1980s, the *Medical and Health Annual*'s coverage of the epidemic's clinical, social, economic, and political aspects has been extensive; this year is no different. The unrelenting toll of AIDS is the subject of the first article, "The Fabric of Their Lives" (pages 6–15)—a compelling photo essay.

Is psychotherapy inevitably a long, costly, drawn-out process? Definitely not. In "Spotlight on Brief Therapy" (pages 290–293), a clinical psychologist, known internationally for his work in treating depression with active, brief methods, offers practical advice for those seeking short-term treatment.

Is it true that a clove of garlic a day will do what the proverbial apple is said to do—only better? In "Is Everything Coming Up Roses for Garlic?" (pages 222–229), a chemist examines the fragrant herb's purported abilities to prevent cancer, lower the risk of cardiovascular disease, and promote longevity. (Garlic is not the only dietary substance considered on the pages that follow. Salt, the carotenoids, cholesterol, selenium, zinc, fluoride, "junk food," and beef from "mad cows" are some of the others.)

Health policy is another area that comes in for scrutiny. Three contributors to this volume examine the health care delivery systems of three countries—the U.S., Canada, and the U.K.—and find that none is in peak health.

Just as this book was going to press, in September, two popular prescription weight-loss drugs, suspected of causing heart-valve problems, were withdrawn from the market. In "Body Weight: Biology, Not Behavior" (pages 307–310), experts examine the whole class of medications now being used in the treatment of obesity. They also describe the recent leaps in the understanding of the problem, including the appreciation that weight gain and loss may be genetically determined.

I have mentioned just a handful of topics that receive considerable attention in the *1998 Annual,* a volume that we (the editors and artists who worked on it) hope will help readers keep pace with the exciting developments in medicine and health. Our goal was to produce a timely and stimulating resource; we hope we have succeeded. Whenever possible, we have listed other sources of information—including lots of Web sites—for those who want to learn more.

—Ellen Bernstein

Contents

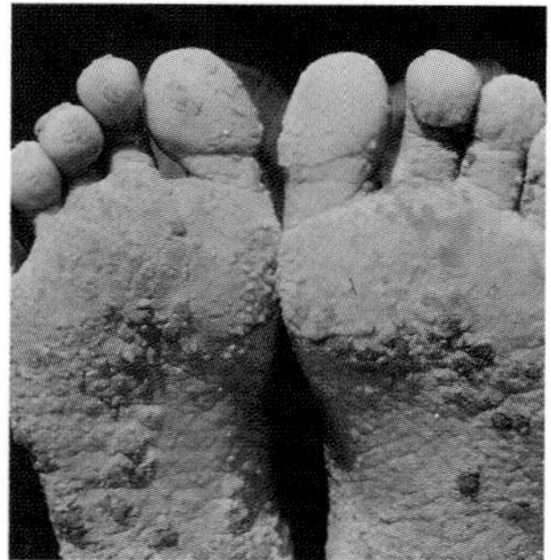

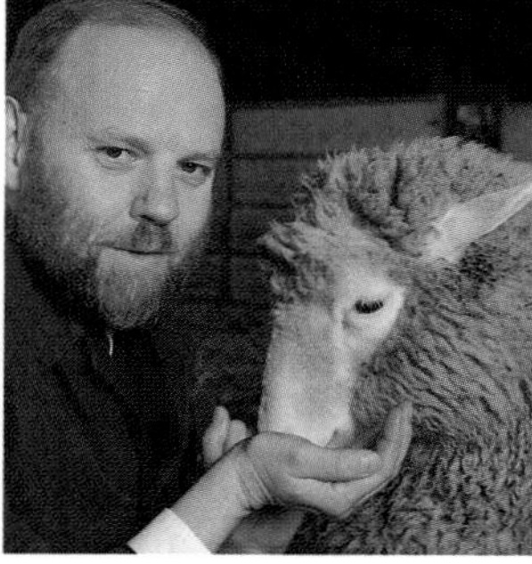

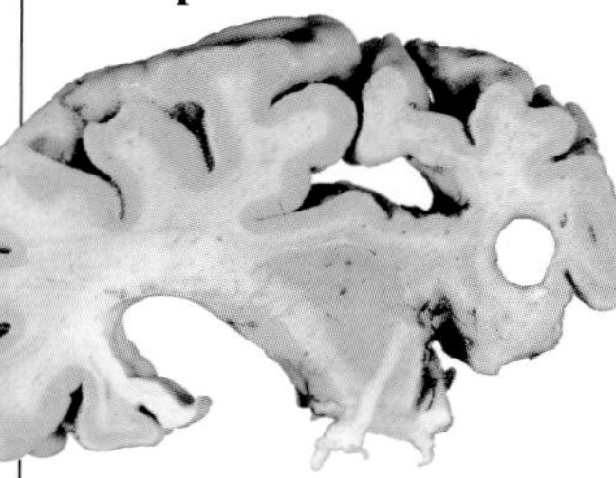

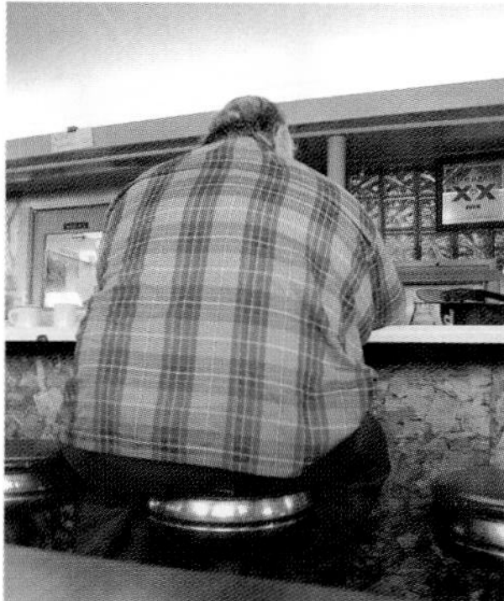

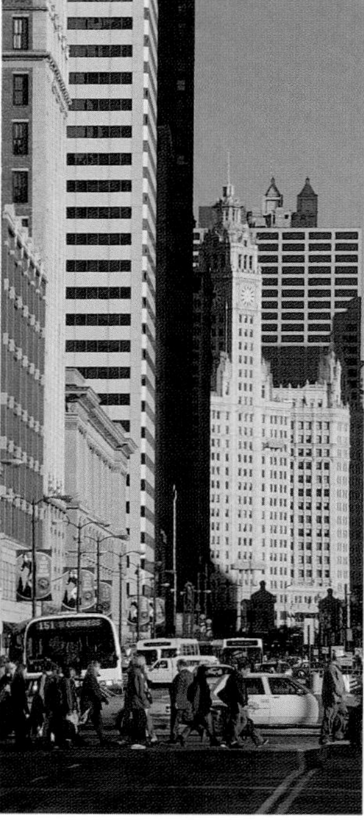

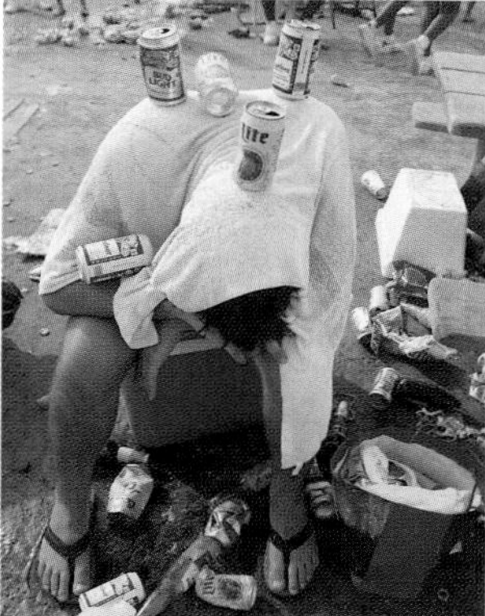

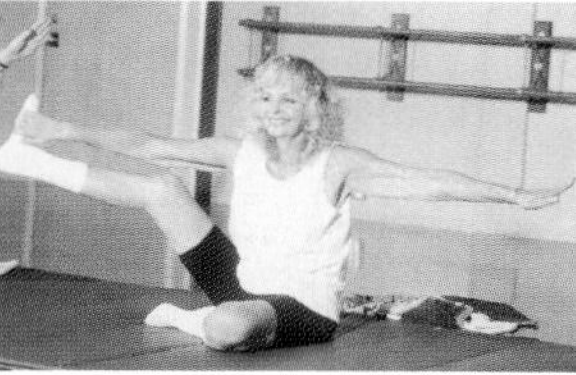

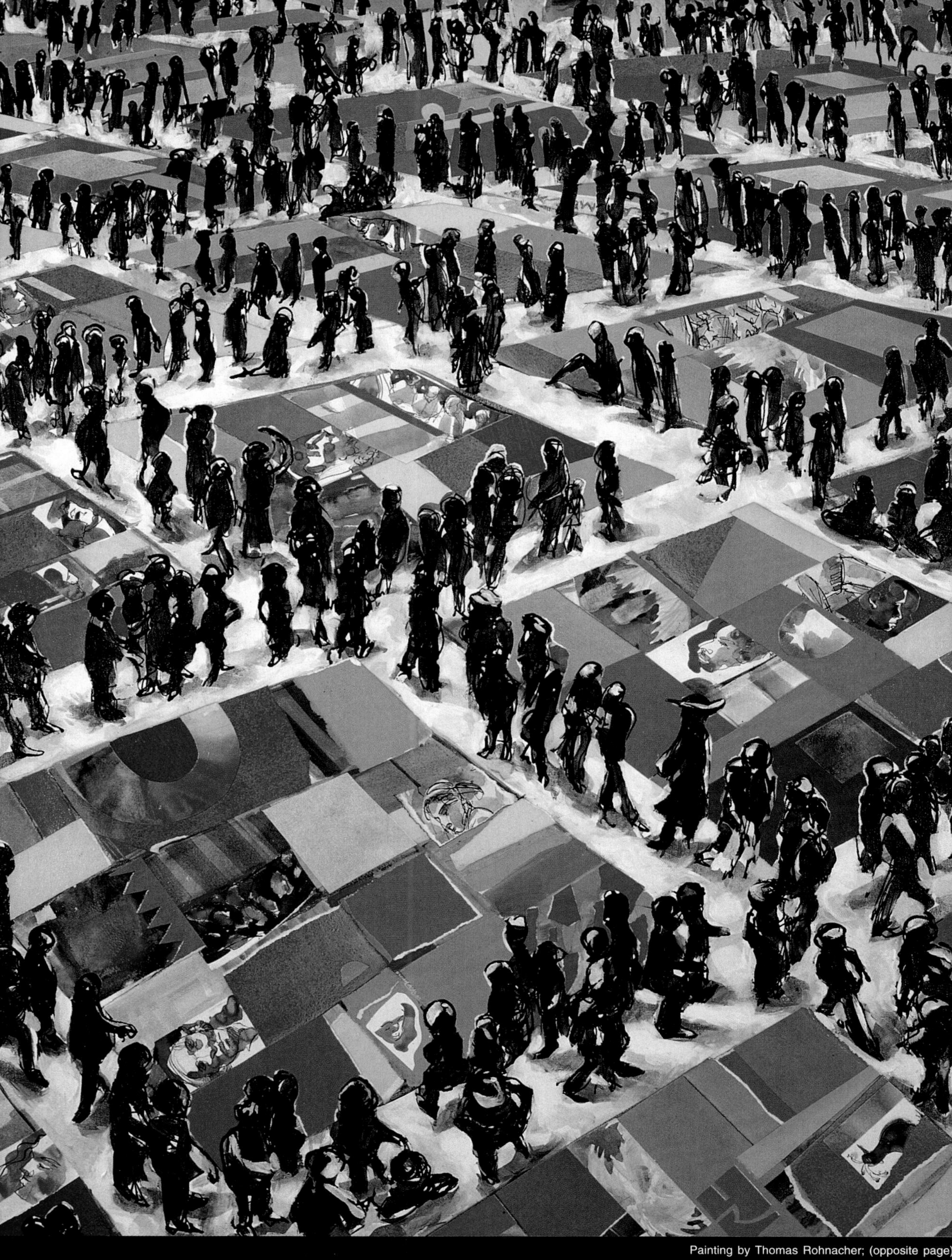

Painting by Thomas Rohnacher; (opposite page) Dennis Brack—Black Star

The Fabric of Their Lives
A Photo Essay

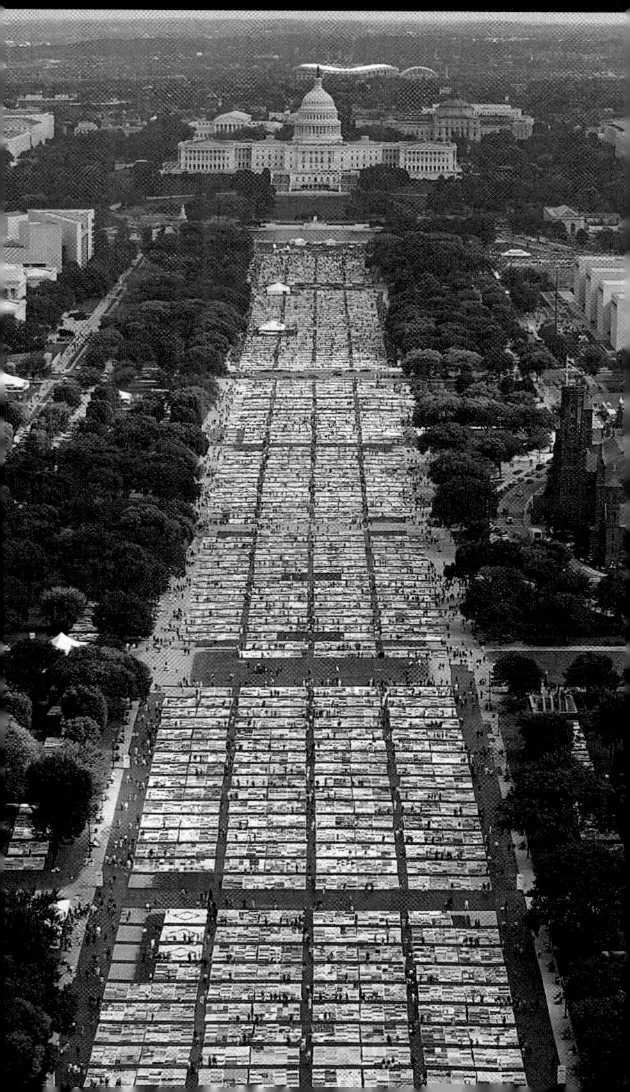

It began a decade ago as two single hand-sewn fabric panels—each measuring about 90 centimeters × 180 centimeters (3 feet × 6 feet)—commemorating two young men, Marvin Feldman and Ed Mock, both San Franciscans who had died of AIDS when it was still a "new" disease. At last count (in March 1997) it had grown to the size of 25 football fields, weighed a whopping 56 tons, and consisted of 42,537 panels created by artists and would-be artists from every corner of the globe. In 1996 alone, no fewer than 1,228,340 volunteer hours were devoted to the creation of this dramatic work in progress. Its messages, paying tribute to hundreds of thousands of individual men, women, and children whose lives have been lost to the AIDS pandemic, are expressed in materials as diverse as burlap, buttons, Barbie dolls, bubble wrap, champagne glasses, condoms, credit cards, love letters, pearls, car keys, cremation ashes, stuffed animals, tennis shoes, and wedding rings.

International visitors remember loved ones during the most recent (1996) showing of the quilt on the Mall in the U.S. capital.

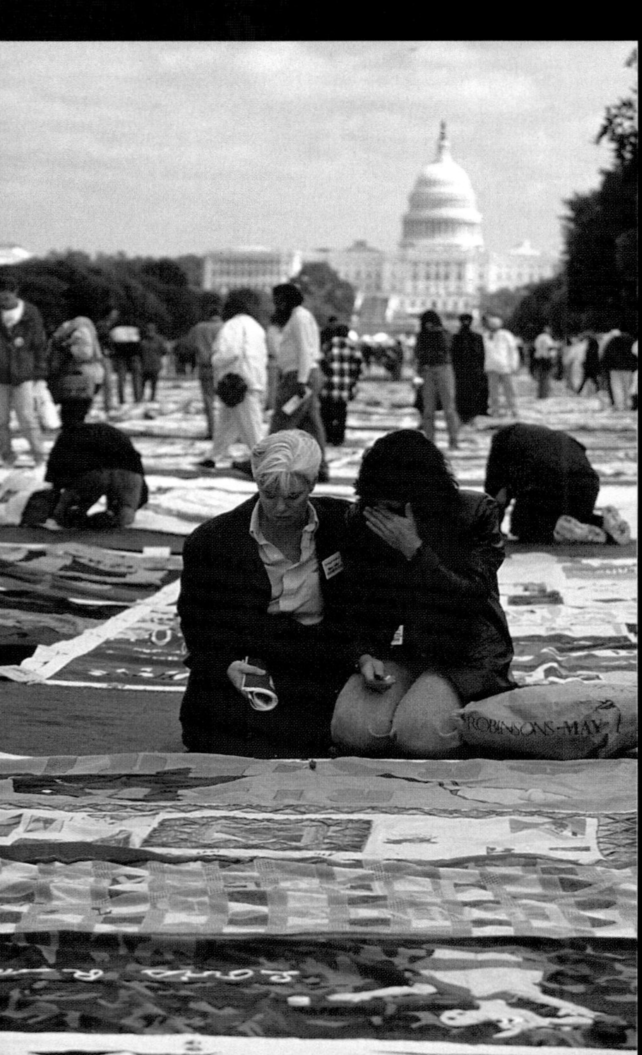

Dirck Halstead—Gamma Liaison

Selected recent additions to the NAMES Project Memorial Quilt appear on these opening pages of the *Annual.* They come from across the U.S. and several continents. Each panel eloquently tells its own story; together they provide a powerful visual reminder of the continuing AIDS tragedy that has left no segment of the global community untouched.

What more is there to say about the largest patchwork community art project in the world that has not been articulated in its individual messages of love and loss? Very little. Just a few facts:

- In the quilt's first public showing (June 1987), 40 of its panels hung from the balcony of the mayor's office in San Francisco.
- The quilt has been shown five times in its entirety on the Mall in Washington, D.C.—the first time in October 1987 and most recently in October 1996.
- Between 1987 and 1997 over eight million people viewed the quilt, which had been displayed in one form or another around the world many hundreds of times.
- In 1989 the quilt was nominated for the Nobel Peace Prize; that same year the film *Common Threads: Stories from the Quilt* won an Academy Award for the best feature-length documentary.
- There are currently 45 NAMES Projects chapters in the U.S. and 36 independent affiliates worldwide.
- Among the better-known individuals to whom panels of the quilt have been dedicated are: tennis player Arthur Ashe; director/choreographer Michael Bennett; Kimberly Bergalis, a young Florida woman who was infected during a dental procedure; fashion designers Tina Chow, Perry Ellis, Willi Smith, and Halston; ballet dancer Rudolf Nureyev; actors Anthony Perkins, Robert Reed, Brad Davis, and Rock Hudson; artist Keith Haring; photographer Robert Mapplethorpe; news anchor Max Robinson; and Washington Redskin Jerry Smith.
- Anyone who wants more information about the memorial quilt or the NAMES organization can write to NAMES Project, 310 Townsend Street, Suite 310, San Francisco CA 94107-1639; E-mail the project at info@aidsquilt.org; or visit its Web site at http://www.aidsquilt.org. MHA

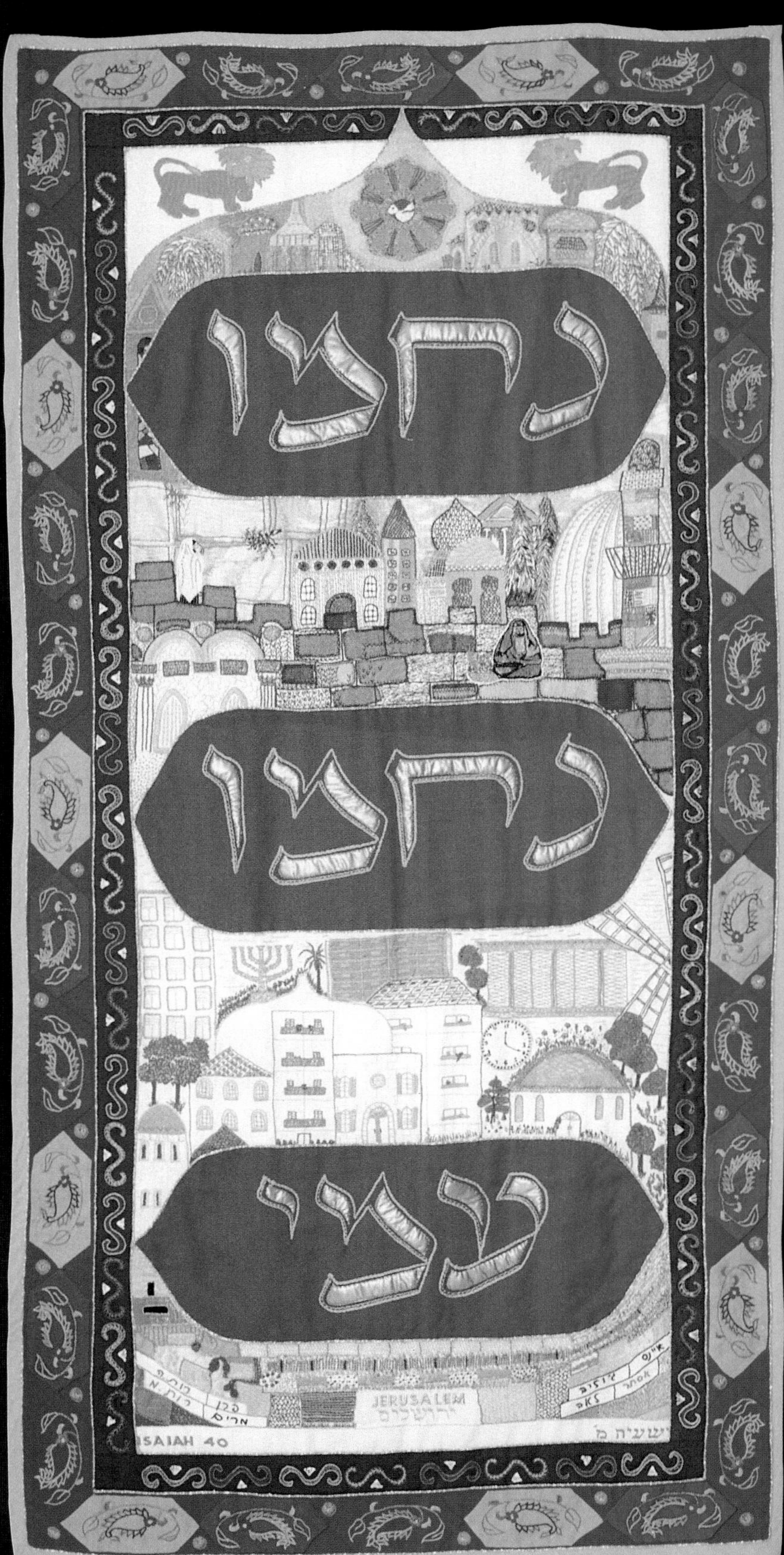

The Jerusalem Panel, the work of the Jerusalem Embroiderers, is dedicated to those who are HIV-positive or living with AIDS as well as to the memory of those who have died. The panel took a year to complete and was first shown in 1995. The text, from Isaiah 40:1, reads, "Comfort, comfort my people."

Proyect HaShemot; photograph, Douglas Guthrie, Jerusalem

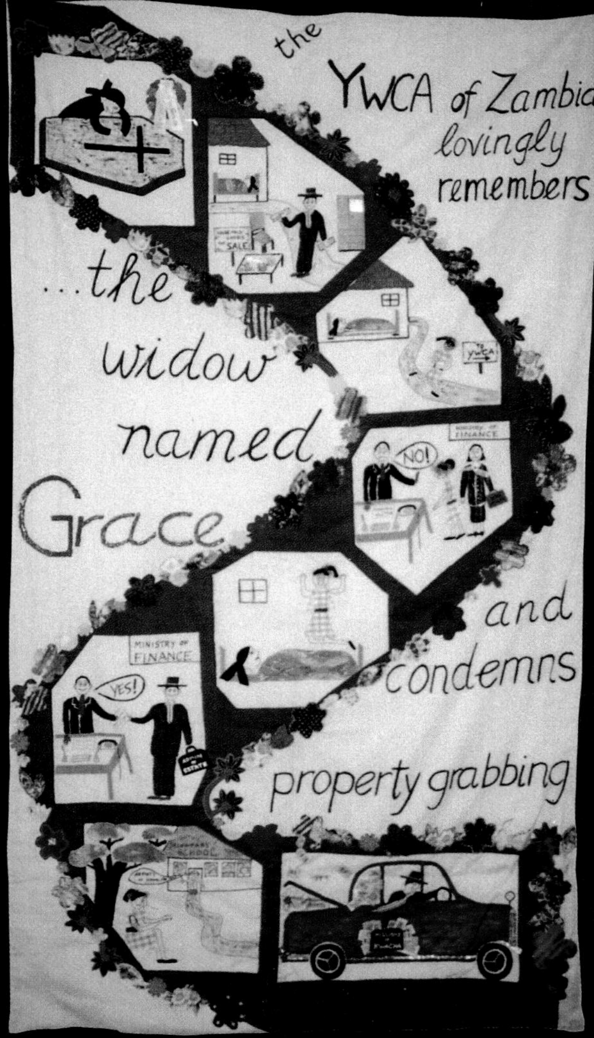

(Right) The AIDS Memorial Panel of the YWCA of Zambia recounts, in eight sequential scenes, the sad story of a woman named Grace. After her husband dies of a disease suspected to be AIDS, his brother, acting as executor, attempts to appropriate the widow's death benefits, which she needs to provide for the couple's only child, a daughter named Precious. Grace dies after a long and futile legal battle with her brother-in-law, and the money goes to him. He keeps most of it, buying himself a new automobile and leaving the orphaned Precious to fend for herself. (Bottom) A beadwork panel in a Zulu design made by the staff of the Western Province AIDS Training, Information and Counselling Centre in Gugulethu, South Africa; the names of the deceased were left off deliberately by family members, who feared possible reprisals.

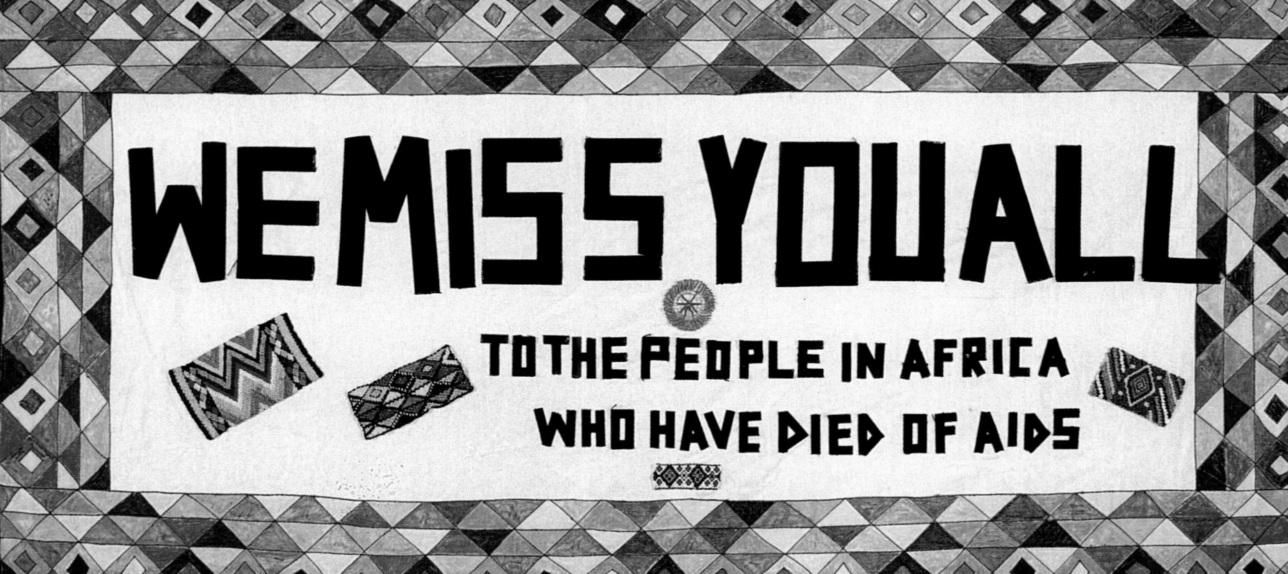

(Top) Zambia AIDS Memorial Quilt; photograph, Ilse Mwanza; (bottom) The NAMES Project: South Africa Cape Town Committee; photograph, Bruce Sutherland

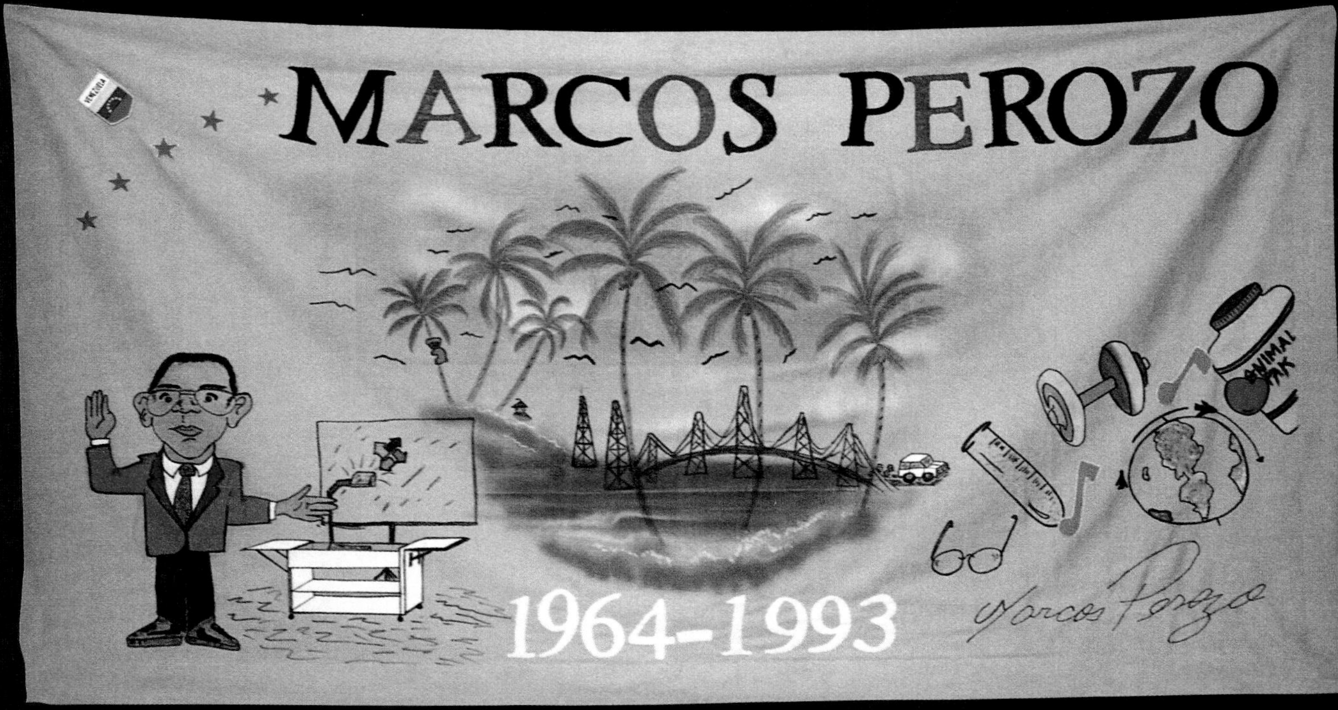

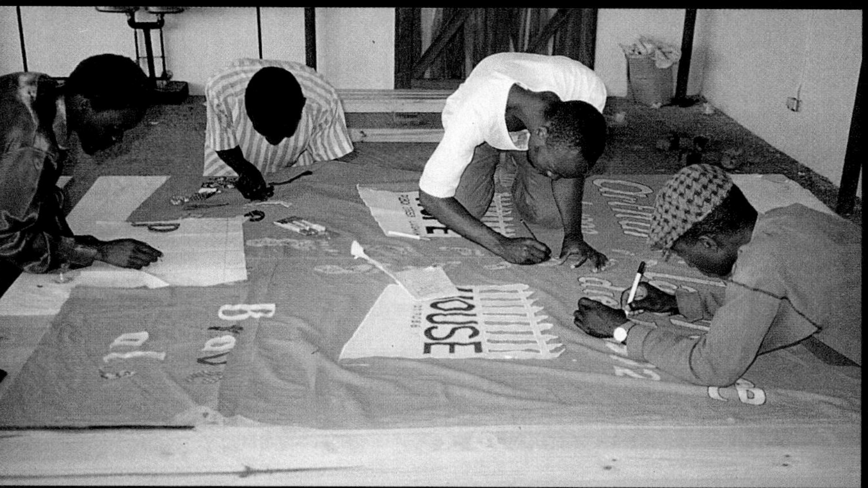

(Top) The quilt panel for Marcos Perozo, put together over a four-month period in 1995 by his colleagues at the English Resource Center in Caracas, Venezuela. (Left) A group in Lusaka, Zambia, prepares a panel in memory of two founders of Hope House—an information and outreach center and shelter for persons living with AIDS. The creators themselves later succumbed to the disease. (Bottom) Members of the Taiwan AIDS Memorial Quilt Project at work.

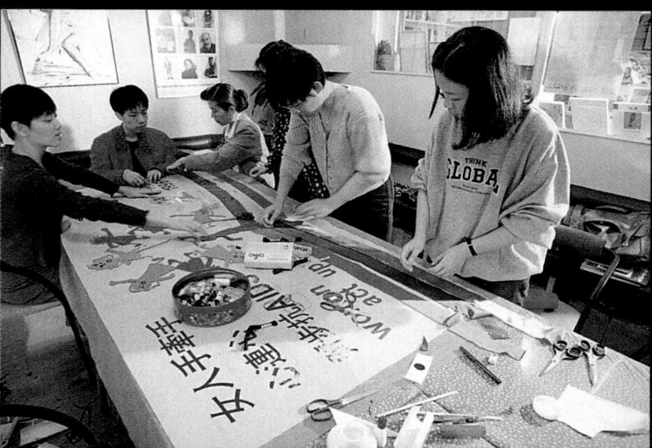

(Top) Fundación MAROZO; (center) Zambia AIDS Memorial Quilt; (bottom) Taiwan AIDS Memorial Quilt Project

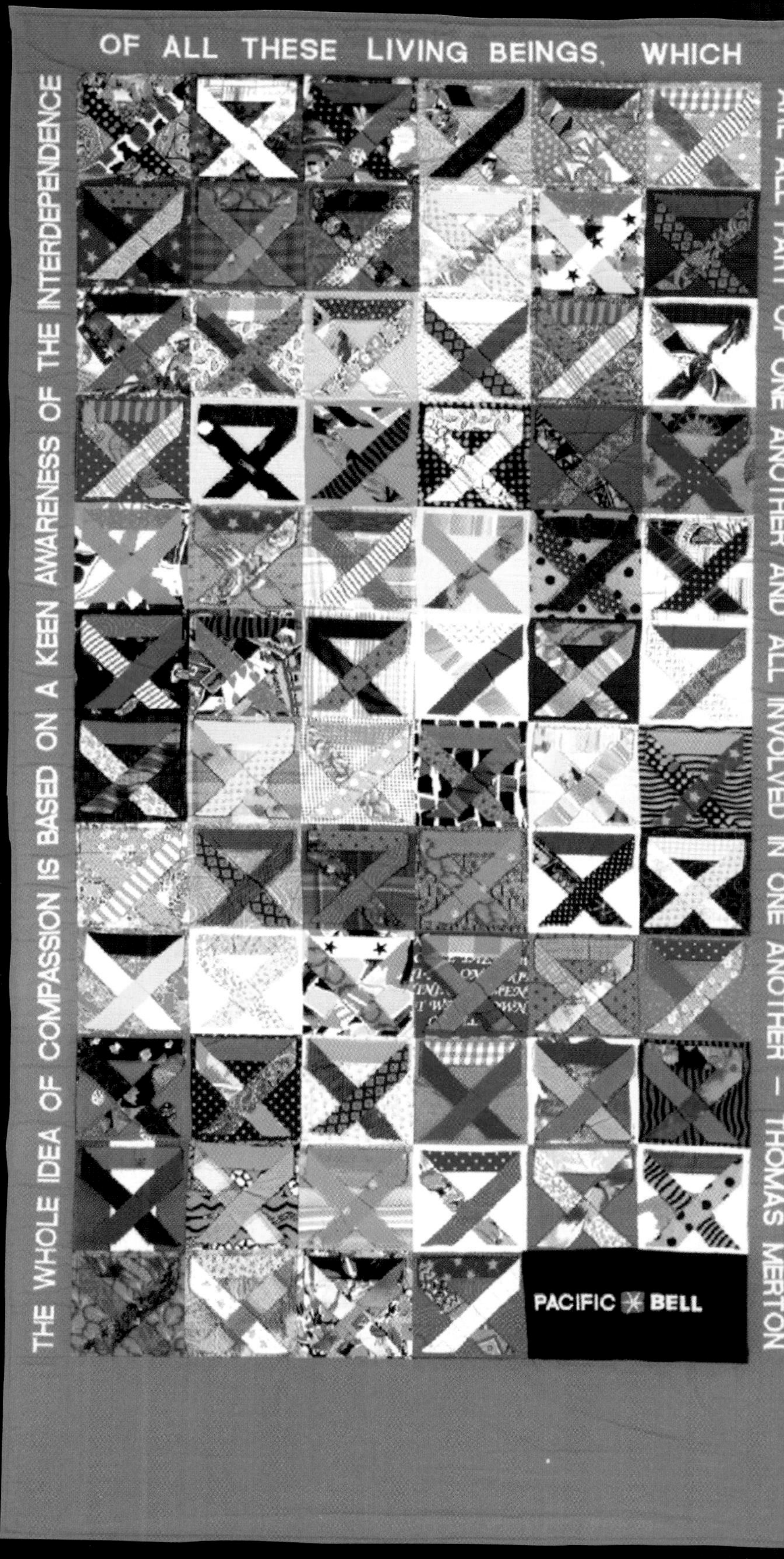

THE WHOLE IDEA OF COMPASSION IS BASED ON A KEEN AWARENESS OF THE INTERDEPENDENCE
OF ALL THESE LIVING BEINGS, WHICH
ARE ALL PART OF ONE ANOTHER AND ALL INVOLVED IN ONE ANOTHER – THOMAS MERTON
PACIFIC BELL

The Pacific Bell AIDS Memorial Quilt, dedicated to company employees who died of AIDS and related illnesses, was designed and stitched together by master quilt makers in California. Each square is made of four pieces of fabric, each piece representing an individual who died. The motif of the AIDS awareness ribbon is repeated in each of the 70 squares.

(Left) The quilt on display in Taipei, Taiwan, on World AIDS Day, Dec. 1, 1995. (Center) "Joining hands is a symbol of solidarity and love for life" is the message of the panel made by volunteers at Centro Solidarietà Genova in Genoa, Italy, a lodging for people with HIV. (Bottom) Panoramic views of Geoffrey Towes's native New York City and Cape Town, South Africa, where he spent his last days, bracket an open sea, upon which sails the *Achille Lauro,* the ship he served on as purser.

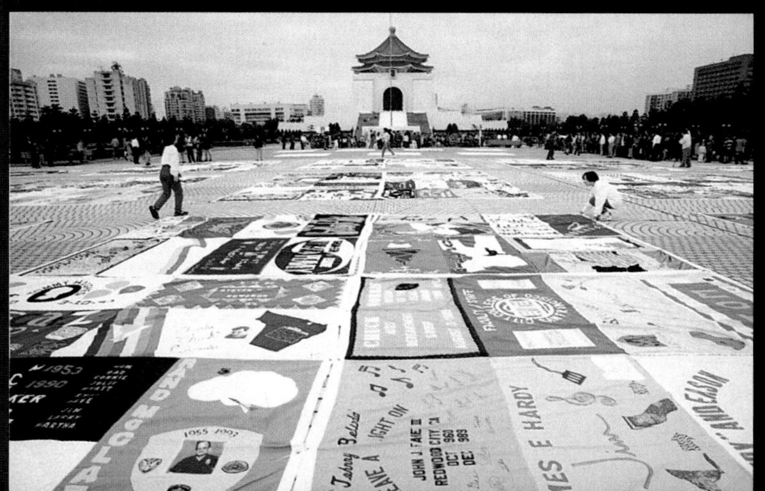

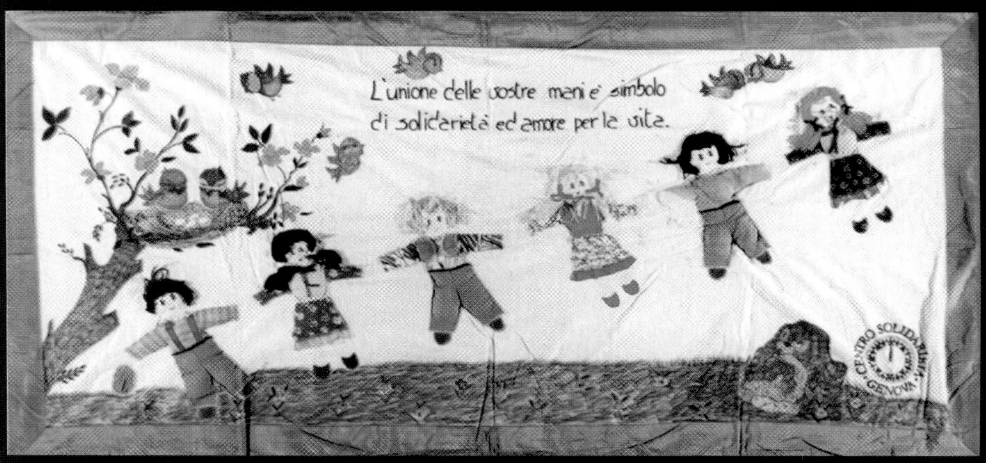

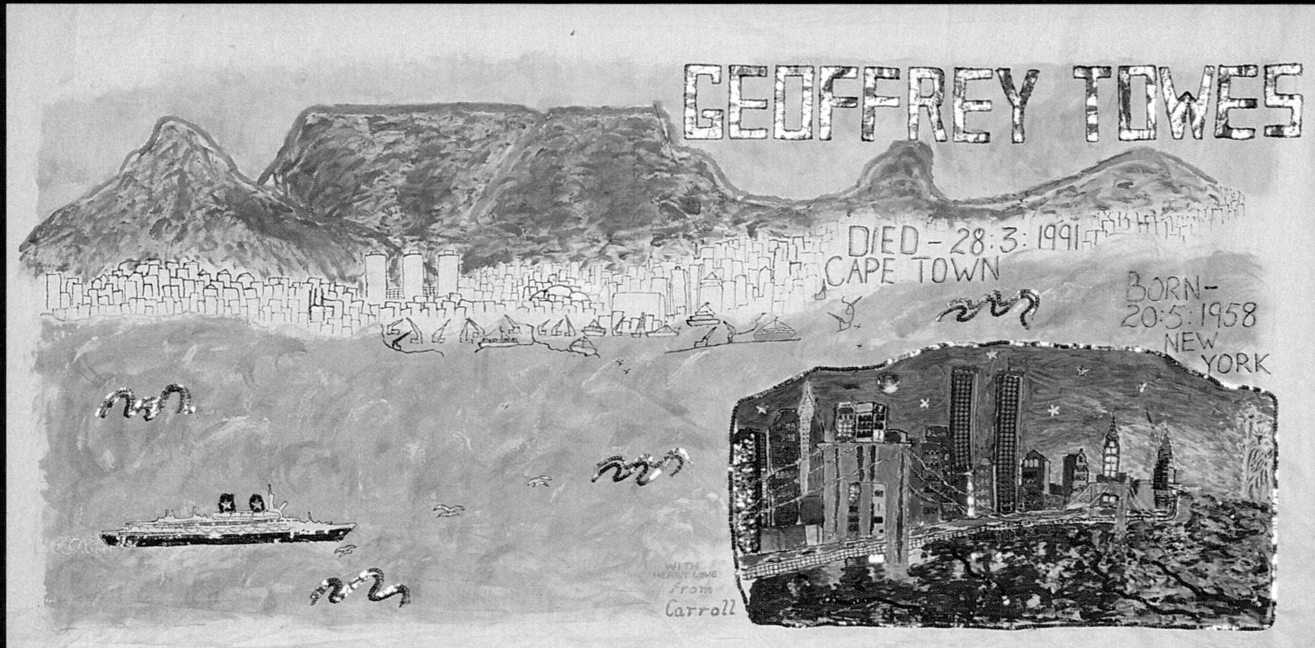

(Top) Taiwan AIDS Memorial Quilt Project; (center) NAMES Project Italy under the sponsorship of ASA, Milan; photograph, Lorenzo Ceva, Milan; (bottom) The NAMES Project: South Africa Cape Town Committee; photographs, Bruce Sutherland

(Right) Antonisia was only five months old when she died of AIDS at Nazareth House in South Africa; her quilt panel incorporates a few of her favorite items, including a dress, a bonnet, a bib, and a teething ring. (Below) The colorful Danish NAMES quilt comprises panels for eight individuals who died of AIDS.

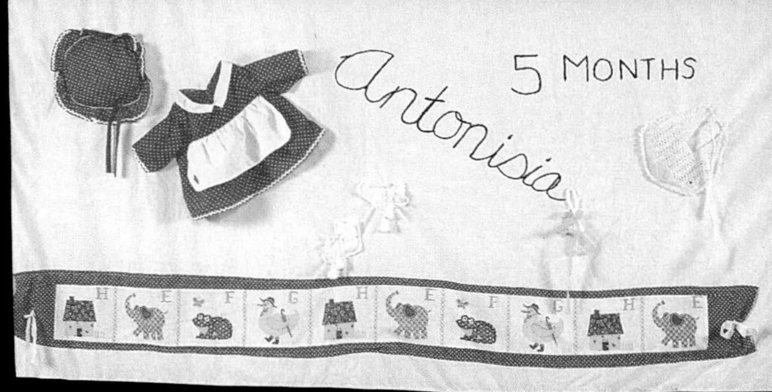

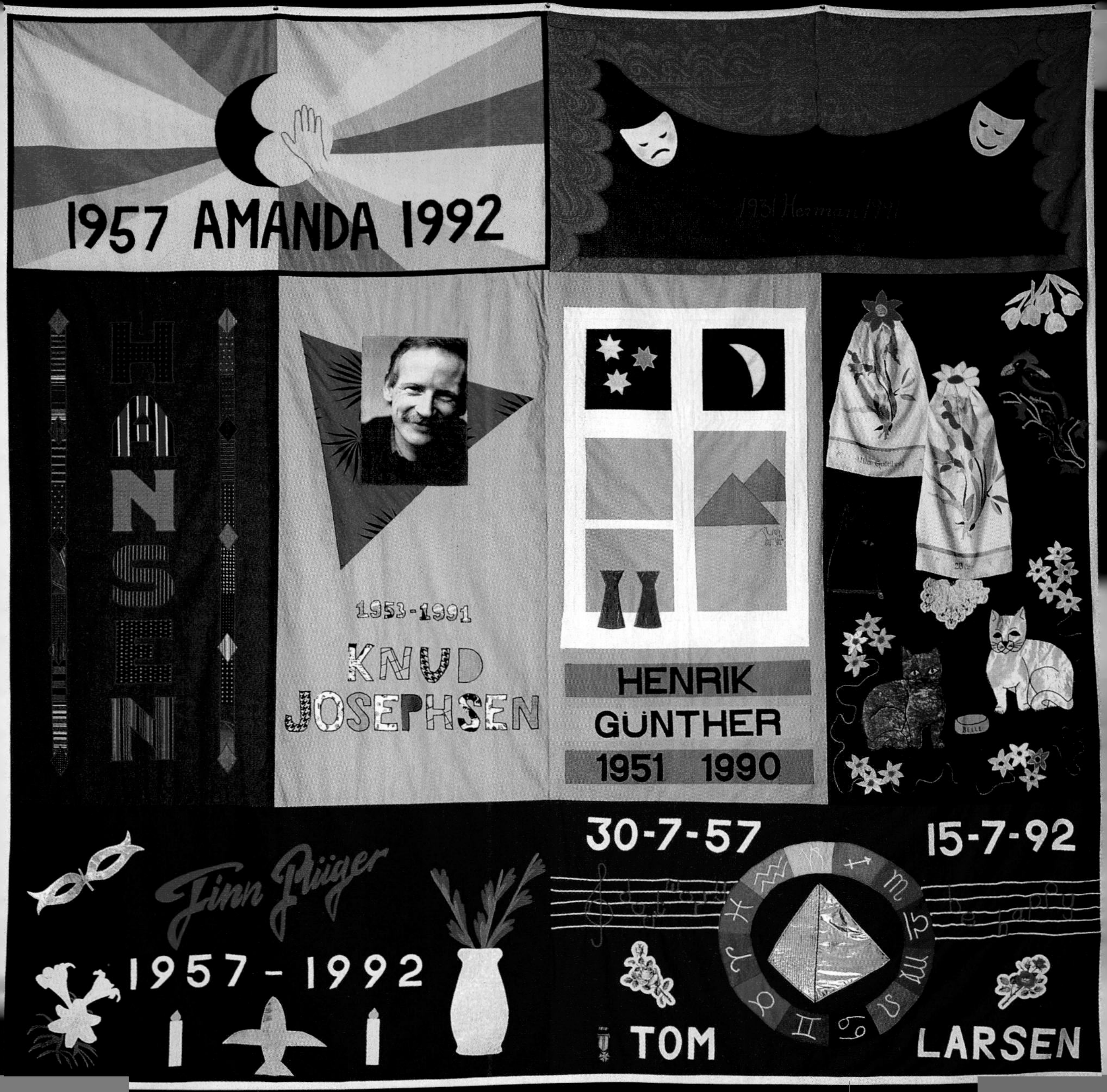

ject: South Africa Ca
therland; (bottom) Da

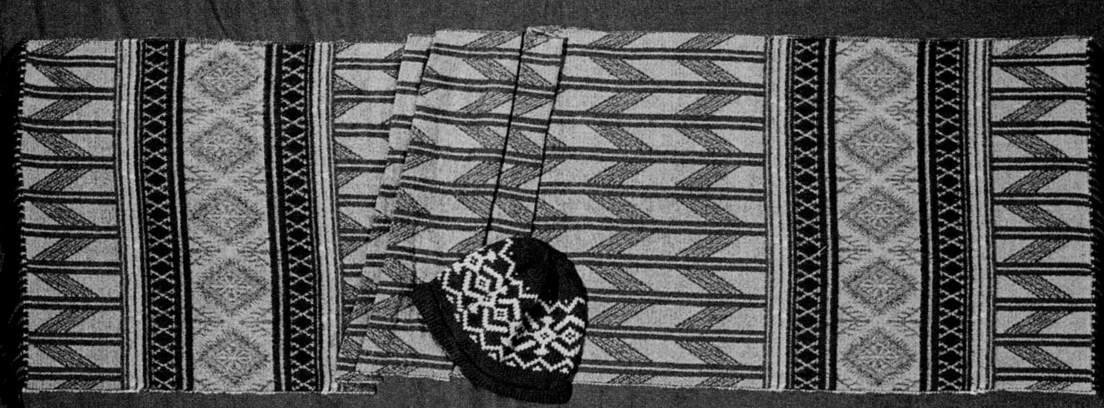

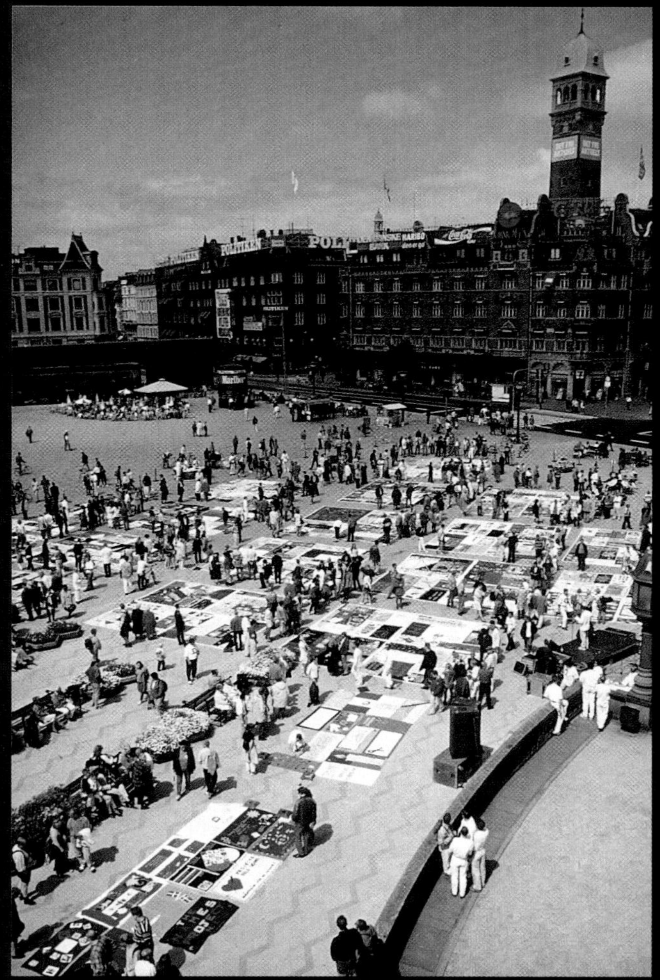

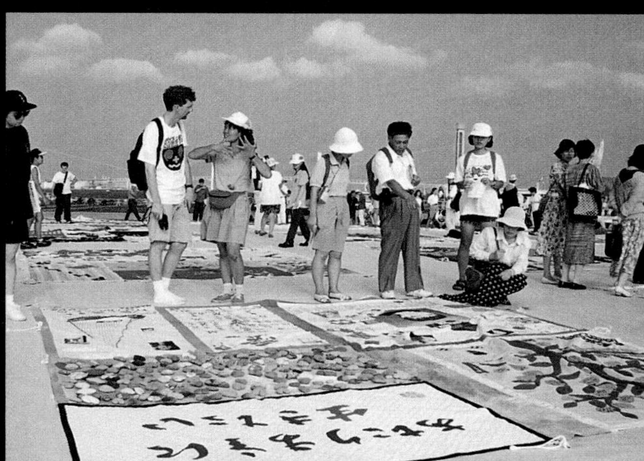

(Top) The panel for a German AIDS victim, Rainer Hawel, was contributed by his companion from England and includes Rainer's favorite cap and scarf. (Left) Quilt panels from affiliates of the NAMES Project in 14 European countries are displayed in Copenhagen's Town Hall Square during the Europride Festival in June 1996. (Above) In conjunction with the X International Conference on AIDS in Yokohama, Japan, in 1994, Memorial Quilt Japan organized a large-scale display that involved 634 panels from 17 countries.

(Top) Münchner AIDS-Hilfe; photograph, Johannes Weiss; (bottom left) Danish NAMES Project; (bottom right) AIDS Memorial Quilt International Display/Yokohama; Memorial Quilt Japan

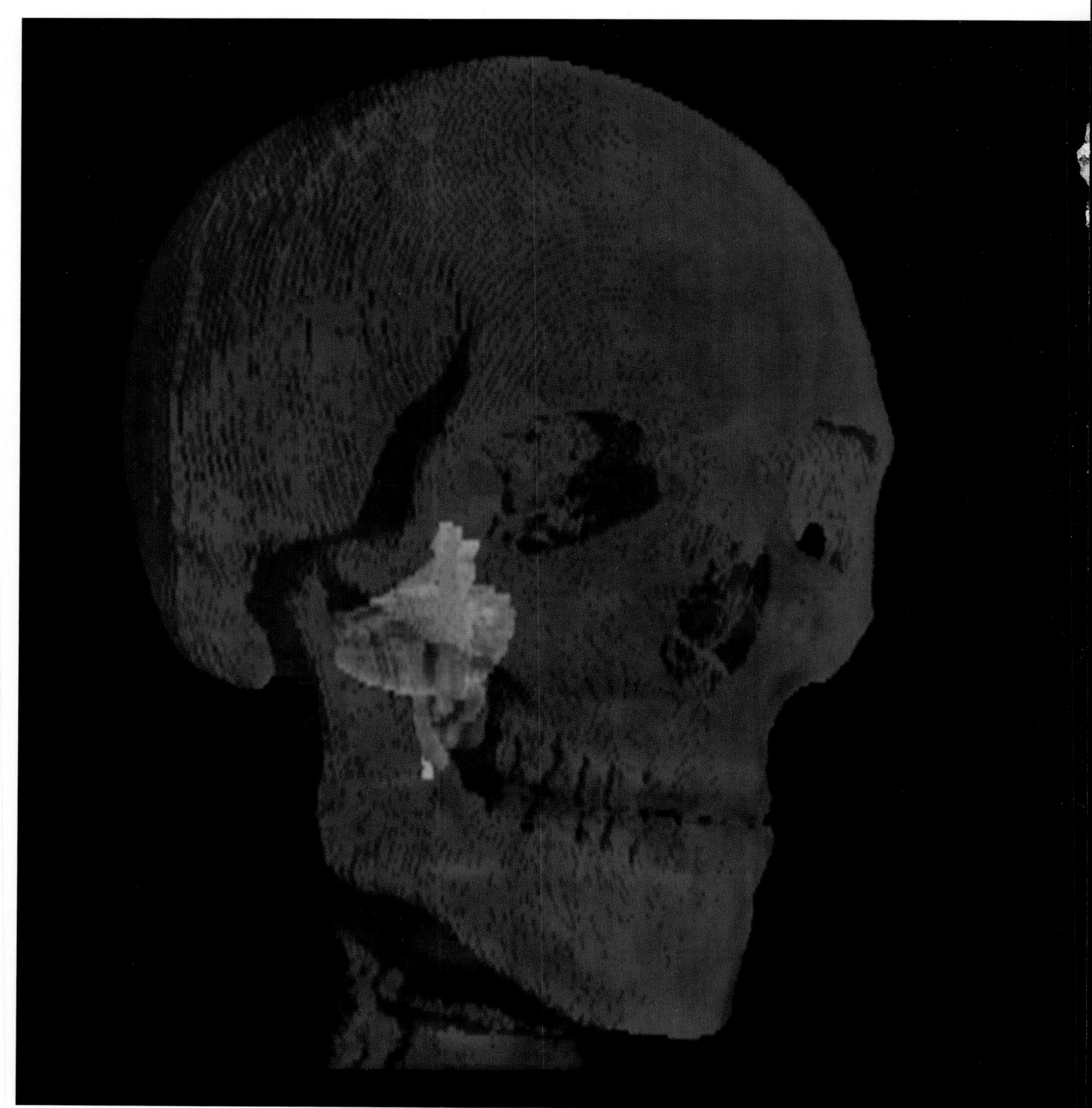

The Anatomist's New Tools

by Gary D. Hack, D.D.S., Gwendolyn Dunn, D.D.S., and Mi Young Toh, M.S., M.A.

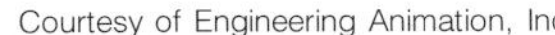

Courtesy of Engineering Animation, Inc.

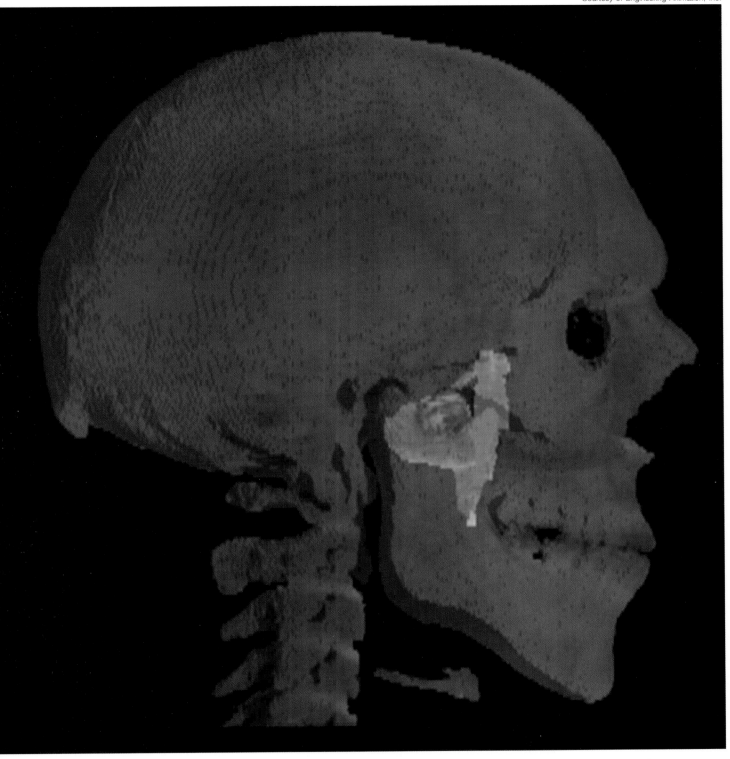

Gentlemen, damn the sphenoid bone!

—Oliver Wendell Holmes (1809–94), at the opening of his anatomy lectures at Harvard Medical School

The announcement of a new anatomic discovery is always astonishing—and it is all the more so at a time when anatomy departments in medical and dental schools around the world are closing their doors. Indeed, many would consider anatomic research a moribund field—or, in any case, one that had long ago reached its limits. Has not every bone, tissue, muscle, joint, organ, and vessel of the human body been not only identified but immortalized on the pages of *Gray's Anatomy,* among other time-honored medical texts?

Yet as recently as 1996, just such an announcement *was* made. Scientists at the University of Maryland at Baltimore (these authors among them) discovered and reported on a physical connection between the muscular system and the central nervous system that had never previously been described in the medical literature. This finding may go a long way toward helping to explain the relationship between headache and muscle tension.

Just an everyday dissection

The discovery was serendipitous, occurring during inspection of a sagittally sectioned cadaver specimen (*i.e.,* one that had been cut from front to back, revealing internal structures on the left and right sides). The scientists, who were interested in examining the muscles of mastication (chewing) from unusual perspectives, noticed that the deep neck musculature was physically attached to the dura, the highly sensitive membranous covering of the brain and spinal cord. The specific muscle that captured their attention—the one that was actually attaching to the dura—was the rectus capitis posterior minor (RCPM) muscle, which extends from the base of the skull to the first cervical vertebra (C_1), or atlas, in the upper region of the neck. A bridge of tissue appeared to be connecting the RCPM muscle to the spinal dura at the atlanto-occipital junction (the space between the occipital bone (C_0) at the base of the skull and the atlas.

Anatomist Andreas Vesalius (1514–64) lectures at Padua. The Renaissance Flemish physician performed dissections with a degree of meticulosity hitherto unknown; his detailed descriptions and illustrations of the human body revolutionized the practice of medicine.

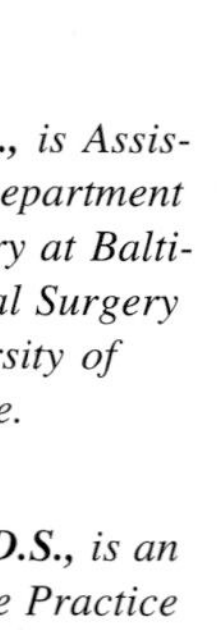

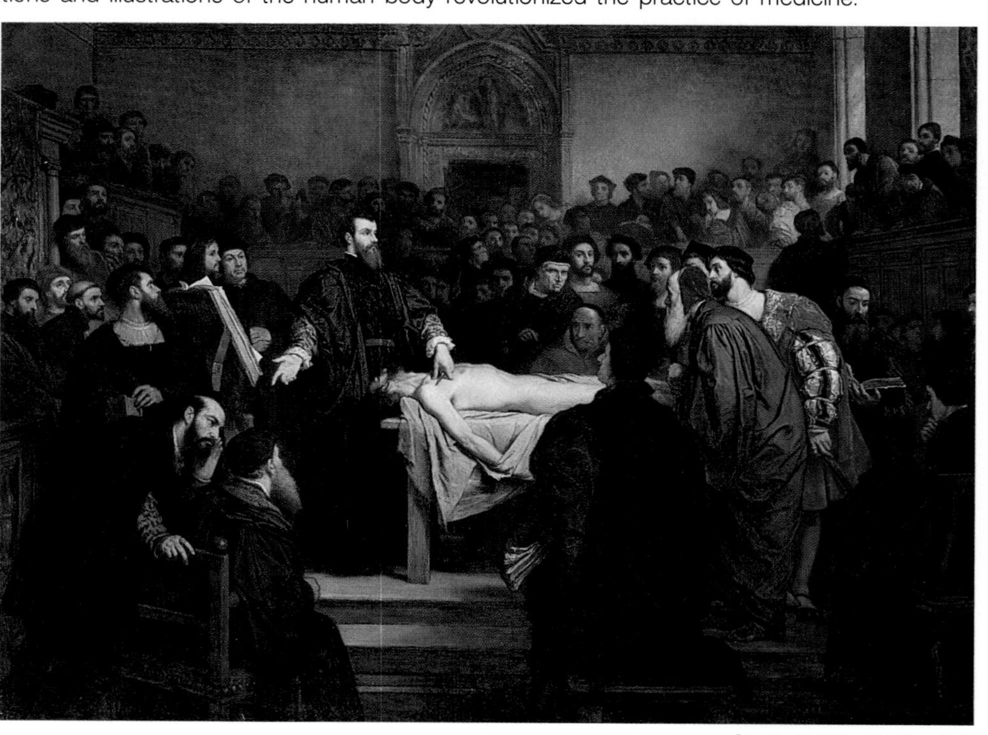

Giraudon/Art Resource, New York

Gary D. Hack, D.D.S., is Assistant Professor in the Department of Restorative Dentistry at Baltimore College of Dental Surgery Dental School, University of Maryland at Baltimore.

Gwendolyn Dunn, D.D.S., is an Orthodontist in Private Practice and Volunteer Dissector in Anatomical Services at the University of Maryland at Baltimore.

Mi Young Toh, M.S., M.A., is a Biomedical Imaging Researcher who has worked on the Visible Human Project at the National Library of Medicine, National Institutes of Health, Bethesda, Maryland.

Courtesy of Gary D. Hack, Gwendolyn Dunn, and Mi Young Toh

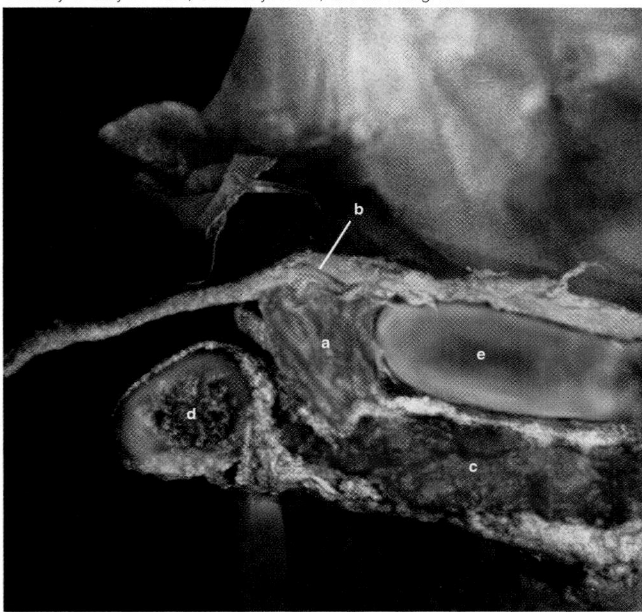

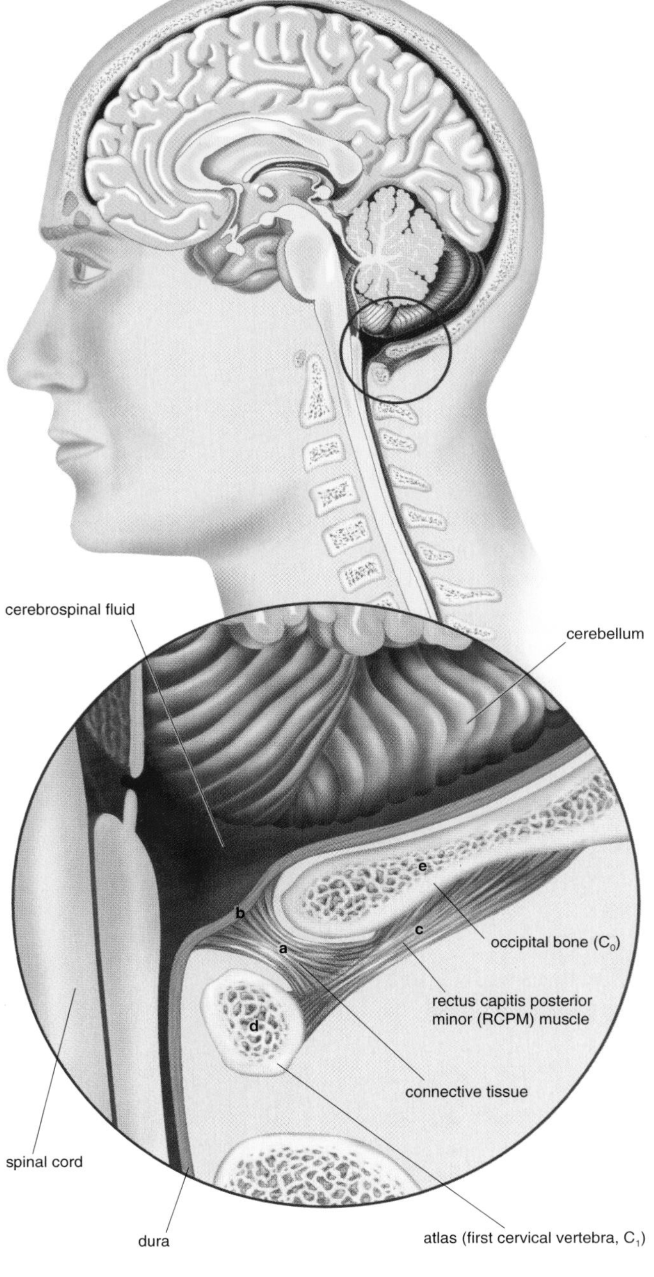

(Right) Illustration revealing a newly discovered tissue bridge (a) connecting the dura, the membranous covering of the brain and spinal cord (b), to the rectus capitis posterior minor (RCPM) muscle (c) at the base of the skull between the atlas (C_1) (d) and occipital bone (C_0) (e). (Above) Cadaver specimen showing the same structures.

While the RCPM muscle is described in considerable anatomic detail in standard textbooks of anatomy, its physical connection to the dura had not been noted.

Since their discovery the Maryland scientists have observed this previously unheralded connection in dissection after dissection in cadaver after cadaver. Additionally, an animal model (the *Macaca fascicularis* monkey) has been identified, which has allowed the scientists to investigate further; in each of more than 10 consecutive *M. fascicularis* dissections, just such a tissue bridge was revealed to them.

The scientists' announcement was initially met with polite skepticism—if not a few raised eyebrows. After all, anatomists had been rigorously studying the human body for over 500 years, and neurosurgeons routinely operate in the region of the "new" tissue. (While gross anatomy, the study of body structures as seen with the naked eye, is an ancient discipline, the science did not flourish until the Renaissance, reaching its culmination between 1500 and 1850, by which time the anatomic structures of the human body and their interrelationships were thought to be well established.) Why, then, had the physical relationship between the RCPM muscle and the spinal dura *not* been previously described? Had it truly been overlooked?

The Maryland team credits the discovery to the unorthodox angle from which the dissection was performed. To fully appreciate the three-dimensional packing of the anatomic structures of the head-neck region, the researchers considered it important to be able to view the area in question from various perspectives; that meant approaching the structures from more than one angle. Whereas the conventional anatomy laboratory approach to the dissection they were performing is from the back of the neck, the scientists in Baltimore made their incision from the side. The former approach does not disclose the muscle-dura tissue bridge, but the unorthodox approach did!

Gross anatomy is not a big field of medical research these days, and when scientists perform dissections, most are not likely to experiment with unusual approaches. Nor do they expect to discover "new" anatomic structures or new relationships between known structures. On that score, it is interesting to note that reports confirming the existence of the muscle-dura connection are now coming from other anatomy laboratories; practicing neurosurgeons, too, are seeing what they had not seen before. In fact, some researchers have reported a thickening in the spinal dura in the region of the recently discovered connective tissue bridge. They postulate that contraction in the RCPM muscle creates tension on the dura via the newly described connection, and such tension is responsible for the observed dural thickening.

Courtesy of Michael Rothman

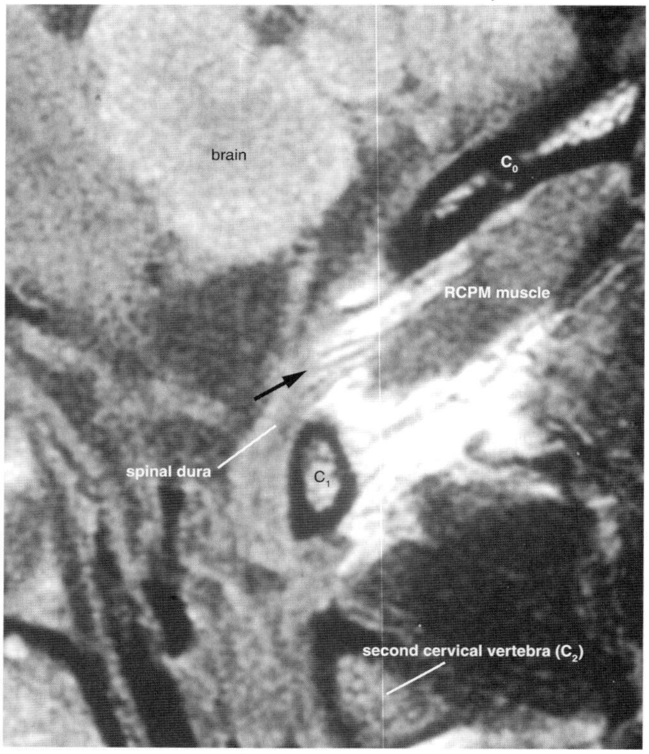

Magnetic resonance image (MRI) of the connective tissue bridge (arrow) attaching the RCPM muscle to the spinal dura; researchers came upon the bridge quite unexpectedly.

Virtual verification

New technologies are allowing these authors and their colleagues to validate their discovery. In cadavers as well as in living patients, the connection has been revealed with magnetic resonance imaging (MRI), a noninvasive technique that relies on the response of hydrogen atoms in body tissues to a magnetic field to produce computerized images of internal body parts. But the most exciting confirmation comes from the U.S. National Library of Medicine's Visible Human Project (VHP). Thus far, the project consists of two digitized cadavers, one male and one female, both individuals who bequeathed their bodies to science. The cadavers, aged 39 and 59, respectively, selected because they were "ideal specimens," were frozen and then cut head to toe into thousands of transverse slices. The male cadaver (Visible Man, or Visible Human Male) was sectioned into 1,871 slices, each one millimeter in thickness. The female cadaver (Visible Woman, or Visible Human Female) was sectioned into over 5,000 slices, each one-third of a millimeter in thickness. Each frozen section (cryosection) was photographed, and the images were then digitally transferred to a computer. These transverse cross-sectional images can be presented in their original form, or they can be reformatted and viewed in a variety of different planes (*e.g.*, coronal, sagittal, and oblique).

All of these cross-sectional images can be readily utilized in medical teaching programs and by scientists familiar with such anatomic detail. The technology allows for the boundaries of identifiable anatomic structures to be precisely defined; such boundary identification is known as segmentation. Once segmented, each distinct anatomic structure can be reassembled to create a three-dimensional (3-D) image. These images can be viewed in isolation or in relation to surrounding structures. They can also be rotated in various directions, which allows for visualization from novel perspectives. Finally, extremely useful biomechanical models can be developed from the 3-D images.

Incredible journeys into the human body are now possible, thanks to the creation of the world's first "virtual cadavers." The VHP represents the first complete electronic image library of "average, normal" human bodies; never before have such comprehensive high-quality medical images been available. This new technology enables researchers to study human anatomy from perspectives and in contexts that were never previously possible. To be sure, in the future this remarkable resource will have a profound effect on medical education and research; its numerous potential applications include simulations that allow surgeons and students to master complex operations without risk to live patients and telemedicine, in which detailed high-resolution pictures of internal body structures can be transmitted in "real time" from one location to another—for example, from a remote clinic in rural West Virginia to a major medical center in Washington, D.C. The VHP data sets are already being applied to a wide range of educational, diagnostic, treatment-planning, virtual reality, artistic, mathematical, and industrial uses by over 700 licensees in 26 countries.

Digital cadaver images from the VHP data sets proved to be just the tool that these authors needed to support their finding of a muscle-dura connection; they were able to view the connection in full-color computerized cross-sections. Future research plans include using the VHP data sets to construct 3-D models of the connection that will enable simulations of its movement and determination of its roles in function and dysfunction.

New piece in the headache puzzle?

What is the clinical significance of this new discovery? The investigators postulate that the normal function of the newfound connection may be to resist the inward folding of the dura, which tends to occur when the neck is extended or the head tipped backward. This inward buckling of the dura could compromise the flow of the cerebrospinal fluid, contained within the dural sac, which nourishes and protects the brain and spinal cord. But what if the connection were to malfunction? Could abnormally increased tension in the RCPM muscle result in increased tension in the dura? Could such tension play a role in headaches?

Sustained contraction of head and neck muscles is known to produce pain that is experienced inside the head—*i.e.,* tension headache. But by what mechanism does contraction of muscles *outside* the skull produce pain *inside?*

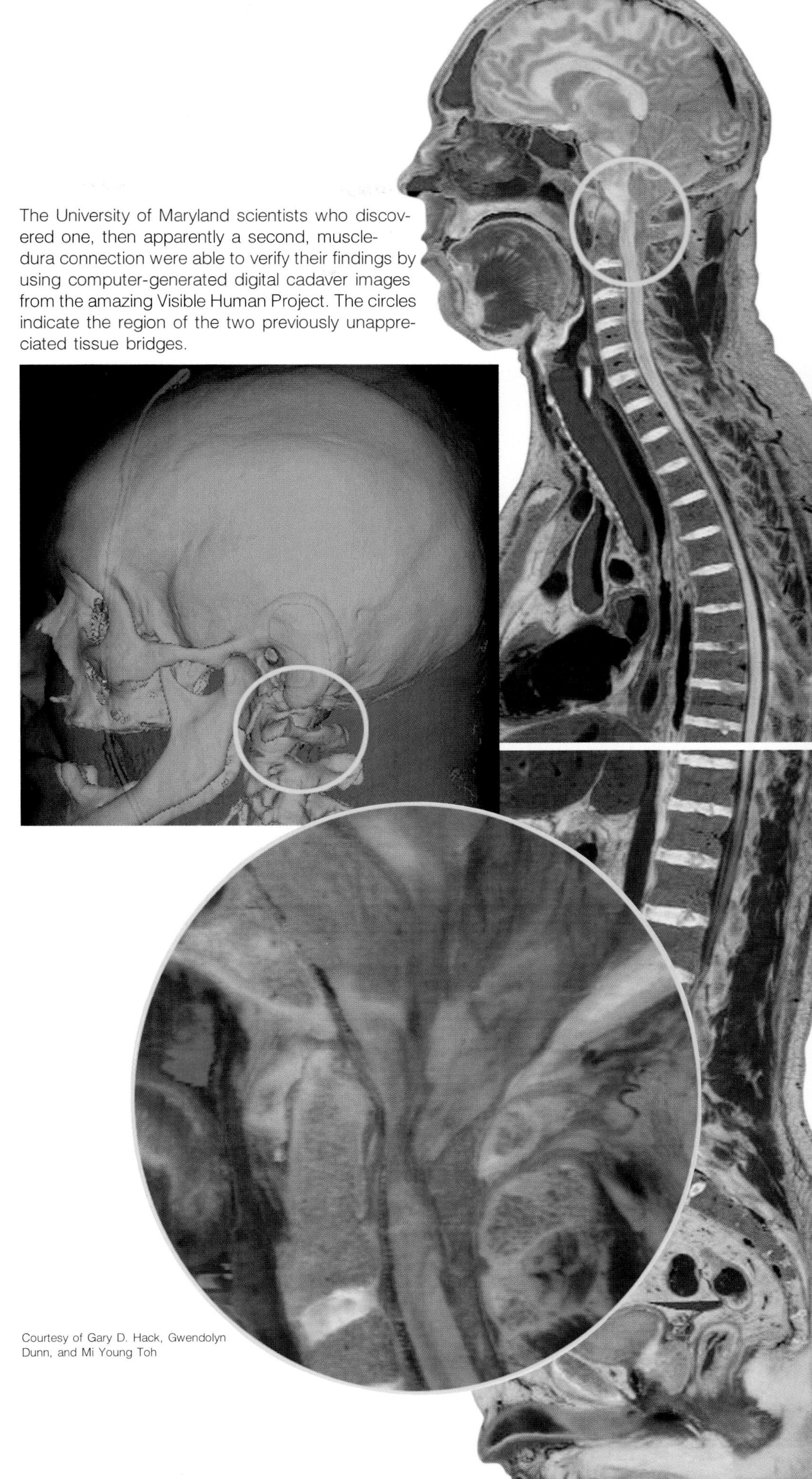

The University of Maryland scientists who discovered one, then apparently a second, muscle-dura connection were able to verify their findings by using computer-generated digital cadaver images from the amazing Visible Human Project. The circles indicate the region of the two previously unappreciated tissue bridges.

Courtesy of Gary D. Hack, Gwendolyn Dunn, and Mi Young Toh

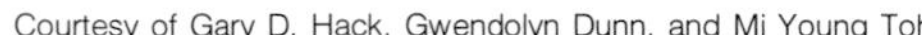
Courtesy of Gary D. Hack, Gwendolyn Dunn, and Mi Young Toh

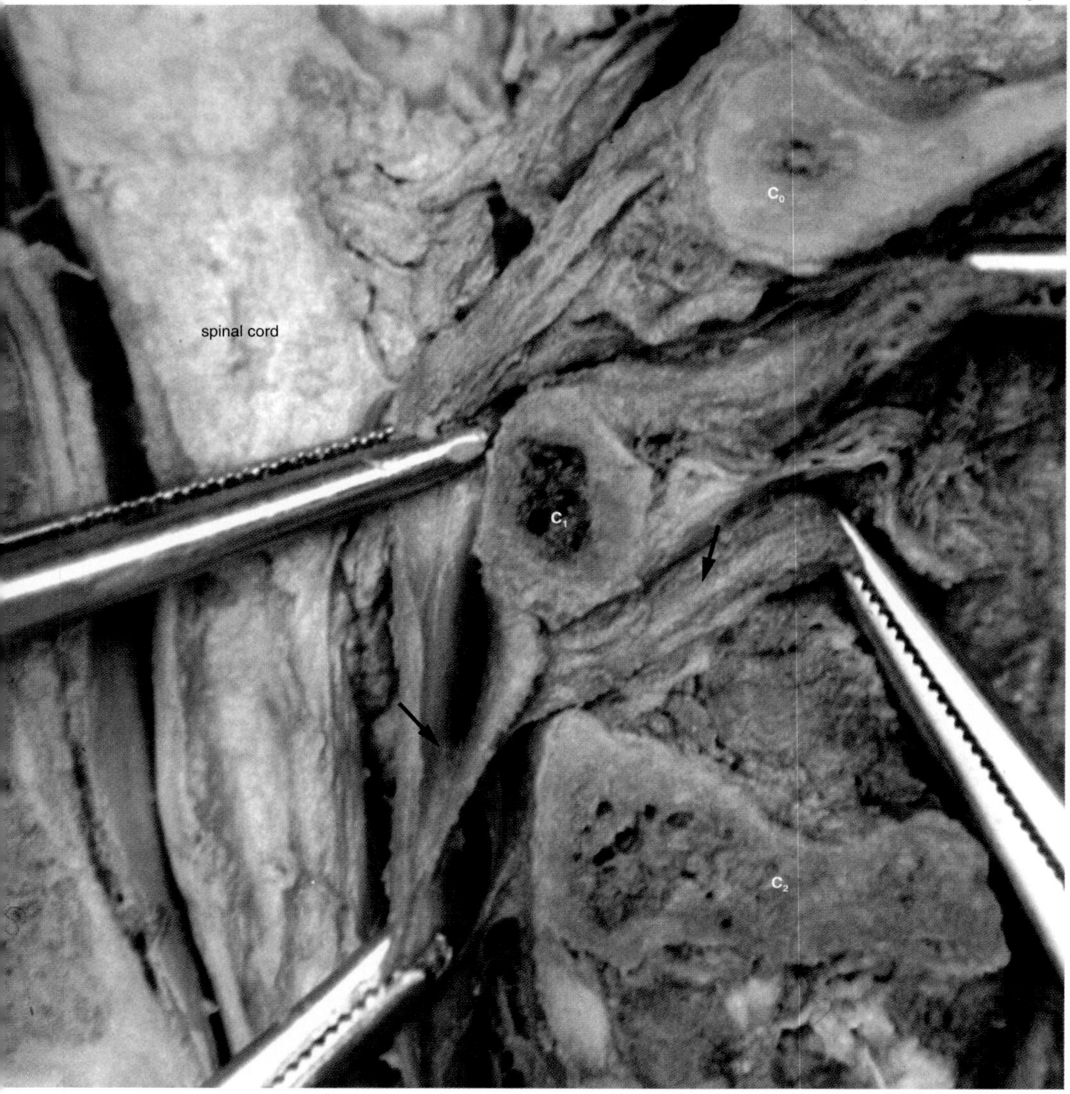

Cadaver specimen showing muscle-dura connections. The arrow on the right points to the muscle-dura bridge at the junction of the atlas (C_1) and axis (C_2); the arrow on the left points to the tissue bridge attachment to the spinal dura. Both connections are suspected of playing a part in tension headaches.

Does the new finding of a physical connection between skeletal muscle and the spinal dura represent the "missing link" that scientists have long sought to explain the pain of so-called muscle-contraction (tension) headaches?

Neurosurgeons describe the brain as "insensitive." It is known, however, that the covering of the brain, the dura, is extremely sensitive, and tension on the dura during neurosurgical procedures can produce pain experienced as headache. The Maryland scientists speculate that the newly described muscle-dura connection may transmit forces from neck muscles to the pain-sensitive dura. As already noted, not all the mechanisms of headaches are fully understood. Some researchers believe that headache pain is primarily caused by changes in brain chemistry that result in a lowering of the threshold at which pain is perceived. An increasing number of researchers postulate that headache pain may be produced by structures located in the neck. While the notion that headache may arise from cervical (neck) structures may be new to some medical practitioners, it is a concept that is widely accepted by chiropractors, osteopaths, and other professionals who regularly perform manipulative procedures involving the cervical spine.

A growing body of literature relates headaches to injury or pathology affecting neck structures. Moreover, a number of clinical trials have suggested that treatments such as massage, spinal manipulation, and biofeedback directed at the neck are valuable for managing muscle-contraction headaches. Spinal manipulation as a treatment for tension headache is predicated upon the assumption that dysfunction in the neck muscles contributes to the head pain; in the U.S. more than 90% of such procedures are performed by chiropractors. The muscle-dura connection may represent—at least in part—the underlying anatomic basis for the effectiveness of this treatment. Such treatment, as performed by a chiropractor, would decrease muscle tension and thereby reduce or eliminate pain by reducing the potential forces exerted on the dura via the muscle-dura connection.

It is interesting to note that surgeons who have severed this connection as part of some other surgical procedure have found that at least some of their patients experience fewer chronic headaches

(Bottom) Based on an original illustration by Brent Bauer

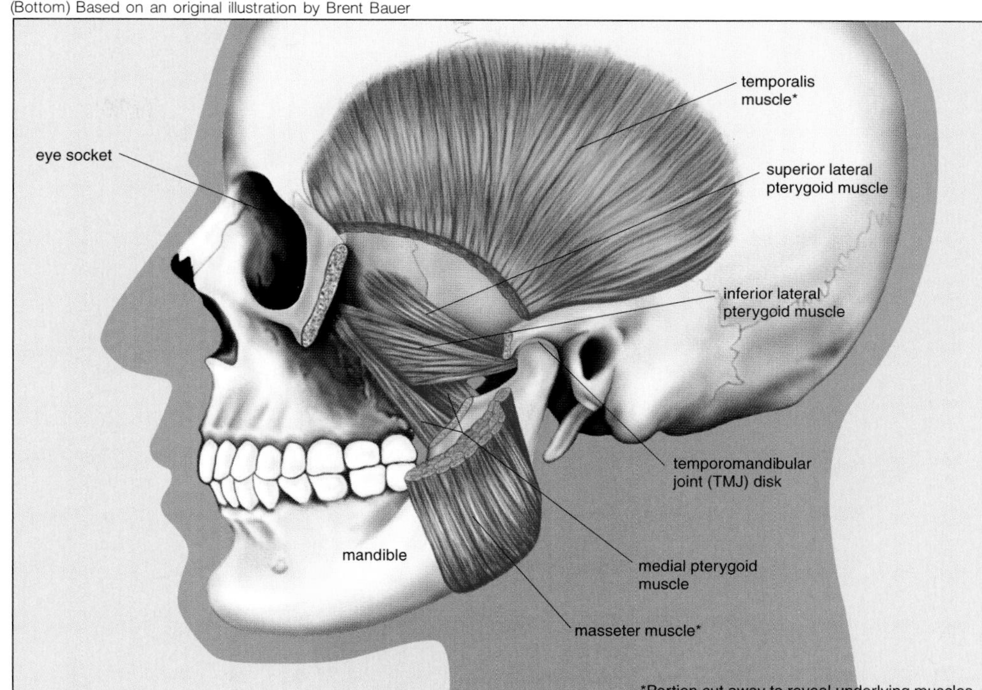

(Right) Until 1996 anatomists were aware of just four chewing muscles: the temporalis, masseter, lateral pterygoid, and medial pterygoid. (Below) A newly discovered fifth mastication muscle—the sphenomandibularis muscle—was previously thought to be a part of the temporalis muscle.

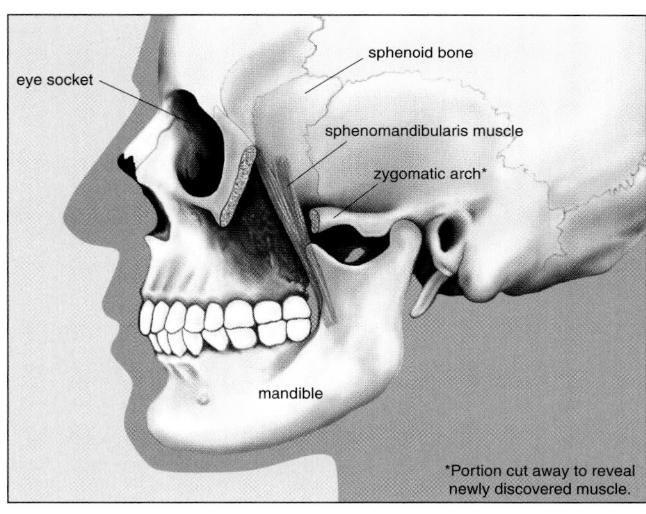

afterward. This would support the concept that neck muscles may pull on the sensitive dura via the newly described connection and thereby produce the pain. Moreover, Herman Edeling, a neurosurgeon in Johannesburg, South Africa, has recently developed a neurosurgical procedure based on the new anatomic discovery. The operation, which Edeling calls “myodural release,” involves cutting the muscle-dura connection to prevent the RCPM muscle from affecting the dura.

Eureka II

Do other muscle-dura connections exist in the human body? The Baltimore team, working in conjunction with staff at the National Library of Medicine in Bethesda, Maryland, is now utilizing the VHP data sets in a unique way. Initially, the VHP was used to help validate the existence of an anatomic structure after it was “discovered.” Presently, the technology is being used to “discover” structures as yet unseen and undescribed. Upon viewing a series of the VHP’s cross-sectional images, the cooperating scientists recently identified what appeared to be another muscle-dura connection—this one located between the first (C_1) and second (C_2) cervical vertebrae and involving two neck muscles—the rectus capitis posterior major and the obliquus capitis inferior. Taking the new information back to their laboratory, the researchers were able to verify the existence of this second muscle-dura connection in cadaver specimens. What are the clinical implications of this additional bridge? Here, too, a role in headache pain is hypothesized, as the mechanics of the two anatomic connections appear to be similar.

Jaws V

Is it possible that other anatomic structures remain “hidden” in the head-neck area? Undoubtedly, yes! In fact, after their discovery of muscle-dura connections, the Maryland team uncovered an unappreciated muscle in the human jaw, extending from a bony process (extension) located behind the eye socket (orbit) to the mandible (lower jaw). Though aspects of this structure had been noted before and viewed on MRI scans, most anatomists assumed that what they were seeing was part of the tempo-

Courtesy of Gary D. Hack, Gwendolyn Dunn, and Mi Young Toh

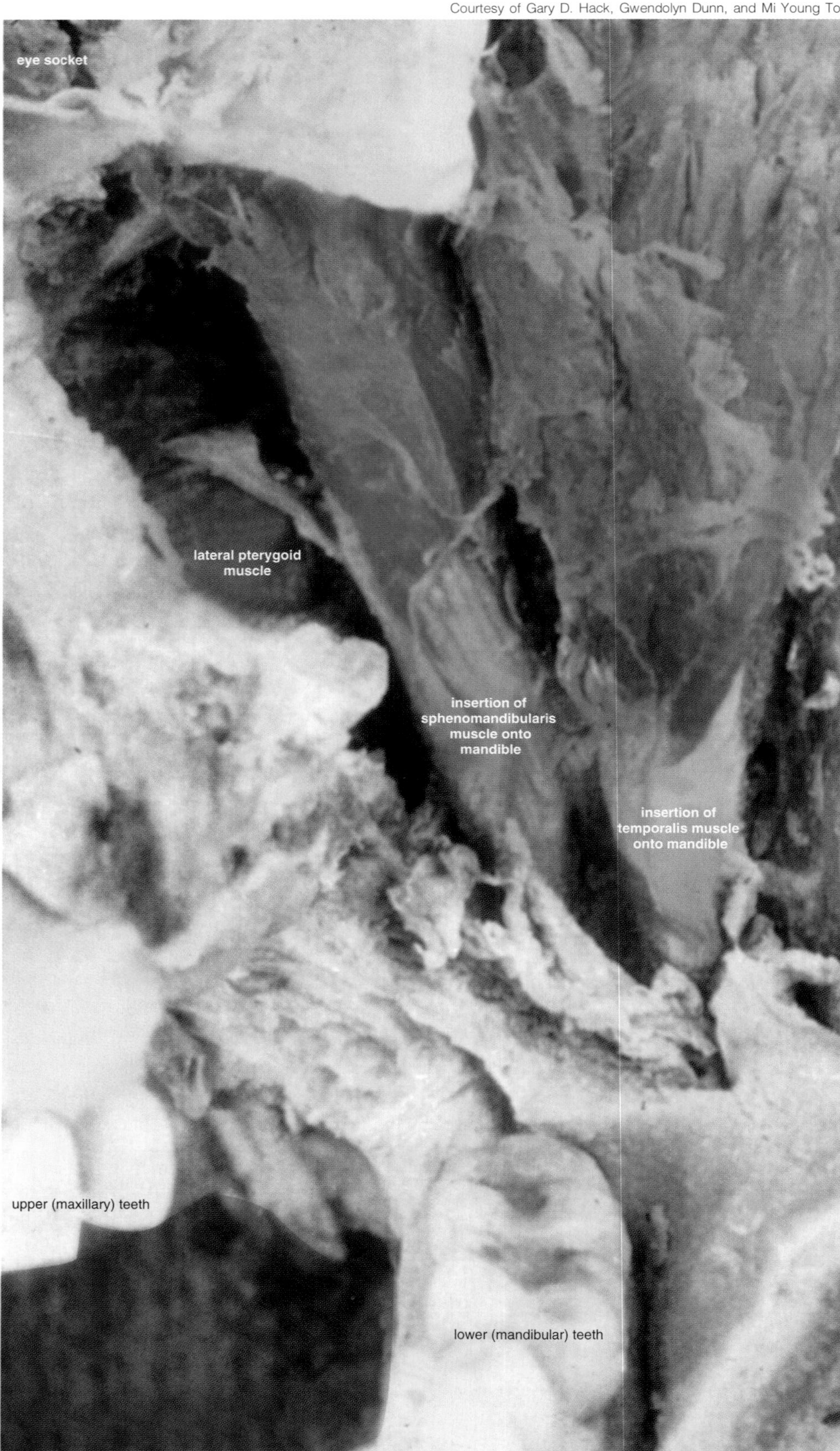

ralis muscle. Only by approaching this structure from a unique perspective were the University of Maryland scientists able to recognize the structure as a distinct entity. Owing to its origin at the sphenoid bone and its insertion onto the mandible, the discoverers named the new muscle the sphenomandibularis.

The standard dissection method for disclosing the jaw muscles is to cut from the side of the head. In so doing, the dissector encounters deep muscle fibers, which appear to be part of the temporalis muscle. When the region in question is approached from the front, however, as it was by the Maryland team, the sphenomandibularis is revealed as an independent muscle (measuring, on average, about 3.5 centimeters [1.8 inches] long, 1.3 centimeters [0.5 inch] wide, and 1.3 centimeters deep), with its own blood and nerve supplies. According to standard atlases of anatomy, there are four chewing muscles—the temporalis, the masseter, and the lateral and medial pterygoid muscles. The sphenomandibularis appears to be the fifth muscle of mastication. There are several hypotheses about its potential functions.

First, its location behind the eye socket may account for

Anterior view of a cadaver specimen showing the sphenomandibularis muscle's position—from its origin in a bony process behind the eye socket to its insertion onto the mandible.

the retro-orbital pain experienced by some patients with dysfunction of the masticatory muscles. It has been reported that hyperactivity of the temporalis muscle can refer, or transfer, pain to the retro-orbital area, mimicking migraine headache. In view of the retro-orbital location of the sphenomandibularis muscle, this so-called referred pain may actually be primary pain. Additionally, it is reported that compression of the maxillary nerve (a division of the fifth cranial nerve) by blood vessels is involved in the pathogenesis of cluster headache, a type of severe, unilateral headache occurring mainly in males and involving the eye, temple, neck, and face. Because the maxillary nerve passes between the sphenomandibularis muscle and the bony posterior wall of the maxillary sinus, it may be that the discovery of the fifth jaw muscle will eventually lead to a keener understanding of the latter variety of headache, often said to be the most excruciating.

These authors speculate that spasm in the sphenomandibularis muscle may compress the maxillary nerve against the posterior wall of the maxillary sinus. Therefore, the maxillary nerve may be irritated and become symptomatic if stressed to an uncommon extent by the newly described muscle. Amelioration of spasm in the sphenomandibularis muscle could assuage the retro-orbital pain. The sphenomandibularis muscle has been identified on

Courtesy of Michael Rothman

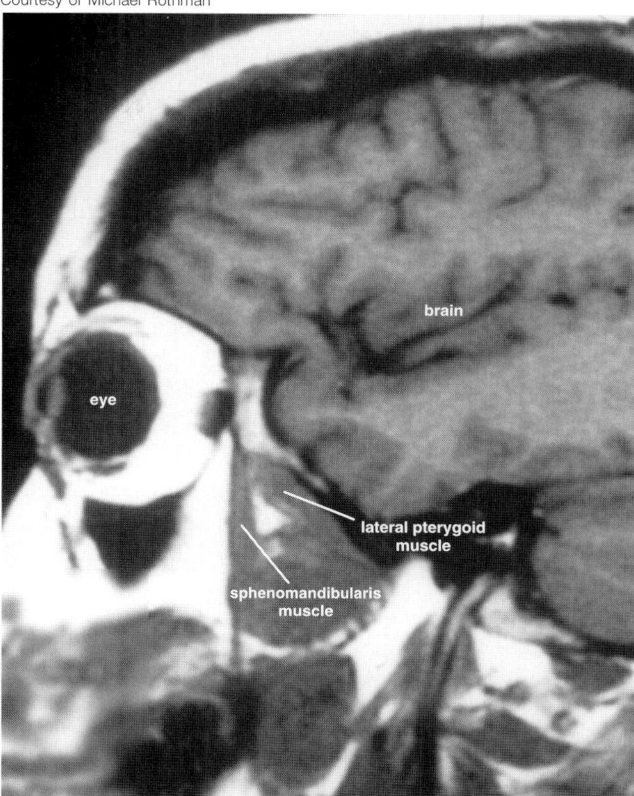

MRI scan showing the sphenomandibularis muscle in relation to the lateral pterygoid muscle, eye, and brain. The "new" muscle's location suggests it may be associated with the excruciating pain of cluster headaches.

MRI scans done by neuroradiologist Michael Rothman at the University of Maryland. These preliminary MRI data support the concept that the sphenomandibularis is distinct from the temporalis muscle. Further support comes from patients with trigeminal nerve damage (injury to either of the largest pair of skull nerves, which are used in chewing and in movement of the mandible). These patients have significant degeneration of the temporalis muscle, whereas the sphenomandibularis muscle is not affected. The temporalis muscle is known to be innervated, or supplied, by branches of the trigeminal nerve. The two trigeminal nerves innervate all the known muscles of mastication. When the trigeminal nerve is damaged, the muscles that it innervates undergo atrophy (wasting). The finding that the sphenomandibularis muscle is resistant to this process suggests that it has a unique (or possibly a dual) nerve supply. In addition to the MRI data, preliminary biochemical evidence also suggests that these two muscles are distinct. Physiologist Peter Reiser at Ohio State University, using biochemical analysis, has noted that the sphenomandibularis muscle appears to contain a higher percentage of slow-contracting muscle fibers than does the temporalis.

Again, the VHP, with its wide applications, is being utilized to verify and elaborate upon this discovery. Having a universally available set of data is crucial not only for confirming the existence and function of a "new" body part but also for comparing the findings of different investigators. Headed by physician Peter Ratiu and engineer John Kerr, visual media specialists at Engineering Animation, Inc., of Ames, Iowa, have created a 3-D image of the sphenomandibularis muscle, revealing its relationship to the skull and the surrounding musculature. The computer imaging company has also devised a computer program that replicates the dissection technique used in the discovery of the muscle.

Once the technology has been refined and becomes less costly, such computerization will allow the discovery process to be repeated in the classroom; thus, the muscle would be revealed to students in much the same way it was first revealed to its discoverers—and this would be achieved without destroying additional cadaver specimens. (The latter is of consequence because there is a chronic shortage of cadavers available for research and instruction.) Further studies on the vascularization and innervation of the new muscle are under way, and 3-D functional biomechanical models are being developed to determine whether the sphenomandibularis muscle can indeed compress the maxillary nerve against the posterior wall of the sinus. Thus far, it would appear that the sphenomandibularis is a postural muscle—one that may play a key role in stabilizing the jaw.

A joint of contention

The Maryland team has challenged the concept that "all is known" concerning gross anatomy. The sphenomandibularis muscle, as described above, may play a vitally important role in the human anatomy—namely, that of stabilizing the jaw—yet its very existence, let alone its function, was not known until a short time ago. The lower jawbone is connected to the temporal bone of the skull by the temporomandibular joint (TMJ). There is, however, considerable controversy concerning the jaw joint's anatomy. TMJ disorders (sometimes called myofacial pain dysfunction syndrome, temporomandibular joint pain dysfunction syndrome, or simply TMJ syndrome) constitute a significant complaint among medical and dental patients. Epidemiological surveys that have examined the prevalence of TMJ disorders in the general population suggest that 40–60% of people have at least one recognizable symptom.

Some common indications of TMJ syndrome are facial pain, headache, ear pain, pain focused in the masticatory muscles or the jaw joint itself, limitation of jaw movement, and dislocation of the joint. How can clinicians effectively treat dysfunction of this joint if its anatomy is not fully understood? The joint is formed where the mandible hinges against the skull. Interposed between the mandible and the skull is a semirigid tissue known as the TMJ disk (*see* top illustration, page 23). Pathology of the jaw joint is often related to displacement of the disk from its normal position. Specifically, it is the relation of the superior lateral pterygoid (SLP) muscle to the TMJ disk that is most hotly disputed. The SLP muscle is a component of the lateral pterygoid, one of the muscles of mastication. Some authorities contend that there is no muscular attachment of the SLP muscle to the disk. Other researchers report a nonfunctional muscular attachment. Still others have found a functional muscular attachment. Among the latter group are those reporting that the SLP muscle pulls and displaces the disk in an anterior (forward) and medial direction (toward the center of the head). A recent report, however, suggests that the majority of disk displacements are away from the center (anterior and lateral). While further investigation of the anatomic and functional relationship of the SLP muscle to the TMJ disk is needed—and there are likely to be other factors involved—preliminary investigations have revealed an anatomic factor that may resolve this confusion.

In their anatomy laboratory, these researchers have observed a hitherto unappreciated but anatomically and

The Visible Human data sets are allowing scientists to study anatomy from perspectives that were never previously possible. (Below) Finely detailed three-dimensional cross-sectional images are magnified and configured to illuminate a portion of the Visible Human Female head.

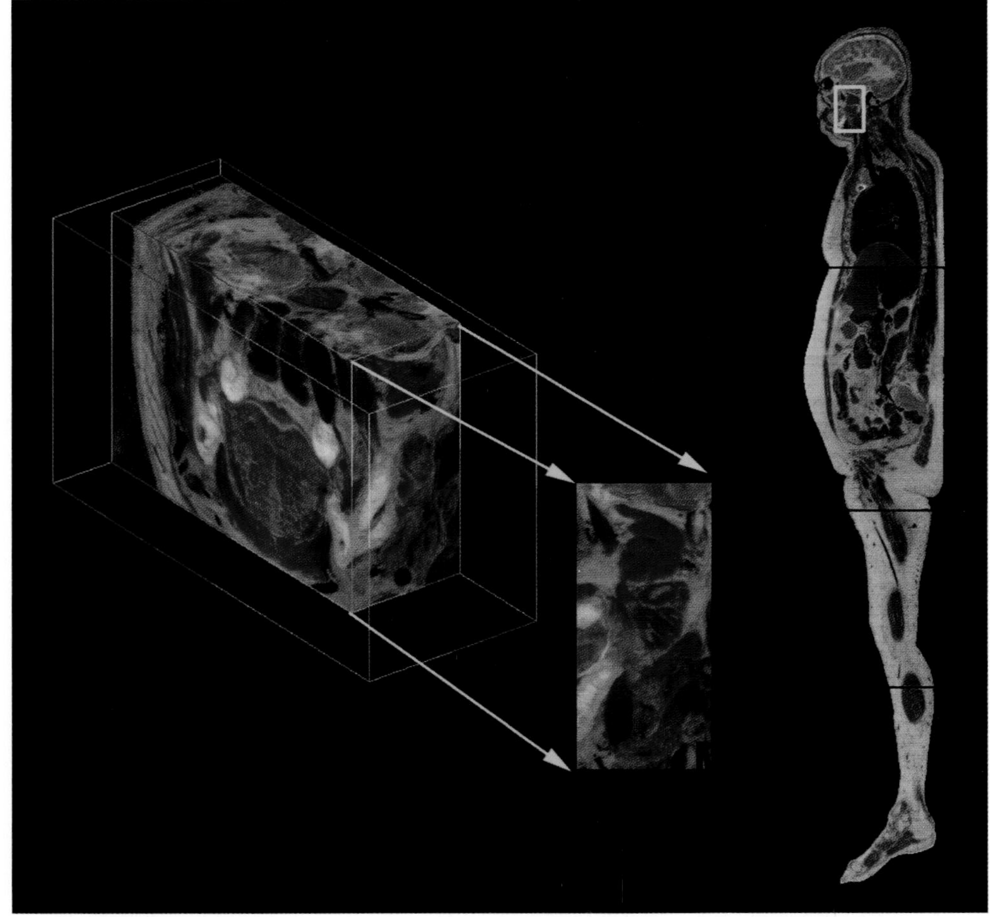

Courtesy of Gary D. Hack, Gwendolyn Dunn, and Mi Young Toh

Courtesy of Gary D. Hack, Gwendolyn Dunn, and Mi Young Toh

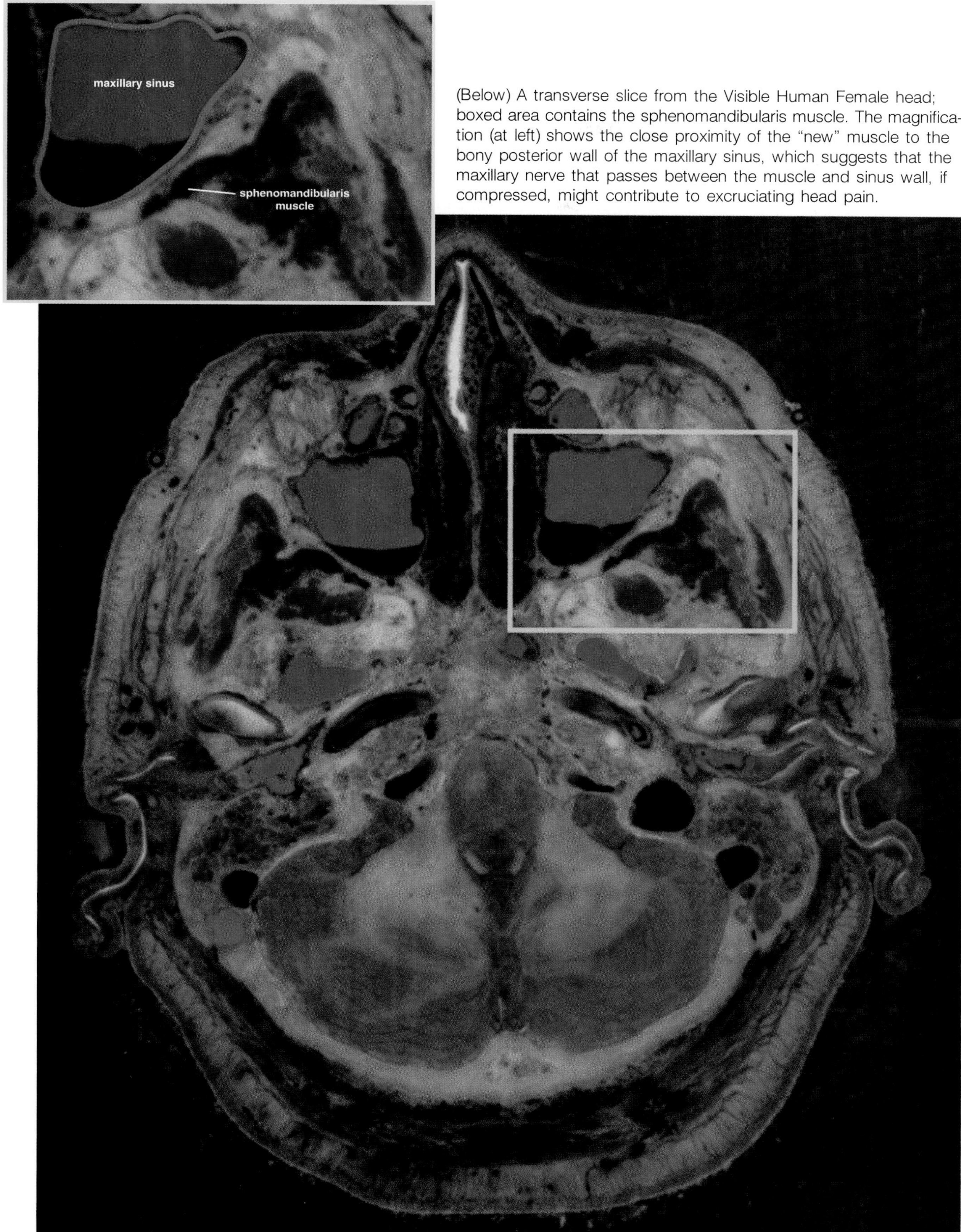

(Below) A transverse slice from the Visible Human Female head; boxed area contains the sphenomandibularis muscle. The magnification (at left) shows the close proximity of the "new" muscle to the bony posterior wall of the maxillary sinus, which suggests that the maxillary nerve that passes between the muscle and sinus wall, if compressed, might contribute to excruciating head pain.

functionally distinct portion of the SLP muscle that attaches to the disk and potentially pulls it in an anterior-lateral direction. Again, it was an unusual angle of dissection that provided a unique view of the structures in question. Anatomy manuals teach a lateral dissection of this particular anatomic area *(i.e.,* cutting from the side of the head); in this case, however, a superior approach (cutting from the top of the head) was used, removing the base of the skull to reveal the structures of interest. The next step will be turning to the VHP data sets to validate this intriguing cadaveric finding and then to develop functional biomechanical models from which more can be learned.

(This page and opposite, top) Courtesy of Engineering Animation, Inc.

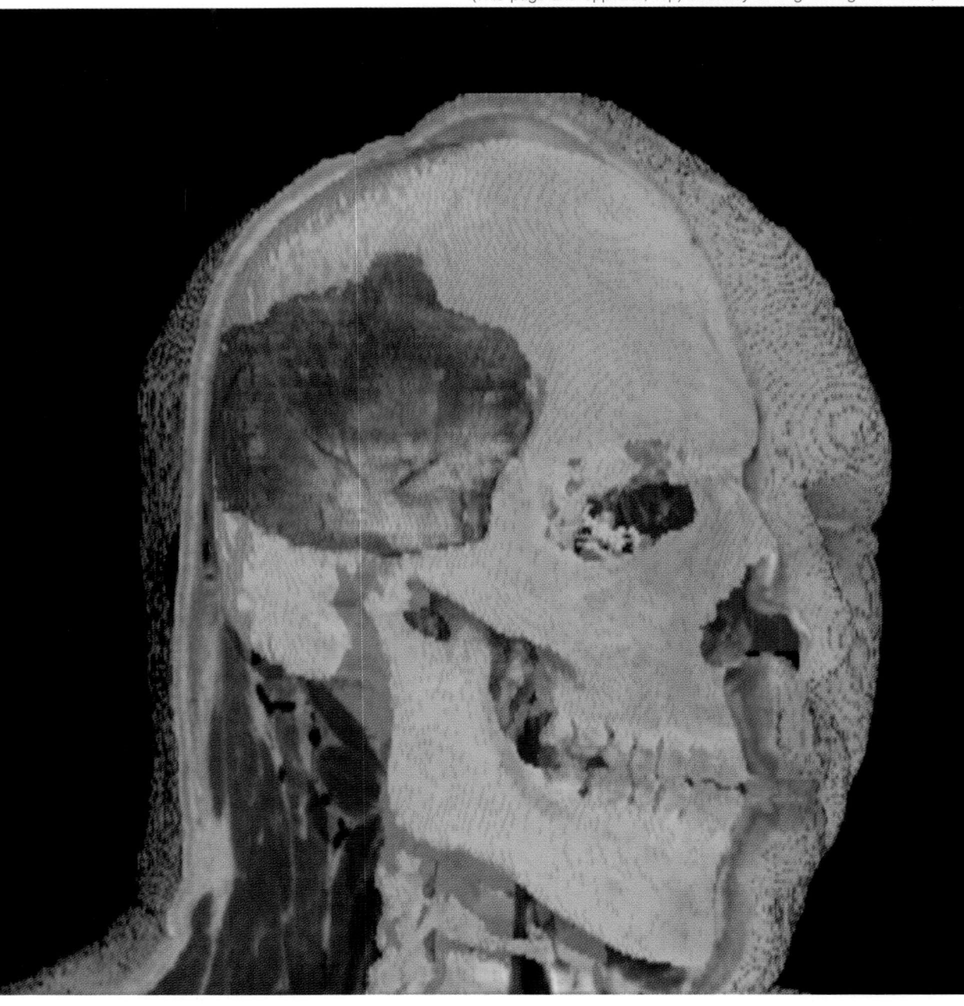

Morbid but not moribund

Giovanni Battista Morgagni (1682–1771) of Padua, Italy,

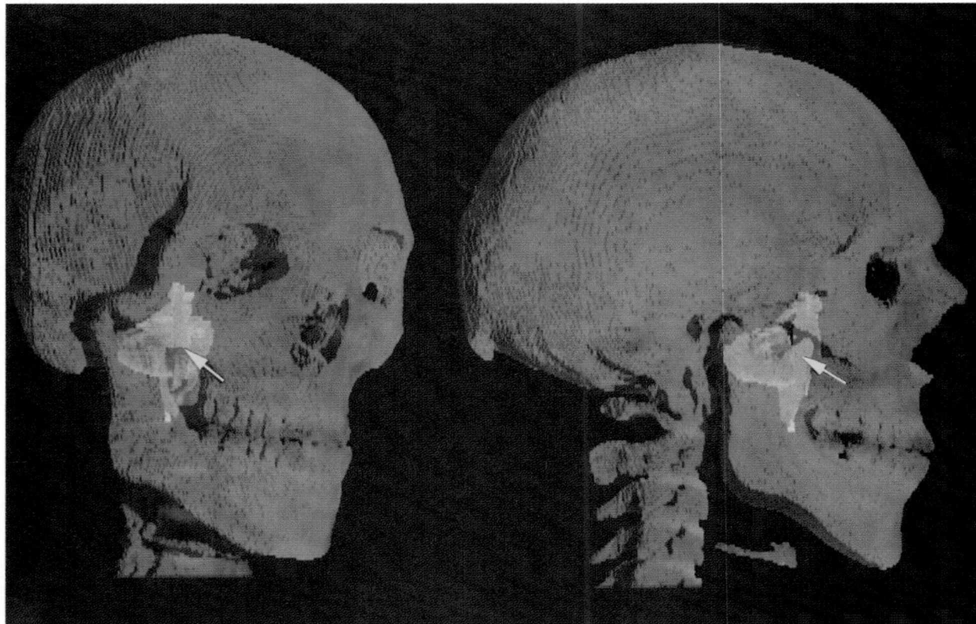

Computer-generated 3-D images derived from the Visible Human Male. (Left) The sphenomandibularis muscle from two perspectives. (Above and opposite page, top) The surgical approach that is needed to reveal the fifth mastication muscle. These images are being used to create sophisticated biomechanical models that will shed even more light on the "new" muscle's function.

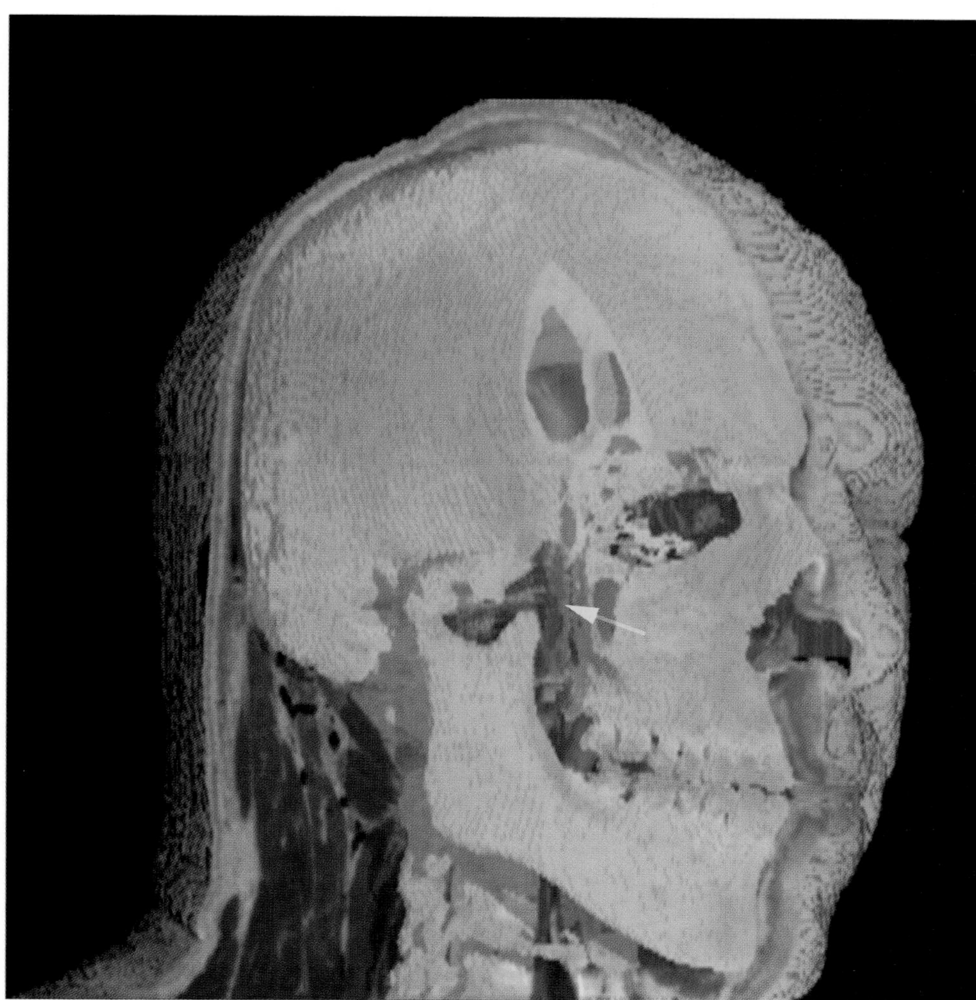

one of the greatest anatomists that ever lived, wrote in his most famous clinical treatise, *De Sedibus et Causis Morborum per Anatomen Indagatis* (*The Seats and Causes of Diseases Investigated by Anatomy*): "For those who have dissected or inspected many, have at least learn'd to doubt when the others, who are ignorant of anatomy, and do not take the trouble to attend to it, are in no doubt at all." The human body is an amazingly complex structure about which—even at the end of the 20th century—not everything is known.

Contrary to popular belief, anatomic research has not yet "seen its day." As is evidenced by the findings described above (of several "new" structures in the head-neck area alone), gross anatomy—aided and abetted by some sensational new tools—is a revitalized science with a future full of promise. MHA

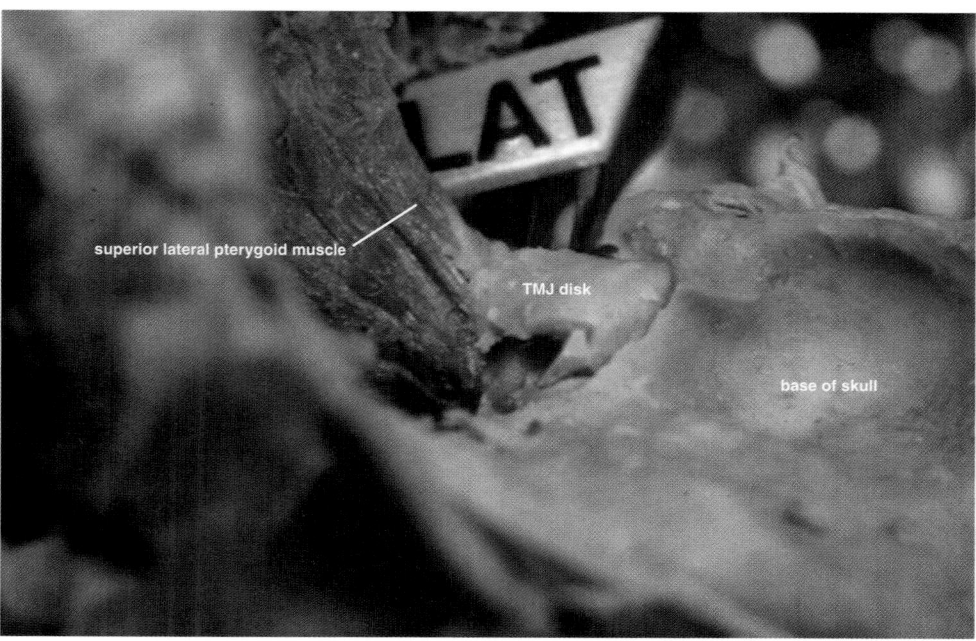

(Right) Cadaver specimen showing the attachment of a portion of the superior lateral pterygoid muscle to the temporomandibular joint disk. Only this unique view from above reveals the previously unappreciated relationship of the muscle to the disk. Better understanding of this part of the head-neck anatomy should lead to new treatments for painful TMJ disorders.

Courtesy of Gary D. Hack, Gwendolyn Dunn, and Mi Young Toh

Panic over Prions

by Fred Brown, Ph.D., F.R.S.

A little more than a decade has passed since bovine spongiform encephalopathy (BSE), a fatal neurological disease of cattle, was first observed in herds in the United Kingdom. Although similar ailments are known in other animals, including sheep and goats, this particular livestock disease had never before been seen in the U.K.—or anywhere else, for that matter.

Cattle suffering from BSE have a heightened sensitivity to touch and sound, are noisier than normal, and engage in excessive licking and grinding of the teeth. Affected animals develop an unsteady gait and exhibit behavioral changes, becoming apprehensive, frenzied, and nervous—hence the name "mad cow" disease. Typically, cows with BSE die

*Virologist **Fred Brown, Ph.D., F.R.S.,** is Visiting Scientist, United States Department of Agriculture, Agricultural Research Service, Plum Island Animal Disease Center, Greenport, New York.*

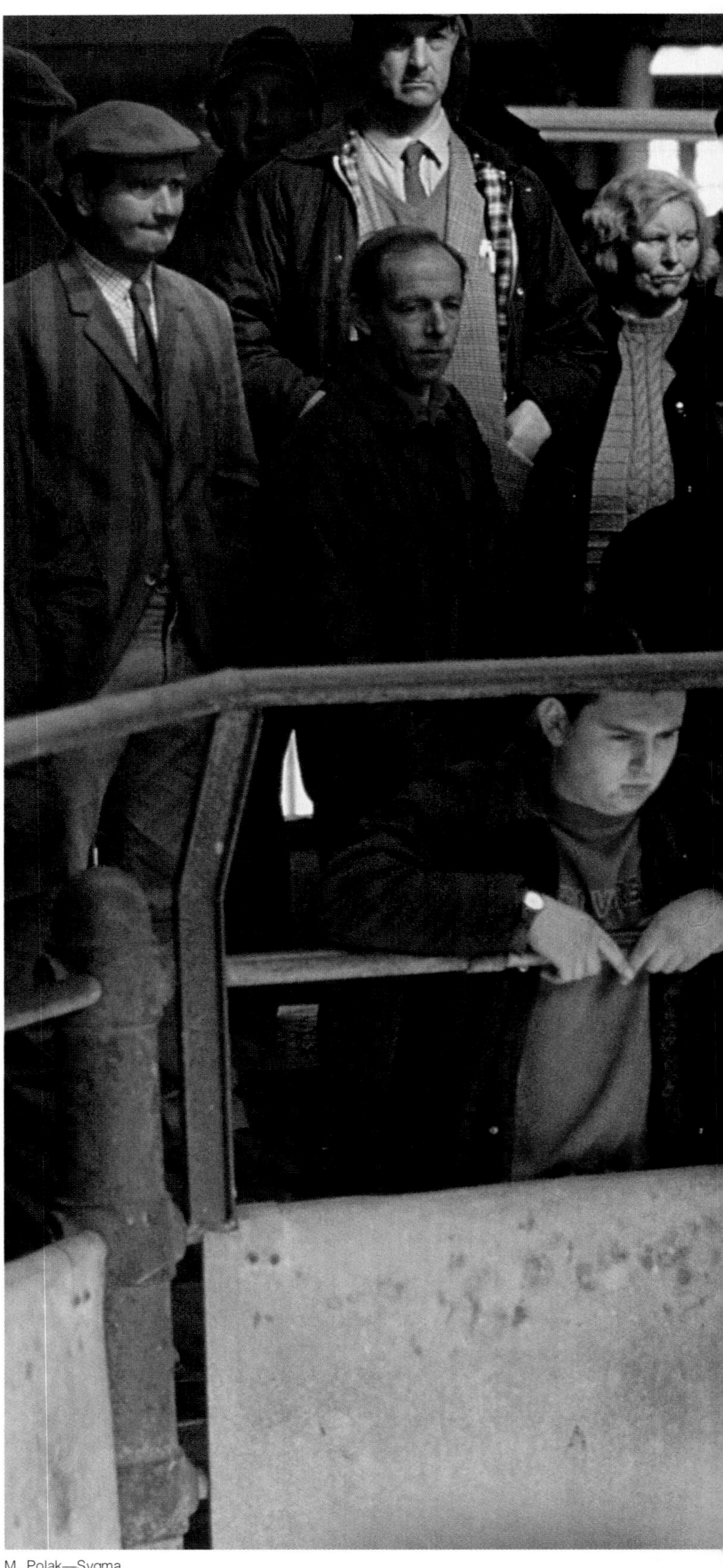

The uncertain future of the British cattle industry is reflected in the grim faces of spectators at the livestock market in Northampton, England, on March 30, 1996.

M. Polak—Sygma

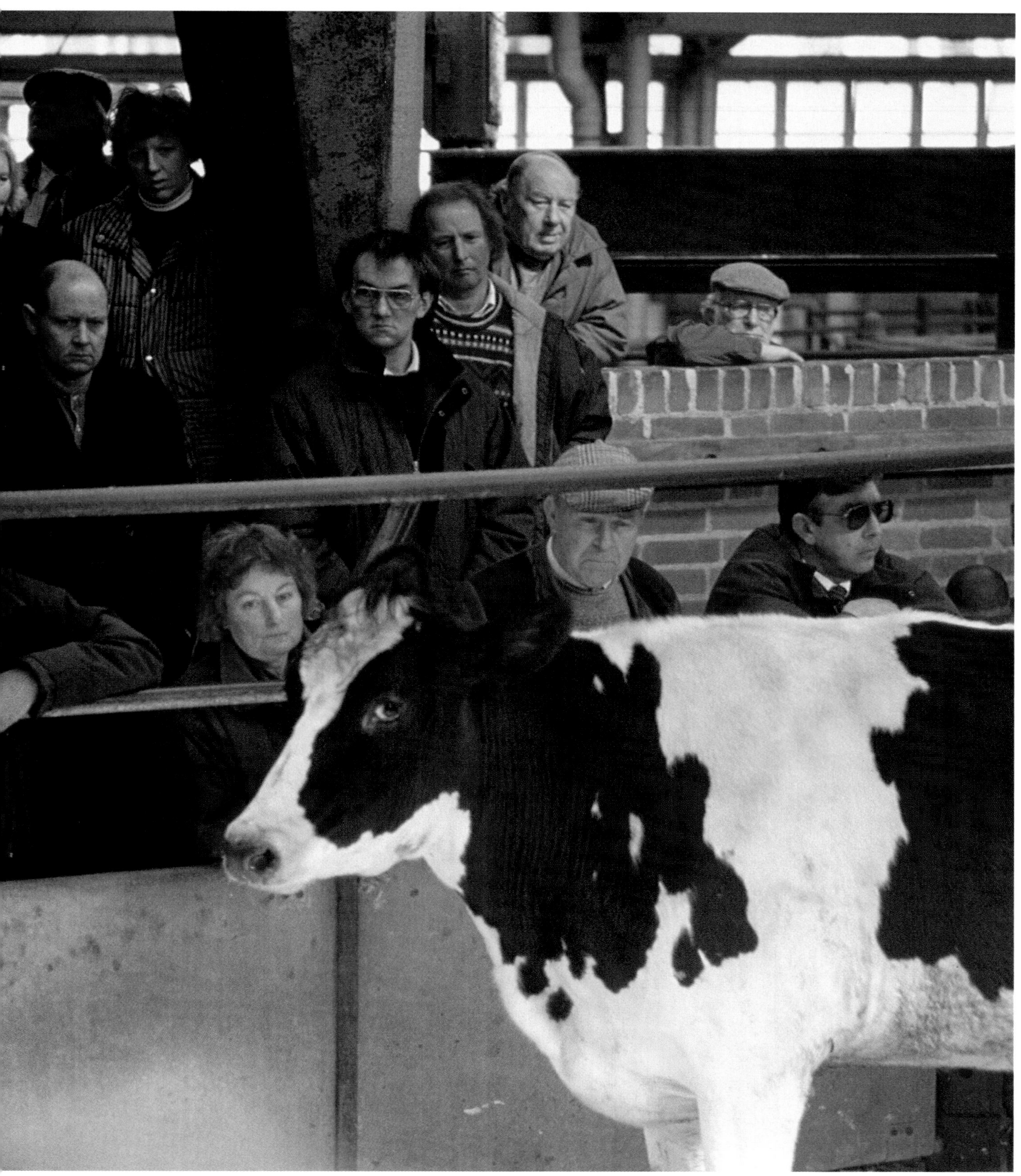

Nigel Dickinson—Still Pictures

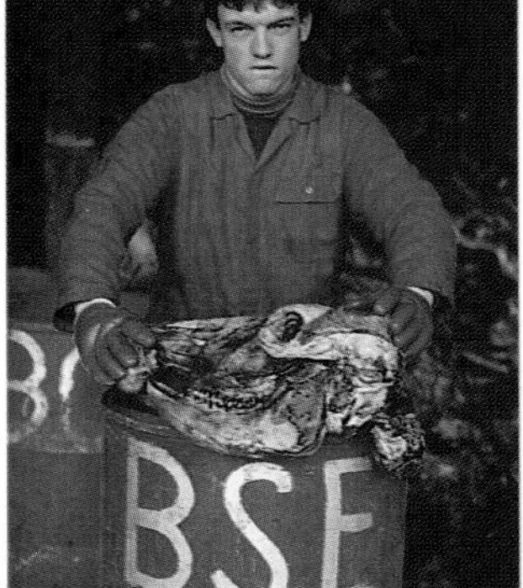

Dyed blue to identify them as contaminated, the remains of cows suspected of being infected with BSE are incinerated at Wrexham, Wales.

within a few months after the appearance of symptoms, although some live only a few weeks and others as long as a year. Postmortem examination of their brains reveals structural abnormalities similar to those found in the brains of sheep that have died from scrapie, a similar fatal neurological illness named for the tendency of affected animals to rub, or scrape, their bodies against stationary objects.

"Beefgate"

Few could have predicted in 1987, when the first case of BSE was reported, that this puzzling ailment would eventually require the slaughter of millions of animals, imperil the British beef industry, raise a public health alarm, and create a national scandal that threatened to undermine the government of the then prime minister John Major. Agriculture and health authorities in the U.K. were concerned by the emergence of this apparently new veterinary disorder; in 1988 a committee was established under the leadership of Sir Richard Southwood, vice-chancellor of the University of Oxford and a respected zoologist, to monitor the progress of the epidemic, examine the implications of BSE for both animal and human health, and advise the government on any necessary measures to control the spread of the disease.

The number of cows with BSE rose alarmingly—from 20 known cases in 1987 to more than 700 by 1988. In 1993 more than 1,000 cases a week were being reported. By the mid-1990s more than 160,000 sick animals had been identified and slaughtered; more than half the dairy herds in the U.K. were involved. Subsequently, cases of BSE were reported in various other countries, including Canada, Ireland, France, Germany, Switzerland, The Netherlands, Denmark, Portugal, Spain, and Oman—although not on the scale seen in the U.K. To date, the disease has not been reported in the United States.

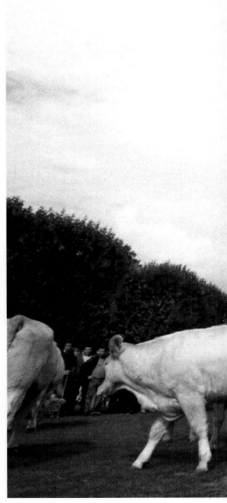

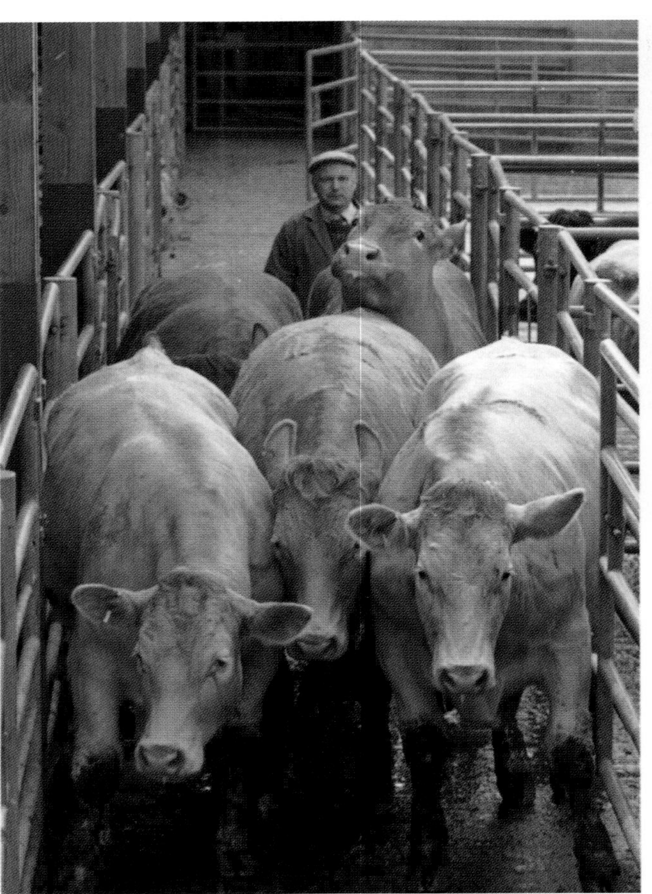

Cows headed for the slaughterhouse are herded onto a truck. The U.K. government decided in 1996 that all cattle older than 30 months would have to be destroyed.

John Redman—Associated Press

Philippe Wojazer—Reuters

The timing of the British outbreak led scientists to suspect that a change in the processing of offal (viscera and other body parts left over after the butchering of animals for meat) might be responsible. Several decades ago British farmers began feeding their cattle a protein supplement

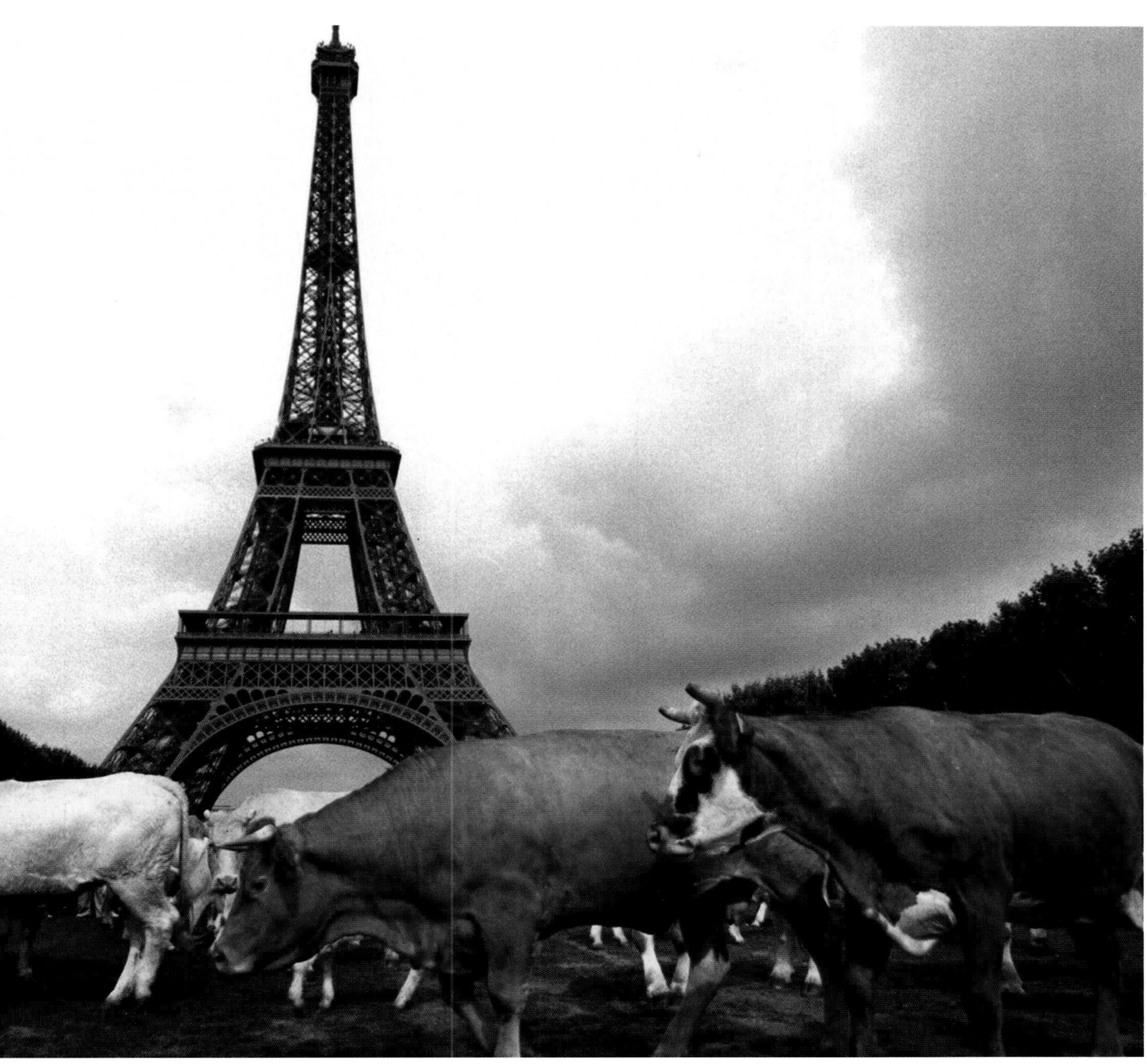

Cattle turned loose by French farmers protesting a drop in beef prices graze in a park in the heart of Paris in August 1996.

made from sheep offal. Later, cattle offal was added. In the early 1980s the rendering process (by which carcasses are converted to various products, including protein supplements for animal feed) was changed, and a step that involved the use of a solvent was eliminated. It is now believed that the solvent had the ability to inactivate the infectious agent that is the cause of BSE. In 1988, in an attempt to stem the tide of the BSE outbreak, the government banned the use of offal in cattle feed. In 1994 the incidence of BSE (number of new cases reported) declined for the first time since the start of the epidemic.

In April 1990 the role of the Southwood Committee was inherited by the Spongiform Encephalopathy Advisory Committee (SEAC), which had a wider mission: to advise the two ministries most directly involved—the Department of Health and the Ministry of Agriculture, Fisheries, and Food—on the whole range of related dis-

Sittler—REA/Saba

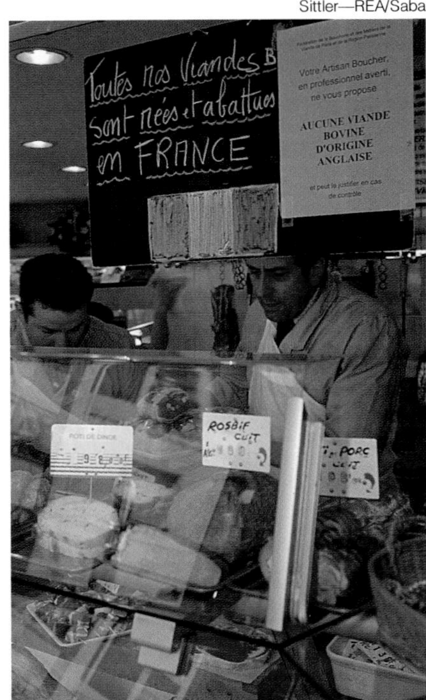

Signs in a Paris butcher shop assure customers that the beef is from French cows. Beef consumption all over Europe plummeted after March 20, 1996.

eases known collectively as the transmissible spongiform encephalopathies, or TSEs, a group of degenerative neurological disorders that affect several different species of mammals, including humans (*see* Table). At autopsy the brains of victims of the TSEs are found to have numerous holes, which give the brain tissue a characteristic spongelike appearance—hence the term *spongiform.*

Humans enter the picture

The best-known human TSE is Creutzfeldt-Jakob disease (CJD), an extremely rare disorder and one whose name was, until very recently, virtually unknown to most people. On March 20, 1996, Stephen Dorrell, the U.K. secretary of state for health, announced in the House of Commons that 10 unusual cases of CJD had been identified in England, Northern Ireland, and Wales and that scientists were investigating the possibility of a link between these human illnesses and BSE. Dorrell's statement was based on ad-

The carcass of a BSE-infected cow is burned in a field in Dorset, England. To contain the outbreak, millions of animals were scheduled to be destroyed.

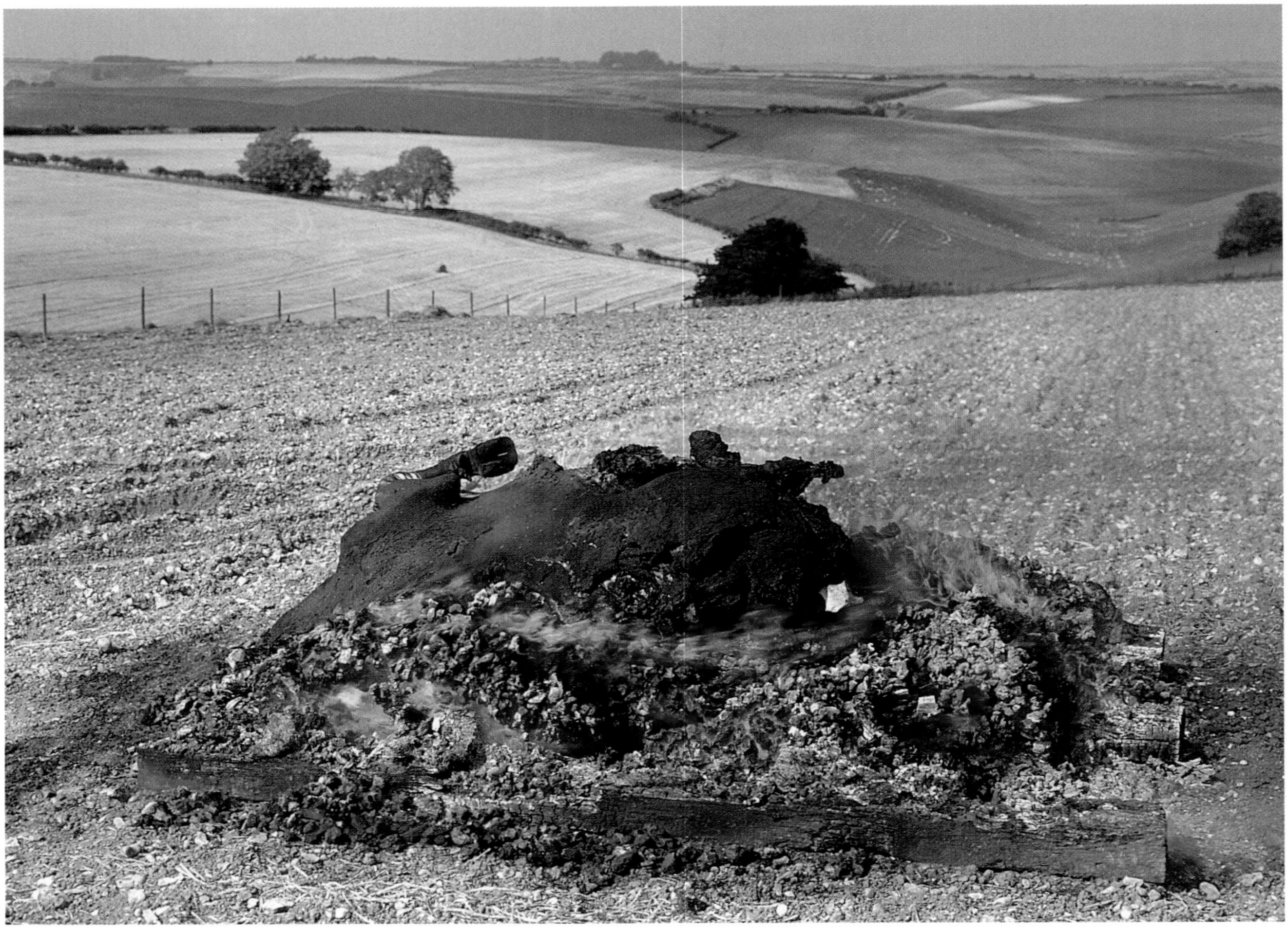

Sinclair Stammers—Science Source/Photo Researchers

vice he had received from the SEAC regarding recent findings by the CJD Surveillance Unit in Edinburgh, an investigative laboratory established in 1990 to track the disease. The unit's scientists had identified 10 cases of CJD in people aged 42 and younger, including several teenagers; the relative youth of the victims was particularly noteworthy, as CJD is usually seen only in older people. Moreover, Dorrell acknowledged that a review of the patients' medical histories and consideration of other possible causes of the illness had "failed to explain these cases adequately." Dorrell noted that there was no scientific proof that BSE could be transmitted to humans in beef (although scientists have demonstrated that other animals can acquire BSE by eating brain tissue from BSE-infected cattle), but, he told the members of Parliament, the advisory committee had concluded that the 10 cases were probably linked to exposure to BSE before the ban on the use of parts of butchered animals in cattle feed.

A British diner enjoys a McDonald's hamburger, safe in the knowledge that the popular fast-food chain is using only imported beef.

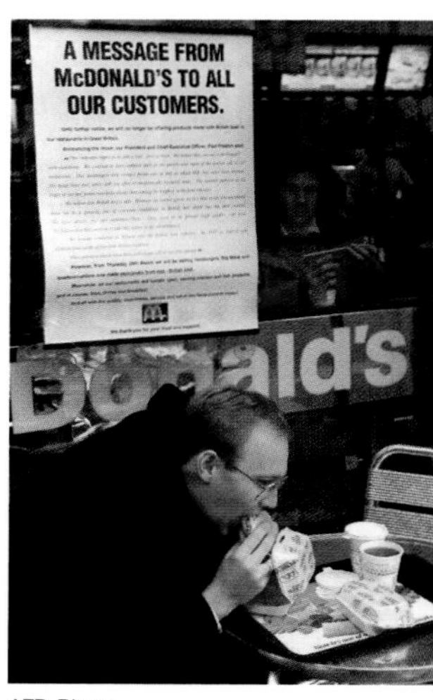

AFP Photo

The findings of the CJD Surveillance Unit were published in the British medical journal *The Lancet* on April 6, 1996:

> *Ten cases of CJD have been identified in the U.K. in recent months with a new neuropathological profile. Other consistent features that are unusual include the young age of the cases, clinical findings, and the absence of the electroencephalogram features typical for CJD.... These cases appear to represent a new variant of CJD, which may be unique to the U.K. This raises the possibility that they are causally linked to BSE. Although this may be the most plausible explanation for this cluster of cases, a link with BSE cannot be confirmed on the basis of this evidence alone. It is essential to obtain further information on the current and past clinical and neuropathological profiles of CJD in the U.K. and elsewhere.*

The British public—which, over the course of a decade, had been repeatedly reassured by government officials that British beef was safe and human health not at risk—was understandably confused and frightened. Was there a direct link between BSE and CJD? Could the cattle disease be transmitted to humans via beef? Did the recently reported unusual cases of CJD represent a new variant of the illness? In October 1996, in an attempt to answer these questions, neurologist John Collinge and his colleagues at St. Mary's Hospital, London, examined brain tissue from patients with typical and atypical CJD, looking for a characteristic protein that builds up in the brains of people (and other mammals) with spongiform encephalopathies. Their analysis confirmed the distinctiveness of the new CJD variant and pointed to a close relationship between this illness and BSE. Nonetheless, more than a year later scientists were still uncertain whether the same infectious

Naturally Occurring Transmissible Spongiform Encephalopathies (TSEs)

Affected animal	Disease name	Date of first report (if after 1986)	Geographic distribution
Cat (domestic)	Spongiform encephalopathy (SE)	1989	British Isles
Cheetah	Feline SE	1992	Australia,* Great Britain, Ireland*
Cow	Bovine SE	1987	U.K., Ireland, France, Denmark, Portugal, Switzerland, Germany, Canada, Falkland Islands, Oman
Eland	SE	1989	England
Elk	Chronic wasting disease	...	North America (localized)
Gemsbok	SE	1988	England
Greater kudu	SE	1989	England
Human	Kuru	...	Papua New Guinea (declining to rarity)
	Creutzfeldt-Jakob disease	...	Worldwide (rare)
	Gerstmann-Sträussler (-Scheinker) syndrome	...	Worldwide (extremely rare)
Mink (farmed)	Transmissible mink encephalopathy	...	North America, mainland Europe (rare)
Moufflon	Scrapie	1992	England
Mule deer	Chronic wasting disease	...	North America (localized)
Nyala	SE	1987	England
Oryx, Arabian	SE	1989	England
Oryx, scimitar-horned	SE	1993	England
Puma	Feline SE	1992	England
Sheep	Scrapie	...	Widely distributed but not reported in Australia, New Zealand, and some European and South American countries

*Animals presumably exposed in Great Britain before export.
Source: Adapted from September 1994 report of U.K. Spongiform Encephalopathy Advisory Committee.

agent was responsible for both disorders.

Normally, the cause of an infectious disease can be identified fairly quickly. Tissue from affected individuals is examined for signs of the agents (such as viruses and bacteria) that transmit the disease. Blood from affected individuals is tested for antibodies that their immune systems may have produced in response to these agents. In the case of BSE and CJD, and all the other spongiform encephalopathies as well, no such antibodies have ever been identified. These disorders appear to be caused by something quite unlike the pathogens familiar to medical scientists. With the exception of scrapie, however, which has been known to farmers and livestock raisers for more than two centuries, these illnesses have been little studied, and support for research in this area has traditionally been meager.

Shivering in New Guinea

Despite the lack of a concerted scientific effort, much information about the TSEs has accumulated over the years. Scrapie has long been a matter of concern because of its potential economic impact on the British wool industry. The TSE that first attracted attention outside veterinary and agricultural circles, however, was a bizarre neurological ailment found only among the inhabitants of the northern highlands of Papua New Guinea. This illness, called kuru (the word in the local language for "shivering" or "trembling"), was first described in the medical literature by the U.S. physician and virologist D. Carleton Gajdusek in 1957.

Kuru had existed in New Guinea for generations when Gajdusek arrived. Affected individuals first developed an unsteady gait; this was followed by tremor and uncontrollable movements. All victims died in less than two years. Although some scientists assumed kuru to be an inherited disorder, to Gajdusek the epidemiological pattern suggested an infectious disease. It was he who discovered that kuru was spread through the ritual eating of human brains, a traditional funerary custom in this part of New Guinea. Gajdusek concluded that the disease developed many years after exposure to the infected tissue, and he postulated that the infectious agent must be an extremely slow-acting virus.

The similarity of the central nervous system effects of kuru and scrapie was first noted in 1959 by U.S. veterinary pathologist Bill Hadlow, then working at the Agricultural Research Council's Institute in Compton, Berkshire, England. While at the Wellcome Institute in London, Hadlow saw an exhibit of photographs taken by Gajdusek in New Guinea. Hadlow suggested that it would be useful to try transmitting the kuru-causing agent from a human to another primate. Along with his colleagues Jo-

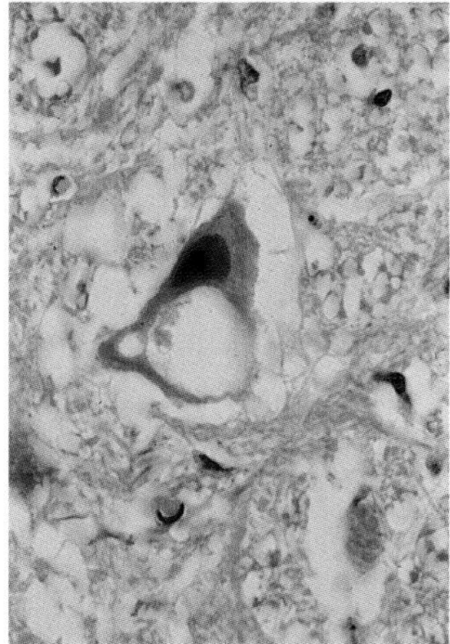

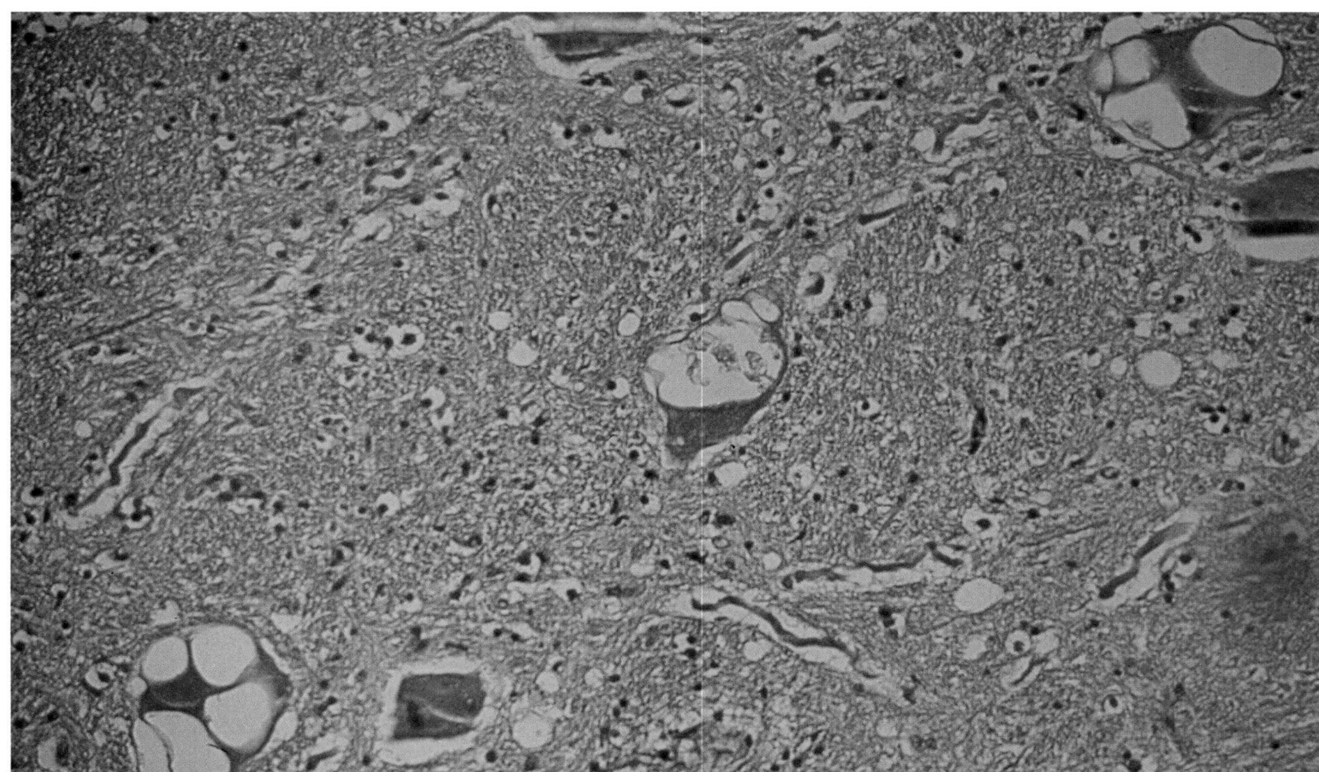

Microscopic views of tissue from the brain of a scrapie-infected sheep (right) and that of a cow that died from BSE (below) show the pathologic features characteristic of the transmissible spongiform encephalopathies, or TSEs.

(Below) Jim James—PA News; (center) Colin Wheeler; (opposite page, top) J.B.P.—Sygma; (opposite page, bottom) Cneva-Lyon/Sipa Press

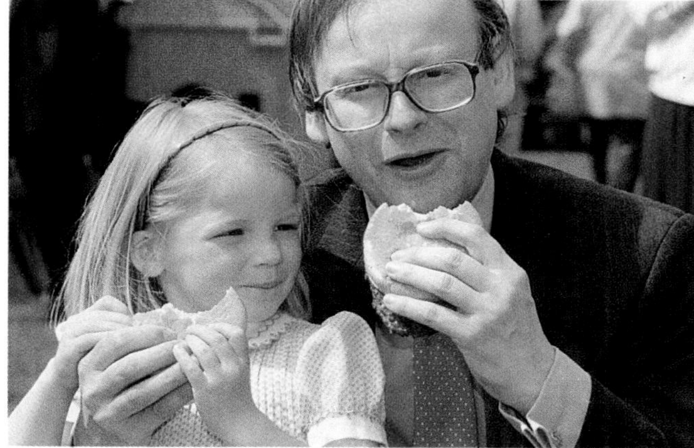

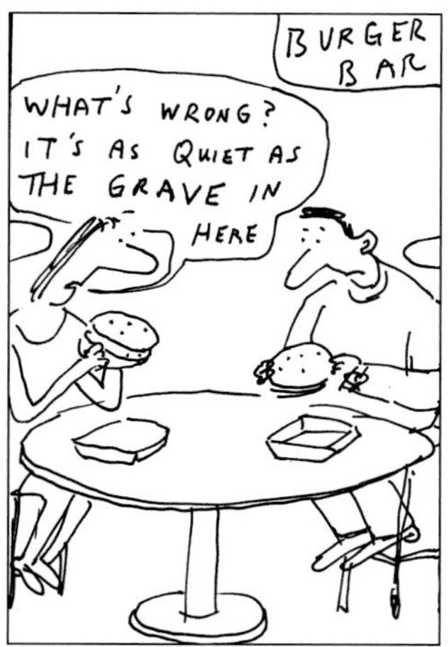

"Our beef is safe," proclaimed the British agriculture minister, John Gummer (above, with his four-year-old daughter), in 1990. (Left) A cartoonist's ironic comment on the government's belated admission of a probable link between BSE and CJD.

seph Gibbs and Mike Alpers, Gajdusek subsequently did this. (For his work on kuru, Gajdusek was awarded the Nobel Prize for Physiology or Medicine in 1976.)

In the meantime, the Fore people of New Guinea have been persuaded to abandon ritual brain eating, and the incidence of kuru is declining. Today the human TSE of greatest interest is CJD. First described in the 1920s by two German psychiatrists, Hans Creutzfeldt and Alfons Jakob, CJD is extremely rare; only an estimated one case per million people is reported annually. The incidence is virtually the same worldwide. The illness usually strikes people in their 50s or older, and in the majority of cases the origin of the disease is unknown. These cases are called sporadic—that is, neither infectious nor inherited. About 14% of cases show a familial pattern, and another 1% or fewer are due to the accidental transmission of the infectious agent by medical or surgical procedures. It should be emphasized that the latter are rare cases, and measures are now in place to prevent their recurrence. (In the 1980s, for example, after reports of CJD cases attributed to growth hormone extracted from the brains of human cadavers, the use of the natural hormone was discontinued.)

If not a virus, what is it?

As mentioned above, using the many technologies available today, scientists are usually able to isolate and classify the cause of an infectious disease. The TSEs, however, have proved extremely resistant to all efforts to identify their causative agents. One thing scientists have discovered through these efforts is that the agents responsible for scrapie, kuru, BSE, and CJD are extremely stable and cannot be rendered noninfectious by the physical and chemical treatments used to destroy most bacteria, fungi, or viruses. Thus, brain tissue from an infected animal, although subjected to temperatures or chemicals that would destroy all known viruses, is still capable of transmitting the infection to a healthy animal. Indeed, quite severe heat treatment is required for ensuring that the TSE agents have been made innocuous.

A second finding is that all of these diseases have remarkably long incubation periods. This makes their study not only slow but extremely difficult. Even in mice and ham-

D. Carleton Gajdusek (left) and a colleague examine a young victim of kuru in 1957. Gajdusek attributed the mysterious neurological disorder to a slow-acting virus.

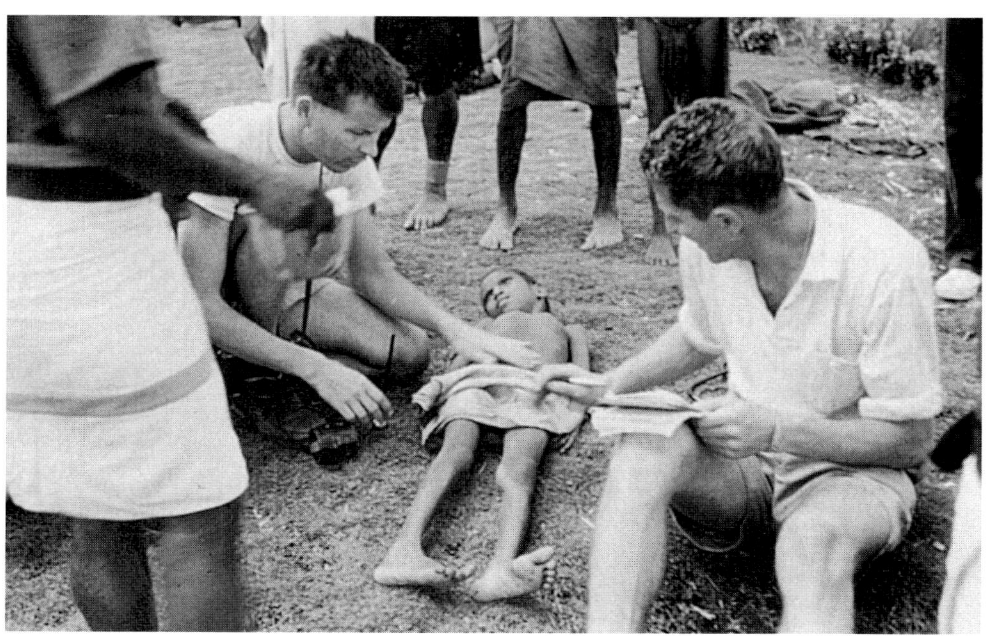

Reproduced with permission of Judith Farquhar and D. Carleton Gajdusek sters, relatively short-lived experimental animals, the incubation period of TSEs is measured in months—long enough to deter all but the most dedicated investigators.

As mentioned above, most of the research in this field has focused on the agent that causes scrapie. The disease was first transmitted experimentally in France in the 1930s, first to sheep and later to goats. It was the development of mouse and hamster models, however, that allowed research to proceed at a reasonable pace. Because the scrapie agent was capable of passing through membranes that were impermeable to bacteria, scientists recognized that it must be very tiny. The obvious conclusion—that it was a virus—was questioned as early as 1964 by Ian Pattison, a veterinarian also working at the institute in Compton, because the scrapie agent possessed several properties that were not typical of viruses.

In 1967 two landmark papers, by Gordon Hunter and Dick Gibbons at Compton and John Griffith, a physicist at Bedford College, London, summarized the evidence for the agent's being something other than a virus. Significantly, these scientists questioned whether this infectious agent contained a nucleic acid—*i.e.,* DNA or RNA.

If the scrapie agent indeed lacked a nucleic acid, it would be unlike all previously identified causes of infectious disease. In order to produce disease, bacteria, viruses, and other agents must be present in the body of the "host" animal (*i.e.,* the one being infected) in vast numbers. To create a sufficiently large population, they rely on the strategy of replicating, or reproducing, themselves inside the body of the host. The nucleic acids, DNA and RNA, are the only known molecules that possess the ability to self-replicate. Virtually every cell in the human body contains these molecules and depends on them for the creation of new cells. Even viruses, which are the simplest known infectious agents, have at least two components, nucleic acid and protein.

The protein-only hypothesis

The protein-only hypothesis—the notion that the infectious agent of scrapie consists solely of protein—was first suggested by Griffith. As expected, most of the scientific community greeted the idea with considerable skepticism. In fact, the hypothesis has been one of the enduring puzzles in molecular biology over the past three decades and has led to many acrimonious debates.

The causal agents of virtually all infections can be seen under either the conventional microscope (bacteria, fungi, protozoans) or the electron microscope (viruses). Until 1981 the agent causing scrapie had eluded microscopic searches. In that year, however, working at the New York State Institute for Basic Research in Developmental Disabilities, Pat Merz, an electron microscopist, and Robert Somerville, a biochemist, described protein particles in the brains of mice infected with scrapie. They named them "scrapie-associ-

Cause of disease—or a result of it? Electron microscopy reveals the structures known as scrapie-associated fibrils in brain tissue from an infected sheep.

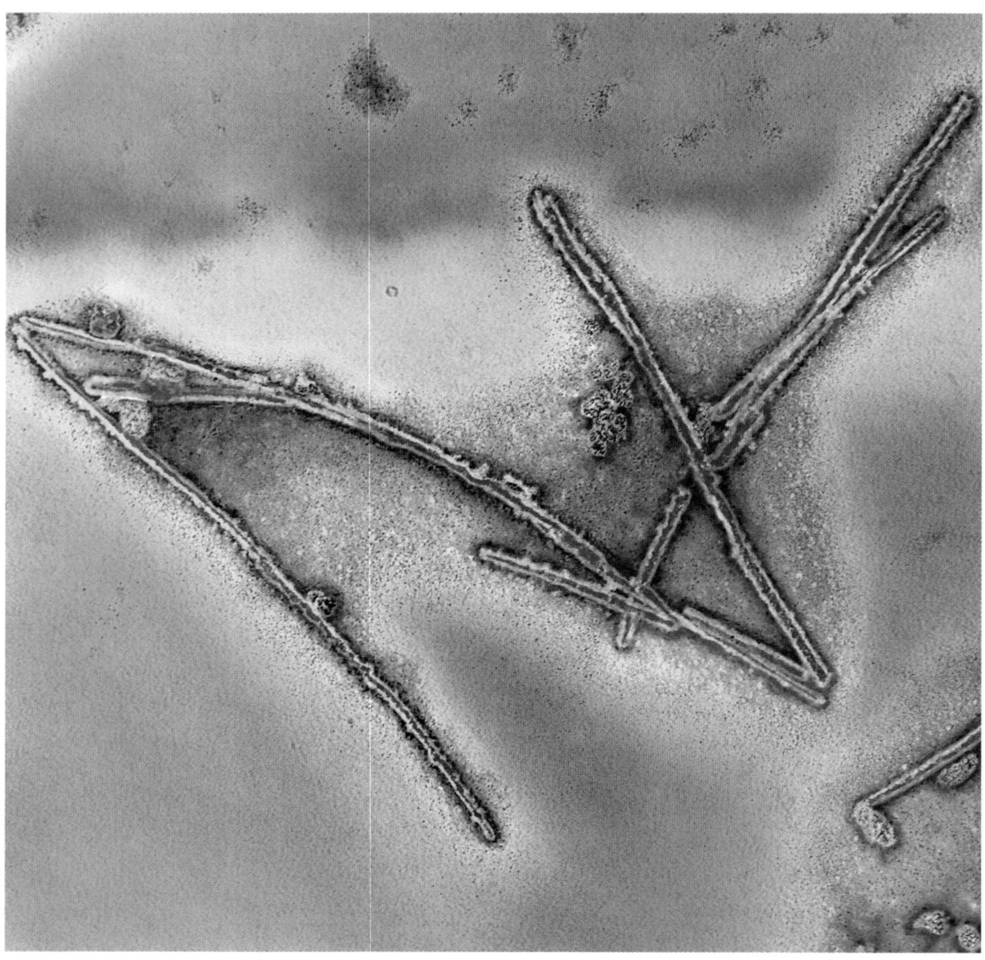

EM Unit, VLA/Science Source/Photo Researchers

Image created by S. Farr-Jones, using MidasPlus, University of California, San Francisco. Adapted from F.E. Cohen and T.L. James, *Proceedings of the National Academy of Sciences USA*, September 1997 (in press)

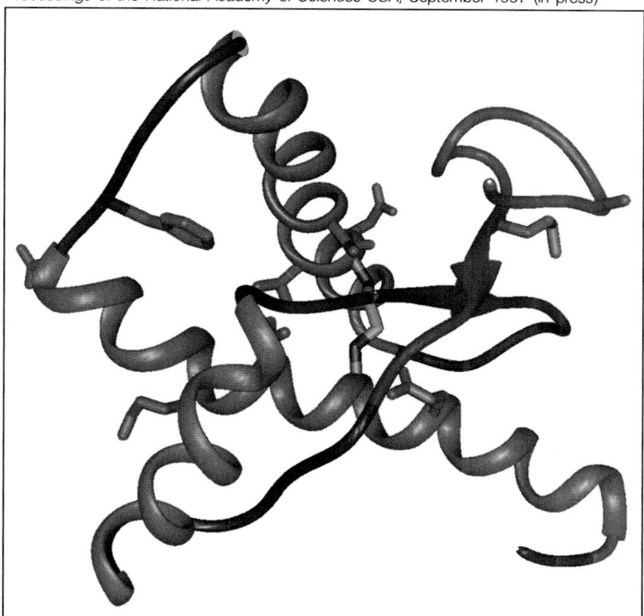

Normal structure of the prion protein, determined by means of nuclear magnetic resonance spectroscopy. In turquoise are the sites of mutations that facilitate shape change, which, according to one theory, is responsible for disease.

ated fibrils." While this discovery represented a major breakthrough, it was still unclear whether these structures were the agent of the disease or a result of it.

Stanley Prusiner, a biochemist and physician at the University of California, San Francisco, took the view that they were the agent. Unable to detect any nucleic acid in his purified fibril preparations, Prusiner renamed them "prions," short for proteinacious infectious particles, and this term, now widely used, is even included in most standard English dictionaries. Prusiner proposed that prions were proteins of abnormal conformation (*i.e.,* shape, or structure). He also proposed that they were themselves capable of causing disease—in the absence of DNA or RNA—by influencing their normal counterparts in the body to develop the same abnormality.

A major problem with this theory rests on the work of a group led by geneticist Alan Dickinson, at the Animal Breeding Research Organization in Edinburgh, and Hugh Fraser, a veterinary pathologist at the nearby Moredun Institute. In their research the Edinburgh scientists had found that different isolates, or samples, of the scrapie agent had different effects—for example, differing incubation periods—in mice of the same strain. In the 1960s the same investigators had also discovered a gene that controls the development of scrapie in mice, and subsequently they found a corresponding gene in sheep. Dickinson coined the term *virino* to describe the presumed infectious agent, which he described as a hybrid composed of protein from the body of the affected animal and another molecule, presumably DNA or RNA, carrying the information that enables the protein to replicate.

A crucial biochemical observation was made in 1985 by Prusiner and researchers in the laboratories of two internationally renowned molecular biologists, Charles Weissmann in Zürich, Switzerland, and Leroy Hood in San Francisco. They found that the scrapie fibrils were, in fact, composed of an abnormal form of a normal cellular protein, which thus confirmed at least part of Dickinson's virino theory. But the debate regarding the presence or absence of a nucleic acid continued. Heino Diringer of the Robert Koch Institute in Berlin and Laura Manuelidis, a neurologist at Yale University, are among those convinced of the presence of a nucleic acid in fibril preparations. Indeed, Manuelidis claims that as the TSEs have been purified in the laboratory, it has become clear that the infectious particles have the physical and molecular

The Prion Hypothesis: How a Protein Might Cause Disease

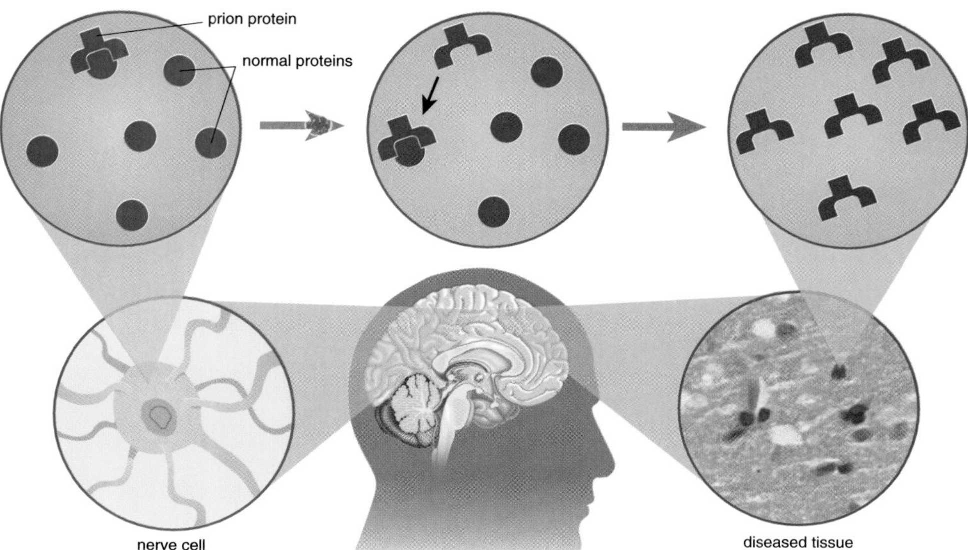

Adapted from information obtained from Dimitry Schildlovsky; (inset) Ralph Eagle Jr.—Photo Researchers

characteristics of a virus and that DNA sequences are present in samples of the infectious material.

If prion protein produced in the laboratory could be made infectious, the protein-only theory would be confirmed. Such proof has not been obtained so far. Nonetheless, in the summer of 1997 Richard Bessen and Byron Caughey at the Rocky Mountain Laboratory in Hamilton, Montana, succeeded in converting the normal prion protein into its abnormal form. It is not outside the bounds of possibility that a second molecule (DNA or RNA) may be required as a nucleus around which the conversion process starts.

The underlying feature of the protein-only model that makes many scientists, including this author, uncomfortable is the fact that even an enormous number of abnormal proteins take a long time to produce disease in recipient mice. Since a high dilution (up to a millionfold) of the same material can produce disease in nearly the same time, it seems logical to these authorities that the agent must be capable of multiplying itself. This observation would suggest the presence of a replicating molecule—*i.e.,* DNA or RNA.

The burning issue

While solving these puzzles is fundamental to an understanding of the TSEs, a more immediate problem is determining the relationship between the agents causing the different TSEs. The burning issue, of course, is whether the infectious agent that causes BSE is also responsible for the unusual cases of CJD recently reported in Britain. The work of Collinge and his team suggests that this is so, but more decisive analysis is still required.

Several years ago Dickinson demonstrated that different strains (*i.e.,* closely related but not identical forms) of the scrapie agent could be distinguished from each other by measuring the time required by different samples of infectious material to cause disease in laboratory mice. On the basis of this observation, some scientists have suggested that it would be possible to determine whether the agents of BSE and the new variant of CJD are the same by comparing their incubation periods in mice.

In Dickinson's work, however, the samples of infectious material had first been adapted by growing the agent in mice until the incubation period of each became "fixed" (*i.e.,* set at a specific, predictable length), which is what usually happens when an infectious agent is adapted to a laboratory setting. It is questionable, therefore, whether much weight could be attached to a comparison of the lengths of the incubation periods of fresh samples derived from different sources, in this instance the brains of a BSE-infected cow and a human patient with the new CJD variant.

An alternative method of determining if BSE is indeed the causal agent of the new form of CJD, and one that has surprisingly met much resistance within the SEAC, would be to inoculate brain material from the human patients with the new form of CJD directly into the brains of cattle. Would the animals then de-

Confiscated beef products await disposal in the United Kingdom. Ensuring the safety of the food supply is now among the government's top priorities.

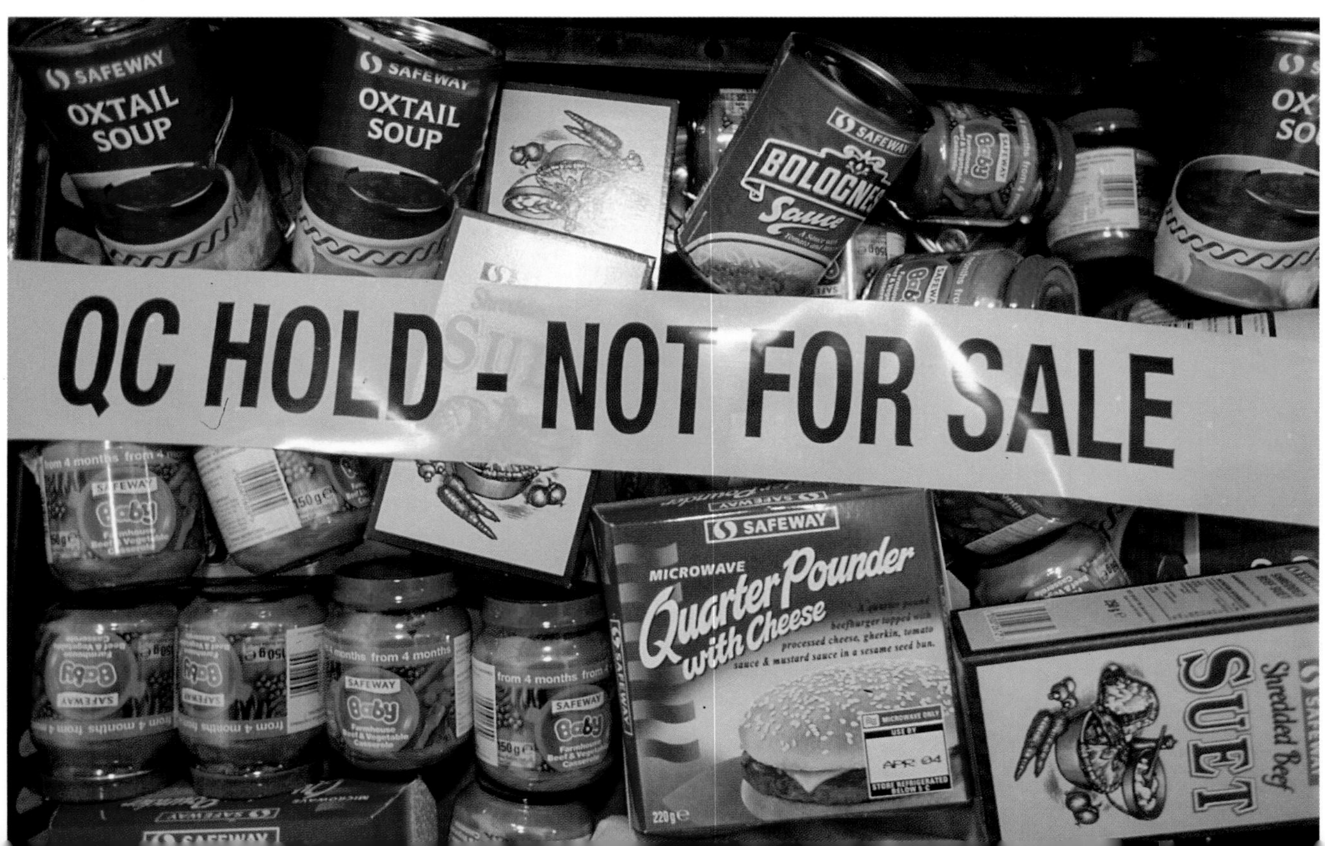

velop BSE? This is the most direct approach and one that would observe the well-respected postulates of the 19th-century German physician Robert Koch—the cofounder (with Louis Pasteur) of the science of bacteriology—for determining the identity of a disease-causing agent.

(Below) Hubert Raguet—Eurelios/Science Source/Photo Researchers; (opposite page) Nigel Dickinson—Still Pictures

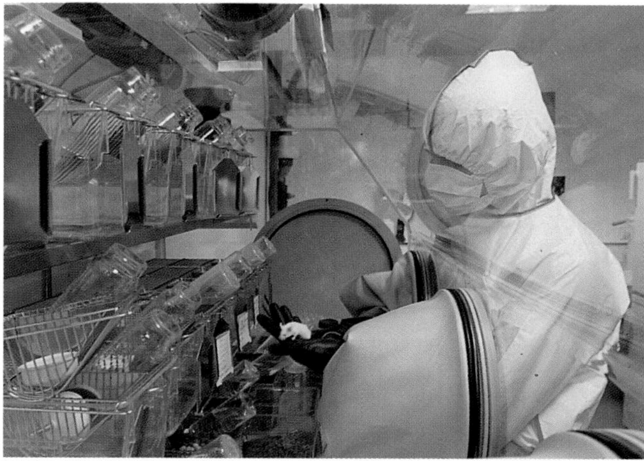

A scientist in protective gear handles a mouse that has been experimentally infected with BSE. Determining the relationship between the cattle disease and its human counterpart is a major focus of current research.

The iceberg—or just the tip?

Irrespective of the fundamental issues regarding the nature of the agent or agents that cause the TSEs, it has become very important to resolve those pertaining to the safety of meat and milk. It should be emphasized that by using the same methods employed to determine infectivity of brain tissue, scientists have not detected the BSE agent in the meat or milk of cattle with the disease or in other products such as gelatin derived from offal.

By the summer of 1997, 21 cases of the so-called new variant CJD had been confirmed in the U.K. and one in France. The crucial question is whether this cluster of cases heralds the beginning of a major outbreak of CJD or will eventually prove to have been an isolated anomaly. According to epidemiologists and statisticians, it is too early to determine if a major upsurge in CJD is under way. In the meantime, only 11 additional cases have been reported since the epochal announcement of March 1996. Should the public take reassurance from this small number? Epidemiologists think that this would be an overly optimistic view. Only time will provide the answer.

As mentioned above, scrapie was known in sheep and goats for more than 200 years, and yet in all that time, no evidence emerged of its posing a threat to human health. Then, in the 1980s, BSE suddenly appeared. Because sheep parts had originally been used in the protein supplement fed to British cattle, it seemed reasonable to assume that the scrapie agent may have crossed the species barrier and infected the brains of cattle. Did it then repeat the process, "jumping species" from cattle to humans?

So far there is no evidence that the scrapie agent can cause human disease. Indeed, there is not even direct evidence that it causes BSE. Nonetheless, from observing the actions of other infectious agents—the poliovirus, for example—scientists know that a single change in the genetic material of the agent can distinguish a virulent strain from one that is harmless. It is conceivable that such a change also could enable an agent to infect a species never before susceptible to it. In fact, a similar process is suggested as the mechanism by which HIV, the virus that causes AIDS, crossed the species barrier from nonhuman primates to humans.

Are the new CJD cases reported in Britain in the past two years the tip of an iceberg? Several issues must be resolved before that question can be answered. The first and most important is to establish whether BSE and the new form of CJD are caused by the same agent. The second is to determine why only one or two animals in a herd develop BSE, while the rest apparently remain healthy. The third is to determine the incubation period of the new variant CJD. These imponderables make predictions simply guesswork.

There is, however, one clear message. Despite enormous progress in medical science and basic understanding of the brain and nervous system, the human neurological diseases remain largely a mystery. Are BSE and CJD perhaps related to Alzheimer's disease, the age-associated dementia that also apparently involves unusual brain proteins?

In 1981 this author was a member of a group of scientists, headed by the University of Cambridge virologist Peter Wildy, that convinced the U.K.'s leading medical and agricultural agencies that research on scrapie and CJD should be undertaken at a single institution. It was clear to these authorities even then that the close relationship of the two diseases demanded that they be studied side by side. The events of the past two years have only underscored the soundness of the recommendation. MHA

Will the "Beefeater"—a symbol of England since Tudor times—become a relic?

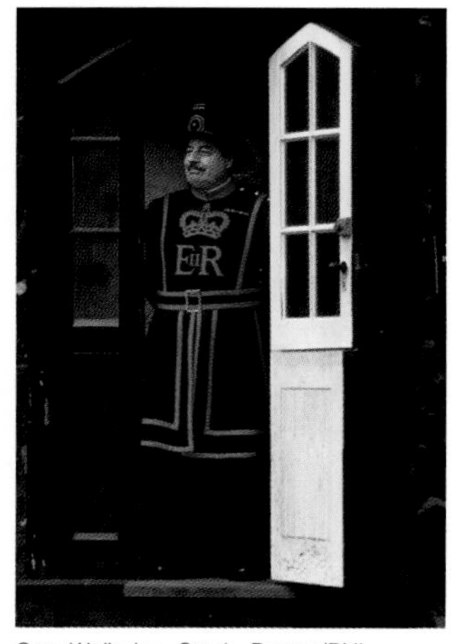

Cary Wolinsky—Stock, Boston/PNI

From Mother to Fetus, from Superstition to Science

by F. González-Crussi, M.D.

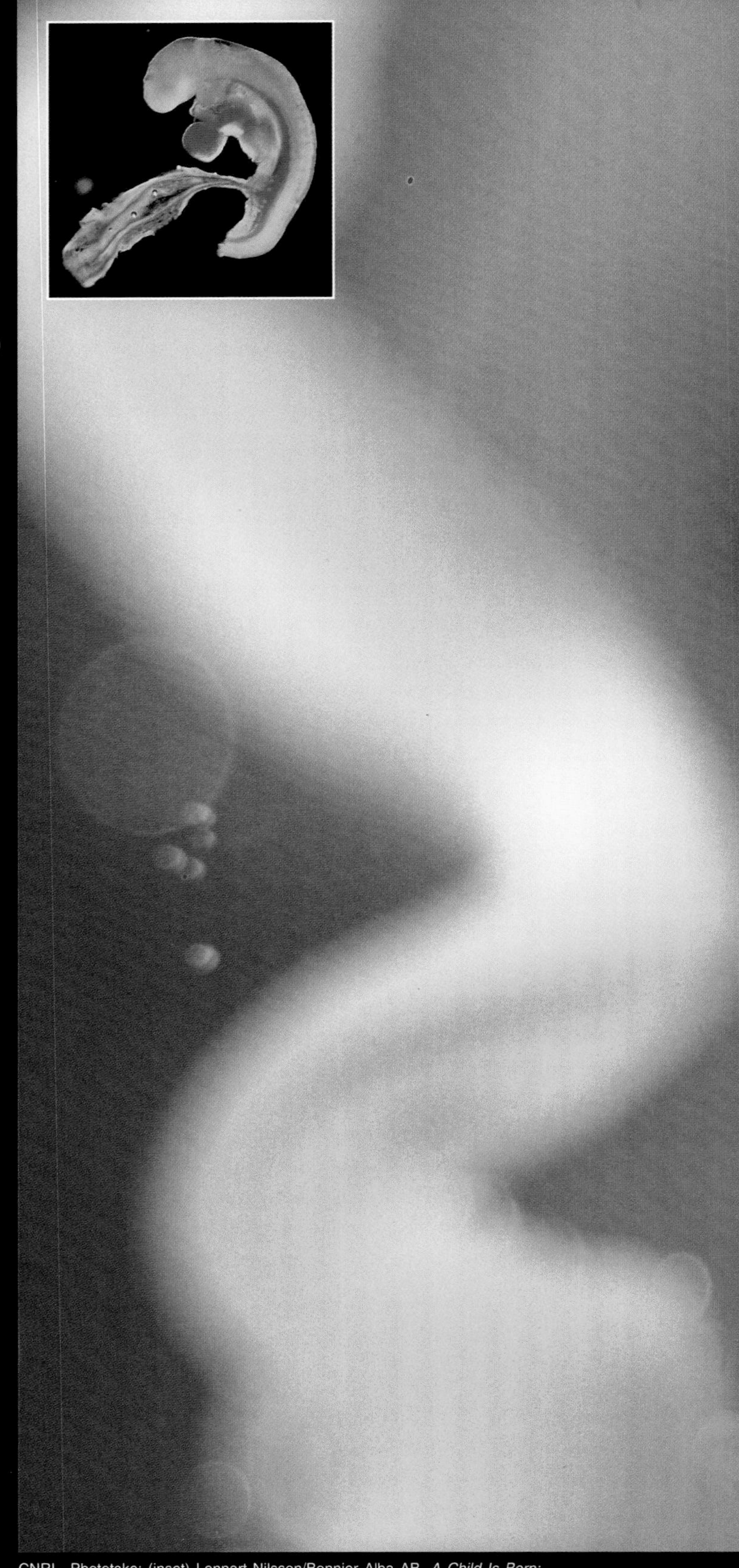

CNRI—Phototake; (inset) Lennart Nilsson/Bonnier Alba AB, *A Child Is Born;* (opposite page, inset) Matt Meadows—Science Source/Photo Researchers

F. González-Crussi, M.D., is Professor of Pathology at Northwestern University Medical School and Head of Laboratories at Children's Memorial Hospital, Chicago. He is the author of many books, including Notes of an Anatomist *(1985),* Three Forms of Sudden Death *(1986),* On the Nature of Things Erotic *(1988),* The Five Senses *(1989),* The Day of the Dead *(1993), and, his most recent,* Suspended Animation: Six Essays on the Preservation of Bodily Parts *(1995). Several of his books have been translated into his native Spanish, as well as French, Italian, Dutch, and Japanese.*

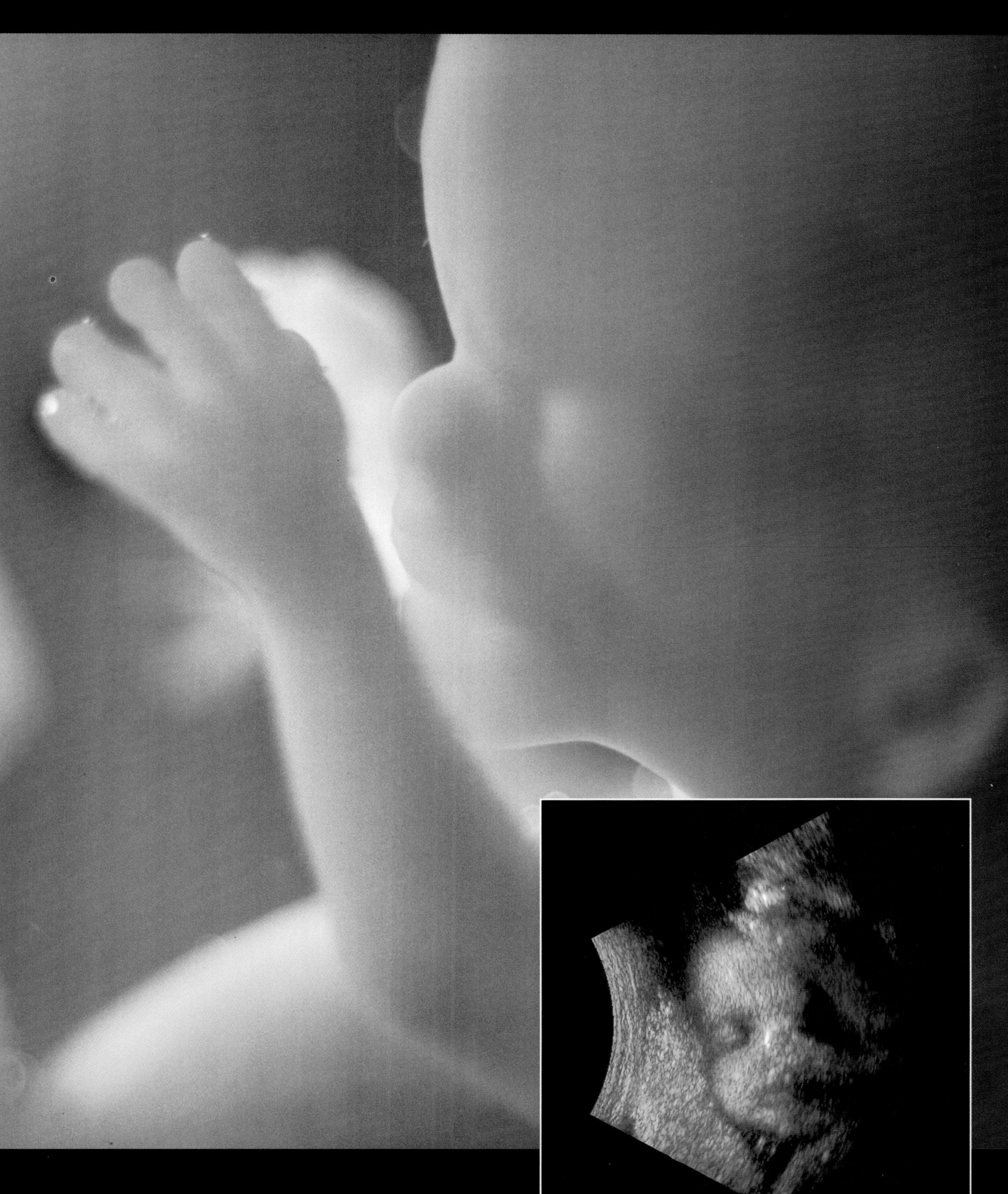

Prospective parents share a universal desire: to engender healthy, handsome progeny. Central to this eugenic aspiration is an appreciation of all that can go wrong—the myriad influences to which the fetus is susceptible. In modern times a great deal has been learned about the situations and agents that can contribute to abnormal embryofetal development and produce congenital defects. Knowing what they do, health professionals today advise women to do everything they can to ensure the well-being of their unborn children. Taking vitamins; refraining from smoking, drinking alcohol, and taking unnecessary medications; exercising within reason; eating a proper diet; avoiding caffeine; resting adequately; and having regular prenatal examinations are all steps a woman can take to optimize the healthy development of her fetus. In earlier times, when very little was known about the actual causes of birth defects, just about anything the mother did during gestation could seem suspect. Thus, superstitions and myths often dictated the "dos" and "don'ts" of pregnancy.

Jim Olive—Peter Arnold, Inc.

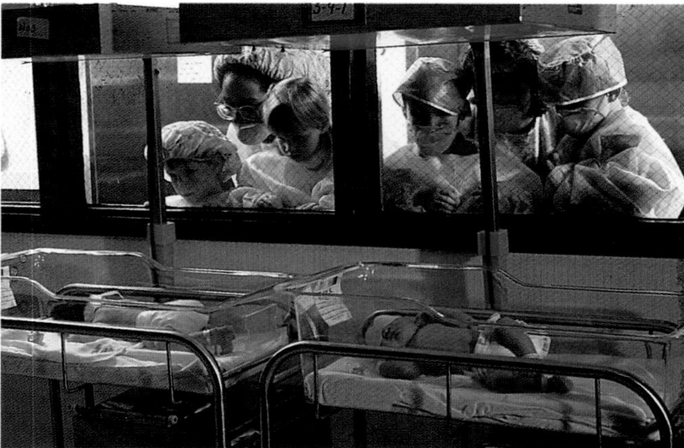

With considerable pride, joy, and awe and undoubtedly some trepidation, new parents and others observe newborns in a hospital nursery soon after their extraordinary transition from the womb to the world.

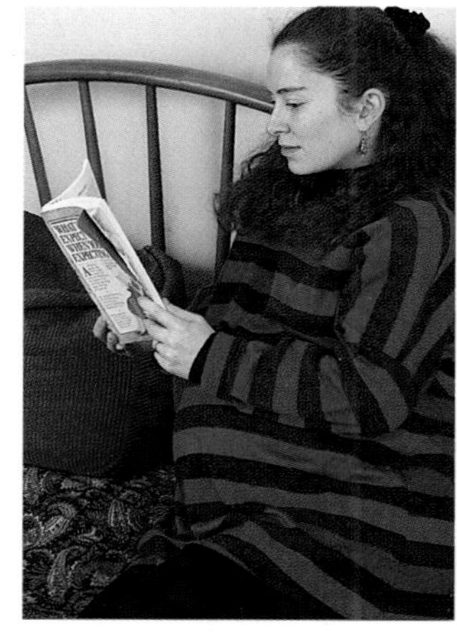

(Right) A woman in her third trimester consults an authority; (below) fitness-conscious moms-to-be take an aqua-aerobics class. Knowing that so many of the things they do will affect their developing fetuses, most women do everything possible to ensure that all is well in the womb.

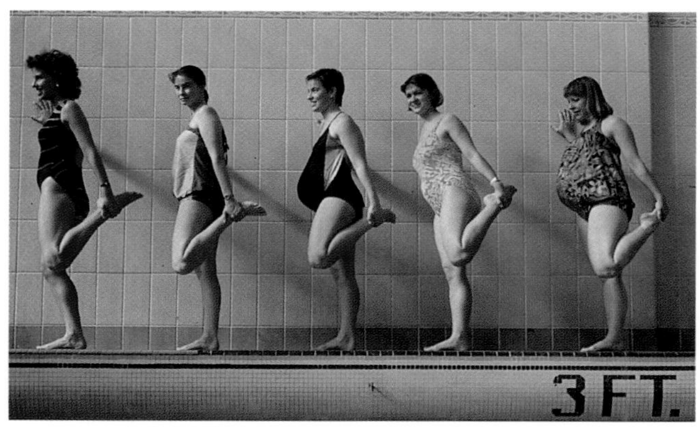

(Top) Laura Dwight—Peter Arnold, Inc.; (above) Annie Griffiths Belt—Aurora

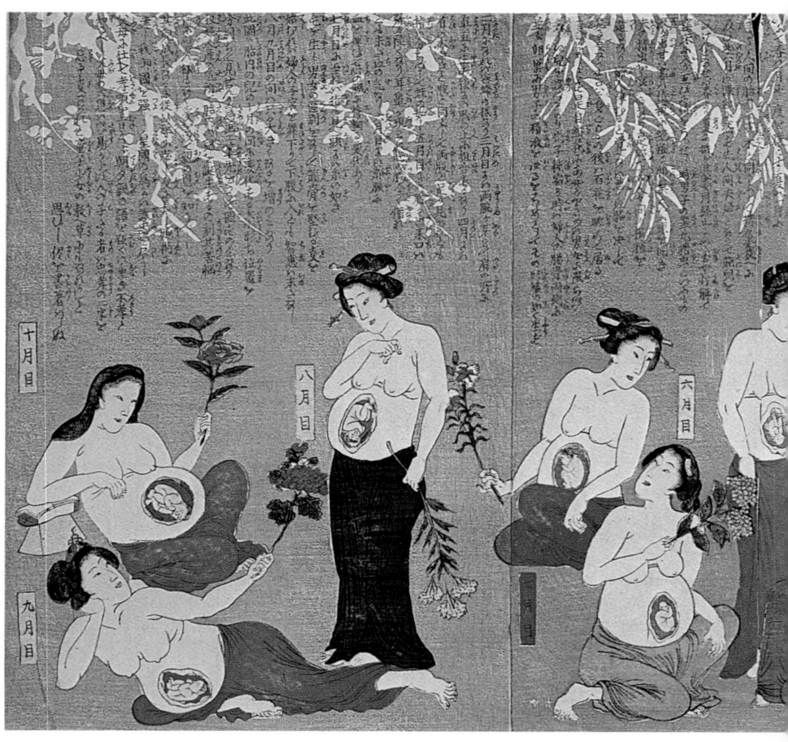

Imagine that!

Consider, for example, the mother-to-be's mental tranquility. It was commonly—and probably quite rightly—believed that a placid state of mind was vital to the development of a healthy conceptus. The Greek physiologist Empedocles (*c.* 490–430 BC), best known for his cosmological theories of personality, propounded the idea that expectant mothers could enhance the comeliness of their unborn children by looking at beautiful art objects. The Spartans of ancient Greece, apparently with the same eugenic end in mind, decreed that pregnant women should look upon statues of the youthful twin deities Castor and Pollux, revered for their good looks and athletic prowess. In the 3rd century AD, Heliodorus of Emesa wrote the long and popular work of fiction *Aethiopica,* in which a child is born with perfectly white skin, despite being the offspring of dark-skinned parents. The author attributed this unusual phenomenon to the mother's having gazed at a particular painting of the fair princess Andromeda.

By the same token, it was widely assumed that tempestuous agitations of the mother's mind would adversely affect her fetus. The "maternal imagination," which could somehow stamp physical markings ("impres-

Pregnant women desire healthy babies; few sentiments are as timeless or universal, as is suggested by a pre-Christian-era Phoenician statuette (right) and a 19th-century Japanese print (below).

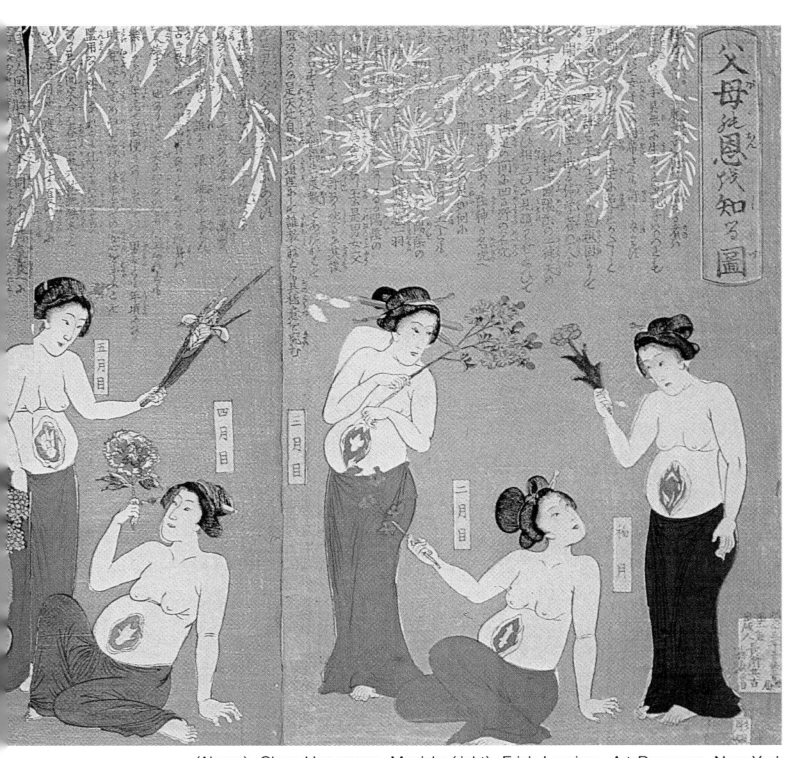

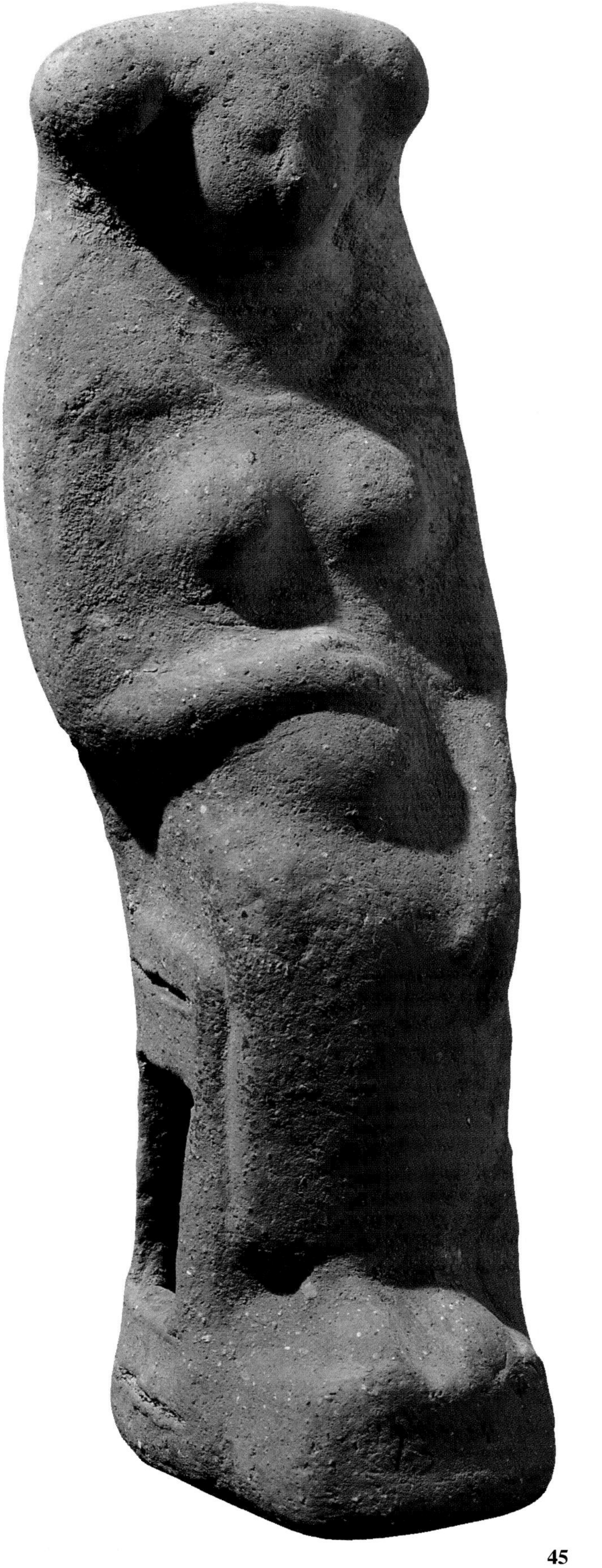

(Above) Claus Hansmann, Munich; (right) Erich Lessing—Art Resource, New York

Giraudon/Art Resource, New York

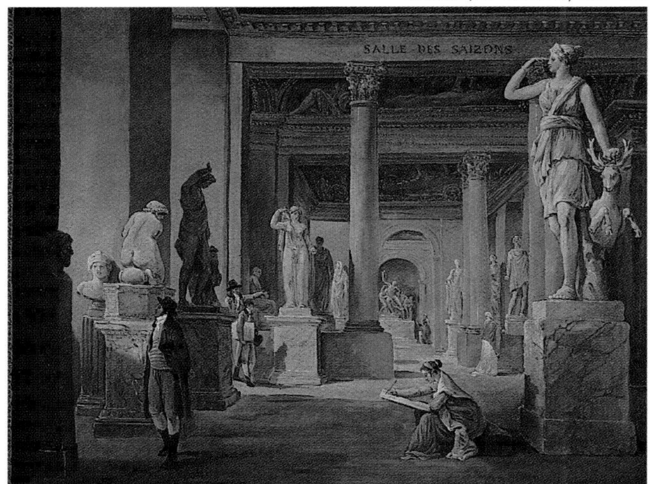

(Above) Viewing statues in the Louvre, Paris. The ancient Greeks believed mothers might enhance the comeliness of their progeny by gazing at beautiful art objects.

sions") upon the fetus, was held responsible for all sorts of deformities.

The branch of embryology concerned with the development and classification of malformed fetuses is known as teratology (*teras* is the Greek word for "monster"). A much-quoted vignette from the annals of teratology concerns the birth of a girl in Austria in the early Renaissance whose hair-covered skin resembled the fur of a bear. This unusual physical attribute was most likely due to the rare condition known as hypertrichosis, or hirsutism, but at the time, the child's excessive body hair was considered proof of the power of the maternal imagination. The accepted explanation for her animal-like appearance was that at precisely the time she was conceived, her mother had looked upon a painting of Saint John the Baptist, clad in an animal skin, doing penance in the wilderness.

Similar reasoning may have led to the ancient Egyptian belief that it was dangerous for mothers to look at monkeys during pregnancy. During an archaeological excavation at the ancient city of Hermopolis, the mummified corpse of an anencephalic infant (born without a brain) was uncovered. The body had been bandaged, protected, and arrayed in the posture commonly reserved for monkey corpses. The close resemblance of anencephalic newborns to monkeys, it seems, convinced the Egyptians that a woman could actually give birth to offspring of another species—assuming she had been startled or deeply impressed by the sight of such a creature while bearing her unborn child.

In a famous passage of scripture, Genesis 30:31–39 (King James Version), Jacob agrees to tend Laban's sheep, cattle, and goats, asking only that he be allowed to keep any animals born "speckled" and "spotted." He then proceeds to peel patches of bark off "rods of green poplar, and of hazel and chestnut tree" and places them before the cattle's watering troughs so "that they should conceive when they came to drink." When many calves are born "ringstraked, speckled, and spotted," the obvious conclusion is that the appearance of the rods had "impressed" the animals. This, of course, was to Ja-

(Opposite) Jacob cleverly acquired lambs, goats, and calves from the flocks of Laban—animals conceived before tree rods that he had intentionally manipulated.

The "hairy virgin" below (1560) was said to have been "conceived by the force of imagination." Many thought the maternal imagination had also caused the abnormal hairiness in the Austrian child at right.

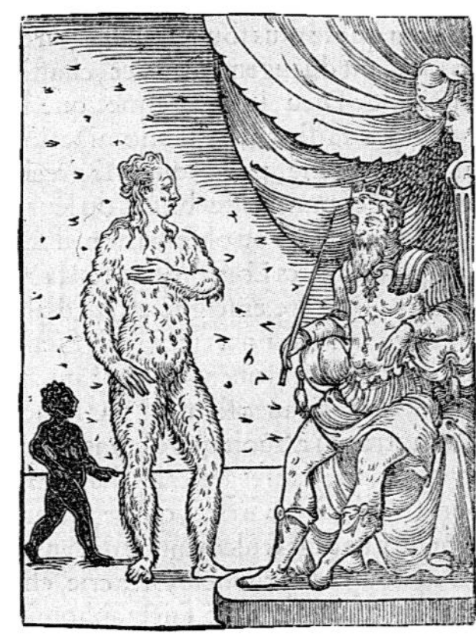

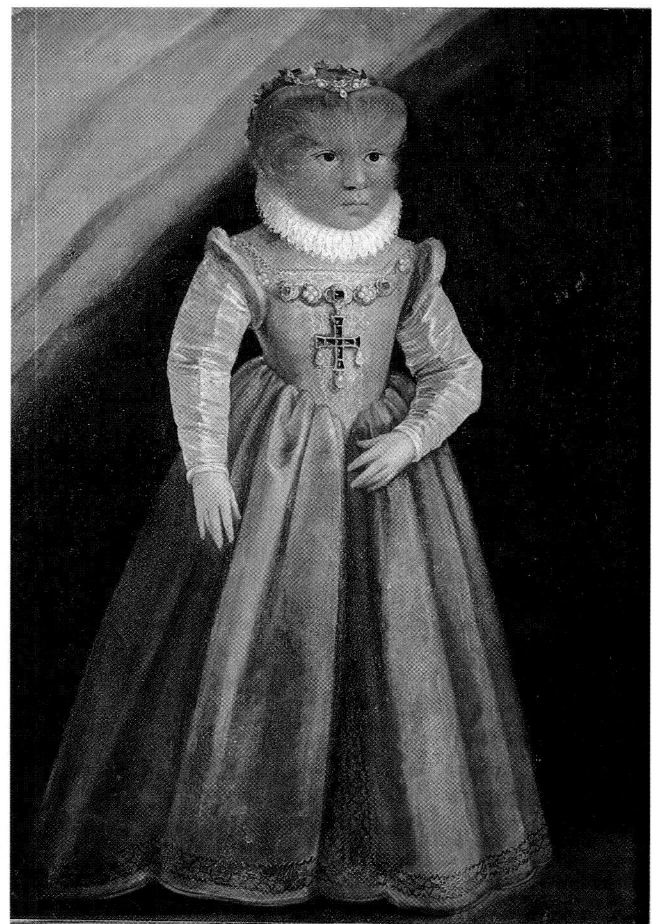

(Left) E.T. Archive; (above) Erich Lessing—Art Resource, New York

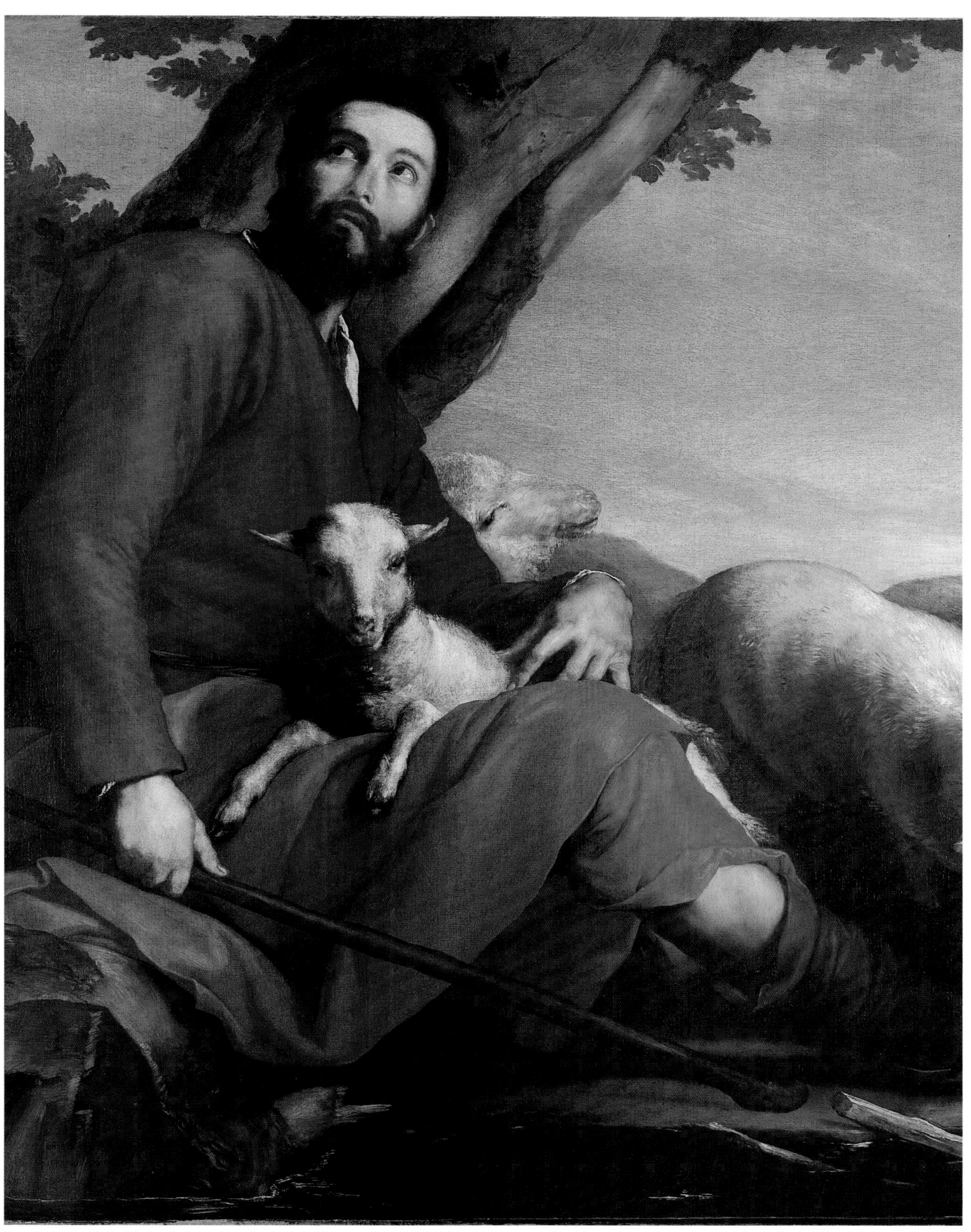

"Jacob with the Flock of Laban," oil on canvas by José de Ribera, probably 1638, 132 x 118 cm; reproduced by courtesy of the trustees of the National Gallery, London

E.T. Archive

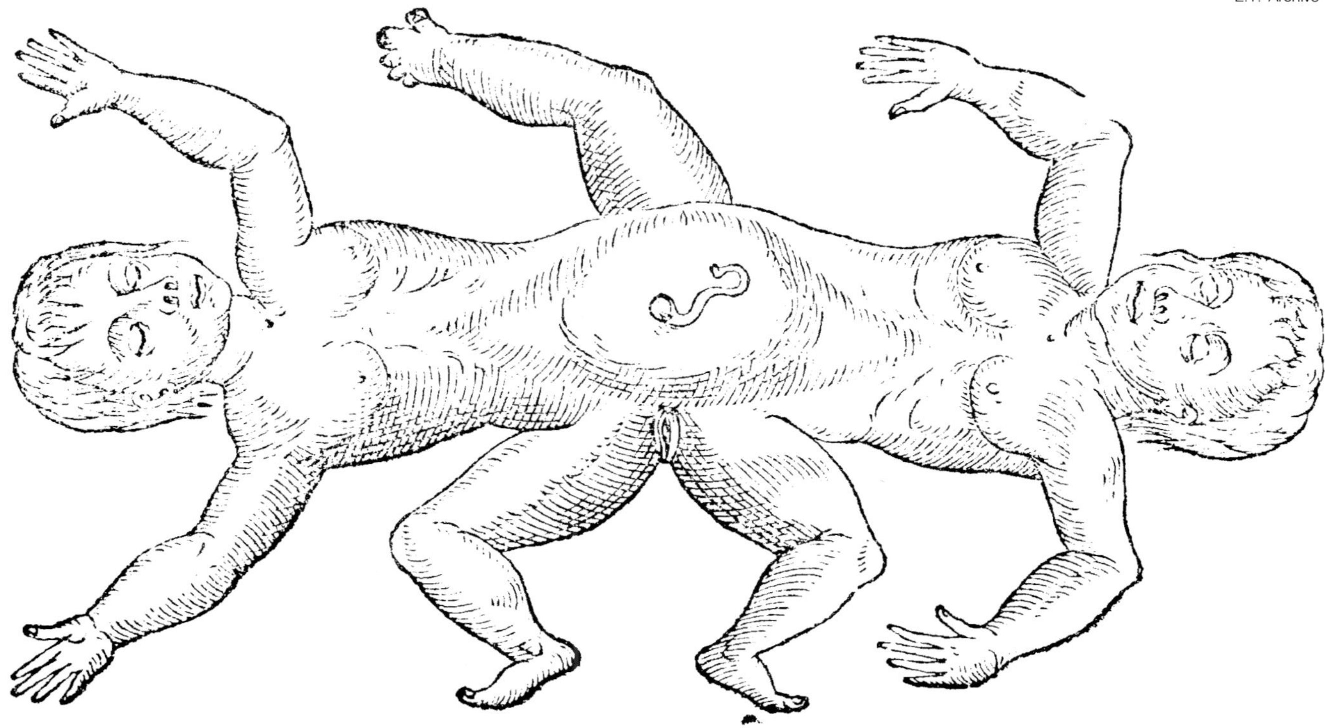

Illustration from a work by Ambroise Paré, who believed monstrous offspring could be conceived during a mother's (or father's) strange dreams or visions.

cob's immense financial benefit. In his ability to direct the outcome of a biological process and then to reap commercial benefits from the results, Jacob can be said to have anticipated today's lucrative biotechnology industry; he might even be regarded as the "father of genetic engineering."

Although belief in the power of the mother's imagination to affect the outcome of her offspring was widespread, such "imagination" was never very clearly defined. In his treatise *De la génération de l'homme, des monstres* (1573; *On Monsters and Prodigies*), the French surgeon Ambroise Paré alluded to that "ardent and obstinate fancy a woman may experience while she is conceiving, owing to some object or fantastic dream, or some nocturnal visions that a man or a woman may have at the time of conception." In the Nov. 14, 1896, issue of the *Journal of the American Medical Association (JAMA),* William F. Batman, a physician from Lebanon, Indiana, defined maternal impression as "a profound and sudden impression made on the mother's mind [that] may pervert or stop the growth, or cause defect in the child with which she is pregnant." Quite a hodgepodge of emotions and phenomena—joys, terrors, whims, surprises, fantasies, dreams, cravings, and so forth—it seems, were included in the category of "imagination." Likewise, a vast range of deformities and oddities in infants were considered "impressions."

In the 18th century it was common to ascribe a unique "erethism," or abnormal irritability, to the maternal (and by extension to the feminine) sensibility. In his *Dictionnaire philosophique* (1764), the French philosopher and writer Voltaire asserted, "This passive imagination of easily unsettled brains sometimes determines the transfer to the children of the impressions that the mother has received. There are innumerable examples; the author has seen some so striking, that he would belie his own eyes if he were to doubt [their existence]." The French physician Jacques-Auguste Blondel reported the strange occurrence of a triple

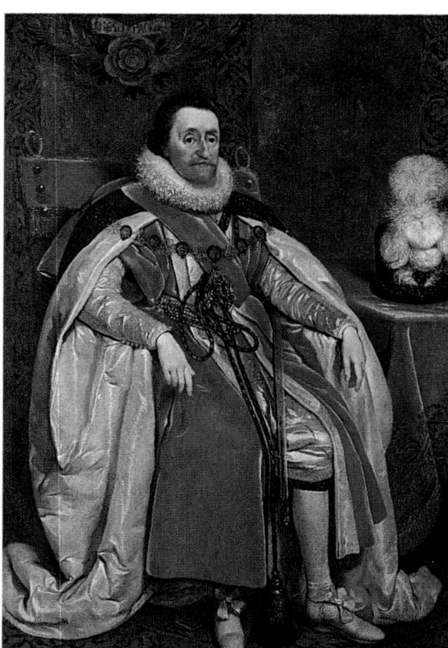

James I of England, oil on canvas by Daniel Mytens, 1621, 148.6 x 100.6 cm; by courtesy of the National Portrait Gallery, London

Certain quirks in the personality of James I, king of England from 1603 to 1625, were attributed to a brutal murder witnessed by his mother, Mary, Queen of Scots, during her pregnancy. More likely, the king's character was shaped by events of his childhood.

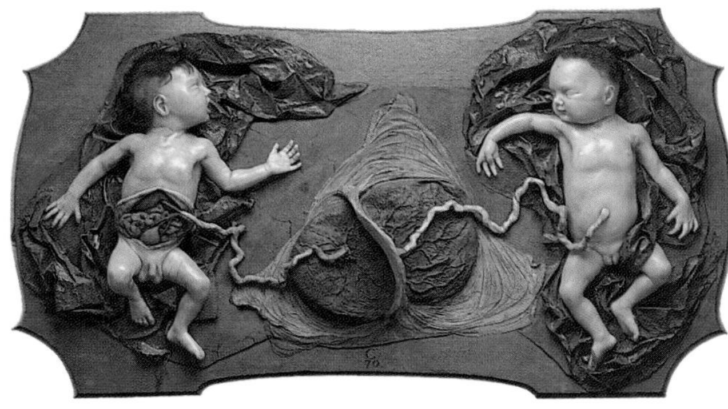

Wax model (18th century) showing the intimate connection of twins in utero to the placenta, the blood-rich structure that mediates all maternal-fetal metabolic exchanges.

birth to a woman who was obsessed with the idea that she would deliver on the day of the Epiphany. Her offspring consisted of two white children and one black child, which was in keeping with the complexions of the three Magi, whose coming is commemorated by the feast of the Epiphany.

Does she dare to eat a peach?

Whereas the mere exercise of the imaginative faculty at almost any time during the period of gestation was believed sufficient to cause *physical* changes in the fetus, the presumed effects of maternal discomposure upon the *mental* state—the character and personality—of the offspring were considered to be of even greater subtlety. Mary, Queen of Scots, was pregnant with the future James I when she witnessed the murder of her Italian secretary at close range. Some thought that the shock of the experience directly affected the temperament of the English king, who was never able to witness the unsheathing of a sword without feeling faint. Blondel, in the 18th century, was among those who refuted that explanation. In 1737 he published a book that ascribed the timidity of James I not to a single terrifying experience suffered by his mother but to the climate of anguish and uncertainty that darkened the whole of his childhood.

Longings, sudden urges, eccentric whims, and perversions of the appetite were all manifestations of this hypothetical irritability inherent in the feminine nature. Sometimes that irritability led to spectacular forms of madness, including episodes of anthropophagy, in which pregnant women were possessed by the invincible desire to bite off the skin of friends or relatives. In *The Adventures of Peregrine Pickle* (1751), the Scottish physician and picaresque novelist Tobias Smollett described the gestational aberrations and irksome demands of the pregnant Mrs. Pickle. At various times in the narrative, she is seized with the desire to pinch her husband's ears, to pluck some hairs from his beard, or, on occasion, to eat peaches. Members of her household rush to satisfy her capricious desires lest the baby be born with deformed

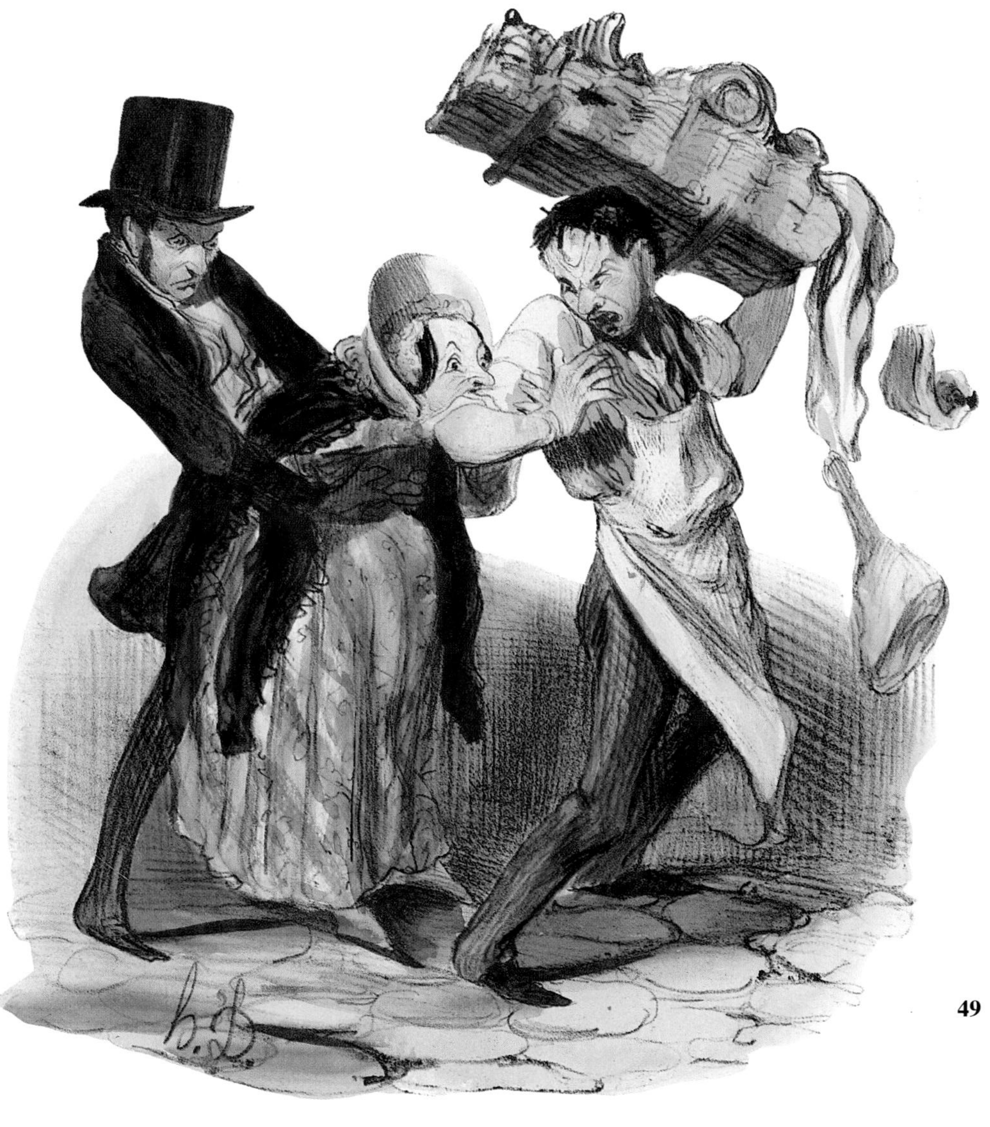

In less-scientific times, many thought that if a pregnant woman's cravings—*e.g.,* for a bite of flesh—were not satisfied, her fetus might be adversely affected.

(Top) Erich Lessing—Art Resource, New York; (bottom) Jean-Loup Charmet, Paris ears, a grey beard, or a fuzzy growth on its body. Her request for peaches is especially worrisome because nutritional wisdom of the day held that peaches were injurious to the health of the mother-to-be. So, at the same time that Mrs. Pickle is exhorted to eat a peach to satisfy her craving, her family frantically prepares an antidote that she also must swallow.

Longings and cravings during pregnancy, however, were certainly not a laughing matter. Members of the medical profession took these pregnancy-induced whims of their female patients very seriously, believing that maternal desires, if not promptly satisfied, would cause the fetus to be born bearing the marks of the thwarted wish. It may be that at a time when women had few "rights" and were considered the "weaker sex," some expectant mothers took advantage of their situation, reaping everything they could from the tender solicitude and obliging protectiveness that their condition inspired. But privileges so cunningly exacted came at a high price. Women were easily startled, readily worried, and often terrified beyond measure by the possibility that an unwitting impression might damage their offspring. An astute 18th-century physician described women in the precarious state of pregnancy this way: "Restless and alarmed, they lose their cheer, their repose, and their sleep. Their blood is altered; fear of an imaginary ill makes them suffer real ills, and becomes noxious to the health of the child."

Unimpressed: skeptics surface

Like his contemporary Blondel, Denis Diderot did not accept that maternal impressions were responsible for either mental or physical attributes of offspring. In his famous *Encyclopédie,* Diderot squarely lays the blame for at least some of the deformities in newborns at the hands of midwives:

> *Prompted by a curiosity that is natural to those who think a little, the curiosity to see man's birth, after having seen his death time and again, I [went] to visit one of these women... who receive young people seeking instruction in the matter of deliveries, & I saw there examples of inhumanity that would defy belief in a land of barbarians.... These midwives, in the hope of attracting the greatest number of spectators, and therefore payors, sent emissaries to announce that they had a woman in labor, whose child in all assurance was coming unnaturally. People arrive; and not to deceive them they returned the child into the womb, and drew it by the feet. I would not dare to say this if I had not been an ocular witness several times, & if the midwife herself had not had the imprudence of confessing it to me, after all the attendees were gone.*

Claus Hansmann, Munich

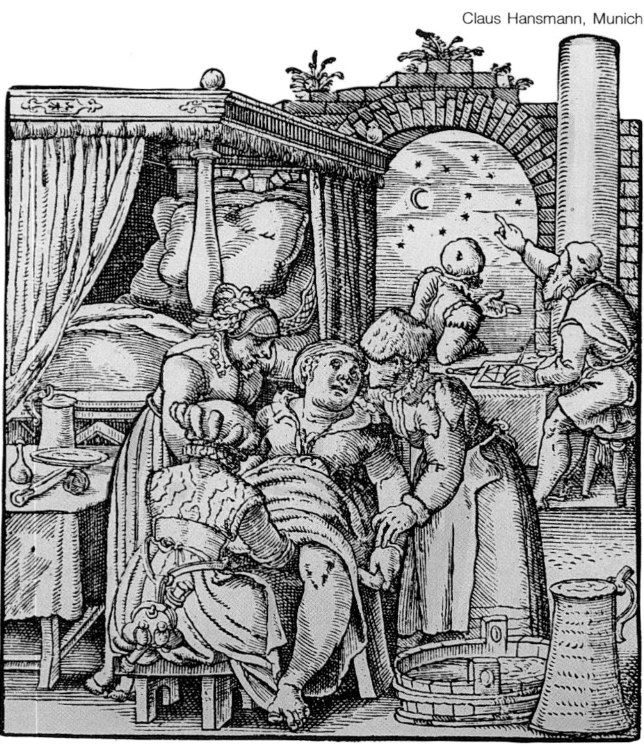

Though many in the 18th century believed that "maternal impressions" could produce fetal deformities, the French encyclopedist Denis Diderot was quite certain that most birth defects were the work of "barbarian" midwives.

By the first half of the 19th century, the belief in the power of maternal impressions to modify the physical traits of the fetus had begun to lose sway as scientists convincingly showed that the concept was without basis in fact. In England pregnant women were questioned prospectively (during gestation) about incidents that impressed them forcefully; most denied any such occurrences. It was only *after* childbirth that mothers came up with all sorts of fanciful explanations to account for anomalies and idiosyncrasies in their offspring.

Such deeply rooted beliefs, however, do not necessarily vanish because their falsity is brought to light. Even at the end of the 19th century, there were prominent physicians who still believed in maternal impressions. The aforementioned article in *JAMA* described an incident in which a pregnant woman was frightened by a dog and gave birth to a daughter "who possessed an uncontrollable fear of dogs" and "anything in the canine race." Later in her life, when the daughter herself was pregnant, she was bitten by a dog. She had a miscarriage, and the shape of the dead fetus's head sharply resembled the dog's skull. The attending physician reported to the Chicago Medical Society:

> *I secured the dog that had been the occasion of such trouble, and to-night I show you the skull of the dog,*

Stephan Elleringmann—Bilderberg/Aurora

which I would like to have you compare with the little monster. Those who believe in the transmission of maternal impressions will get some consolation from examining these specimens, and those who believe such results happen as mere coincidence will have to account for this freak as best they can.

The article concluded with a ringing affirmation of the noble role that doctors could play in eugenics: "We as scientific physicians, who... are one hundred years in advance of the politician, should teach our patrons how to care for our pregnant women, and the danger from maternal influences. This... will strengthen the human race."

Music to fetal ears

Though today the medical profession has discarded uncritical superstitious beliefs about maternal impressions, this does not mean that the mother-to-be's state of mind is irrelevant during gestation The fetus is no longer considered a strictly insentient being. Rather, the developing child in the womb is keenly sensitive to a variety of stimuli. Researchers are just beginning to define the ways in which the fetal organism responds to such stimuli. One way they are doing so is to study infants born prematurely.

The process of birth represents an extraordinary transition. Normally the newborn confronts this radical change from the intrauterine to the extrauterine world with uncanny efficiency. Such instantaneous physiological adjustments on the part of the infant have been as much a source of wonder as a focus of scientific investigation. Physicians who care for premature newborns are aware that the success of their ministrations is largely subordinate to the fact that their patients are, in many ways, still fetuses. Because their organs are not as fully developed either structurally or functionally as those of full-term babies, very premature babies are ill-equipped to make the necessary outside-the-womb adaptations.

The fetal environment is often characterized as vaguely "dark, quiet, warm, and humid." It is, however, much more than that. Newborn specialists know that a delicate premature infant does not have the capacity to survive in an environment that is jarringly discrepant from the one it was accustomed to. For the infant to thrive, conditions must be as close as possible to those of the womb. Thus, experts have studied not only the best ways to handle, position, feed, and cover them but also the temperature, level of humidity, and other stimuli to subject them to.

The auditory stimulation of the fetus is one very intriguing domain that is currently receiving considerable attention. It is well established that the fetus can hear, although the specific mechanisms of sound transmission and auditory perception in the womb have yet to be fully delineated. Researchers maintain that newborns have an unconscious but important memory of the maternal heartbeat; this explains the ease with which babies are lulled to sleep by the ticking of a clock or by being held closely against another person's chest.

As early as the 24th week

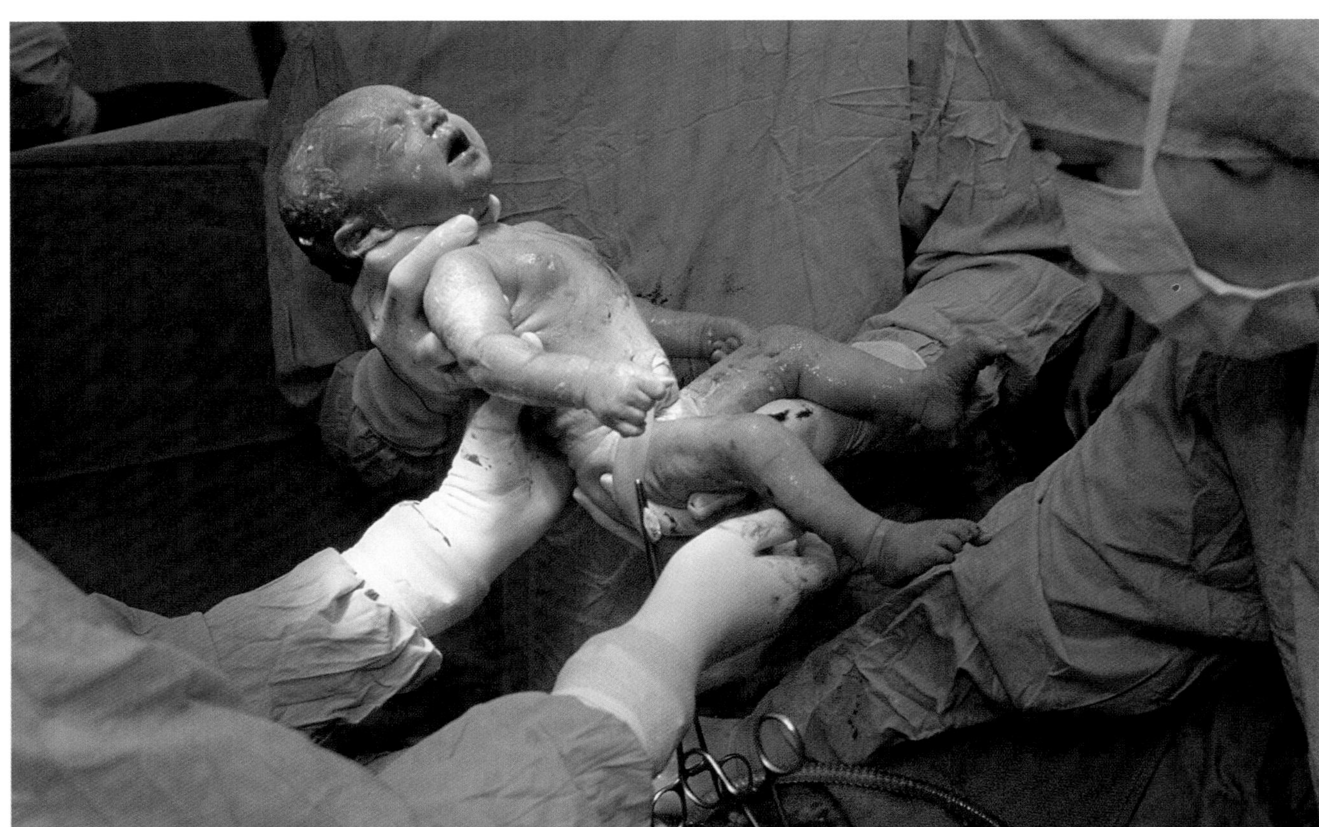

Fresh from the womb, the newborn infant must make extraordinary adjustments to the extrauterine world. In fact, most babies adapt to their radically unfamiliar circumstances with an uncanny degree of facility.

(Below left and right) Annie Griffiths Belt—Aurora; (bottom) Stephan Elleringmann—Bilderberg/Aurora; (opposite page) Petit Format/Nestle/Science Source/Photo Researchers

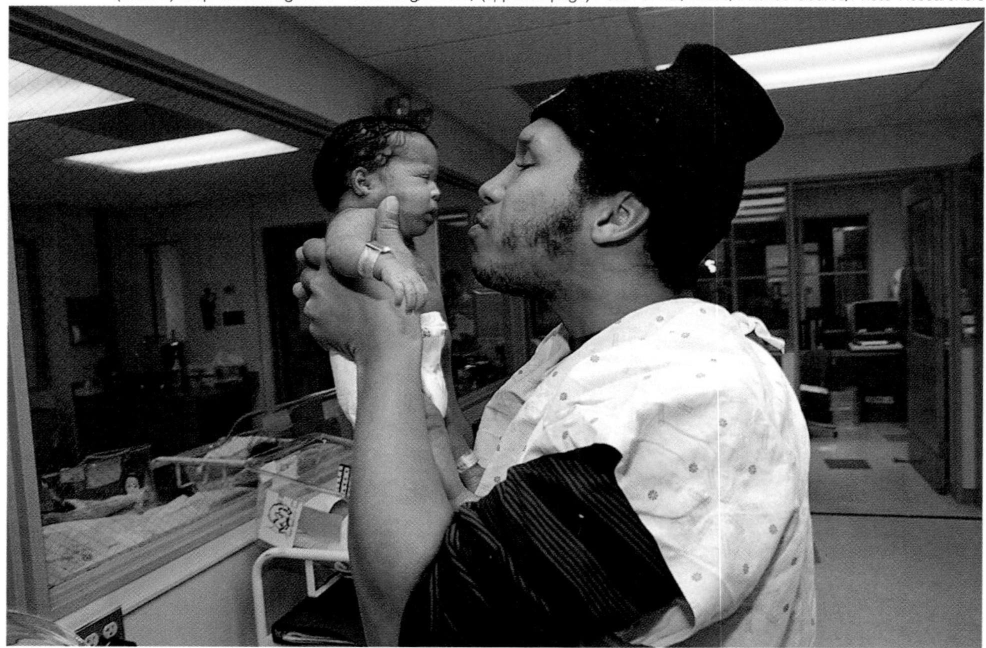

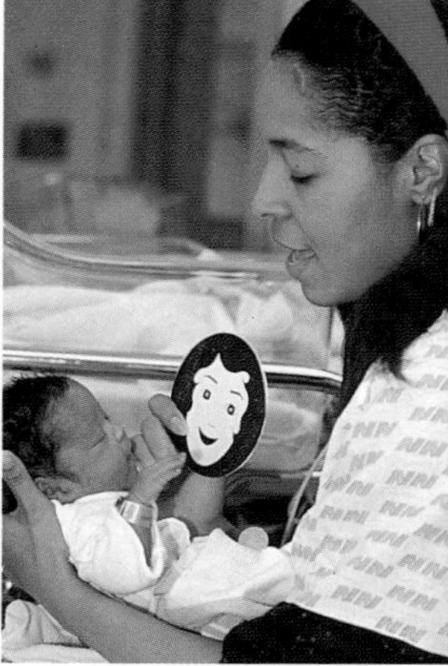

Because they are essentially still fetuses with underdeveloped nervous systems, premature infants have an especially uphill battle. "Preemies" may be kept in womblike incubators in special-care units for weeks or months. They also need lots of human contact and stimulation, which parents are best suited to provide.

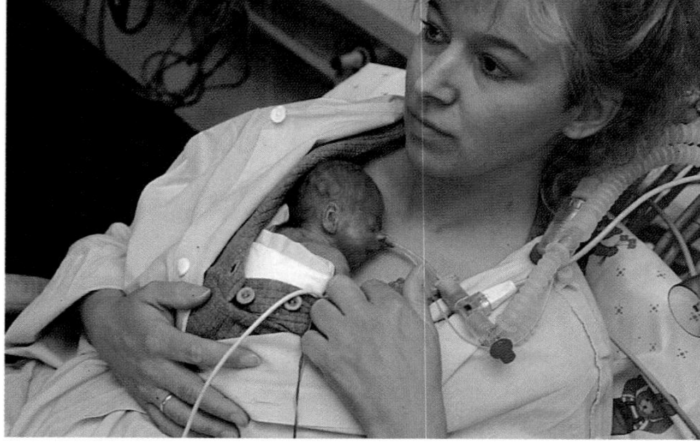

of gestation, the fetus is sensitive to a "uterine symphony" composed of intrauterine sounds (such as those generated by the intestinal, cardiovascular, and respiratory activities of the mother) and extrauterine noise. The "symphony" plays constantly at an intensity in the range of 80 to 95 decibels, which is about 5 to 30 decibels louder than normal conversation. In utero sound perception, however, is quite different from hearing in the external world. Researchers are just beginning to appreciate those qualitative differences. Investigators have placed underwater microphones ("hydrophones") inside the uteri of pregnant women to obtain sound recordings. Analysis of the information has yielded some insights into what the fetus hears. The sounds most readily detected by the fetus are those of low frequency—under 500 Hertz—the mother's rhythmic heartbeat being dominant.

In an effort to determine whether the fetus was affected by the mother's response to different kinds of music, investigators had pregnant women wear headphones into which music was piped. The study found that the fetal heartbeats showed no detectable change when the mother was hearing the music. It could be that the fetus had its own musical preferences, which did not necessarily coincide with those of the mother.

On the other hand, if a woman is exposed to hazardous noise levels during pregnancy, as many women undoubtedly are—from a wide variety of environmental sources—it seems likely that the baby's hearing could be damaged in utero. Noise-induced hearing loss is a well-characterized occurrence, but whether hearing is damaged during fetal life and under what circumstances this happens are still unanswered questions. While research into sense perception during fetal life is in a relatively preliminary stage, some scientists predict that in the future it may be possible to influence the neonatal outcome by decreasing stress during gestational life with various forms of sensory stimulation—perhaps even "music therapy."

Clear and present dangers

The medical profession is as yet unsure how well the fetus

(Opposite page) Fetus at four months. Scientists are just beginning to comprehend the range of stimuli to which the unborn are supremely sensitive.

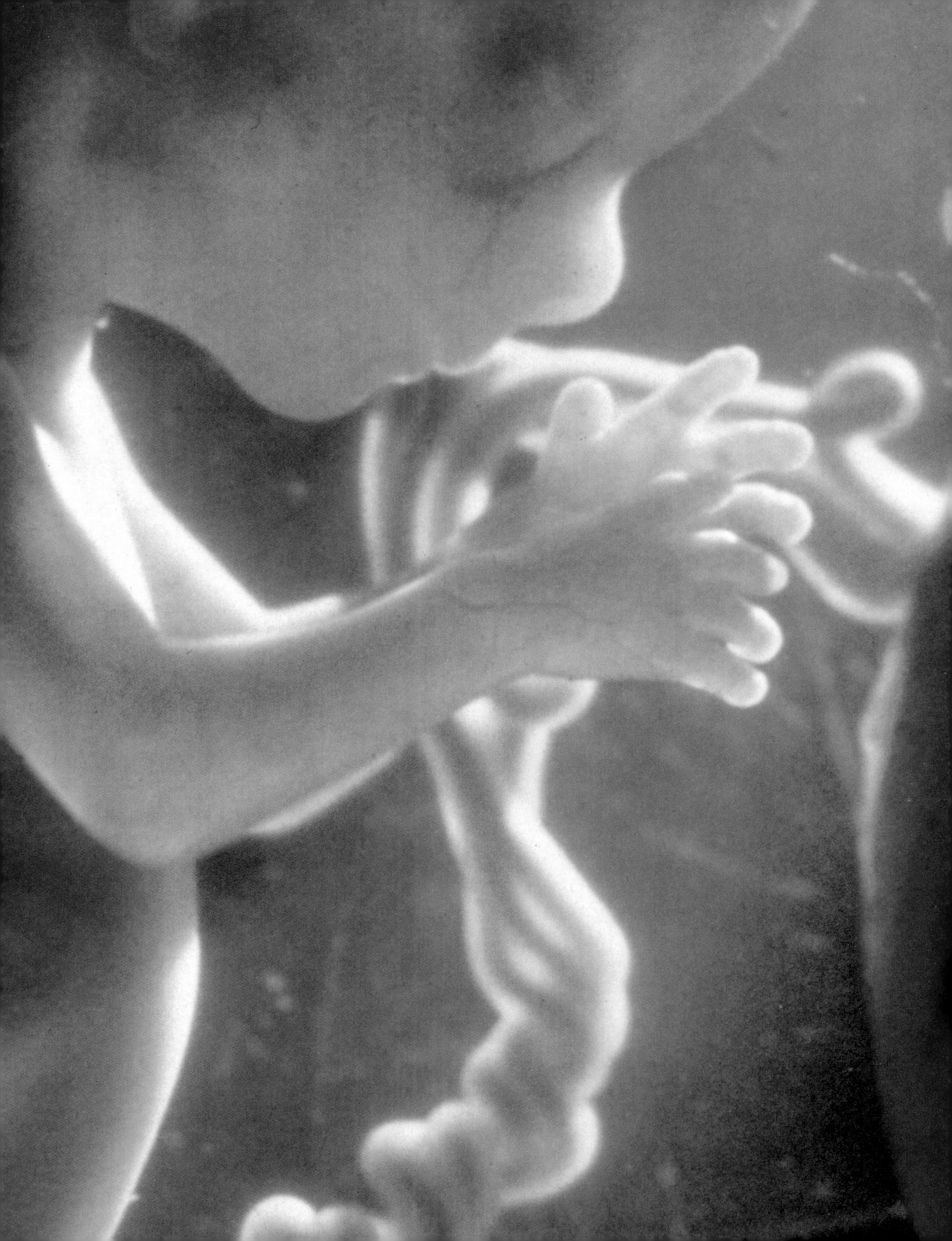

(Below) Owen Franken—Tony Stone Images; (bottom) Annie Griffiths Belt—Aurora

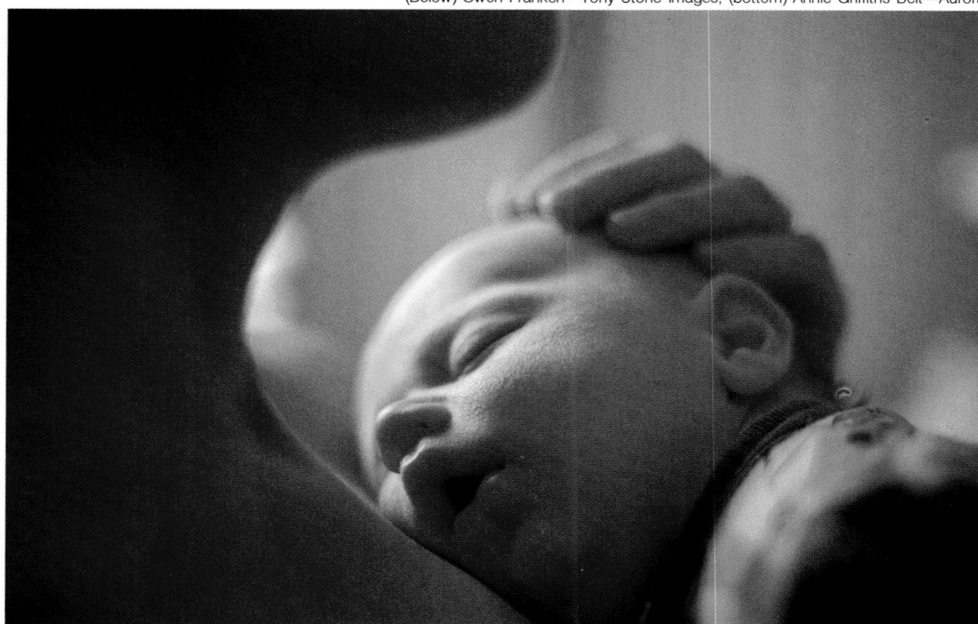

Researchers suspect that newborns "remember" the maternal heartbeat, which may be one reason babies are so easily lulled to sleep upon their mothers' chests.

can hear, taste, remember, or integrate perceptions. But there is no longer any doubt about the harm associated with some maternal actions. Now that superstitious and absurd notions about the influence of maternal impressions have been scientifically quashed, the dictates of common sense are generally applicable to the mother's lifestyle. Pregnancy is a time for healthy moderation. It is not a time for venturing into the unknown or taking risks. There is compelling evidence that two practices—namely, consuming alcohol and smoking cigarettes—can cause irreparable fetal damage, yet even in recent years, both forms of substance abuse have enjoyed social acceptability.

Apparently, the message that is a required warning on all alcoholic beverage containers sold in the U.S.—"GOVERNMENT WARNING: ACCORDING TO THE SURGEON GENERAL, WOMEN SHOULD NOT DRINK ALCOHOLIC BEVERAGES DURING PREGNANCY BECAUSE OF THE RISK OF BIRTH DEFECTS"—is little heeded. In April 1997 the Centers for Disease Control and Prevention (CDC) issued an alarming report that showed a "substantial increase" in alcohol

"Hel-loo!" Can fetuses hear? Investigators suggest that by the 24th week of gestation, babies are attuned to a virtual "symphony" of sounds in the uterus and that newborns are likely to "recognize" familiar voices. The mothers-to-be below are so convinced that their unborn children can hear that they have already begun communicating with them.

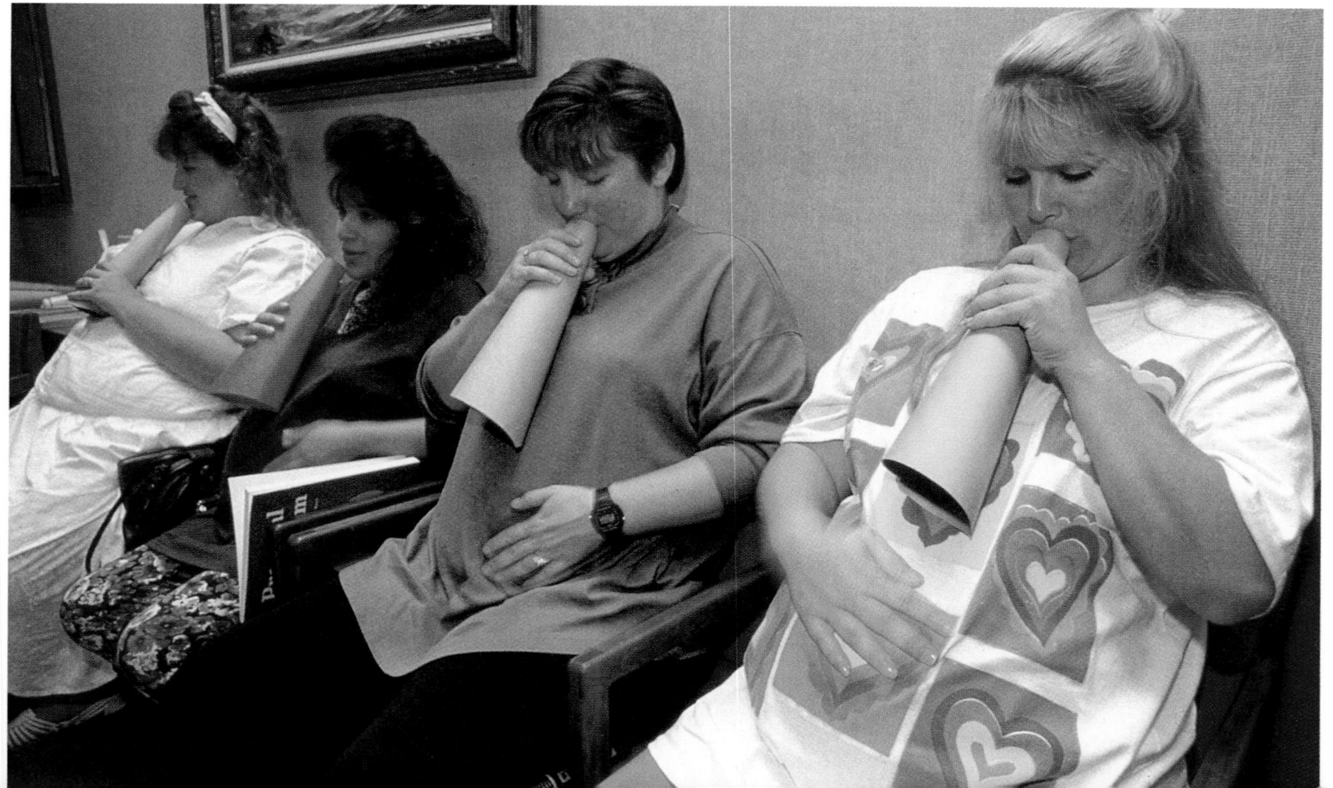

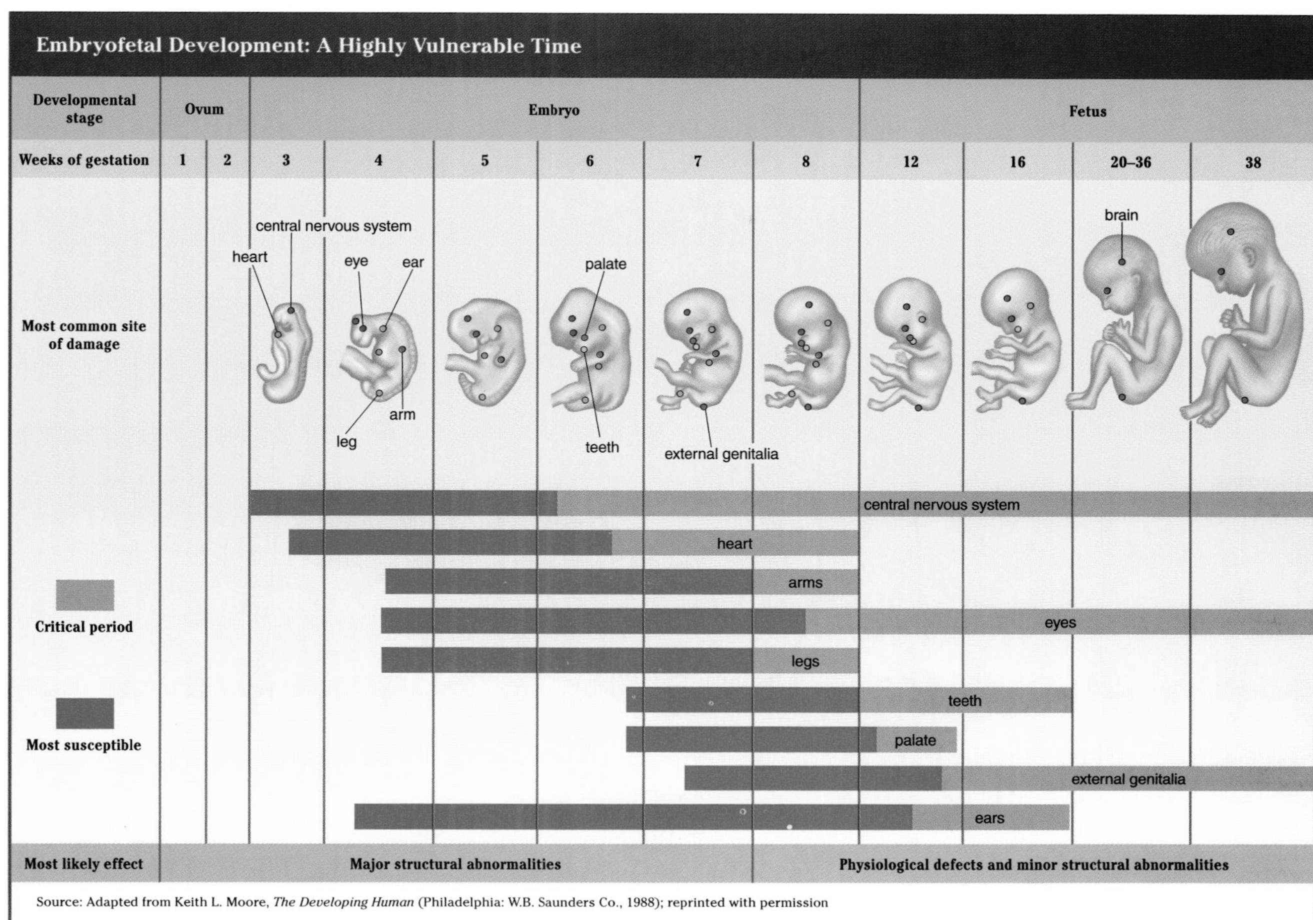

Source: Adapted from Keith L. Moore, *The Developing Human* (Philadelphia: W.B. Saunders Co., 1988); reprinted with permission

use among pregnant women in the U.S. between 1991 and 1995. Of women aged 18–44 who were pregnant at the time of the 1995 interviews, 16.3% reported having consumed alcohol during the preceding month, compared with 12.4% in 1991. The self-reported rate of "frequent drinking" was more than four times higher in 1995 than in 1991.

Alcohol exerts its effects upon the embryo most prominently during the time the nervous system is forming; consequently, exposure to alcohol during the first trimester may have devastating effects upon the child. Recently, autopsies of offspring of alcoholic mothers have shown incomplete brain development and a disorientation of nerve cells within the brain and spinal cord. In at least one documented case, specific cerebral structures, such as the corpus callosum, never formed, which suggests that the damage started before the 80th day of gestation. In some cases the infant may not show any outward physical evidence of damage but will have a number of ill-defined neurological deficits, including poor memory, hyperactive behavior, and short attention span.

The physical and mental defects that result from chronic maternal alcohol consumption are known as fetal alcohol syndrome (FAS). Children with FAS suffer from growth retardation; physical, mental, and behavioral abnormalities; central nervous system impairment, including developmental delay, small head size, and speech or language delay; and distinct facial abnormalities. The CDC reports that approximately 2,000 U.S. children are born annually with FAS, and another 4,000 may expe-rience significant cognitive and behavioral impairment as a result of fetal exposure to alcohol. According to the National Organization on Fetal Alcohol Syndrome, the medical and institutional costs for *one* child with FAS are $1.4 million over a lifetime!

Women who conceive are often unaware of their own pregnancies in the first two weeks; consequently, many do not avoid alcohol consumption. A level of alcohol that may be considered "safe" has not been established; although it has been suggested that the risk is relatively low in the preimplantation phase

A great deal is known about the situations and agents that contribute to embryofetal development. Susceptibilities are different at different gestational stages.

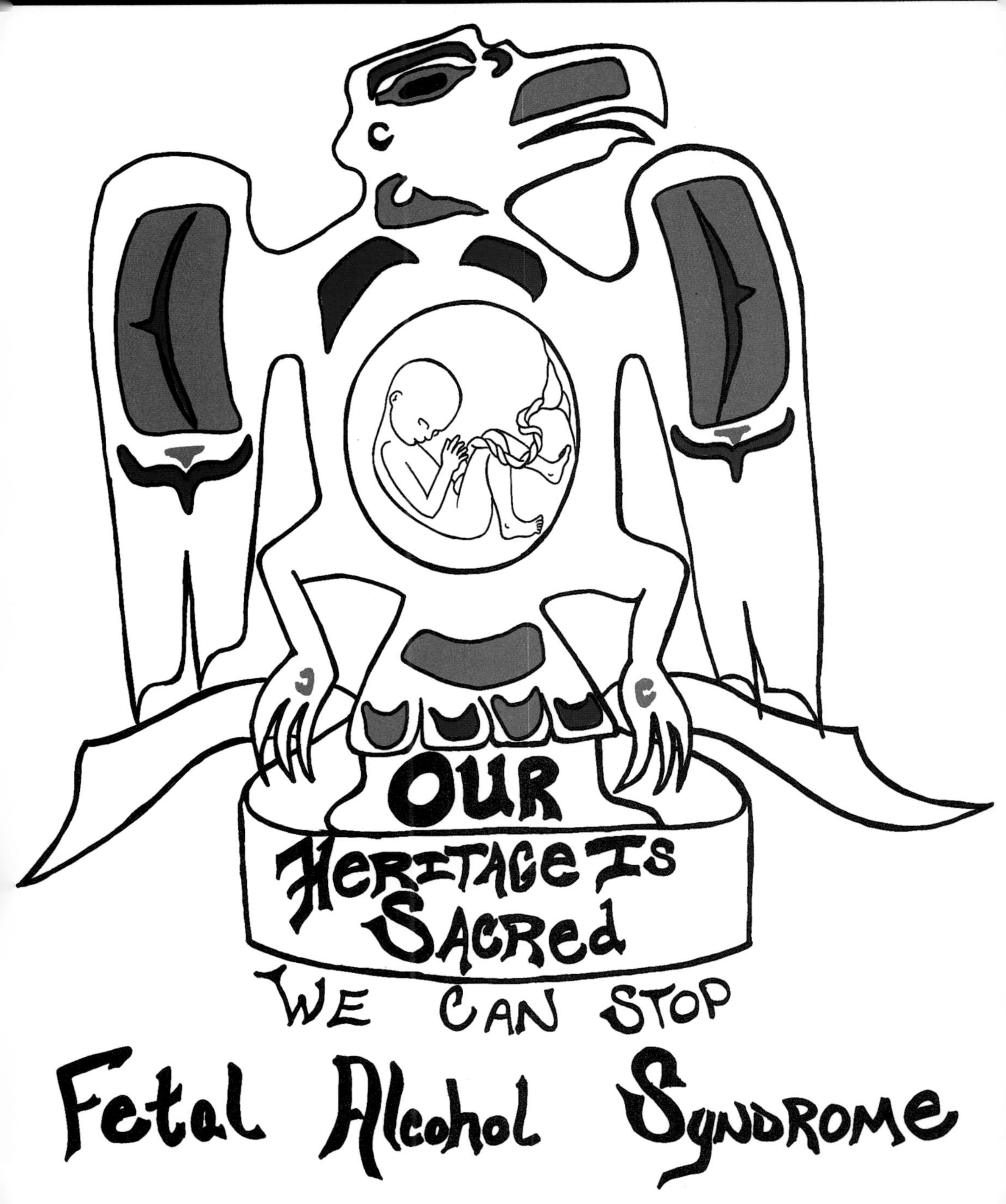

IST: ERIC CHANCE, 13 (LUMMI)

1815 H Street NW, Suite 750 • Washington DC 20006 • (202)785-4585

American Indian children are disproportionately affected by fetal alcohol syndrome. The poster (opposite page) was designed by a 13-year-old FAS victim.

(the first 10 or so days following conception), women contemplating pregnancy are advised to abstain completely. As already noted, there are different susceptibilities at different stages of gestation; the time of formation of the nervous system is one of great vulnerability. As in all pathological states, there may be various degrees of alcohol tolerance among individual women. Furthermore, women who abuse alcohol may have other unhealthy habits, which makes it difficult to dissociate the effects of alcohol from other noxious influences.

"SURGEON GENERAL'S WARNING: Smoking by Pregnant Women May Result in Fetal Injury, Premature Birth, And Low Birth Weight." Warnings such as this have been on cigarette packets sold in the U.S. for about a quarter of a century. Yet smoking continues to be a major public health concern. In the U.S., despite three decades of antismoking campaigns and unflagging efforts on the part of medical and public health professionals and government authorities to curb the habit, one-third of the population still smokes. And though rates among both men and women are declining, they are doing so much less sharply among the latter group—especially young women. Not only is the number of American women with smoking-related diseases on the increase, but according to CDC figures released in June 1997, 14% of teenage women are continuing to smoke throughout their pregnancies.

The most striking effect of smoking on the fetus is the stunting of its growth, resulting in a low birth weight. This happens primarily by slowing fetal growth after the 30th week of gestation. On average, maternal smoking predisposes infants to be born at weights 200 grams (about 7 ounces) below normal. Birth weight is determined by gestational age and rate of fetal growth, and nicotine has a negative effect on both. Nicotine readily crosses the placenta and concentrates in amniotic fluid, fetal blood, and breast milk. Nowadays, to determine whether a fetus has been exposed to tobacco smoke inside the uterus, hairs from the head of the newborn can be evaluated in a laboratory for the presence of cotinine, a metabolite of nicotine. Low birth weight appears to be a product of complex interactions of nicotine, cotinine, and carbon monoxide. The latter interferes with the release of oxygen to the tissues. The risk of perinatal mortality is as much as 20–40% higher for infants whose mothers smoke. On the other hand, women who quit smoking early in pregnancy deliver infants whose weights are comparable to those of children of mothers who never smoked.

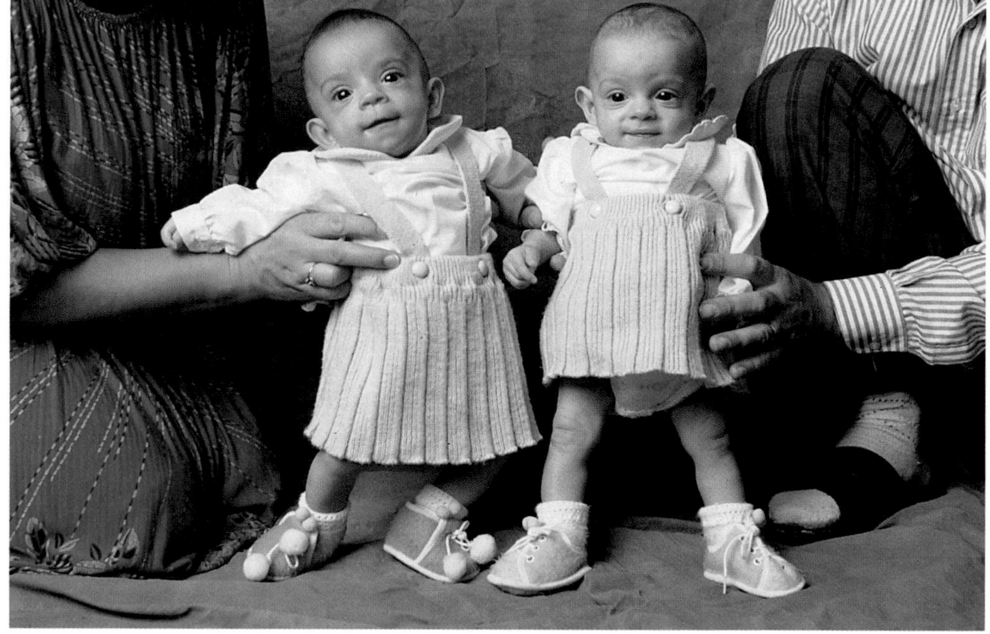

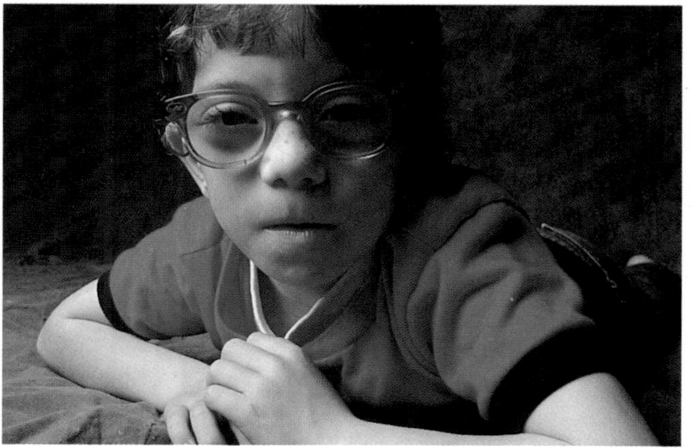

Tragic, visible, and irreversible, FAS—a condition that knows no geographic bounds—is manifested by severe physical, mental, and behavioral retardation. (Above and left) FAS victims: five-month-old fraternal twin girls from France and a six-year-old from Seattle, Washington.

(Opposite page) Courtesy of the National Organization on Fetal Alcohol Syndrome; (above) photographs, © 1997 George Steinmetz

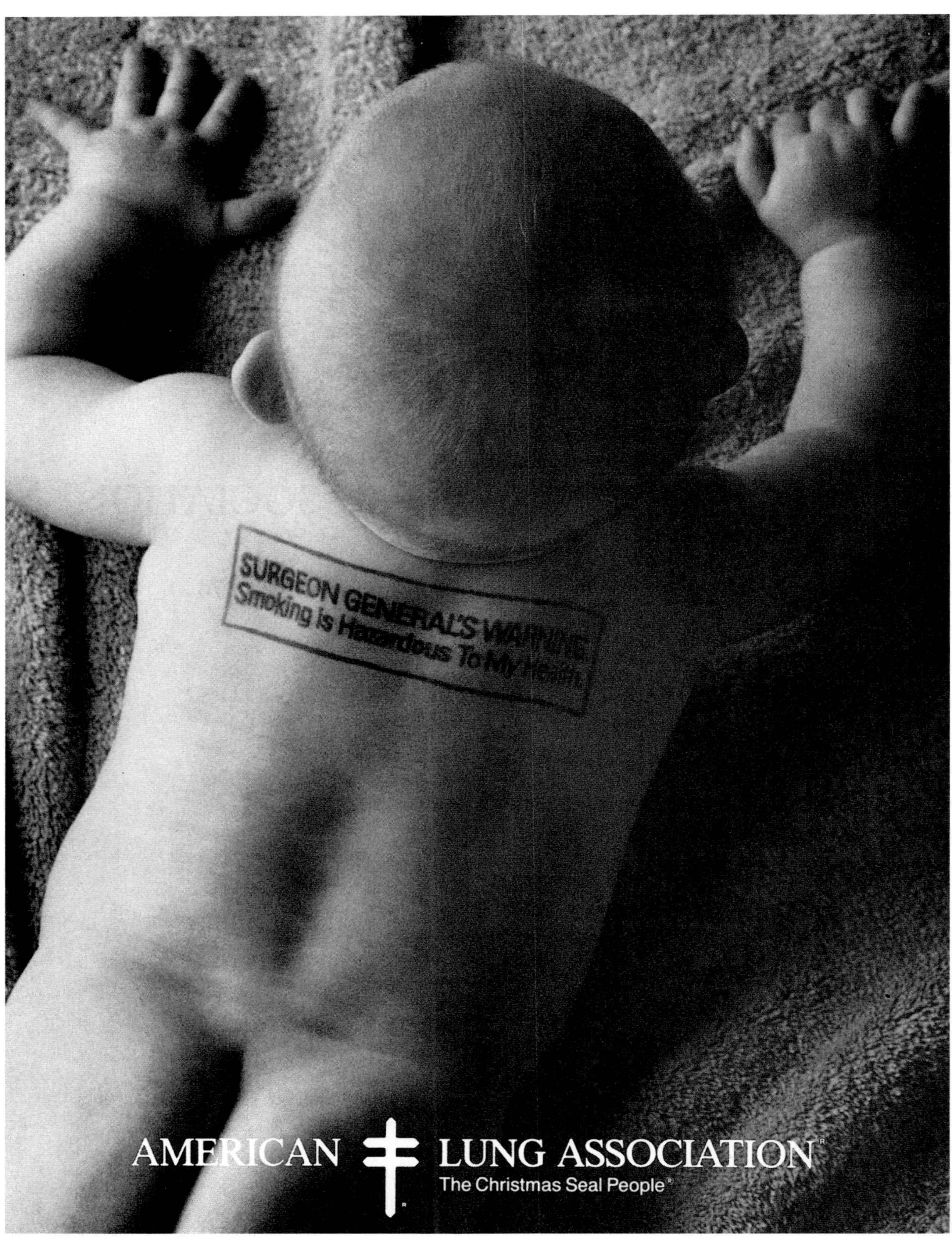
SURGEON GENERAL'S WARNING:
Smoking is Hazardous To My Health.
AMERICAN LUNG ASSOCIATION®
The Christmas Seal People®

(Opposite page) Courtesy of the American Lung Association, New York; (below) Annie Griffiths Belt—Aurora

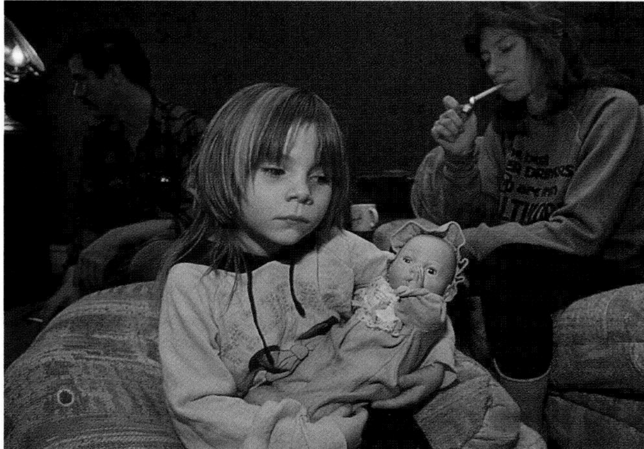

(Opposite page) A sharp message from the American Lung Association to women who smoke—all too many of whom do so throughout gestation. (Above) Every time a pregnant woman lights up, she hurts herself and endangers her fetus. If she has growing children at home, their health, too, is compromised by her habit.

Old myths, new realities

> *From the earliest time, medicine has been a curious blend of superstition, empiricism, and that kind of sagacious observation, which is the stuff out of which ultimately science is made. Of these three strands—superstition, empiricism, and observation—medicine was constituted in the days of the priest-physicians of Egypt and Babylonia; of the same three strands it is still composed. The proportions have, however, varied significantly; an increasingly alert and determined effort, running through the ages, has endeavored to expel superstition, to narrow the range of empiricism, and to enlarge, refine, and systematize the scope of observation.*
>
> —Abraham Flexner, *Medical Education, 1925*

Belief in the power of "maternal impressions," as formerly understood, has largely vanished from the popular imagination and medical wisdom. It is now quite clear that a fetus can feel, hear, respond to stimuli, and demonstrate cerebral cortical activity of a sophistication sufficient to produce memory. Therefore, it is probably not unaffected by the mental state of the mother. If she becomes disconsolate, frightened, elated, giddy, exhausted, intoxicated, or confused, there are likely to be concomitant physiological and behavioral changes that have some measurable repercussion in the fetus. In this sense "maternal impressions" may indeed be a reality whose effects will someday be understood by observant scientists as distinctly as the effects of smoking cigarettes and drinking alcohol. MHA

The "dos" and "don'ts" of pregnancy used to be guided by superstitions and myths. Now medical scientists know a great deal about the many agents and habits that can harm a fetus; being "in the family way" calls for healthy moderation.

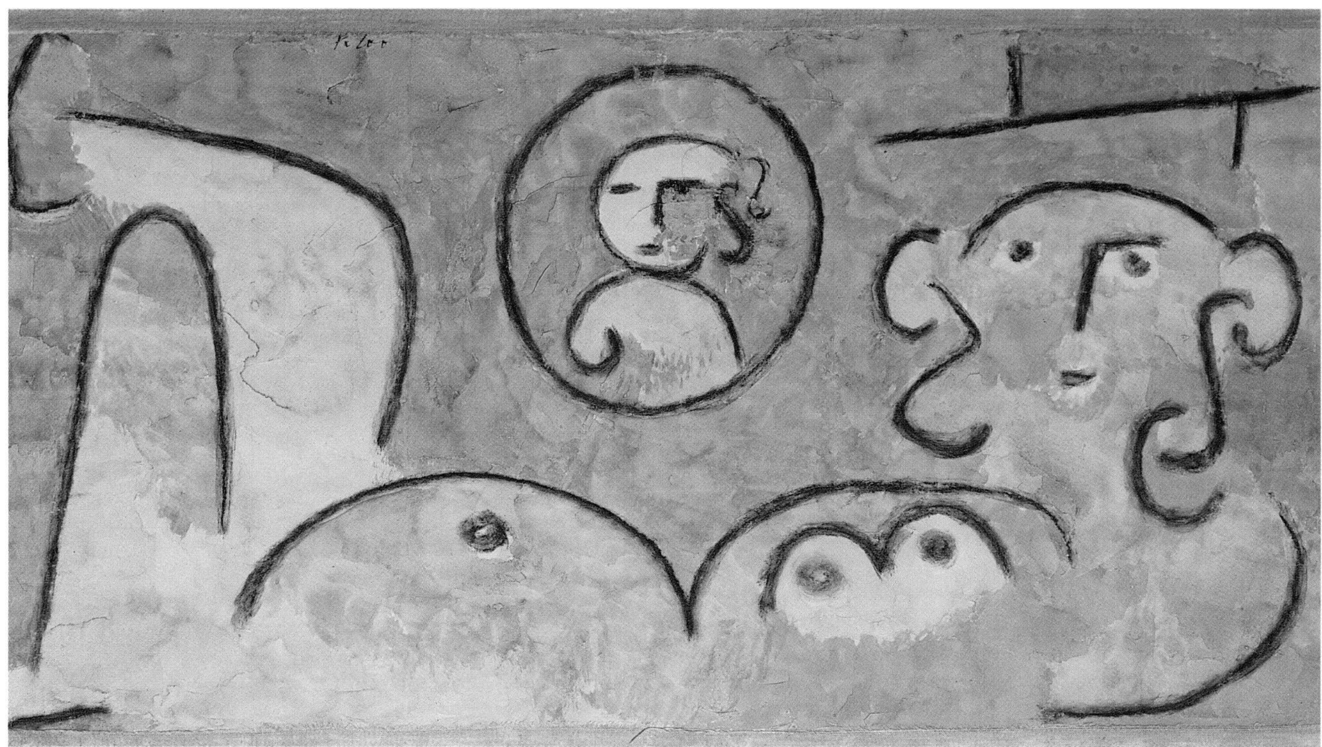

"Thinking of Offspring," watercolor by Paul Klee, 1937; private collection, Milan; photograph, Erich Lessing—Art Resource, New York

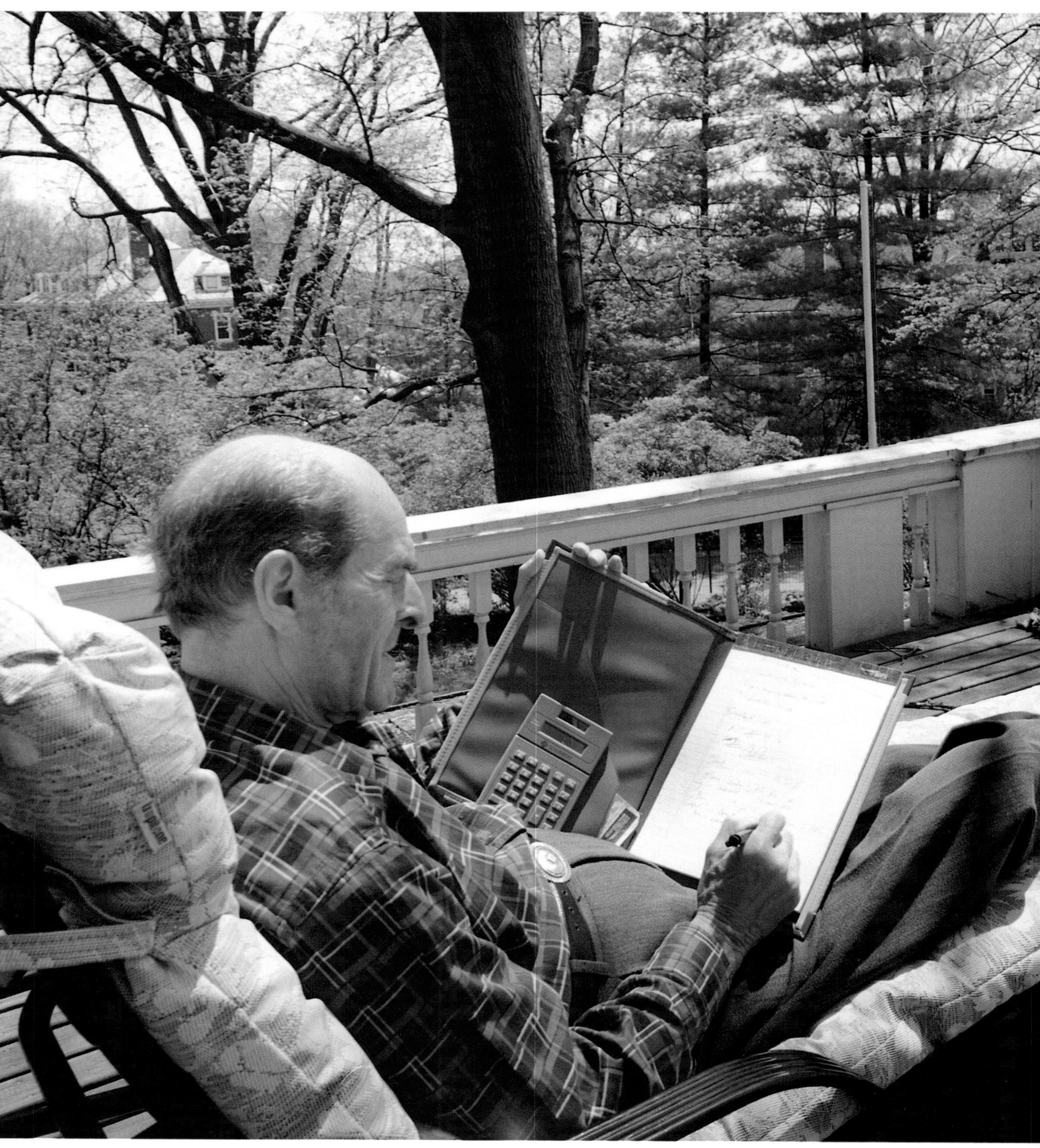

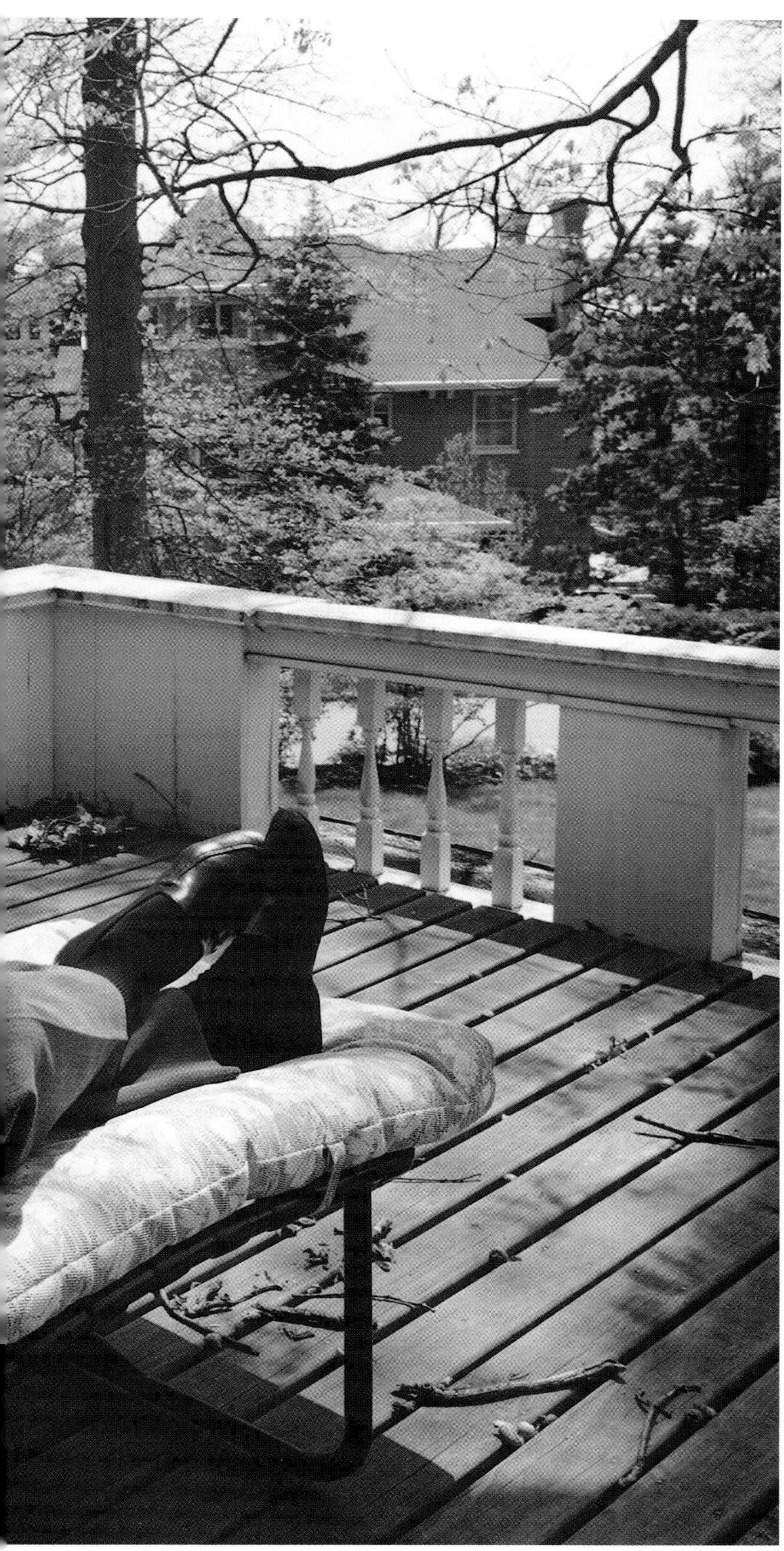

Photograph by Dennis Marsico

Rebel with a Cause: Saving Lives

by Henry J. Heimlich, M.D., Sc.D.

Creative ideas are often attacked because people oppose change or do not understand new concepts. When a prominent discovery is revealed, particularly if it provides an obvious and simple answer to an important question, experts who have worked for years unsuccessfully on the same problem may lash out at the creator and the idea because they themselves did not find the solution or because it exposes flaws in their own theories. Sometimes their resentment toward the innovator has a financial basis.

Creativity requires courage. My role model was the English physician Edward Jenner (1749–1823). At the age of 13, Jenner learned that milkmaids in the countryside who got cowpox, a mild infection contracted from cattle, never developed the dreaded human illness smallpox. (In Jenner's day smallpox was a merciless disease that killed and disfigured millions worldwide.) In 1796, as a country physician with a practice in Gloucestershire, Jenner performed a bold experiment. He inoculated eight-year-old James Phipps with cowpox matter taken from the pus-filled lesions on the finger of a milkmaid, Sarah Nelmes. A month and a half later, Jenner exposed young Phipps to smallpox. The boy did not become sick.

When Jenner reported his result at a London medical society meeting, heated discussions ensued, and other doctors who studied his evidence found it hard to believe. Likewise, the Royal Society refused to publish his findings and advised the author "not to risk his reputation by presenting to the learned body anything which appears so much at variance with established knowledge." When he was unable to find volunteers for his "vaccine" (from the Latin *vacca,* for "cow") in England, he took the procedure to other countries in Europe, where vaccination was widely adopted. Even while English doctors continued to spurn his discovery, Jenner never stopped his crusade to protect the population from "the most dreadful scourge of the human species."

The German-Hungarian physician Ignaz Semmelweis (1818–65) realized that women died from childbed (puerperal) fever because doctors performed autopsies and then, without washing their hands, delivered babies. Semmelweis's medical superiors, however, were unwilling to recognize the significance of his discovery. When an epidemic of puerperal fever broke out in the obstetrics department at St. Rochus Hospital in Pest, Hungary, in the late 1850s, Semmelweis took

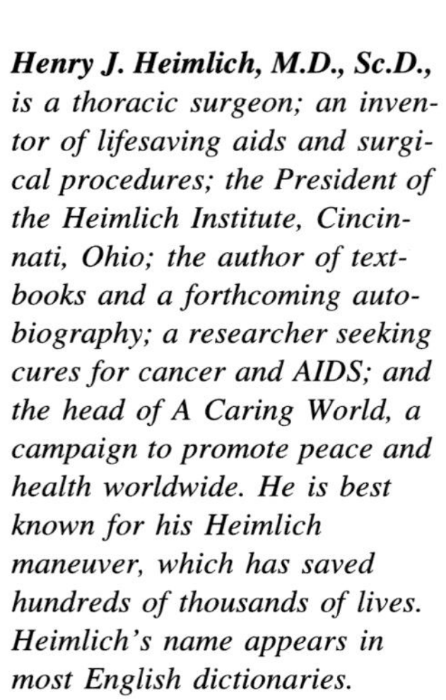

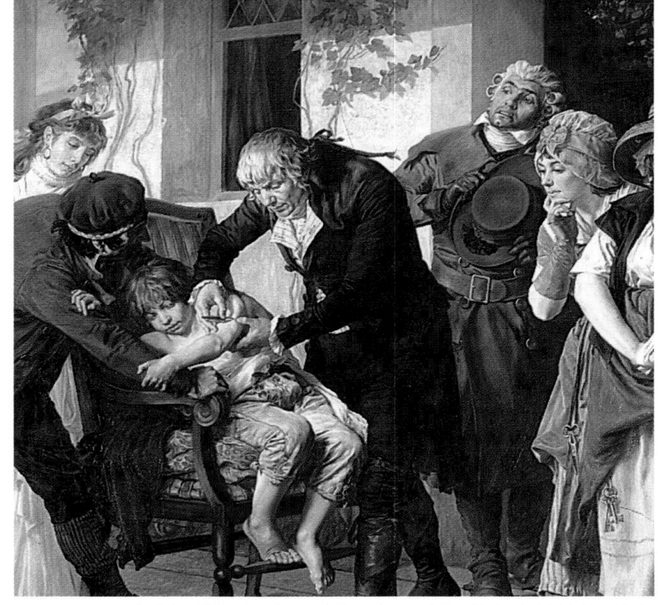

(Left) Edward Jenner vaccinates his first patient against smallpox in 1796. Ignaz Semmelweis (top) discovered the cause of childbed fever and introduced antisepsis into medical practice. Both figures were rebels in their day—and heroes to the author.

(Top) Ann Ronan at Image Select; (bottom) Académie de Médecine, Paris; photograph, Jean-Loup Charmet

Henry J. Heimlich, M.D., Sc.D., *is a thoracic surgeon; an inventor of lifesaving aids and surgical procedures; the President of the Heimlich Institute, Cincinnati, Ohio; the author of textbooks and a forthcoming autobiography; a researcher seeking cures for cancer and AIDS; and the head of A Caring World, a campaign to promote peace and health worldwide. He is best known for his Heimlich maneuver, which has saved hundreds of thousands of lives. Heimlich's name appears in most English dictionaries.*

(Below) Courtesy of March of Dimes Birth Defects Foundation; (bottom left and right) courtesy of the Heimlich Institute

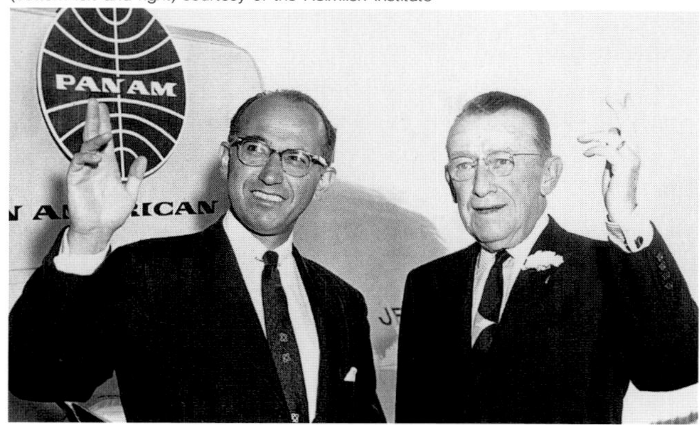

Jonas Salk (left) with Basil O'Connor, the attorney and director of the National Foundation for Infantile Paralysis who paved the way for trials of Salk's polio vaccine to begin.

charge. He sharply reduced maternal mortality simply by getting most of the staff to wash their hands in a solution of chlorinated lime. Despite this demonstration, many doctors still stubbornly refused to wash their hands, and women continued to die. In 1865, his spirit undermined, Semmelweis died, ironically, of the same infection he struggled all his professional life to prevent.

In the early 1950s medical authorities tried to prevent the U.S. medical pioneer Jonas Salk (1914–95) from testing his inactivated polio vaccine. Clinical trials were finally undertaken only because Basil O'Connor, then director of the National Foundation for Infantile Paralysis, an organization devoted to the fight against poliomyelitis, was a powerful attorney and fought the medical establishment on Salk's behalf.

Like others with new ideas, when I first encountered attacks on my work, I thought something must be wrong with *me*. After three of my medical discoveries proved successful, I knew it was *they* who were wrong. Over the years I have come to expect skepticism if not outright rejection; I now often say, "If all of your peers understand what you have done, you haven't been creative," and "Until you are challenged, you don't know you're right." (Others might say, "They don't kick a dead dog.")

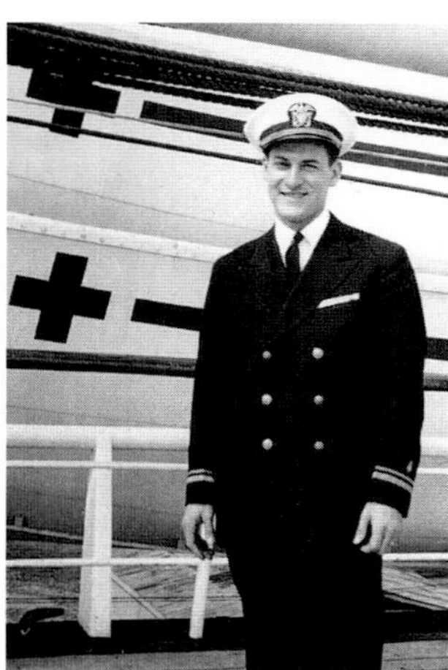

(Above) In 1945 Lieutenant Junior Grade Henry Heimlich, assigned to the U.S. Naval Group China, built a medical corps to serve Gen. Fu Tso Yi. (Right) In 1988, revisiting his Inner Mongolian post, he and Fu's granddaughter, Xiao Dong, pose for a picture, holding a snapshot of the general.

The '40s: the shaving-cream solution

In January 1945, at age 24, I had a nine-month surgical internship. World War II was on. I joined the navy and was assigned to U.S. Naval Group China. I was one of 12 Americans in the Gobi Desert of Inner Mongolia attached to a 250-man Chinese guerrilla army. Gen. Fu Tso Yi had a Chinese Nationalist army of 100,000 men nearby, and my orders were to keep him on the U.S. side against the Japanese. So I built him a medical corps. I trained some 25 Chinese soldiers to care for the sick and the wounded—and to instruct others to do so.

The Chinese I encountered did not trust Western medicine—that is, until I operated on an 18-year-old peasant girl, draining a huge abscess in her abdomen, and she recovered. Hundreds of patients then lined up outside our clinic every day. We treated diseases that most U.S. doctors never see, including smallpox and bubonic plague.

Trachoma, a bacterial infection of the eyelids transmitted by flies, was rampant in China. Inflammation scarred the eyelids, which slowly turned inward. The patients' eyelashes then scratched the cornea, making it opaque and resulting in blindness. As there was no known treatment at that time, I took a chance on treating victims of the eye disease. I ground sulfadiazine pills into

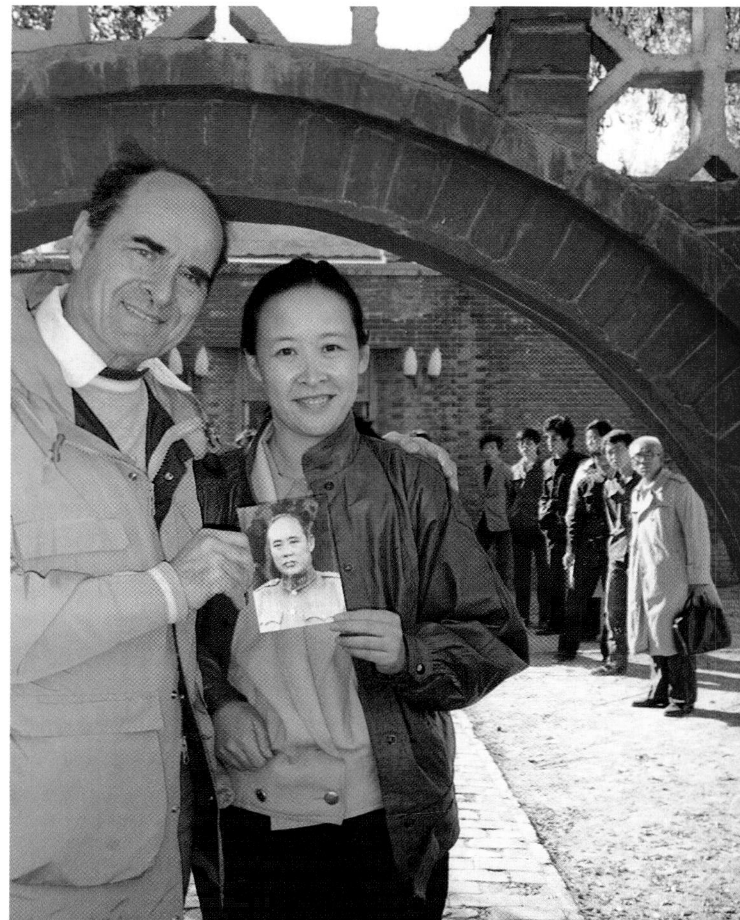

powder and mixed it with Barbasol shaving cream, the only ointment available. (Sulfadiazine is a broad-spectrum antimicrobial agent that was introduced in the early 1940s and was one of the few drugs available at the time for treating bacterial infections.) Chinese corpsmen first applied the Barbasol/sulfa ointment to the infected eyes of a few soldiers, who groaned in considerable agony. Their eyelid inflammations cleared, however, so we proceeded to treat hundreds of trachoma patients.

After the war a medical journal for military physicians independently reported that sulfadiazine cured trachoma. My reward came in 1988 when, accompanied by General Fu's granddaughter, I returned to Inner Mongolia, where I met people I had treated in 1945 who might not have been alive—or able to see—if I had been less bold as a young naval doctor. This confirmation of the success of my first experiment introduced me to the unique kind of satisfaction that comes from carrying out and proving a logical concept.

The '50s: making the most of the stomach

In December 1949 I completed my training in general and chest surgery. A month later I conceived of an operation to replace the esophagus. After successfully performing the procedure on a series of patients, I presented the results at an American Medical Association (AMA) meeting in New York City in 1961. Shortly thereafter, *Life* magazine published a story headlined "Heated Discussions and a Hot Medical Discovery," which included a photograph of me demonstrating the operation on a cloth model of the stomach. The operation gained recognition as the first total organ replacement.

The esophagus carries food from the throat to the stomach. When the esophagus is destroyed by cancer, scarred as a result of repeated regurgitation of stomach acid, or undeveloped at birth, food cannot be swallowed. Prior to the 1950s patients had to be fed for their entire lives through a tube inserted into the stomach.

The stomach is a large tube. I fashioned a small tube from a portion of it; because the blood supply to this new "esophagus" was preserved, it survived and functioned in adults and actually grew as a fully functional organ in children. The tube is reversed, brought upward through the chest, and its end connected to the throat, which enables patients to eat normally.

Ken Heyman—Woodfin Camp & Associates

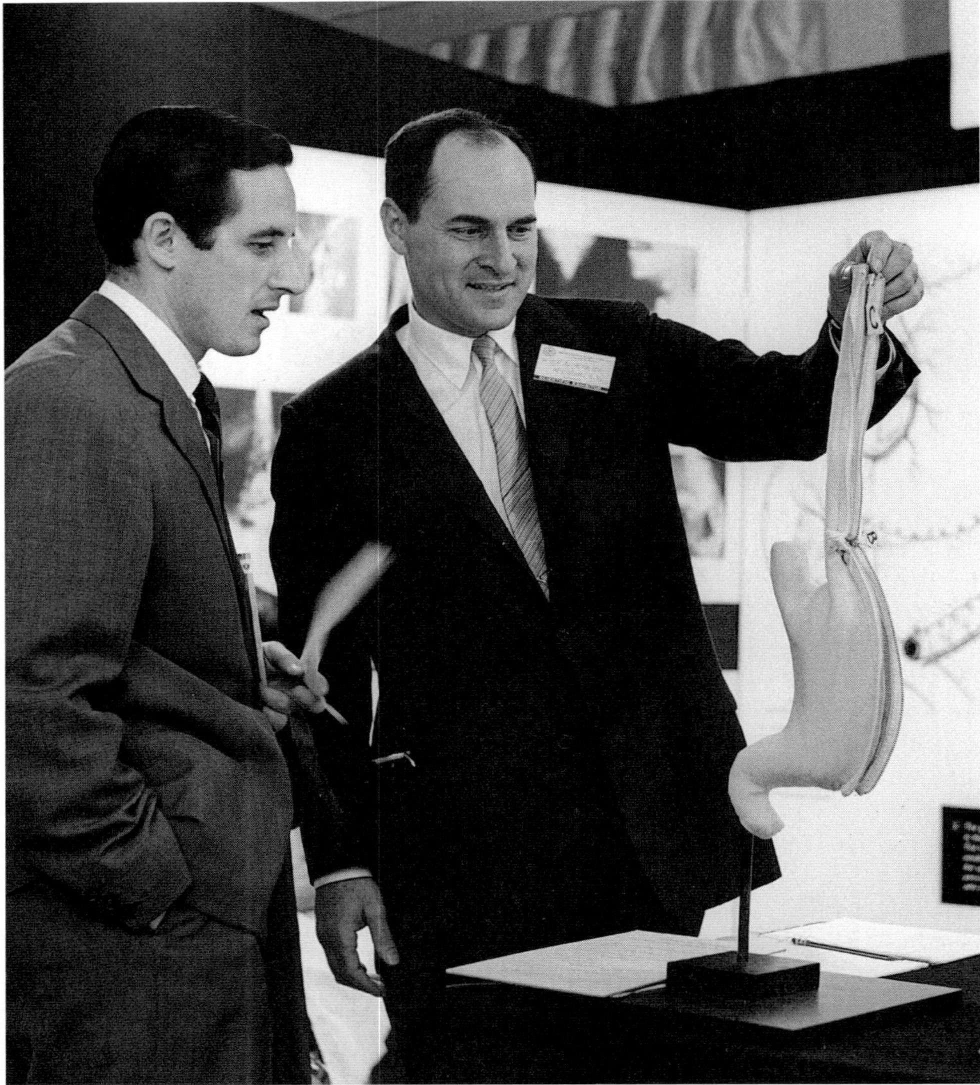

Using a cloth "stomach," Heimlich demonstrates his operation to replace the esophagus. The procedure was dubbed "a hot medical discovery" by *Life* magazine in its June 26, 1961, issue.

I performed my operation in three different hospitals and published a description of it in a medical journal in 1955.

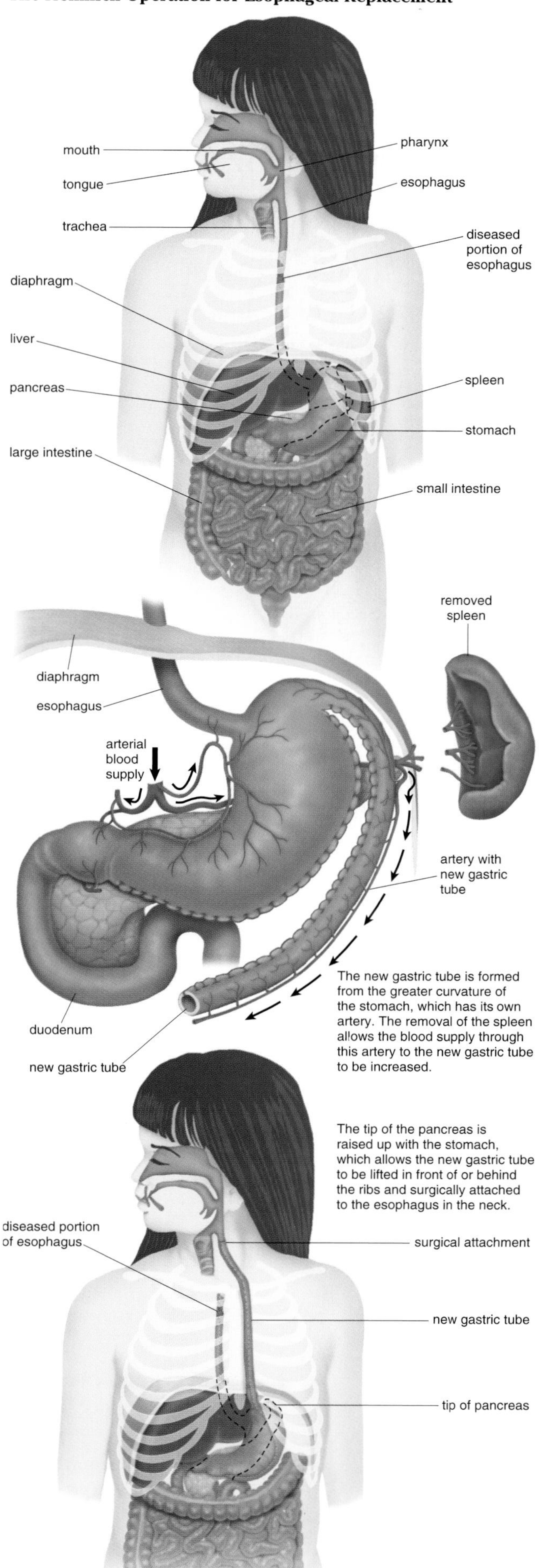

The new gastric tube is formed from the greater curvature of the stomach, which has its own artery. The removal of the spleen allows the blood supply through this artery to the new gastric tube to be increased.

The tip of the pancreas is raised up with the stomach, which allows the new gastric tube to be lifted in front of or behind the ribs and surgically attached to the esophagus in the neck.

The procedure became known as the Heimlich operation for esophageal replacement and is still widely used, primarily on children born with esophageal defects. I was recently greeted by a surgeon in a pediatric hospital who said, "Dr. Heimlich, I performed your operation just last week." Reward enough!

The '60s: why not a valve?

> *A small device barely five inches long is saving lives of hundreds of Vietnam wounded—civilian as well as military. Called the Heimlich Chest Drain Valve, the new device, developed by Dr. Henry Heimlich, is used to drain fluids which accumulate in the chest cavity following heart and lung surgery, during certain illnesses, or as a result of a chest wound. Failure to drain can be fatal.*
>
> —*Reader's Digest,* September 1967

In Inner Mongolia in 1945, one of the Chinese soldiers in our naval group was shot in the chest. He died on the table while I was operating. I have never forgotten the soldier's coffin being carried away on an oxcart.

There are a number of situations that can cause blood and air to fill the chest, collapsing the lung (or lungs). These include being stabbed or shot in the chest, having chest surgery, and suffering from the condition known as pneumothorax, in which an air bubble on the lung bursts. When lungs are collapsed, the patient cannot breathe and may die. One means of handling a collapsed lung is to insert a tube into the chest, which drains fluid and air from it. Such a tube was connected to an extremely complicated suction apparatus.

In 1962 I published a book, *Postoperative Care in Thoracic Surgery,* in which I explained how suction devices for draining the chest work. The devices act like valves, I pointed out; *i.e.,* once blood and air have been suctioned out of the chest, the lung expands. Drainage of the chest must continue until leakage of air or blood has ceased. The principle behind a valve is that it permits fluid or air to run in one direction only. "Well, why not a valve?" I thought, so I proceeded to consider various types of valves.

I ruled out a *ball valve,* in which a ball sits at the opening of a tube. Fluid or air passing through the tube pushes the ball upward. When the flow stops, the ball falls back against the opening, preventing fluid and air from reentering the tube. But if the tube were to fall sideways, the ball would be separated from the tube, and air would flow back into the chest. Next I considered a *flap valve,* whose hinged lid is held against the opening of a tube by a spring. Air or fluid pressure opens the lid; the lid closes regardless of the position of the tube. But if a flap valve was draining blood, and a clot was lodged under the lid, air would flow back into the chest.

A third type of valve, a *flutter valve,* is made of flattened soft tubing, which remains closed until light pressure causes fluid and air to pass through it. At the five-and-ten-cent store, I purchased a noisemaker that consisted of a mouthpiece attached to a flattened piece of thin rubber tubing. Blowing through it made the not-very-melodious sound called a "Bronx cheer," or "raspberry." A man with a collapsed lung due to pneumothorax was admitted to the hospital in New Rochelle, New York, where I was working at the time. I put a tube into his chest, connected its open end to the noisemaker "flutter valve," and sat by his side the entire day. Chest X-rays repeatedly showed the lung expanded. In 1964 Becton Dickinson & Co. (BD) of Franklin Lakes, New Jersey, agreed to manufacture the Heimlich Chest Drain Valve. Pneumothorax patients formerly spent two weeks in the hospital hooked up to a suction apparatus. Now a tube connected to a Heimlich valve is inserted in the emergency room; the patient goes home immediately, and the tube and valve are removed a week later.

That year, I introduced the valve at another AMA meeting, again held in New York City. Four navy officers came up to see me afterward and said they were from the United States Navy Medical Research Institute in Bethesda, Maryland, and that they had to have "six Heimlich valves tomorrow." The commander among them flew into Floyd Bennet Field in New York City the next day. I handed him six valves, which he promptly put in his pocket before reboarding his plane and flying directly to Vietnam. One week later I received a telegram that read: "The Heimlich valve is a lifesaving item. Must have 100 immediately." BD expedited a shipment and subsequently received orders for "unlimited quantities."

(Below) Courtesy of the Becton Dickinson Archives Museum; (bottom) courtesy of the Heimlich Institute

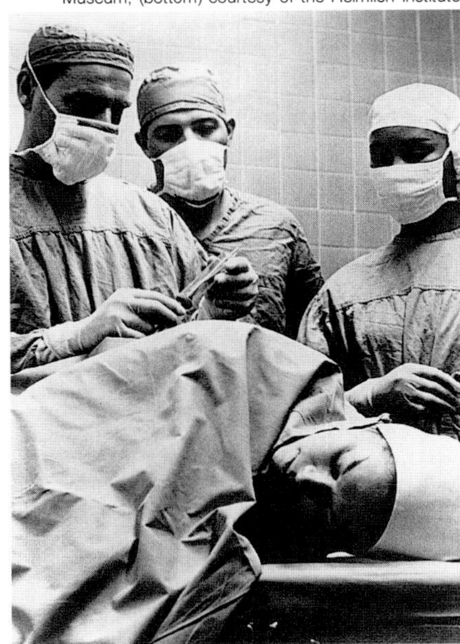

(Right) Heimlich prepares to insert a tube connected to a drainage valve in a patient's chest. (Below) He visits a post-surgical patient who has two tubes with two valves in place. This lifesaving invention evolved from a dime-store noisemaker.

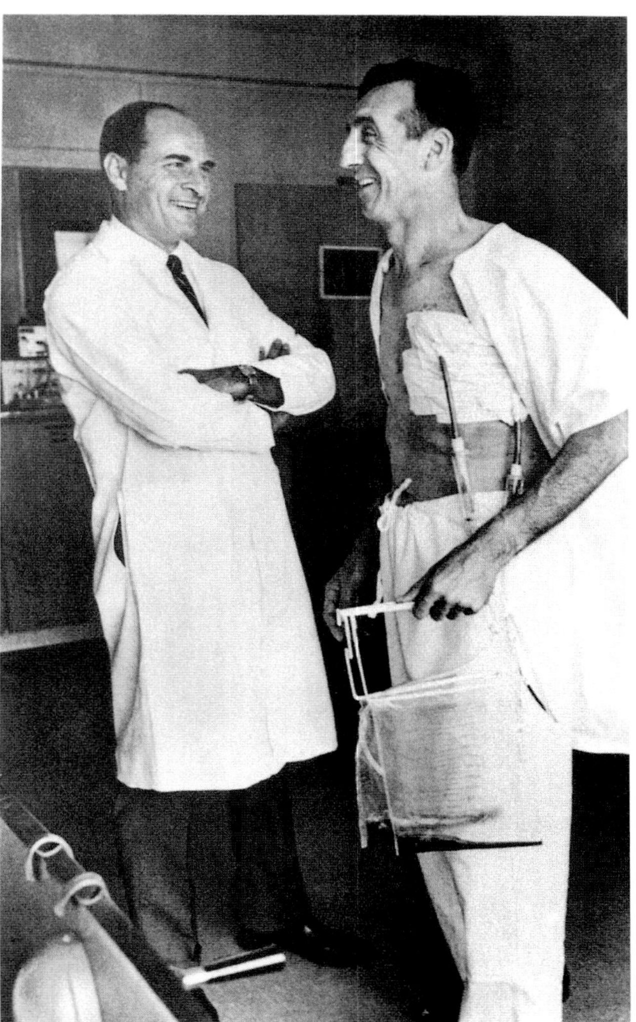

In Vietnam the lives of soldiers who were shot in the chest on the battlefield were saved—for the first time in history—when a drainage tube with a valve attached was inserted through a bullet wound. The valve is disposable and in the 1960s cost but $1 to make. Think of it: $1 to save a life! The valves were also used to save lives during the 1967 Arab-Israeli war. BD and I frequently knew a war was imminent when a country ordered a large supply of valves. We knew three months before the Persian Gulf War of 1990–91 that it would take place. Today more than 250,000 Heimlich valves are used worldwide every year to treat civilian and military patients with chest wounds or following chest surgery.

In the 1980s I spoke at a banquet in Florida; a doctor in the audience stood up and shared this story: "I was on Hill 881 in Vietnam," he said.

"Thirty-four of my men were shot in the chest. Thirty-two of them got off the Hill alive with the Heimlich valve inserted." One of the greatest moments in my life came in February 1993 when I traveled to Vietnam with a delegation of chest surgeons, a visit sponsored by the Citizen Ambassador Program of People to People International. At the Hanoi airport we were greeted by North Vietnamese chest surgeons. When I was introduced, their head doctor said, "Dr. Heimlich, you need no introduction. Everyone in Vietnam knows your name." My immediate assumption was that I would hear a story about the invention for which I am best known: the Heimlich maneuver for saving choking victims (discussed below). But the surgeon proceeded to describe how Heimlich Chest Drain Valves, supplied by the Society of Friends (Quakers), "saved tens of thousands of our people during the war. The American Friends Service Committee kept us supplied with Heimlich valves throughout the war." The physician chairman who opened our meetings always began by saying, "Dr. Heimlich will live in the hearts of the Vietnamese people forever." The first time I heard those words, I cried. Very few things in my life have given me as much satisfaction as knowing that the Heimlich Chest Drain Valve saved countless lives on *both sides* of that horrible war.

The '70s: hands on, the Heimlich way

The Heimlich maneuver has saved more than 50,000 drowning and choking victims to date in the United States alone. It is used throughout the world.

Choking: common and costly. At one time I thought choking to death on a piece of food or an object was a rare occurrence. In 1972 I learned choking was the sixth leading cause of accidental death and that children often choked on toys and by inhaling balloons that exploded during the blowing-up process. I immediately began to do research on the subject. Since 1933 the American Red Cross had taught that back slaps were the appropriate first aid for choking victims. Back slaps became the accepted, indeed the natural, thing to do. Yet in my studies I learned that the recommendation of back slaps was contrary to all scientific evidence.

Reports dating back to 1854 warned that holding a choking person head downward causes suffocation because objects in the trachea (windpipe) fall against the space between the vocal cords, blocking the airway. In addition, since 1854 every study on choking had shown that back slaps can *cause death* by driving a choking object downward, tighter into the airway, and thereby converting a partial blockage to a complete—and fatal—ob-

The Heimlich Chest Drain Valve

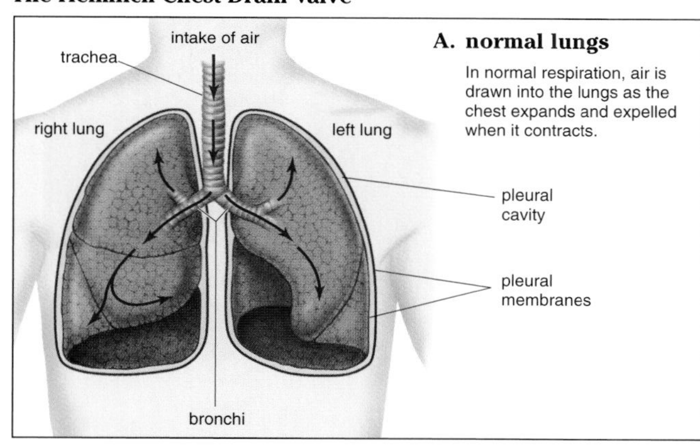

A. normal lungs

In normal respiration, air is drawn into the lungs as the chest expands and expelled when it contracts.

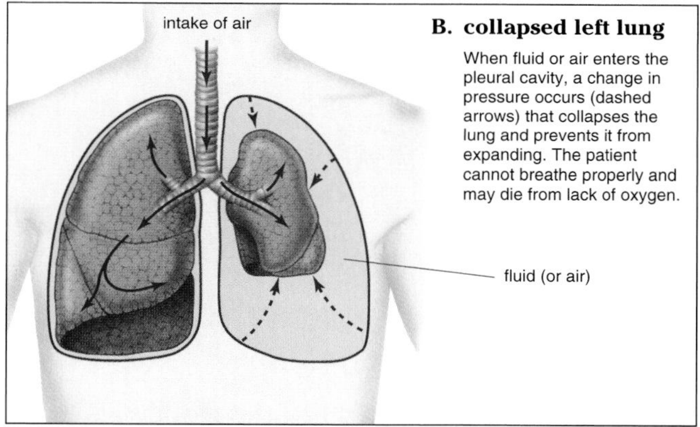

B. collapsed left lung

When fluid or air enters the pleural cavity, a change in pressure occurs (dashed arrows) that collapses the lung and prevents it from expanding. The patient cannot breathe properly and may die from lack of oxygen.

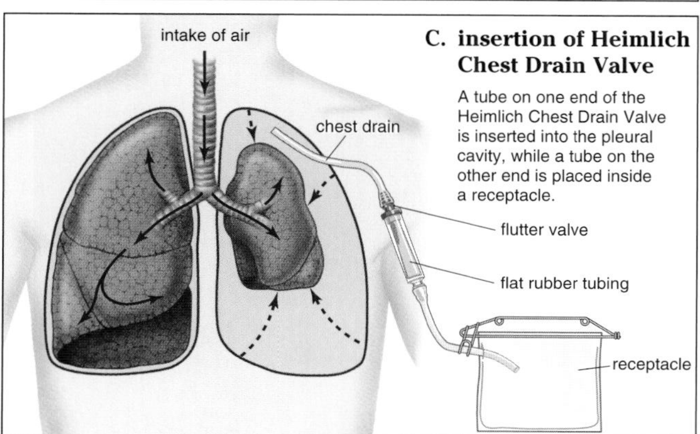

C. insertion of Heimlich Chest Drain Valve

A tube on one end of the Heimlich Chest Drain Valve is inserted into the pleural cavity, while a tube on the other end is placed inside a receptacle.

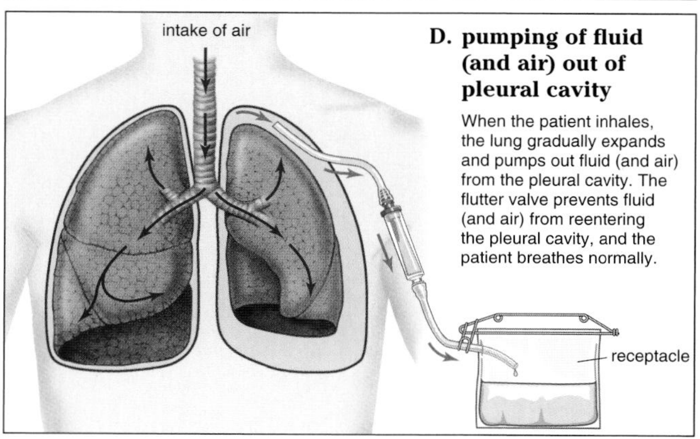

D. pumping of fluid (and air) out of pleural cavity

When the patient inhales, the lung gradually expands and pumps out fluid (and air) from the pleural cavity. The flutter valve prevents fluid (and air) from reentering the pleural cavity, and the patient breathes normally.

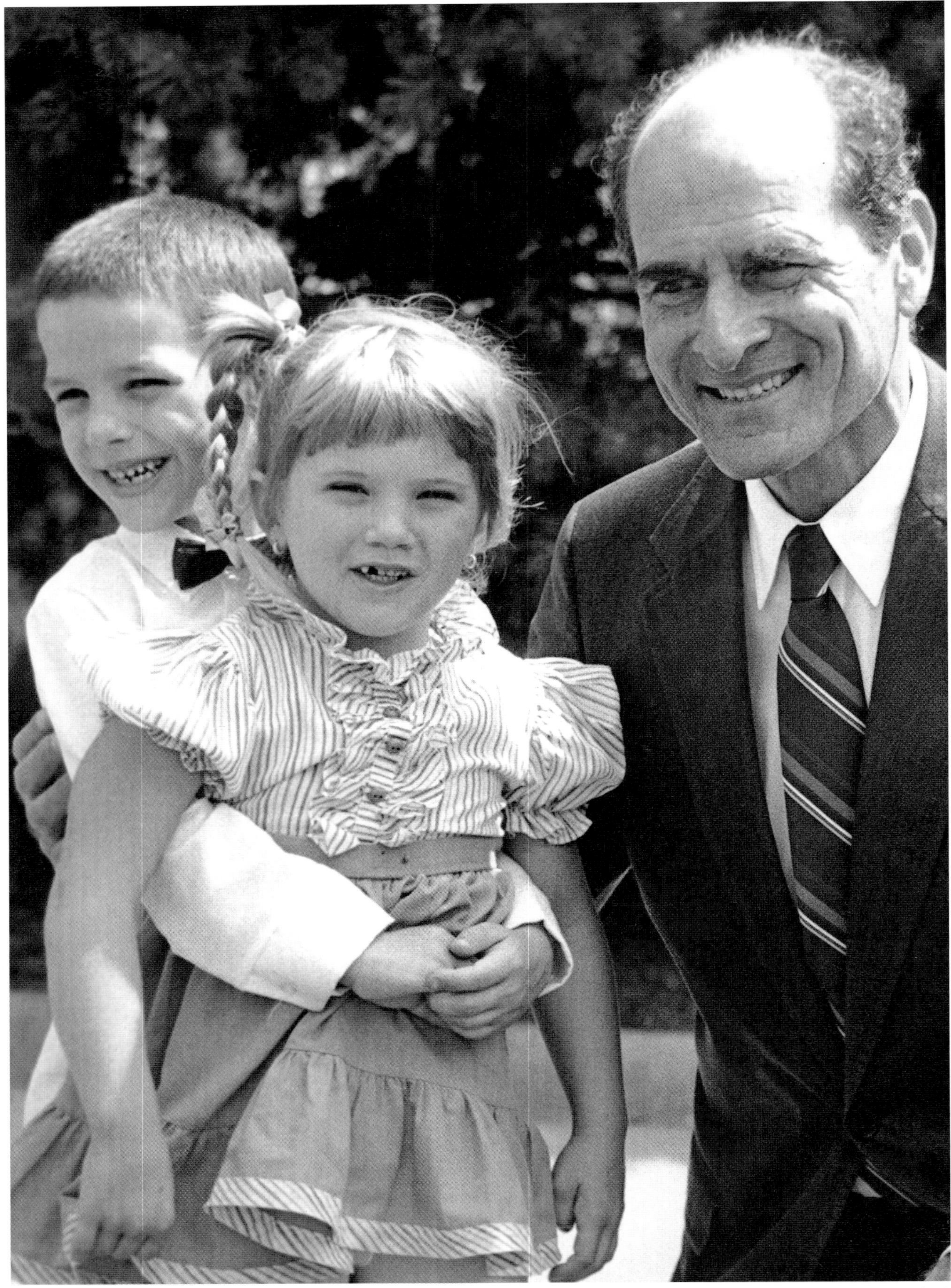

UPI/Bettmann–Corbis

struction. Studies done at the prestigious Chevalier Jackson Clinic in Philadelphia investigating the treatment and outcomes of close to 6,000 choking incidents not only confirmed the hazards of back slaps but advised that putting fingers into the throat of a choking victim can cause the same deadly complication.

A Yale University study (reported in *Pediatrics* in 1982) determined that back slaps drive an object in the throat downward at a force of three g's, or three times the force of gravity (one g is equal to the amount of force exerted by gravity on a body at rest). The chest moves forward, but the obstructing object does not. This follows Newton's law: To every action, there is an equal and opposite reaction.

A solution seemed obvious; what was needed was a way of causing a sufficient flow of air from the lungs toward the mouth to carry away the obstruction. Choking is a true emergency. Brain damage, followed by death, occurs in four minutes. There is no time to look for a device to remove the object from a victim's throat or to call an ambulance. For the life of a choking victim to be saved, there must be an easily learned hands-on method.

I began my work in a laboratory. First I inserted a tube with a balloon on one end into the airway of an anesthetized beagle and attempted to expel it by compressing the lungs. Pressing on the chest was not effective. Pressing upward on the diaphragm with a fist, however, expelled the tube every time. Subsequent tests on myself and colleagues confirmed this effect. Those tests found that subdiaphragmatic pressure generates a powerful airflow of 940 cubic centimeters in a quarter of a second (205 liters per minute).

Brent Meldrum demonstrates how he saved his "sweetheart," Tanya Brandon, from choking on a piece of candy by using the Heimlich maneuver.

I published these findings in June 1974 (in *Emergency Medicine*). A week later the first choking victim was saved by the "Heimlich maneuver" (so named by editors of the *Journal of the American Medical Association,* Aug. 12, 1974, because it had saved so many lives in just two months). I knew that the goal of devising a technique that was both easy to learn and easy to perform had been met when I learned that a four-year-old, who had been taught the Heimlich maneuver by his firefighter father, had saved his two-year-old sister as their helpless, terrified mother looked on.

I soon started receiving letters from choking victims whose lives had been saved by the maneuver; these provided new ideas about the procedure and better understanding of the mechanism by which it works. The director of medical services at Albert Einstein Medical Center, Philadelphia, wrote about his wife's choking experience. The Heimlich maneuver caused a chicken bone, 3.8 centimeters (1.5 inches) long and pointed at both ends, stuck in her windpipe, to shoot out of her mouth. This observation confirmed that it is not the *pressure effect* that expels objects (like a cork popping out of a champagne bottle) but the *flow of air* that drives the foreign object up and out; thus, pressing upward compresses the lungs, expelling a flow of air (similar to the action of squeezing a bellows).

One woman was alone when she choked on a piece of meat. She pressed her upper abdomen against a porch railing and saved herself. People can save themselves by pressing against the back of a chair, the edge of a sink, or the side of a table. Others have reported saving themselves by performing the maneuver with their own fist.

In *Clinical Symposia* (1979), I documented the success of the maneuver in 1,134 instances of choking. In 174 of them back slaps were tried first without success. The important thing was that 35 of those 174 victims had already fallen unconscious, owing to the delay caused by using back slaps, before the Heimlich maneuver was applied. This meant they were seconds from brain damage and death, yet the maneuver still saved them.

For more than a decade, the American Red Cross continued to teach backs slaps for choking. Finally, in 1985, U.S. Surgeon General C. Everett Koop declared that abdominal thrusts, chest thrusts, and back slaps were "hazardous, even lethal" and that only the Heimlich maneuver should be used to save choking persons. Although there is no scientific evidence that either back slaps, chest thrusts, or holding the head downward will save any choking victim, the Red Cross and other groups still teach these methods for rescuing choking infants.

Drowned but not doomed. In the Middle Ages rolling a drowning victim face down over a barrel was a common and often successful treatment. In 17th- and 18th-century Germany, persons rescued after drowning were draped face down over the back of a trotting horse. In the early 1900s a method known as Schafer artificial respiration was introduced; this treatment for drowning had the victim lying face down as the rescuer pressed repeatedly on the lower ribs, saying, "Out goes the bad air, in comes the good air." The barrel, the horse, and the Schafer prone-pressure techniques were crude Heimlich maneuvers. They saved drowning victims because they pushed upward on the diaphragm, which removed the water from the lungs.

Drowning victims die when their lungs fill with water. Air cannot get into water-filled lungs. The Heimlich maneuver removes water from the lungs in four to six seconds. Many drowning victims have been saved by rescuers performing Heimlich maneuvers,

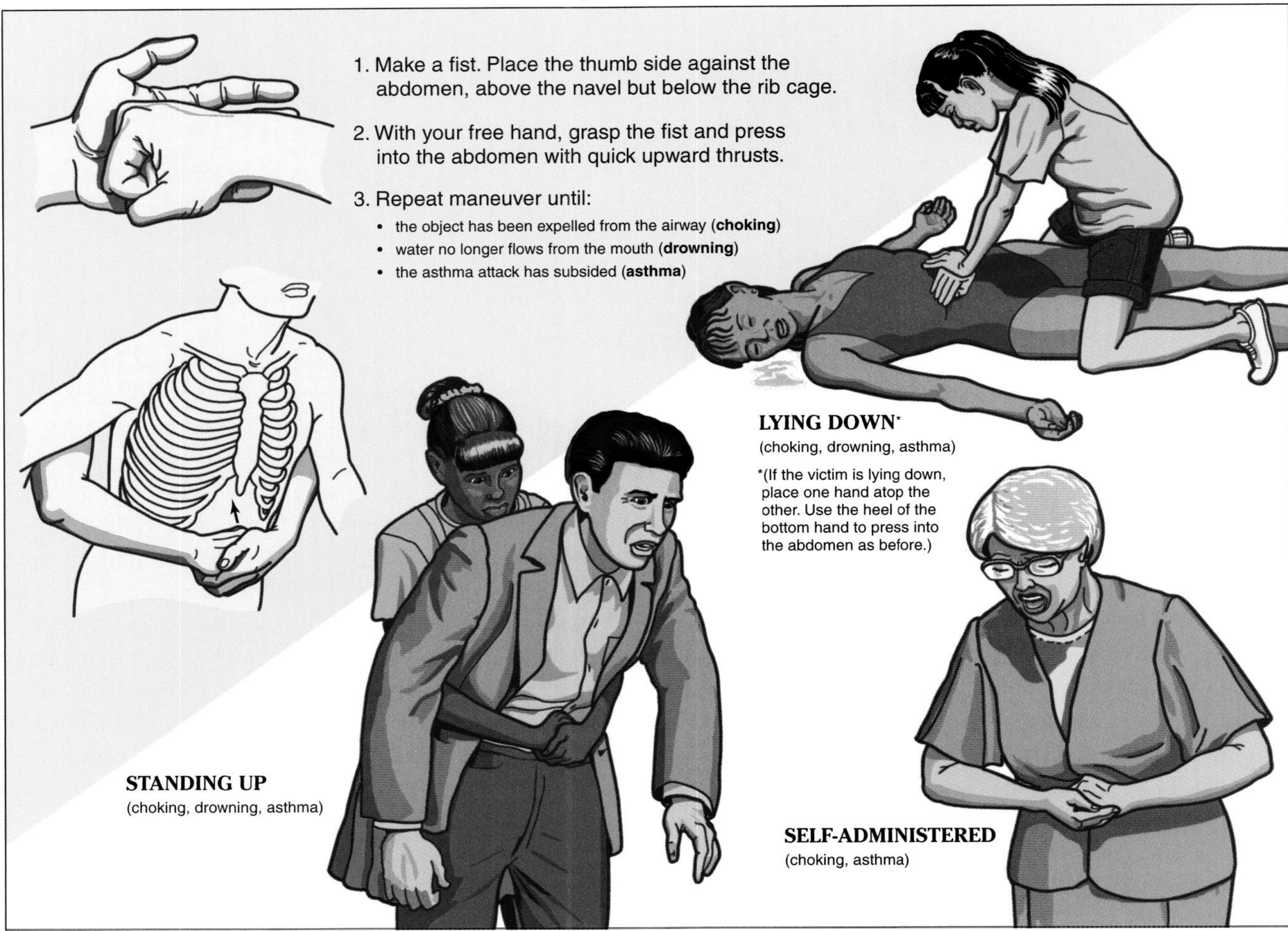

even after cardiopulmonary resuscitation (CPR) has failed.

1. Make a fist. Place the thumb side against the abdomen, above the navel but below the rib cage.
2. With your free hand, grasp the fist and press into the abdomen with quick upward thrusts.
3. Repeat maneuver until:
• the object has been expelled from the airway (choking)
• water no longer flows from the mouth (drowning)
• the asthma attack has subsided (asthma)
LYING DOWN*
(choking, drowning, asthma)
*(If the victim is lying down, place one hand atop the other. Use the heel of the bottom hand to press into the abdomen as before.)
STANDING UP
(choking, drowning, asthma)
SELF-ADMINISTERED
(choking, asthma)

In 1960 mouth-to-mouth resuscitation replaced less-effective techniques of artificial respiration, such as the Schafer method, as the first-aid procedure of choice for heart attack victims. Unfortunately, enthusiastic mouth-to-mouth resuscitation advocates also recommended the method for drowning victims. No study, however, has shown that mouth-to-mouth resuscitation without prior drainage of inhaled water is effective. When lungs are filled with water, air blown into the mouth is forced into the stomach, which distends, causing vomiting; vomit is aspirated into the lungs, causing death. Also, the distended stomach exerts upward pressure on the diaphragm and interferes with breathing. The presence of water in the lungs, even after the victim is on the shore, is equivalent to the victim's still being under the water.

It was Victor Esch, chief surgeon for the Washington, D.C., fire department, who discovered that the Heimlich maneuver would save a drowning victim. In 1974 he was at Rehoboth Beach in Delaware when a lifeguard pulled a drowned man from the water and declared him dead. Esch performed the Heimlich maneuver. Water gushed from the man's lungs, and he recovered instantly.

As Terry Watkins, emergency medical technician and chief of the Destin, Florida, fire department, pulled his fishing boat ashore, his 15-year-old son, who had been fishing with him, pointed to a man who was in the midst of performing mouth-to-mouth resuscitation on a four-year-old boy onshore. The child, Shawn Alexander, was unconscious and blue. Watkins had read that the Heimlich maneuver could save drowning victims, so he promptly grabbed Shawn from the man and performed the maneuver three times. Each time a cupful of water came out of Shawn's lungs. After the third maneuver Shawn coughed up white foam, started to cry, and fully recovered.

Susan Hill of Des Moines, Iowa, had been looking for her 18-month-old grandson, Steven, for about 15 minutes. When she found him lifeless under the cover of her outdoor pool, she remembered having seen illustrations of the Heimlich maneuver—the only first-aid method she knew. She performed the procedure, and water spewed out of the youngster's mouth. Steven showed immediate signs of life and proceeded to recover fully. (While millions know the Heimlich maneuver, few know that the same maneuver that saves choking victims also saves drowning victims.)

A study at the Patrick Institute, Anderson, Ohio, published in *Legal Medicine*

Canadian Ted Young (center) used the Heimlich maneuver to save a drowning victim. The technique's originator (left) traveled to British Columbia to present the rescuer an award.

(1995), found that in a series of unconscious, nonbreathing, pulseless drowning victims, 87% survived when the Heimlich maneuver was performed, whereas only 27% survived when CPR was performed without the Heimlich maneuver. Many rescuers report that the Heimlich maneuver, by causing water to gush out of the mouth, appears to "jump start" breathing. In fact, the maneuver's upward pressure on the diaphragm induces breathing and also massages the heart. A study published in the *American Heart Journal* in 1994 showed that twice as many heart attack victims survived when Heimlich maneuvers were alternated with CPR chest compressions as when chest compressions were used alone. Since 1995 the Heimlich Institute, Cincinnati, Ohio, has received more reports of "drowning saves" with the Heimlich maneuver than of "choking saves."

Actions taken by the first persons on the scene often make the difference between full recovery, death, or brain damage in drowning accidents. Drowning is the third leading cause of accidental death in people of all ages and the leading cause in one-to-four-year-olds in 18 U.S. states. Practical, expedient approaches are needed to save the lives of drowning victims. The American Academy of Pediatrics reports that most child drownings occur in residential swimming pools; the first person on the scene, therefore, is likely to be a parent or neighbor. Some 250 million American adults are *not* trained in first aid but know how to perform the Heimlich maneuver (or else can learn it in about one minute). If the public were to become aware of the maneuver as the "treatment of choice" for drowning victims, every year the lives of an additional 1,000 Americans, most of them children, would be saved.

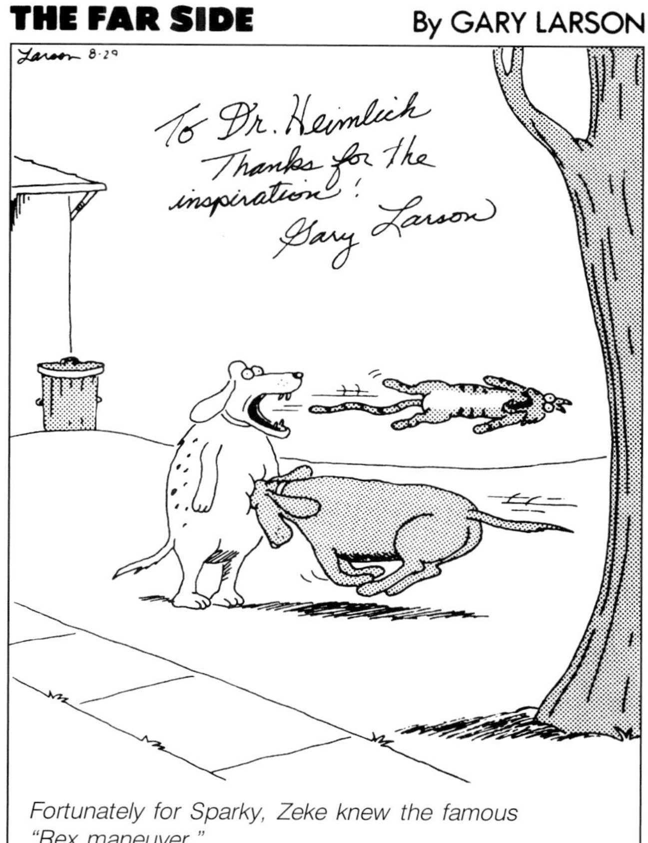

THE FAR SIDE
By GARY LARSON
Larson 8-29
To Dr. Heimlich
Thanks for the inspiration!
Gary Larson

Fortunately for Sparky, Zeke knew the famous "Rex maneuver."

Upon receiving this personally autographed spoof of his acclaimed maneuver as a gift from the cartoonist, Heimlich was duly amused.

The '80s: emphasis on the quality of life

By the 1980s the Heimlich maneuver was saving lives around the world, and my name was well on the way to becoming a household word—not to mention grist for the cartoon mill! My devotion to preventing deaths had not waned, nor could I sit still knowing people were suffering from needless debilitation.

Breathing made a whole lot easier. Patients with chronic breathing difficulties once had to put up with irritating plastic prongs in the nose, through which oxygen (stored in cumbersome tanks) was delivered. Wheelchair-bound patients who required oxygen were connected to a large tank; sucking oxygen from the nose down into the lungs caused them to gasp for air with every breath.

In 1980 I conceived of a tiny tube the diameter of a pencil lead that could be easily inserted into the trachea at the base of the neck in a simple procedure performed under local anesthesia. With this device (named the Heimlich MicroTrach) in place, oxygen jets into the lungs and patients instantly breathe normally. The MicroTrach, which was immediately approved by the Food and Drug Administration, has many advantages. It is held in place by a simple jewelry chain worn invisibly

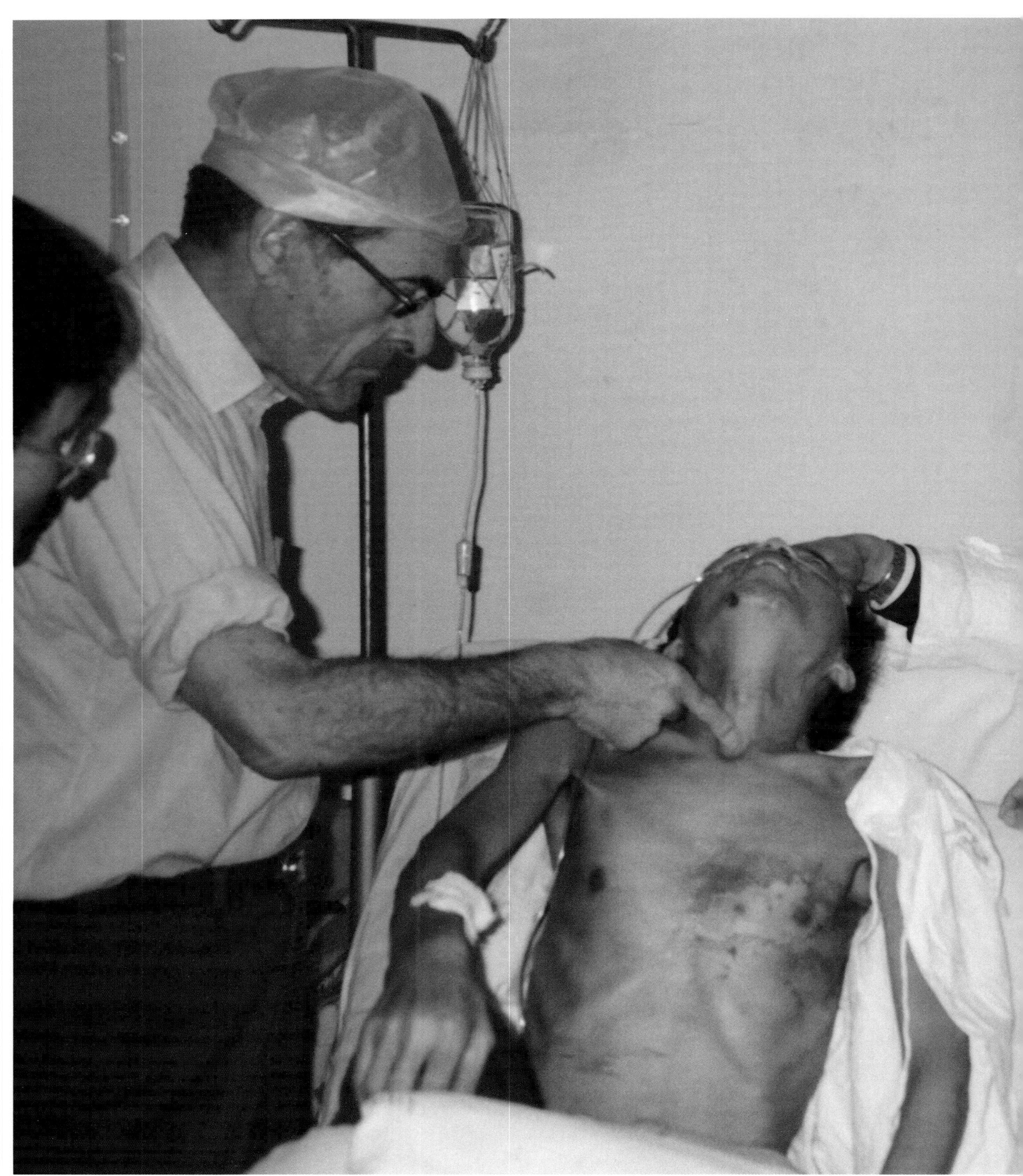

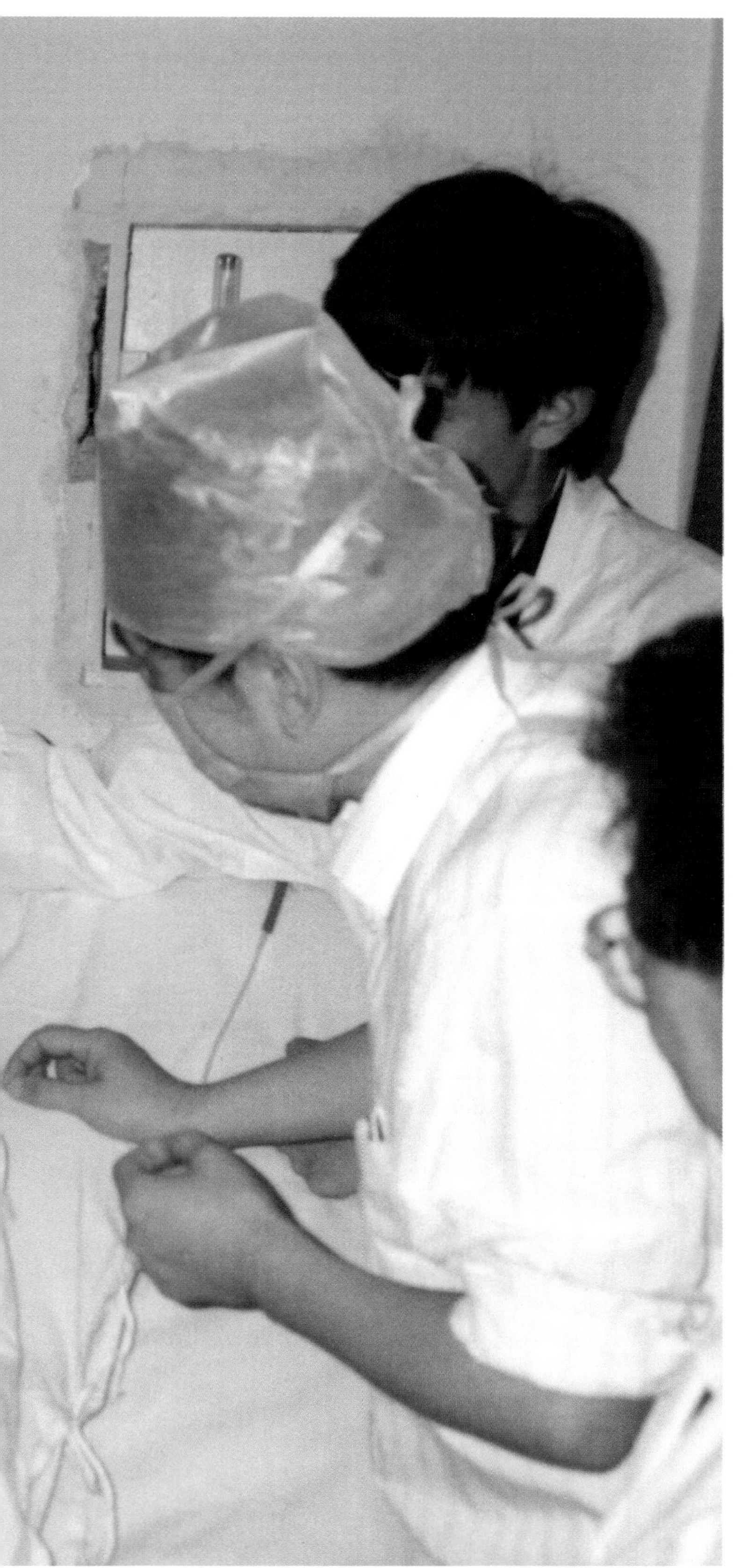

Courtesy of the Heimlich Institute

The inventor guides the insertion of a Heimlich MicroTrach into the trachea of a patient in China. The simple operation is carried out under local anesthesia.

under the collar. Oxygen from a portable container is delivered via tubing that runs under the clothes. Patients with emphysema and chronic heart failure, formerly housebound, now get out and about as much as they desire. Without large, cumbersome oxygen tanks, unsightly nasal devices, or full-time attendants, they now walk into restaurants, stores, and theaters independently, and there is nothing to stop them from playing a game of golf if that is what they fancy.

The advantages do not stop there. It used to be that 50% or more of the oxygen delivered by older methods was lost flowing out the nose and mouth. Now, with the MicroTrach, all of the oxygen is delivered into the lungs, and the therapy costs hundreds of dollars less per patient per month; a lightweight oxygen container that can be carried in a purse or a shoulder bag lasts a half day instead of hours. Sterile saline solution can be instilled through the MicroTrach by the patient to dissolve mucus and stimulate coughing, which then expels the mucus; this process keeps the lungs clear and prevents lung infections that otherwise plague emphysema patients. With the MicroTrach oxygen does not flow through the nose and mouth; therefore, taste and smell are not impaired, which means the patient's appetite returns and nutrition improves. When the tube is removed, the opening is as small as a hole in a pierced ear.

Swallowing restored after stroke. Creative acts result from accumulated knowledge. This is seen in the treatment I developed for swallowing problems associated with stroke.

At age six Muhammad Ben Driss Hayani-Mechkouri swallowed a caustic substance that destroyed his esophagus, pharynx (throat), larynx (voice box), and trachea. Until age 14 he could not swallow or speak. Ben was fed through a tube inserted through the abdomen into his stomach, and he breathed through a tube in his neck leading into his trachea. He lived in the Cheshire Foundation Home, in Tangier. Consultants from France and England considered Ben's case hopeless. A Moroccan physician, however, had heard of the Heimlich operation for esophageal replacement. In October 1970, with the help of Variety Clubs International, the U.S. consul general in Morocco, and transportation provided by Air France, Ben was taken to Ohio, where I operated on him at Jewish Hospital in Cincinnati.

Ben's throat was blocked at the base of the tongue. For eight years he had expectorated saliva into a cup every 15 minutes; at night he drooled onto his pillow. In performing my operation, I joined a new "esophagus," fashioned from a portion of

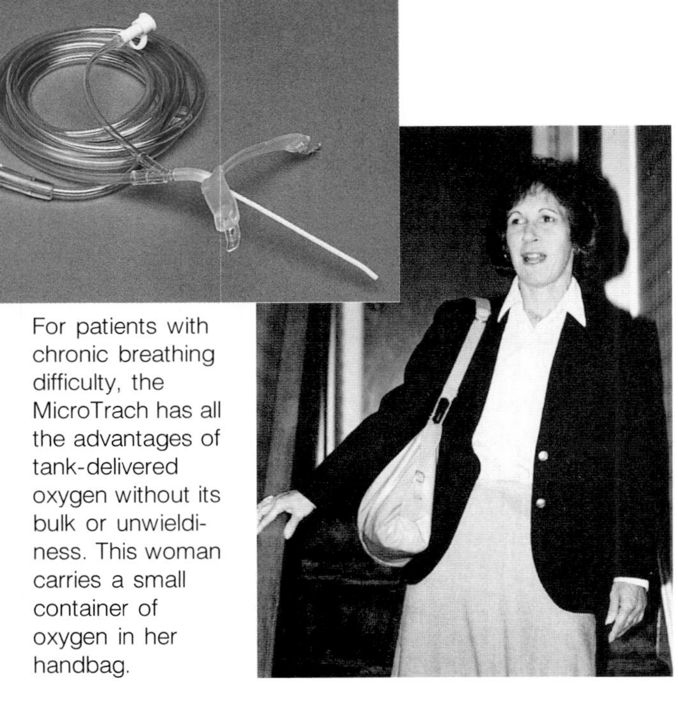

For patients with chronic breathing difficulty, the MicroTrach has all the advantages of tank-delivered oxygen without its bulk or unwieldiness. This woman carries a small container of oxygen in her handbag.

his stomach, to the throat at the base of the tongue.

After Ben recovered, he still could not swallow, even though the opening between the throat and the reversed gastric tube was large enough for food to pass into his stomach. As already noted, from age 6 to 14, he had not eaten. "Has he forgotten how?" I wondered.

Sucking is the first step in swallowing. When premature infants cannot suck, they are taught to do so. An adult demonstrates by sucking on the baby's finger, then putting the finger into the child's mouth. The infant imitates the action.

Ben probably thought I was crazy when I insisted on sucking his finger! But I got him to duplicate my action in a matter of a few days. Very shortly he was not only sucking and swallowing but eating voraciously. Since Ben was of the Islamic faith and could not eat pork, he was put on a kosher diet, which he seemed to relish. I will never forget watching him enjoy his first ice-cream pop! (Ben also learned to speak. We taught him a method for speaking used in patients who have had a cancerous larynx removed—he swallowed air into his stomach and regurgitated the air while moving his lips.) I subsequently tested the sucking treatment on other patients who had not swallowed for as few as 4 and as many as 24 years, with similar results.

Stroke patients who lose the ability to swallow food are tube fed. Paralysis from stroke is unilateral *(i.e.,* confined to one side of the body). I wondered if strengthening the unaffected half of the mouth and throat might restore swallowing, just as exercising healthy muscles of a paralyzed arm restores its function. I began working with poststroke patients in the early 1980s and published the first scientific study in 1983.

First, I got the patients to suck their fingers in order to strengthen the muscles of the mouth. Indeed, many hospital staff were intrigued to discover elderly patients, in wheelchairs lined up in hospital corridors, sucking their fingers all day long! Then I had them put their fingers on my Adam's apple to feel its upward, then downward, movement as I swallowed. Repeating this exercise on themselves strengthened their nonparalyzed throat muscles. Soon they could coordinate their muscle actions so that sucking was followed by swallowing. Within a week, patients who had not eaten for 10 years swallowed ice chips; shortly thereafter, they were eating a regular diet and able to have their feeding tubes removed permanently.

In 1991 physicians at Johns Hopkins University, Baltimore, Maryland, reported in *The New England Journal of Medicine* that people with postpolio syndrome (paralysis occurring 20 or more years after polio) may have swallowing difficulty due to paralysis of one side of the throat. The authors recommended that family members learn the Heimlich maneuver because patients with swallowing problems have frequent choking emergencies. In a letter published in the Oct. 10, 1991, issue of the *Journal,* I informed the editors that as in stroke victims, the healthy muscles in patients with postpolio syndrome are amenable to strengthening, and when normal swallowing has been restored, chances are that the Heimlich maneuver will be unnecessary.

The '90s: AIDS, cancer, and asthma

In the present decade I have turned my attention to devastating illnesses for which medicine has yet to find cures. AIDS was identified in 1981; by 1996, 37.8 million HIV/AIDS cases had been reported to the World Health Organization, and 6.4 million had died. The war on cancer was declared in 1971 but has yet to be won. In 1996, 1,359,000 new cases in the U.S. alone were diagnosed and some

Muhammad Ben Driss Hayani-Mechkouri, after his esophagus was replaced; it was hard to tell who enjoyed his first bite of ice cream more—Ben or his doctor!

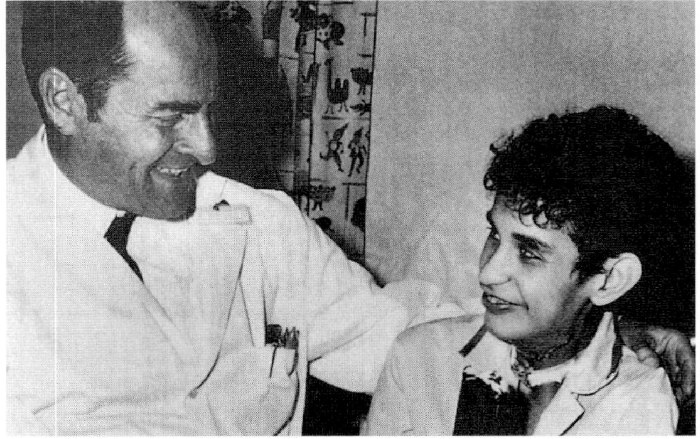

(Top) Life Medical Technologies, Inc.; (center and bottom) courtesy of the Heimlich Institute

554,740 cancer patients died from their disease.

Inducing one disease to cure another. Early stages of syphilis are curable with arsenic injections or antibiotics. When syphilis invades the brain (neurosyphilis), the blood-brain barrier prevents drugs from reaching their target in the brain, so cure is not possible. The Austrian psychiatrist and neurologist Julius Wagner-Jauregg received the 1927 Nobel Prize for Physiology or Medicine for discovering that malariotherapy (artificial induction of malaria) cured neurosyphilis. A curable form of malaria (*Plasmodium vivax*) inoculated into neurosyphilitic patients caused malaria; three weeks later medication (quinine) cured the malaria—and at the same time brought neurosyphilis, a previously fatal disease, under control. Giving a disease to cure (or prevent) disease was not an unfamiliar concept. Jenner's cowpox vaccination to prevent smallpox is one example; Albert B. Sabin's live poliovirus vaccine to prevent poliomyelitis is another.

From 1931 to 1965 the U.S. Public Health Service provided blood taken from malaria patients for malariotherapy, which cured tens of thousands of cases of neurosyphilis. Malariotherapy was discontinued in 1965 in the U.S. and in 1975 in England because neurosyphilis had been largely wiped out (and because penicillin, which cured early syphilis, prevented neurosyphilis from developing). In a comprehensive review of malariotherapy published in the *Journal of Parasitology* in 1984, Eli Chernin, at the Harvard School of Public Health, concluded:

Courtesy of the Heimlich Institute

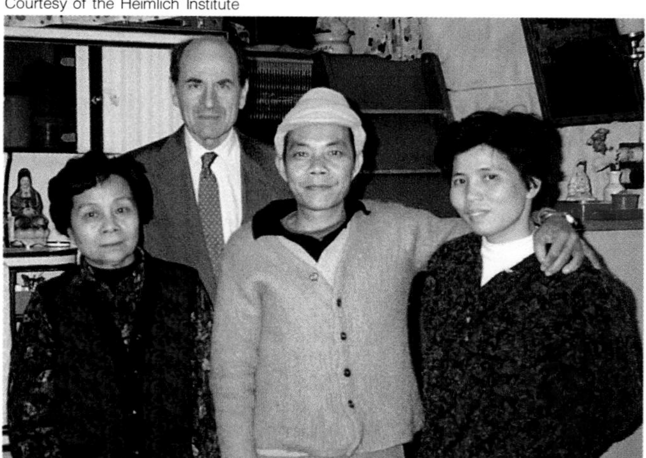

Heimlich (rear) in China with a cancer patient (center) who was treated with experimental malariotherapy. The therapy is now being tested on patients with AIDS.

> ***Malariotherapy was less expensive and produced clinical improvement more frequently and more rapidly than did the best drug treatment [and]... records of treatment-related deaths or extreme debility are few relative to the thousands of patients treated.... It is not hard to imagine the almost certain fate of the thousands of paretics [neurosyphilitics] who would have sickened horribly and died but for malariotherapy.***

Physicians thought that it was the malarial fever that cured neurosyphilis. In the 1980s, however, studies showed that malaria infections boost the immune system, stimulating production of immune substances, including interferons, interleukins, and tumor necrosis factor. I realized that because AIDS and cancer patients lack vital immune substances, they might benefit from malariotherapy. The Heimlich Institute is treating AIDS and cancer patients with malariotherapy in China (because malaria blood is not available in the U.S., and my World War II contacts there have made such an arrangement possible). A three-week course of malariotherapy was tested against metastasized cancers (tumors that had spread) in 10 patients. It was effective against breast cancer, melanoma, and Kaposi's sarcoma but produced no improvement in cancers of the lung, pancreas, or nasal pharynx.

My colleagues and I reported our experience treating patients infected with HIV, first at the National Institutes of Health in Bethesda, Maryland (in June 1996), and then at the XI International Conference on AIDS in Vancouver (in July of the same year), and the results were published in the medical journal *Mechanics of Ageing and Development* (1997). In our first eight patients, CD4+ lymphocytes (a specific type of immune-system cell targeted by the AIDS virus) rose to normal levels (a standard measure of success in treating AIDS) after three weeks of malariotherapy. Patients in this group are clinically well, and their CD4+ counts have remained elevated for two years without further treatment of any kind. One died in 22 months of unrelated causes. Ten HIV patients are now undergoing malariotherapy—the first of a group of 100 patients to be treated.

Heimlich maneuver redux. About five years ago I heard this story from a woman at a conference I was attending: "My sister, an asthmatic, couldn't breathe and turned blue. I performed the Heimlich maneuver; she immediately took a deep breath and recovered." Shortly thereafter, I received a letter from the mother of a four-year-old reporting that during a deadly asthma attack her daughter was so breathless she could not even inhale her medication. "I was about to rush her to the emergency room but knew there wasn't time." Instead, she performed the Heimlich maneuver, and the child breathed normally.

Asthma attacks—wheezing and shortness of breath that can be fatal—occur when muscles surrounding airways contract, narrowing inflamed air passages. Mucus fills the airways and acts as a valve;

i.e., when asthmatics inhale, air has to slither around thick mucous plugs, but because airways are both clogged and narrowed, the air cannot get out. Trapped air distends the lungs, preventing inhalation and exhalation. Pushing up on the diaphragm with the Heimlich maneuver compresses the lungs, which causes trapped air to be expelled and mucous plugs to be carried along with it and thereby ends an asthma attack. The maneuver is performed gently on asthmatics because only air and mucus must be expelled; by contrast, solid objects and water require a sufficient amount of force to be driven out.

According to the National Institute of Allergy and Infectious Diseases, 15 million to 16 million Americans suffer from asthma. Fourteen Americans die during asthma attacks every day, and in 1996 asthma deaths in the U.S. alone exceeded 5,000. Many are children. Despite the availability of new drugs, asthma death rates increase every year.

The Heimlich maneuver both stops and *prevents* deadly asthma attacks by prophylactically removing mucus. Asthmatics do the maneuver on themselves, and mothers perform it on children several times weekly. I have received report after report from asthma sufferers and parents of children with asthma confirming that the Heimlich maneuver prevents episodes of wheezing; patients, ranging in age from 4 to 82, are no longer having attacks. Moreover, as patients learn this technique, their reliance on potent drugs (which themselves often cause deadly reactions) is greatly reduced.

In cystic fibrosis the accumulation of thick mucus causes obstruction and infection of the lungs. Patients are repeatedly tilted and pounded on the back and the chest to remove mucus. It would be a great boon for these patients, too, if the Heimlich maneuver could help remove this mucus; moreover, since patients can perform the technique on themselves, they would enjoy independence that they do not presently have. Because the maneuver may have still further applications, the Heimlich Institute is encouraging studies that will determine its full potential.

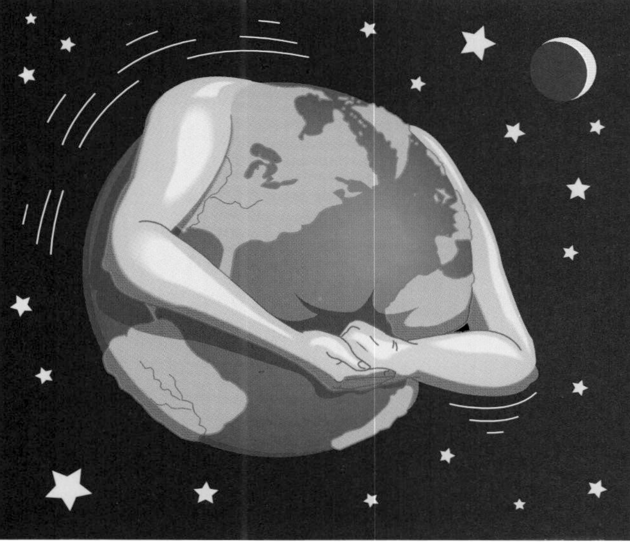

The future: who cares?

Does a creative tendency in one field predict similar tendencies in other fields? Not necessarily. Nonetheless, in my 77th year I have every intention of making a contribution in a field that some might deem outside my bailiwick. I firmly believe there can be creative solutions to even the most gargantuan and formidable problems. Take world peace, for example.

Today's headlines may describe a world of gross injustices, bitterness and hatred, and death and destruction, but is this truly such an *uncaring* world? I believe not. Consider these historic changes in human behavior:

- For the first time in history, major enemy nations attained peace without first resorting to world war.
- In Eastern Europe millions of people faced tanks and overthrew tyrants, with relatively few casualties.
- The United States invaded Somalia solely to feed starving people and establish democracy.
- South Africans voted against apartheid and all the repression it stood for in a democratic election that few would have thought possible.
- Even after having faltered more than once, peace negotiations between Israelis and Palestinians have gotten back on track.

Peaceful transitions are occurring across the globe; no war has achieved some of the triumphs that the world is now seeing. The Heimlich Institute has established the program A Caring World to foster peace and health in the world and bring people together. Factors such as television, computers, air travel, and interdependence of economies and environment bring people together, but their potential to do so has not yet been appreciated.

Caring can spread more rapidly than any cancer. A Caring World encourages the media to publicize the magnanimous acts of those who do not usually make headlines, just as it does the philanthropic gestures of athletes, entertainers, and politicians. The Heimlich Institute is establishing Caring World programs in cities across the United States and hopes eventually to do so abroad. Through this program I hope to teach others what I have learned so well: that true happiness comes from truly giving of oneself. Just as anyone can perform the Heimlich maneuver, everyone can learn to care. Of that I am utterly convinced! MHA

(Above) Based on a sketch by Henry J. Heimlich; (opposite) Dennis Marsico

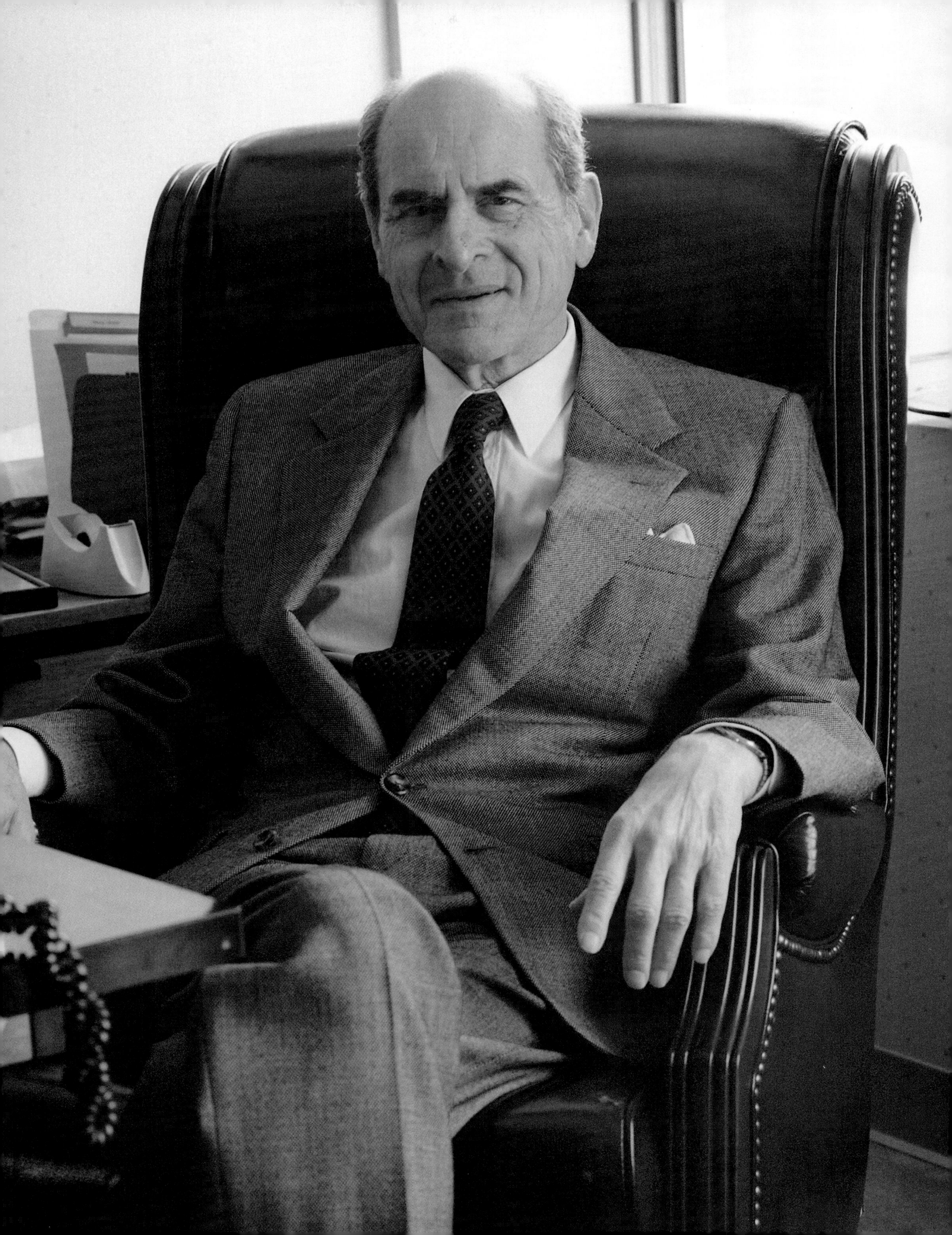

The Body Synchronic

by James Waterhouse, D.Phil.,
and Torbjörn Åkerstedt, Ph.D.

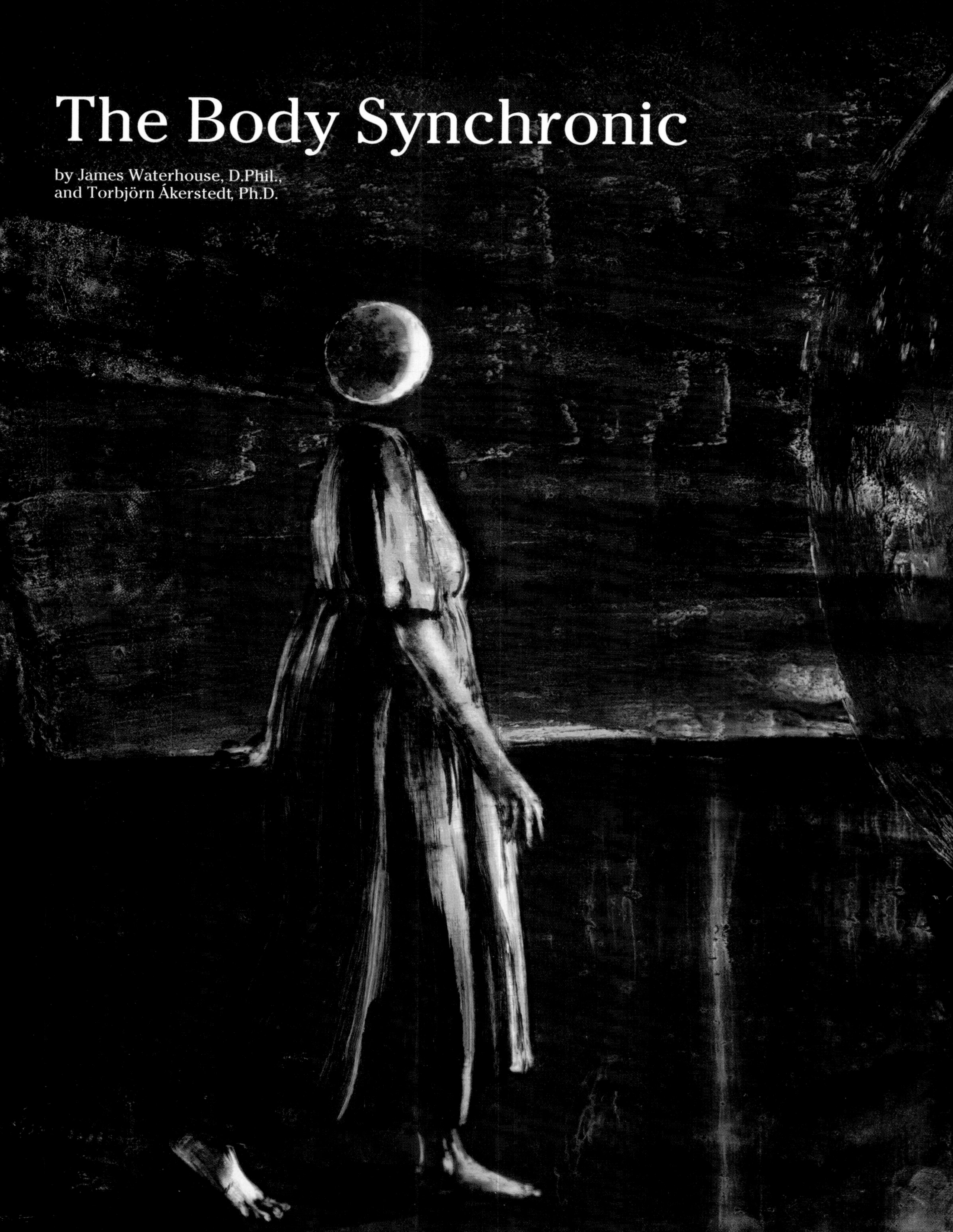

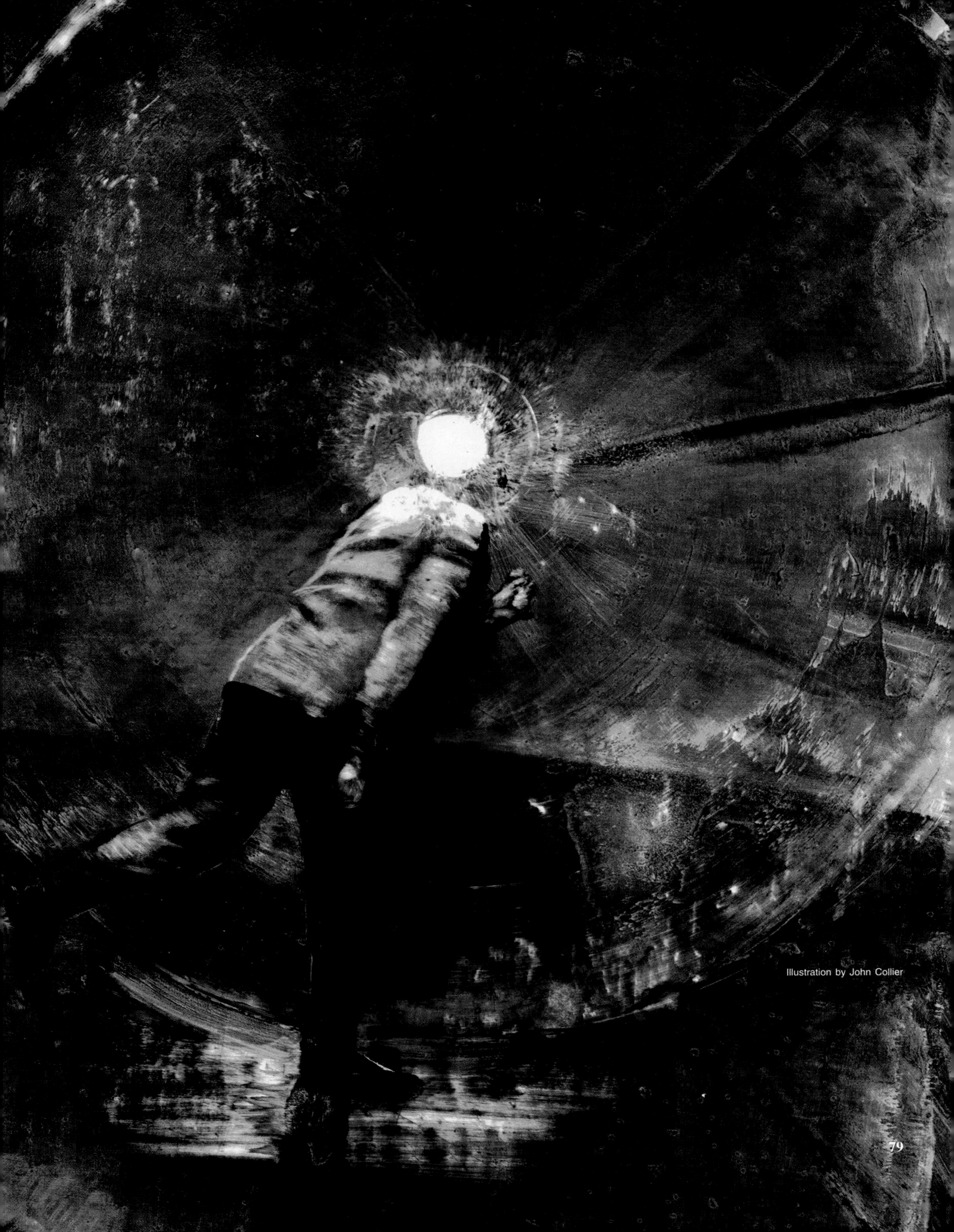

Illustration by John Collier

James Waterhouse, D.Phil., is Lecturer, School of Human Sciences, Liverpool John Moores University, Liverpool, England, and President-elect, International Society of Chronobiology.

Torbjörn Åkerstedt, Ph.D., is Professor, National Institute for Psychosocial Factors and Health, Stockholm, and Past President, European Society for Sleep Research.

The cyclic rhythms of time—the alternation of light and dark, the changing of the seasons—have an impact on all forms of life. The earliest human ancestors would have hunted by daylight and rested during the hours of darkness. They undoubtedly would have observed seasonal changes in the habits of their prey. Certainly an intimate knowledge of the seasons—of when to sow seed, for example—would have been necessary for the development of agriculture. The orientation of Stonehenge and similar megalithic structures in Europe, dating from about 2000 BC, suggests that prehistoric humans were aware of the cyclic and indeed predictable movement of the Sun during the course of the year.

From the Greek and Roman classics onward, literature abounds with descriptions of how plants, animals, and humans, in health and disease, exhibit changes in biochemistry, physiology, and psychology (as these processes are now called) that are in phase with the passage of the hours or the seasons. The 18th-century Swedish botanist Carolus Linnaeus produced one of the most charming such descriptions in the form of a "flower clock"—a diagram showing the times of day at which various flowers open and close. Throughout most of history it seems to have been generally believed that the biological changes taking place in plants and animals, and in humans as well, were responses to the environment or, perhaps, the gods. The causes were thought to be wholly exogenous—*i.e.,* external—and the response of the living organism passive.

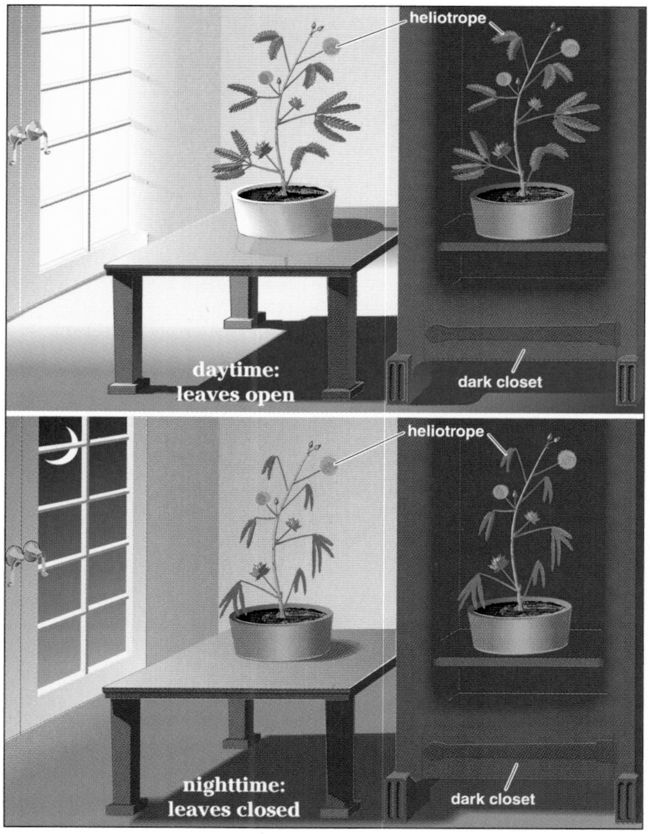

Plants do it, bees do it

The earliest investigations of the response of living things to the passage of time focused on plants. In 1729 the French scientist Jean-Jacques de Mairan demonstrated that the cyclic changes in leaf positions (from open during the day to closed at night) continue even when plants are kept in the dark. This and similar observations began to cast doubt on the long-held view that living organisms were merely passive recipients of information about time. Later, experiments with human subjects revealed that body temperature, which is normally higher during the daytime than at night, continues to fluctuate cyclically even if an individual stays in bed all day and even if he or she remains in the dark. In other words, at least some of the rhythmicity observed in plants and animals is endogenous—originating from within the organism—which implies some form of internal "body clock."

In 1832 the Swiss botanist Augustin Pyrame de Candolle established that even though

In a simple experiment the 18th-century French scientist Jean-Jacques de Mairan showed that the cyclic movements of the leaves of the light-sensitive heliotrope plant are independent of the cycle of light and dark.

(Below) Tom Foley, Minneapolis, Minn.; (bottom) adapted from M. Renner, "The Contribution of the Honey Bee to the Study of Time Sense and Astronomical Orientation," Cold Spring Harbor Symposium on Quantitative Biology, vol. 25 (1960), pp. 361–367

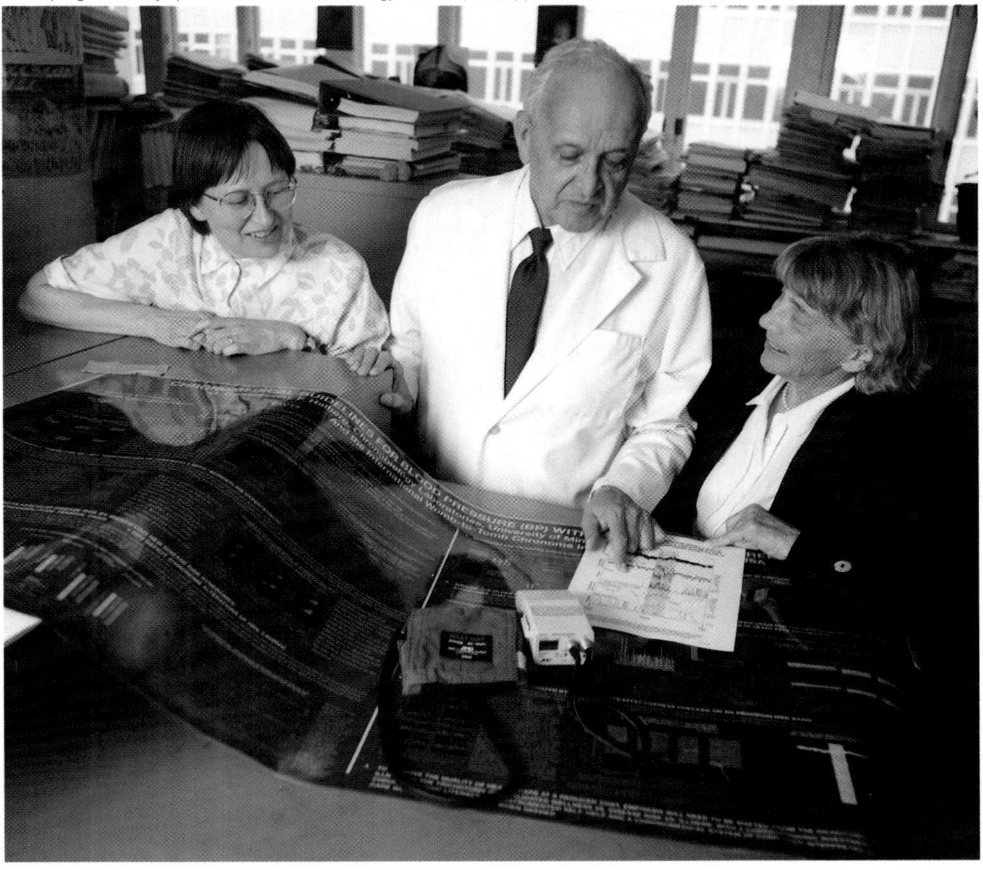

The "father of chronobiology": Franz Halberg in his laboratory with his wife, Othild Schwartzkopff (right), and a fellow researcher.

leaf movements continue in plants deprived of alternating cycles of light and dark, the cycle of movements is repeated not over a period of 24 hours—the length of a solar day—but rather over 22–23 hours. This finding indicated that the internal clock of plants (at least under these conditions) is not an accurate timekeeper. It was not until more than a century later, however, that the Austrian-born scientist Franz Halberg of the University of Minnesota coined the term *circadian* (Latin, "about a day") to refer to the period of approximately but not exactly 24 hours. The persistence in plants of a rhythmic cycle other than 24 hours in length is unlikely to be the consequence of external influences in the environment (*e.g.,* the alternation of day and night, cyclic changes in temperature and humidity). For one thing, no such influence with a cycle of another length is known. For another, different plants have different cycles.

In the 1940s studies of the feeding habits of bees indicated that the internal clock could indeed be an accurate timekeeping device, prompting the insects to visit a particular source of food at the same time each day. The successful replication of these experiments underground in the controlled environment of a salt mine confirmed that the bees' biological rhythms—like those of plants kept in the dark—are not dependent on external cues, such as changes in light or temperature, but rather are innate. Another set of experiments showed that if bees trained in Paris to visit a source of food at a set time were then transferred rapidly to New York, a shift westward of five time zones, the bees would initially visit the food source in their new locale at a time predicted by the

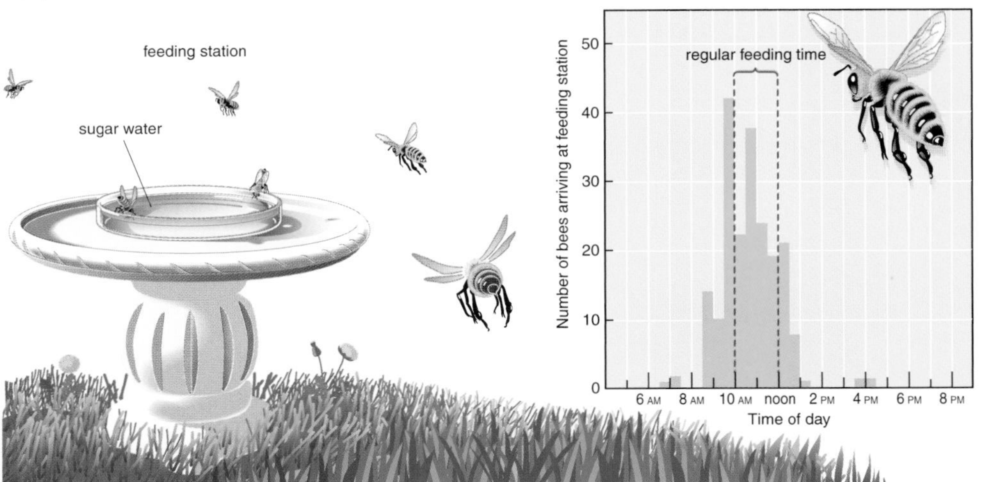

Experiments with bees indicate that they can time their visits to a food source to coincide with a regular daily feeding.

Photographs courtesy of Cambridge Neurotechnology Ltd.

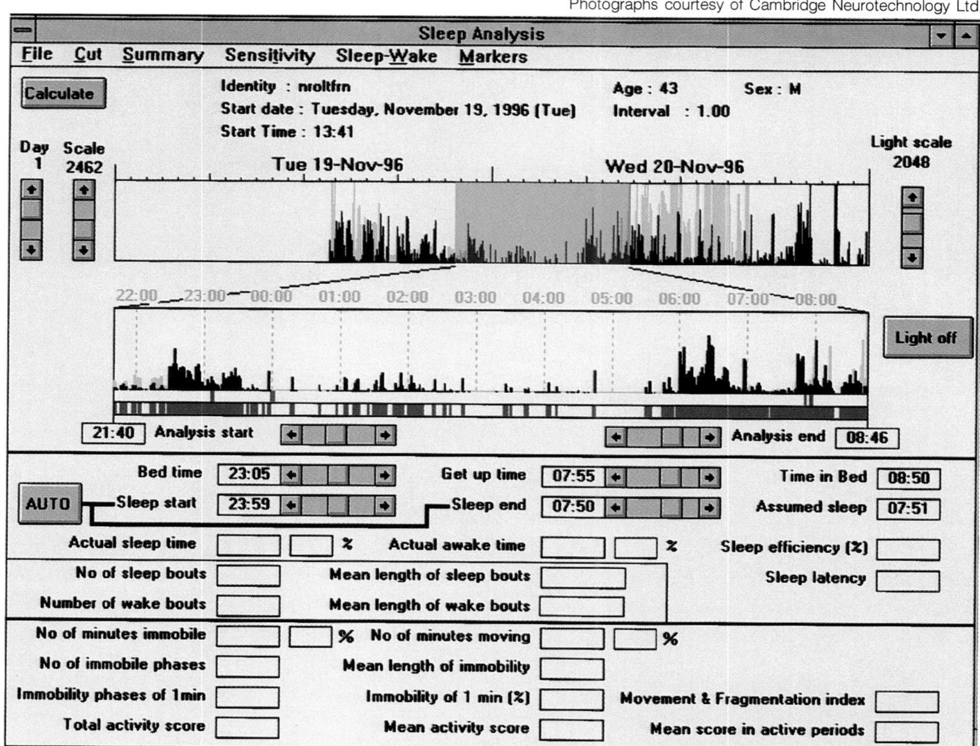

Sophisticated technology for gathering data on human biological rhythms enables scientists to monitor a variety of body functions noninvasively and nonintrusively. The "wristwatch" above is actually a device for monitoring an individual's daily pattern of physical activity. The data it collects are transmitted to a computer, analyzed by a special software program, and displayed (left) on-screen.

French rather than the New York time. In other words, the insects' body clocks were slow to adjust to a sudden change in time zones.

Looking back at those findings, it is clear that by the mid-20th century scientists had either established or inferred all the main properties of the body clock—namely, the presence in living organisms of some sort of internal timekeeping mechanism running on a cycle of about, but not equal to, 24 hours; the need for adjustment of the mechanism to a 24-hour day (or a 24.8-hour tidal day for shore-dwelling creatures); and a tendency of the mechanism toward stability, making the process of adjustment relatively slow.

Volunteers like Stefania Follini, who spent four months in a "time-free" underground environment (below left), have been instrumental in the study of human circadian rhythms. (Below right) Follini emerges from isolation in May 1989.

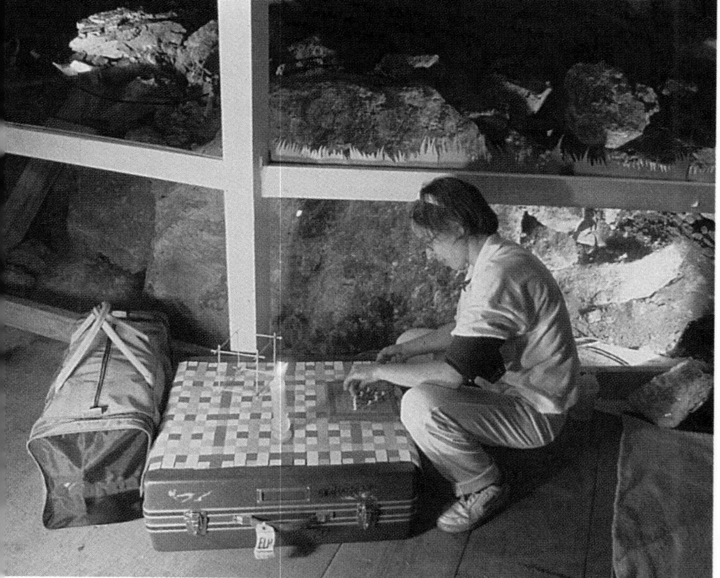

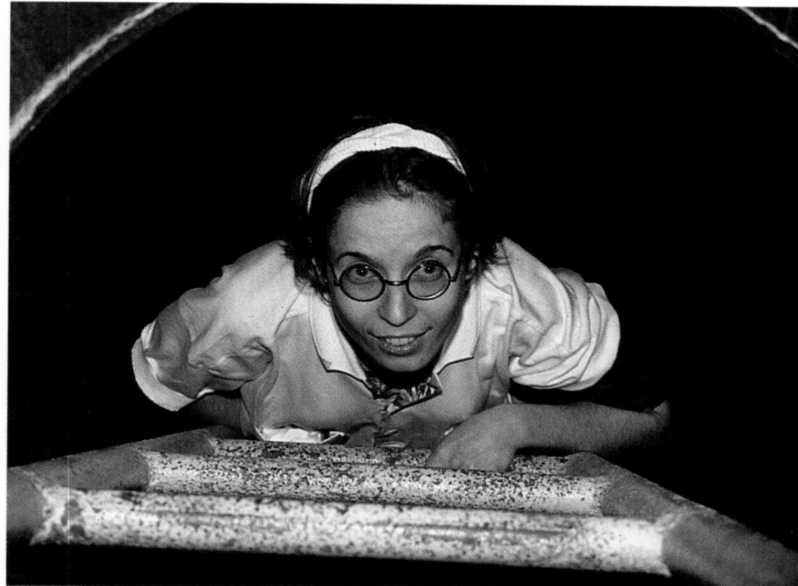

Photographs, Andrea Galvagno—Gamma Liaison

Living "time free"

In the second half of the 20th century, technologies developed in disciplines such as genetics, molecular biology, and pharmacology were applied to the study of biological clocks. The field of study itself was given the name chronobiology.

Because of the difficulties inherent in human experimentation, such work necessarily concentrated on animal species that proved easy to study for these purposes—algae, fungi, sea slugs, fruit flies, and rodents. Fortunately, the assumption made when a particular species is studied—that it acts as a model for species *in general*—has, so far, been found to be essentially correct.

Not that the human species has been ignored. In recent years techniques for obtaining data from humans have become more sophisticated, which has made it possible to gather data more frequently than in the past and, often, noninvasively. Thus, scientists can now continuously monitor subjects' heart rate, blood pressure, and brain electrical activity, sleeping and waking, from a distance. They can measure the levels of many hormones from samples of saliva or urine or as little as a drop of blood. Handheld computers make it possible for volunteers to self-administer tests of mental function (such as short-term memory, reaction time, and logical reasoning) at different times of day.

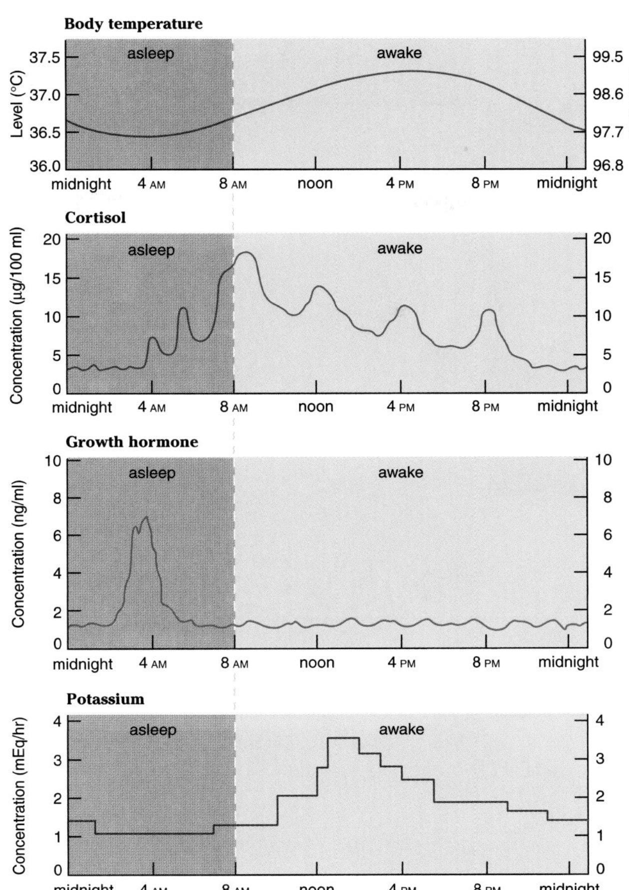

Human chronobiology research has shown that most physiological variables exhibit regular daily rhythms that run roughly in synchrony with the sleep-wake cycle.

Moreover, as test subjects in chronobiology research, humans offer one distinct advantage over other organisms—they can alter their habits as required by the researchers. During the past three decades, in experiments paralleling those conducted in plants over 200 years ago, human volunteers have been placed in "time-free" environments in an attempt to understand the functioning of the body clock. Most of these experiments were originally carried out in underground caves, which effectively insulated the subjects from external time cues, although environments built for this purpose have recently been used.

To date, a few hundred volunteers have been studied for periods ranging from two weeks to as long as nine months, in the absence of all time cues—clocks, of course, but also radios, televisions, regular social contacts and mealtimes, etc. The results have shown that rhythmicity does not disappear in isolation, and with only minor changes, cyclic daily patterns of temperature, heart rate, blood pressure, etc., continue in phase with the sleep-activity cycle. In more than 90% of subjects in these studies, however, the cycle runs longer than 24 hours—averaging, in fact, closer to 25. Thus, in what seems to the volunteer to have been about 24 days in isolation, 25 actual days will have elapsed. The body clock's tendency to follow a circadian cycle rather than adhere to a strict 24-hour cycle is strong evidence that an internal timekeeper is responsible for the observed biological rhythms.

Lives of our days

With the aid of computers and other measuring and recording devices, scientists have been able to study humans as they go about their daily routines. Such research has demonstrated that almost all physiological and biochemical variables do indeed have regular daily rhythms. For many of these variables—among them, heart rate, mental and physical activity, feelings of alertness, digestive processes, and plasma adrenaline levels—the daily rhythm peaks during the daytime and reaches a low ebb during sleep. For other variables—including levels of several hormones (*e.g.,* melatonin, growth hormone, and the sex hormones) and the ability to fall asleep and remain asleep—the peak is during the hours of darkness. Still other functions—such as allergic and immune responses and output of the hormone cortisol—tend to peak at the time of retiring or rising. Taken together, these rhythms yield a picture of the human being as a diurnal rather than a nocturnal creature.

Clearly, though, it is possible that this pattern of human functioning could be nothing

(Left) Brian Smith—Stock, Boston; (right) Ben Edwards—Impact Photos

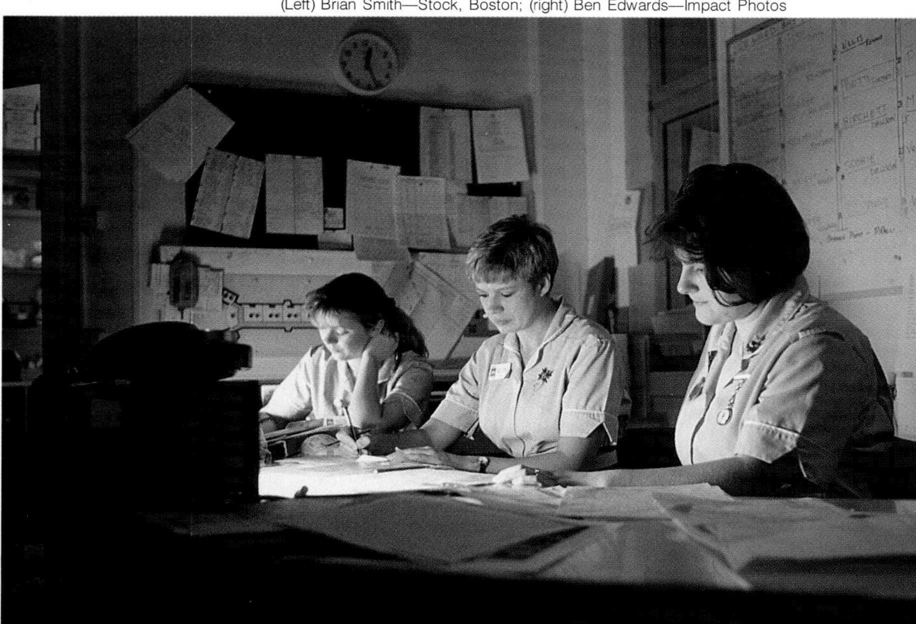

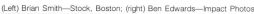

The correlation of human circadian rhythms with the sleep-wake cycle is evidence that the human species is diurnal rather than nocturnal. Still, many occupations require that people function optimally during the nighttime hours.

more than a consequence of daily activities that, owing to social norms, are oriented toward a diurnal existence. A large body of data indicates, however, that such an explanation is inadequate. Consider the following findings:

- Human subjects who remain awake and sedentary in a constant environment (*i.e.,* one without fluctuations in lighting, temperature, noise, or social factors) for at least 24 hours and who consume equally spaced, identical meals do not experience a disappearance of the above-cited rhythms, although some changes may occur.
- The traveler on an intercontinental flight (from New York to Frankfurt, for example, or Los Angeles to Tokyo) will feel tired during the first few days after arrival, particularly during the hours that correspond to night in the "old" time zone, and may not be able to sleep during the "new" nighttime (which often coincides with daytime in the "old" time zone).
- The shift worker on a night shift will feel more tired while on the job and tend to work more slowly, make more mistakes, and suffer more from indigestion than during a regular workday. During the daytime, these same exhausted shift workers will have shorter and more fractionated sleep than normal.

The explanation common to these examples is that the daily rhythms of human life are due at least in part to an internal body clock that continues to run in synchrony with the established timing for some days after a change in habits or time zones. That is, the body clock is stable in its timing and, in order to change at all rapidly, normally requires special manipulation. Lifestyle, however, does have an impact on biological rhythms; physical activity raises an individual's heart rate, adrenaline levels, and alertness, while sleep decreases these and increases growth hormone levels.

The timekeeper in the brain

Once scientists reached general agreement that an internal timekeeping mechanism does indeed exist, the next step was to find it. Most of the research in this area has involved nonhuman organisms, specifically slime molds, fruit flies, and rodents. Studies in rodents have clearly pointed to paired tiny groups of brain cells, called the suprachiasmatic nuclei (SCN), located on either side of the midline of the brain at the base of the hypothalamus and just above where the optic nerves cross over at their entry into the brain. Of all the different kinds of brain cells scientists have studied, those of the SCN alone continue to show circadian rhythms in electrical and secretory activity even when removed from the experimental animal's body and maintained in a laboratory culture in constant conditions. In the living body, cells of the SCN are known to send signals to widely different areas of the brain and neuroendocrine system, which presumably accounts for the widespread influence of circadian rhythms on all bodily processes. These cells also receive both chemical and neural signals from the body as a whole.

The next logical question, then, is what governs the activity of the SCN? Genetic and molecular biochemical studies indicate that the underlying mechanism of the body clock is a set of genes that appear to be activated in a cascadelike sequence. The majority of human genes are located in the nuclei of cells. The genes "encode" (carry instructions for the synthesis of) proteins. Once a gene has been activated, or "turned on," its instructions are carried from the nucleus to other parts of the cell, where the specific protein is produced.

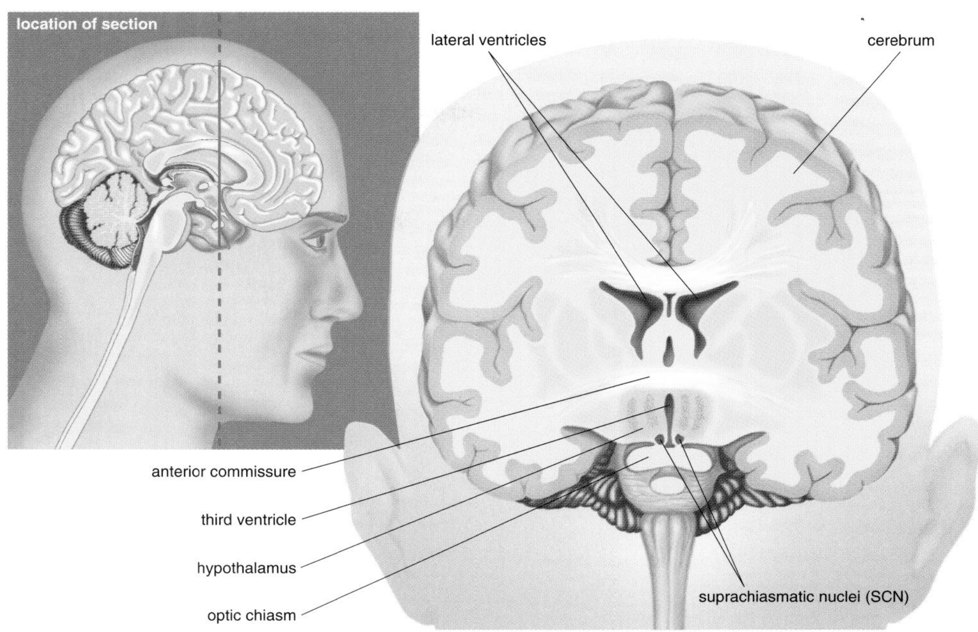

Diagram of the human brain shows the location of the suprachiasmatic nuclei, the paired clusters of cells that function as the body's timekeeping mechanism.

The body clock genes—which thus far have been studied only in fruit flies, bread molds, and mice—encode a special group of proteins called "clock proteins," which are activated in a precise sequence. The protein encoded by the first gene in the sequence is produced in cellular structures called ribosomes. This protein is then transported to the nucleus, where it activates the next gene in the sequence and inhibits its own gene, and so forth.

Current evidence indicates that even though each cell of the SCN can act on its own, for the SCN to function effectively, the individual cells' activity must be linked. This linkage takes place in humans during the first year or so of life (*see* below). By comparing genetic material from many different species, scientists have found that even species very far apart on the evolutionary scale share much of the same genetic information for the body clock—an indication of the fundamental importance of the clock for survival.

Setting—and resetting—the clock

Although in the absence of time cues the human body clock "runs slow" (*i.e.,* runs longer than the solar day) by only about 1–4%—or less than an hour a day—even this slight inaccuracy would render it useless as a timekeeper for daily life. And yet, as described above, most living organisms do possess an accurate inner clock. This accuracy is achieved by continual adjustment of the body clock by time cues in the external environment called zeitgebers (German, "time givers"). The main zeitgeber for a given species is generally the external rhythm that is ecologically most important to that species. For most green plants and many animals, both diurnal and nocturnal, it is the alternation of light and dark; for many shore-dwelling creatures, which are adjusted to the tidal day, it is periodic buffeting by waves or immersion in water. In humans it has been established that light—particularly bright outdoor light—will advance the body clock (*i.e.,* cause the biological rhythms to occur earlier than usual) if a person is exposed to the light after his or her body has reached its temperature minimum, which normally occurs about 5 AM. Light will delay the clock (*i.e.,* cause the biological rhythms to occur later than usual), however, if exposure occurs before the minimum temperature has been reached.

The hormone melatonin, produced by a tiny structure in the brain called the pineal gland, also appears to play a key part in adjusting the human body clock. Melatonin tends to advance the body clock in the evening and delay it in the morning; that is, it works in the opposite way of bright light. Melatonin is normally secreted between evening and morning, when bright light is absent. The opposition of timing and effects of light and melatonin is made even more complete by the tendency of bright light to suppress melatonin secretion.

The two mechanisms thus work together. In the evening melatonin secretion will advance the body clock. If the clock is running fast, however, then melatonin secretion will occur earlier than usual, during daylight hours. The clock will be delayed because of (1) the direct effect of light at this time (as the temperature minimum occurs earlier than usual) and (2) the suppression of melatonin by light (*i.e.,* the melatonin-induced advance will not occur). Conversely, if the body clock is running slow and body temperature falls to minimum levels after 5 AM, then morning light and its suppression of melatonin will combine to advance the clock.

In the environments of most living things, more than one potential zeitgeber is present at any time. For humans in the industrialized world—separated as they are from natural zeitgebers—there are the artificial zeitgebers of electric light and regularly scheduled meals, work, and social and physical activities. The combination of these factors is probably normally responsible for the appropriate adjustment of the human clock.

Scientists theorize that zeitgebers act on the clock by stimulating neural and chemical signals that eventually reach the SCN. It is known, for example, that mammals possess a direct pathway, the retinohypothalamic tract, from the retina of the eye to the SCN. Light entering via the eyes and passing along this pathway activates a group of genes within the SCN, the "immediate early genes." In some way not yet understood, these genes or their protein products impinge upon the cyclic mechanisms that constitute the clock itself. The effect depends upon the stage of the circadian cycle at the time of sensory stimulation (*i.e.,* light exposure). At some stages the immediate early genes act to advance the clock, at others they delay it, and at yet others they have no effect.

Courtesy of Joseph Takahashi, Northwestern University; photograph, Joel DeGrand

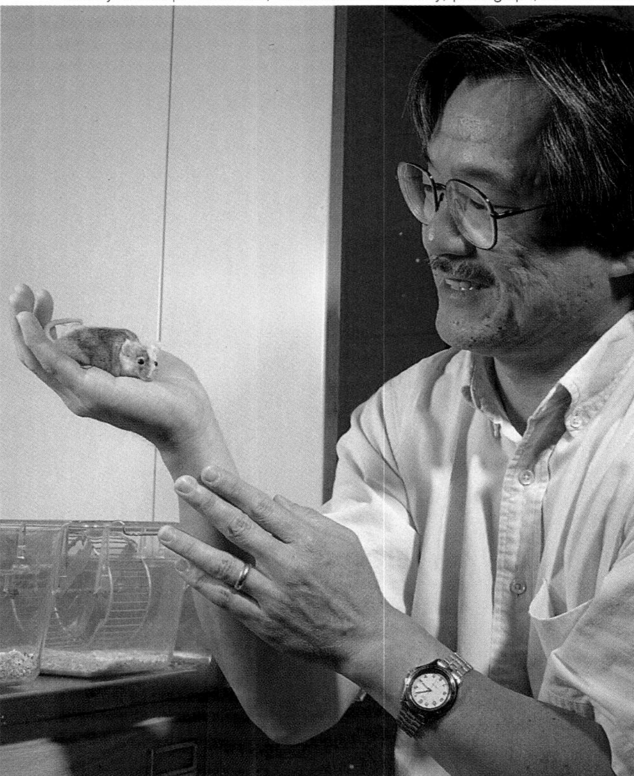

In 1997 Joseph Takahashi, at Northwestern University, Evanston, Illinois, helped identify the first mammalian body-clock gene.

The clock's role

The role of the body clock is twofold. First, it enables the body to alternate between active and inactive modes. Second, it prepares the body to switch from the one mode to the other. In the evening the human clock prepares the body for sleep by reducing adrenaline, blood pressure, and body temperature and increasing melatonin and the sense of fatigue; from about 5 AM onward, the clock prepares the body to awaken by reversing these processes. Normally, lifestyle and zeitgebers act in accord with the body clock.

The clock does not function in exactly the same way

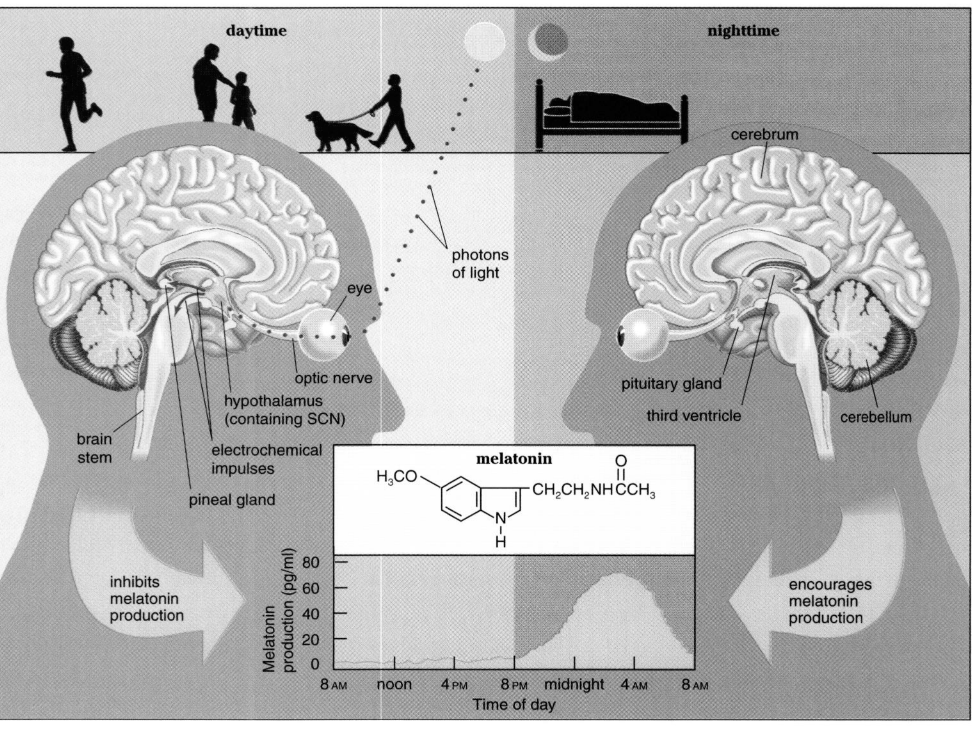

A complex feedback mechanism governs the production and suppression of the hormone melatonin.

(Below) Larry Mulvehill—The Image Works;
(bottom) adapted from Martin Hughes (ed.), *Body Clock* (New York: Facts on File, 1989)

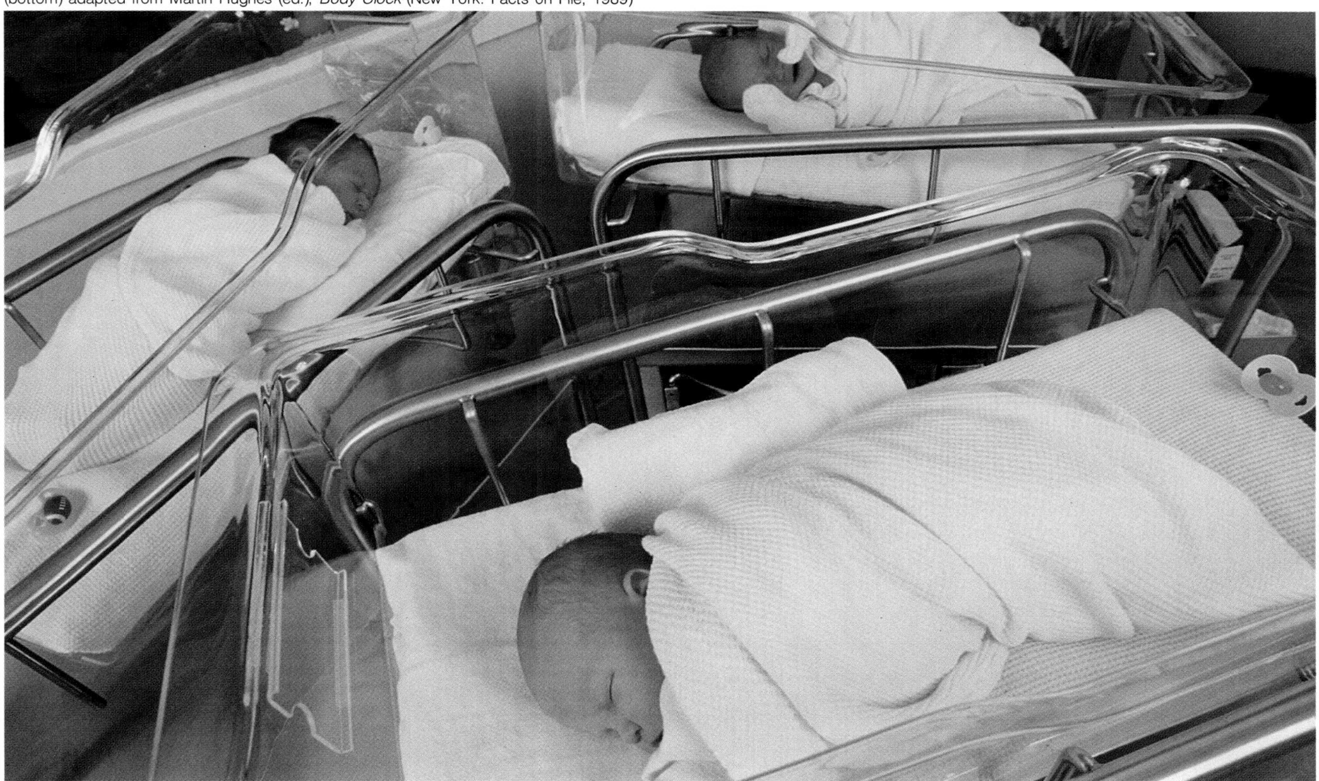

In the first few weeks of life, babies exhibit irregular periods of sleep and wakefulness. Circadian rhythms do not begin to be established until about the fourth month. The length of each sleep period is indicated by black lines on the graph (right); white lines represent periods of wakefulness.

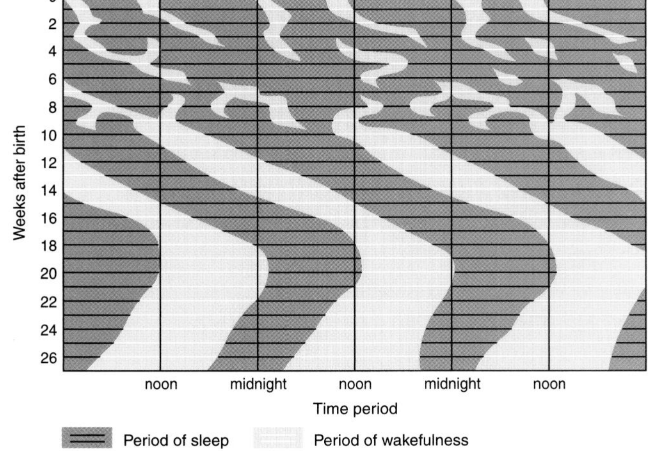

throughout life, however. At birth, for example, humans do not possess a fully developed clock. The most obvious indication of this immaturity is the lack of a circadian rhythm in the sleep and activity cycles of babies. Other rhythms such as the rising and falling of body temperature and cortisol levels are also poorly established in infants. Circadian rhythmicity normally develops in the first months of life but, as might be expected, is delayed in premature babies.

In part, these phenomena are explained by the fact that the SCN are rather small at birth. In addition, the individual cells of the SCN need to fire synchronously, and it is believed that interaction between them is also poorly developed in infancy. Lack of synchrony between cells might explain the observation that babies' daily rhythms, in feeding, for example, are much faster (running in periods of 3–4 hours) than those of adults. The development of normal circadian rhythms is probably dependent on the development of functional connections between the cells of the SCN, coupled with exposure—and the capacity to respond—to external influences.

In the elderly, too, circadian rhythms are weaker and more variable. This change is most apparent in the progressive difficulty older people experience in getting an uninterrupted night's sleep and in their tendency to nap in the daytime. These age-related sleep problems are exacerbated by the failure of the aging body to reduce urine production sufficiently at night, which results in frequent awakening.

Both internal and external factors contribute to these changes. Thus, the SCN appear to decrease in size as people age, and for most people, especially after retirement from work, there is a decrease in the formerly marked contrast between high levels of daytime activity and relative inactivity at night. Moreover, the cessation of work reduces the need for people to follow a structured routine, and aging is often accompanied by mental and/or physical infirmity—all factors that affect circadian rhythms.

(Below) Patrick Ward—Stock, Boston; (right) Hank Morgan—Science Source/Photo Researchers

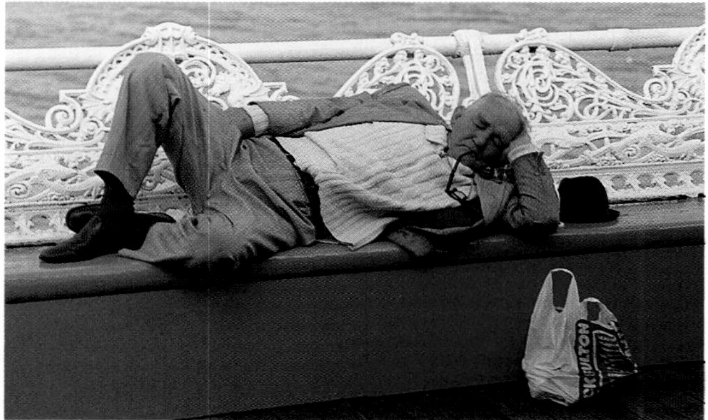

Circadian rhythms become weaker with age, which accounts for the tendency of the elderly to nap during the day.

Out of sync

In certain clinical disorders of adults, including senile dementia and some forms of depression, circadian rhythms and the regular alternation of nocturnal sleep and diurnal activity are disrupted. Abnormal circadian rhythms can be present in younger people as well, again generally manifested as sleep difficulties at night and daytime fatigue. In the form of insomnia called delayed sleep phase syndrome (DSPS), sufferers have no difficulty achieving a refreshing sleep as long as they are allowed to delay sleep until around 5 AM and to rise about 1 PM. Such a schedule is, of course, completely incompatible with the functioning of the world at large.

"Owls" versus "larks." DSPS can be regarded as an extreme form of a much more common condition, one that affects up to 10% of the population and is not a cause for concern—that of being a "night person," or "owl." Such individuals prefer to go to bed late and rise late (sleeping from, say, 1 AM to 8 AM) and to be physically and mentally most active late in the day rather than early. It is believed that owls and, to a greater extent, people with DSPS possess body clocks that run with a later timing than the average for the general population.

By contrast, some healthy individuals characterize themselves as morning types, or "larks." These are people who prefer going to bed early and rising early (sleeping from about 10 PM to 5 AM) and doing important things early in the day. A much more extreme and quite rare form of this preference is advanced sleep phase syndrome, a condition in which an individual desires to go to sleep unusually early, so much so that it results in social strains on the person and his or her family members. In such a case, the body clock runs with an earlier timing than the average for the general population, but, as with DSPS and night and morning types, the body clock is adjusted to a 24-hour cycle.

Problems of the blind. Some individuals, including a large proportion of blind persons, seem not to be able to adjust their body rhythms to a 24-hour cycle; instead, their rhythms continue to run on a longer cycle, as if not subject to adjustment by zeitgebers. For these people sleep loss and fatigue are problems, but they become apparent only periodically. Thus, as the person's body rhythms drift farther out of phase with a normal lifestyle, their sleep problems worsen, becoming most marked when body rhythms and lifestyle are out of phase by 12 hours (with peak body temperature occurring during the night and melatonin secretion starting about 9 AM, for example). A continuing drift of the body clock eventually brings it back into phase, and the individual's nighttime sleep and daytime activity become, once again, temporarily normal.

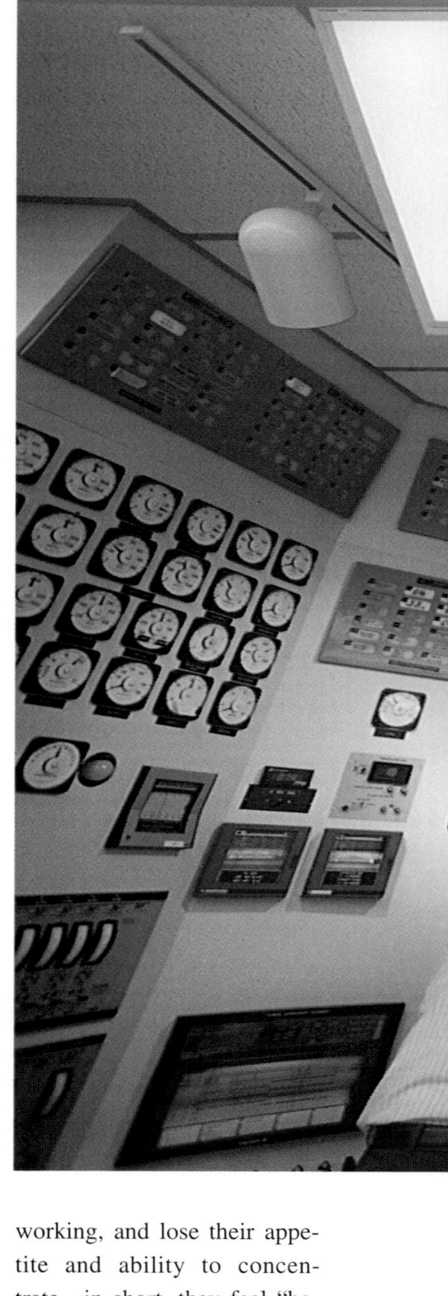

Special cases: jet lag and shift work. Two other examples show the difficulties that arise when body clock and lifestyle do not match—jet lag and the malaise commonly experienced by shift workers. These differ from disorders like DSPS, however, in that they are a *normal* response to an imposed, *abnormal* lifestyle. They arise, in fact, precisely because of the inherent stability of the body clock. Thus, for some days after an international flight and often throughout a rotation on the night shift, individuals have difficulties with sleep, feel tired when they should be working, and lose their appetite and ability to concentrate—in short, they feel "below par."

The increased fatigue in shift work is frequently associated with an increased risk of accidents, particularly in the transport sector but also in industry. Indeed, some of the "mega-accidents" of recent decades, such as the nuclear catastrophes at Three Mile Is-

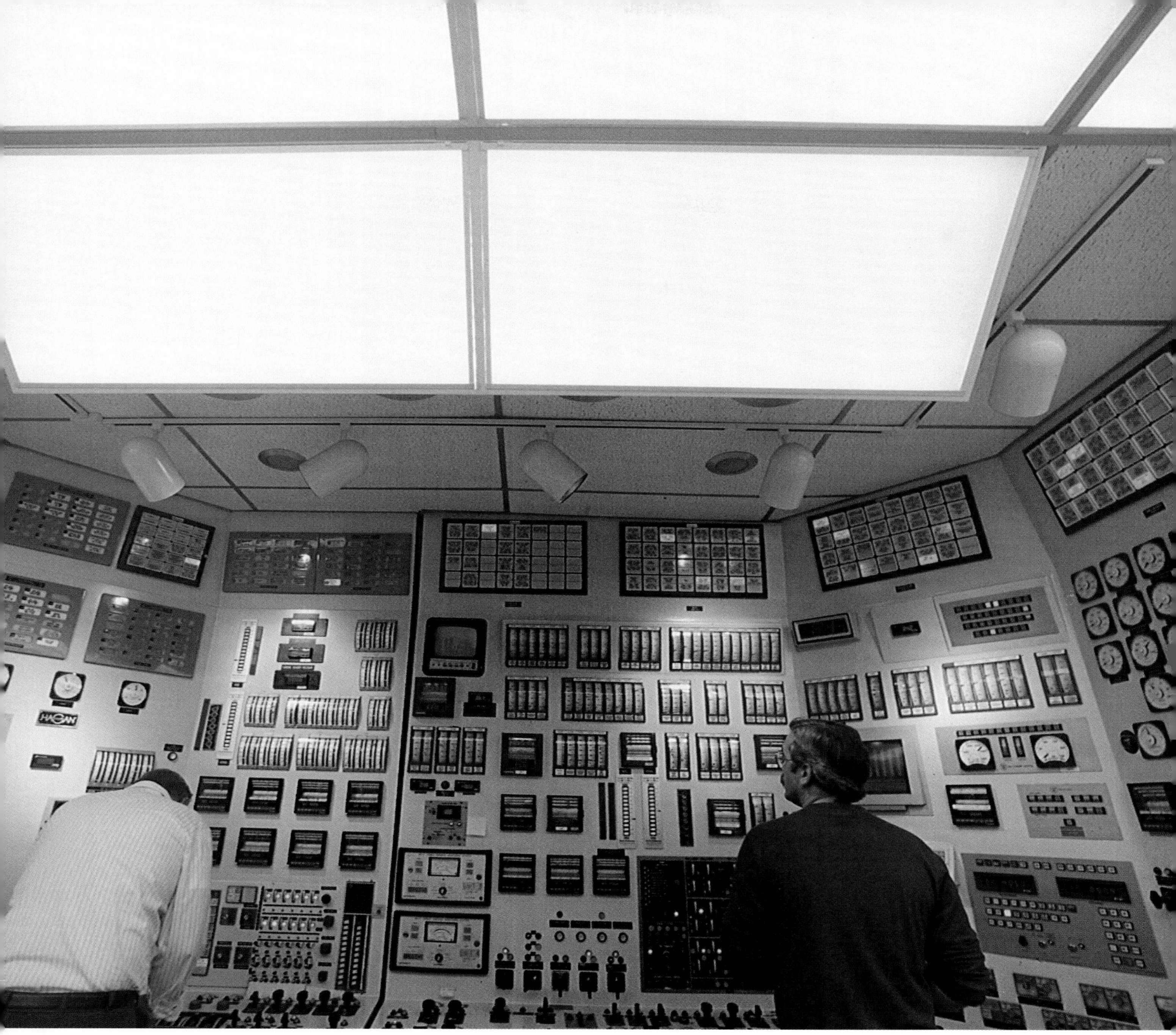

Probability of Errors During Shift Work

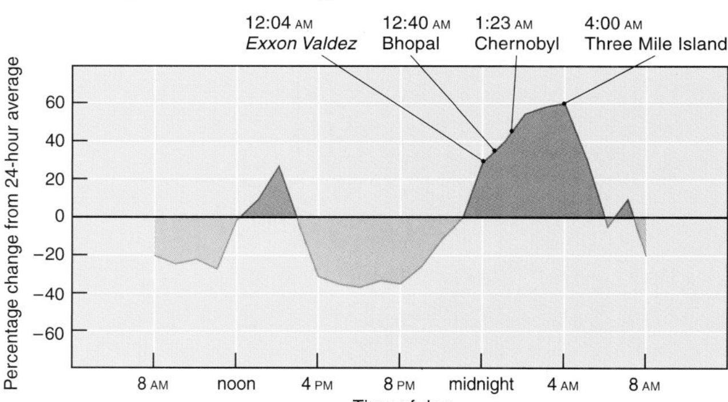

Adapted from information obtained from *Bodyrhythms: Chronobiology and Peak Perfomance,* © 1994 Lynne Lamberg, p. 197, William Morrow and Co., Inc., New York.

(Above) Exposure to bright lights helps adjust the body clocks of workers on the 11 PM to 7 AM shift in a California power plant. The graph at left plots the probability of error by shift workers over a 24-hour day.

land and Chernobyl and the running aground of the *Exxon Valdez,* appear to have been associated with night work and long work hours.

Remedy: enhancing the zeitgebers. Can any of these problems—whether clinically significant or merely inconvenient, whether due to inadequacies of the circadian system or imposed by one's lifestyle—be combated? The answer is that to some extent they can. The remedy involves manipulating the zeitgebers that normally adjust the body clock. The following

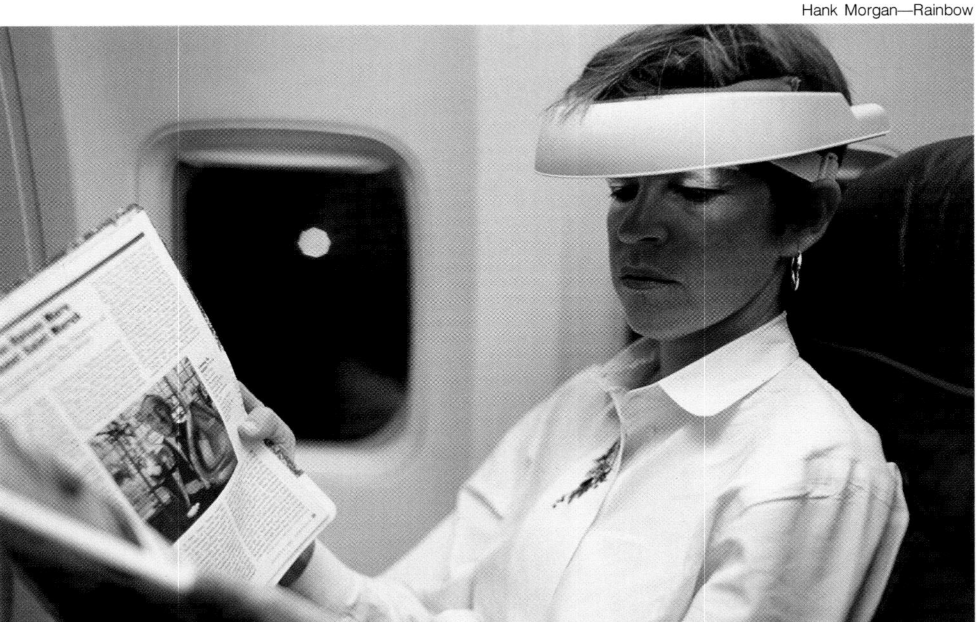

Hank Morgan—Rainbow

A passenger on an international flight uses a light visor to "reset" her body clock and thus mitigate the effects of jet lag, a common problem for those crossing time zones.

are examples of some successful interventions:

- In neonatal intensive care wards, where the environment is kept relatively constant around the clock, newborns who were placed in dimmed light at night and given more of their routine care during the day than at night gained weight more rapidly and made greater progress in neurological development than others treated conventionally.
- In persons with jet lag melatonin capsules, exposure to light at the appropriate time, or both have been shown to adjust the body clock; in shift workers light treatment alone has been effective in treating malaise.
- Healthy blind or aged individuals and patients with depression, senile dementia, or DSPS may be able to achieve a normal night's sleep by methods that include, either singly or in combination, being exposed to bright light each morning, adopting a schedule of organized daytime activities, taking melatonin in the evening, or making an effort to remain in bed all night.

Morning stiffness, afternoon aches

If circadian rhythms are essential to normal functioning, it seems logical to assume that they might affect illnesses. In fact, the consideration of circadian rhythms can be important in both the diagnosis and treatment of disease.

Obviously, the time of day when blood is drawn can affect a diagnosis made on the basis of that blood sample. A given level of substances that show marked circadian variation—*e.g.,* cortisol or growth hormone—may be pathologically high or low when measured in the morning but indicative of good health in the evening.

In some illnesses the frequency of attacks shows marked daily variation. Stroke and heart attack, for example, occur more frequently between 6 AM and noon than during any other six-hour period. The incidence of asthma attacks, on the other hand, peaks in the evening and overnight.

Severity of symptoms also may vary with the time of the day. People with rheumatoid arthritis find that their symptoms are worst on waking in the morning, whereas the joint pain of osteoarthritis is exacerbated toward the end of the day.

These patterns are clearly reflective of normal circadian rhythms in physiology and biochemistry. Thus, it is known that in the morning the following occur: (1) an increase in physical activity and, consequently, increased demand on the heart, (2) an elevation of nervous system activity, which raises blood pressure but also decreases blood supply to the heart, (3) an increase in the aggregability ("stickiness") of the platelets (a type of blood cell), which enhances their capacity to form clots, and (4) a reduction in the activity of the body's natural mechanisms for inhibiting clotting. This combination of factors clearly could increase heart attack and stroke risk.

In the evening, on the other hand, breathing problems may be exacerbated by a combination of factors. Not only is the level of adrenaline—which acts, among other things, to dilate the airways—falling, but so too is the level of the natural anti-inflammatory hormone cortisol. Everyone's airways normally constrict in the evening, but in people with asthma, who have hypersensitive airways, this constriction can lead to labored breathing and even lethal asthmatic attacks.

Cortisol is also implicated in the circadian rhythm of rheumatoid arthritis. The low evening levels of blood cortisol lead, after a delay of some hours, to the increased autoimmune responses in the joints. By contrast, the afternoon and evening pain in osteoarthritis is likely to reflect the pattern of daytime activity and nocturnal rest.

Harnessing circadian rhythms for healing

In addition to seeking ways to reduce the stress of travel and unusual work schedules, researchers have also begun to apply their newly gained understanding of circadian rhythms to the treatment of disease. It is now recognized that treatments for certain conditions can be maximized by being timed to take effect when symptoms are likely to be at their worst. In the past, for example, treatment for high blood pressure often involved taking beta-blocker drugs once a day, typically in the morning. It was reasoned that patients would be unlikely to forget the medication if they took it as part of their regular routine upon rising. This regimen proved to be unsatisfactory, however, as the effects of the drug would start to wear off after about 5 AM, at the very time when they were most needed. More recently, therefore, divided doses of the drug have been recommended, to be taken morning and evening. With this regimen, drug effectiveness is maintained over 24 hours. An alternative approach has been to develop a drug whose effectiveness can span the 24 hours, either because it is released very slowly or because it is not broken down or removed from the body too rapidly. A recent example of this approach is the slow-release formulation of the antihypertensive drug verapamil.

Hormone replacement therapy for conditions such as delayed puberty or stunted growth has also been timed in an attempt to improve effectiveness. A potential problem of conventional hormone replacement regimens is that they produce constant high blood levels of hormone, which can induce receptors in the body to develop resistance to the hormone. Over time, as resistance grows, the efficacy of the therapy decreases. The problem can be overcome by duplicating the normal daily changes in hormone levels; this can be accomplished by administering the therapy once a day, at bedtime, to mimic the normal pattern of high overnight and low daytime levels. This regimen not only is effective in advancing puberty or producing a "growth spurt" but also is more economical than conventional methods as it requires lower hormone doses.

Currently, much interest is focused on applying the lessons of chronobiology to reducing the side effects of cancer chemotherapy while increasing the therapeutic effect. Typically, side effects include severe nausea and damage to the kidneys and bone marrow—problems that often make it necessary to reduce dosage or even to interrupt a scheduled course of treatment. An ideal mode of administering anticancer drugs would minimize toxicity—*i.e.,* damage to the patient's healthy organs and tissues—while having the greatest efficacy—*i.e.,* capacity for killing the cancerous cells.

In fact, the growing interest in the timing of drugs has created an entirely new discipline—chronopharmacology. Early research in this emerging field has demonstrated that identical doses of a drug will be absorbed, metabolized (broken down), and excreted differently according to the time of administration; moreover, efficacy and toxic side effects also can be time-dependent. Recent studies of the underlying mechanisms have determined the following:

- The absorption of a drug in the intestine depends upon the circadian rhythm of blood flow to this organ.
- The rate of drug metabolism depends upon the circadian rhythms in the liver's production of detoxification enzymes.
- The excretion of a drug depends upon circadian changes in kidney function.

In the case of cancer chemotherapy, the efficacy of the treatment depends on finding a time when the body's healthy cells are less sensitive than the cancerous cells to the drugs. Most anticancer drugs work by intervening at a particular stage in the cycle of cell division. Normally, circadian rhythms are present in cell division in healthy tissue, whereas cancerous tissue tends to divide without rhythmicity. The aim, therefore, is to find a time when the healthy cells of the target tissues will be less likely than the cancerous cells to be dividing—and thus less sensitive to the drugs. Moreover, because the toxic effects on kidney function depend upon accumulation of the drug in the kidneys, it is necessary to determine the time of day when urine flow can be maximized, which would thereby reduce drug concentration in the kidneys. Early trials indicate that carefully timed drug delivery may make it possible for higher doses of drug to be given with fewer toxic effects and, more important, a better outcome for the patient.

The future

The great mass of data accumulated in recent years has established the universality of circadian rhythms and their importance in humans as well as in other species. Scientists have demonstrated that circadian rhythms continue in outer space and beyond any known rhythmic influence of the Earth. What is next for this emerging field?

The development of therapies to combat jet lag and the problems of shift workers undoubtedly will continue. The fact that abnormalities of circadian rhythm lead to sleep disorders will be more widely accepted in sleep clinics and in geriatric medicine. Ultimately, detailed genetic, molecular, and electrical studies will further explain the mechanisms living organisms have evolved to deal with that all-pervasive aspect of the Earth's environment—time. MHA

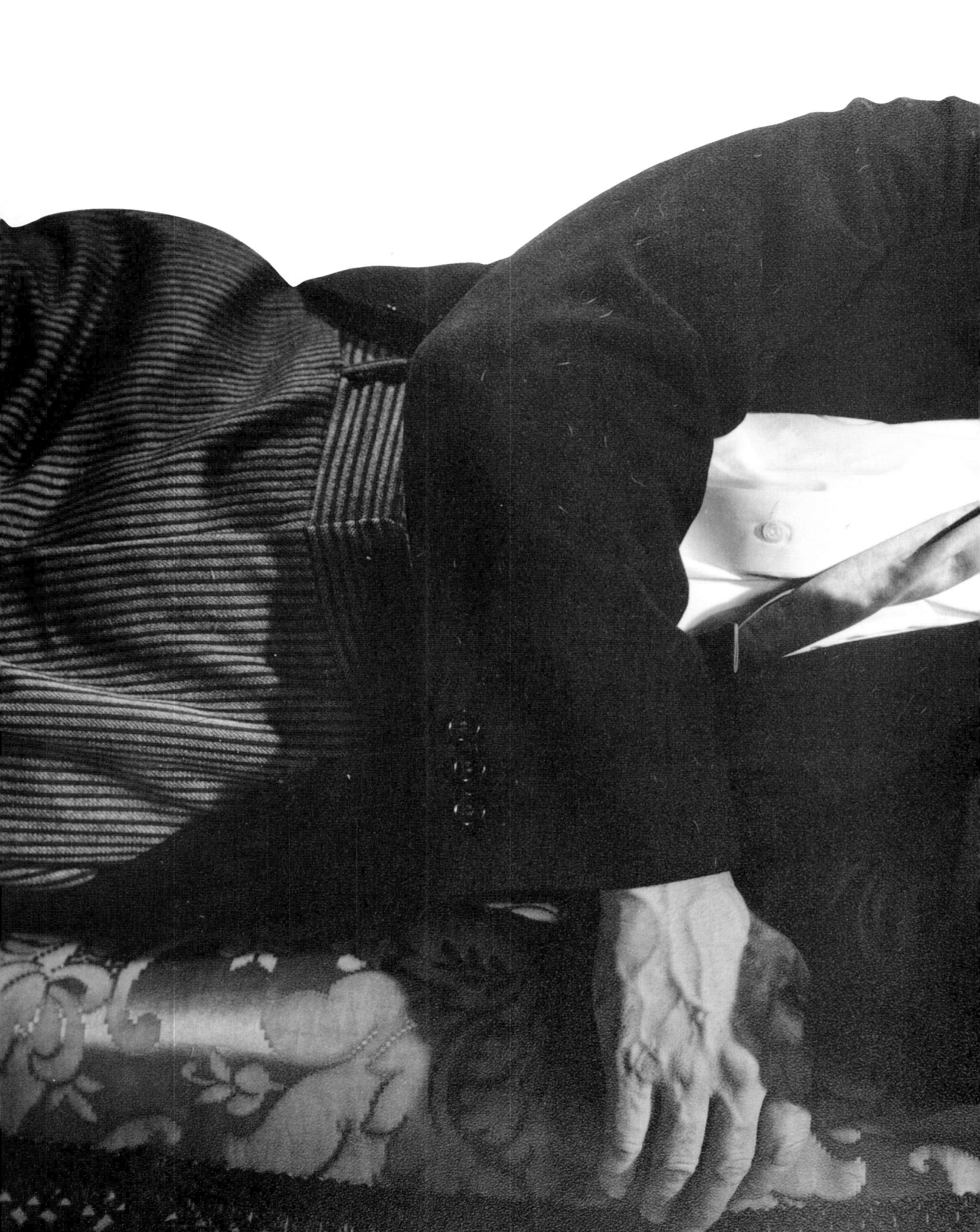

A Good Night's Sleep: Celebrities' Strategies

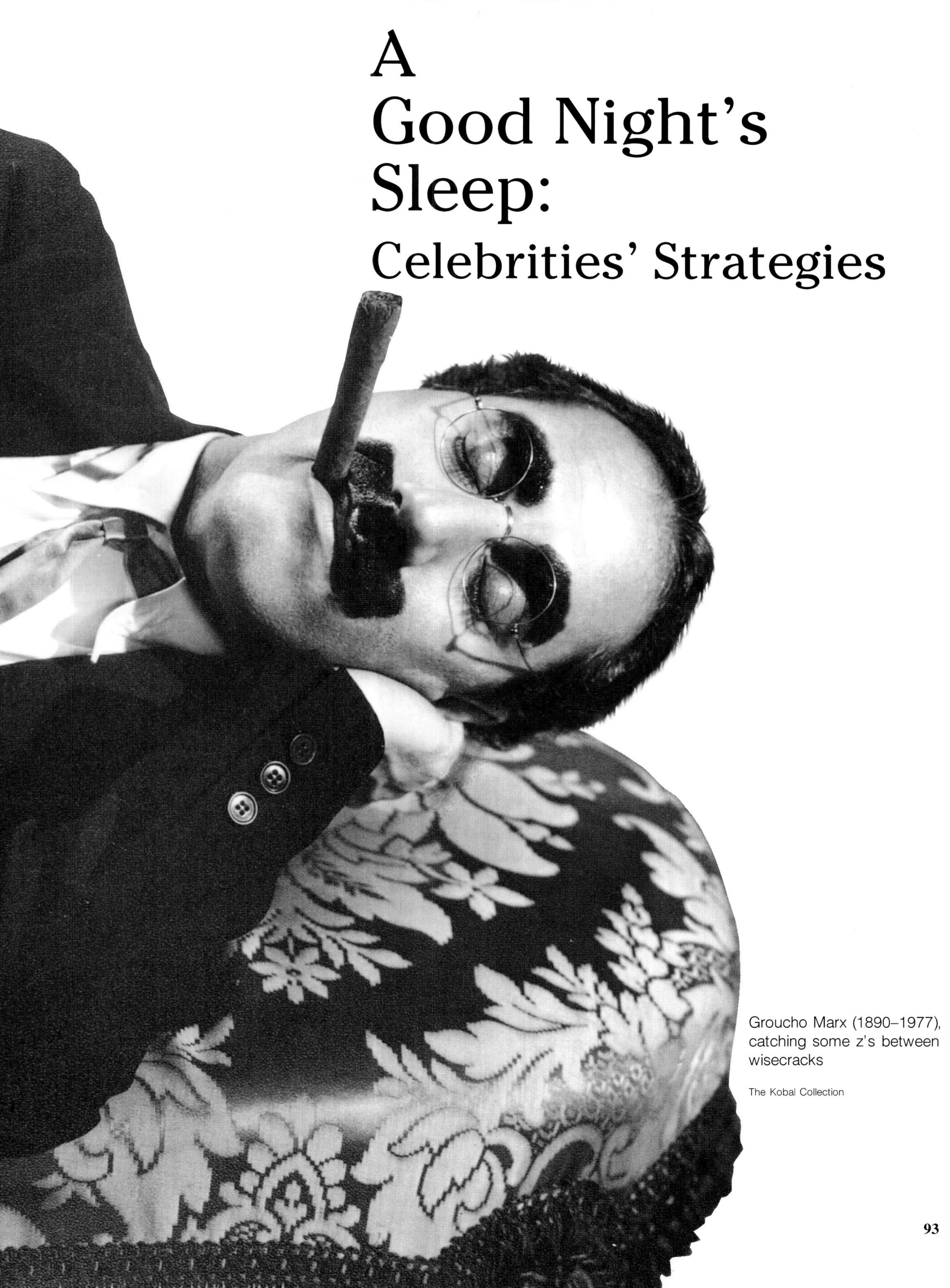

Groucho Marx (1890–1977), catching some z's between wisecracks

The Kobal Collection

As the editors of the *Medical and Health Annual* were planning the present volume and contemplating the mysteries of the body's rhythms (the topic of the preceding article), they began to wonder about the sleep habits of people who have attained "celebrity" status for their accomplishments—whether in medicine, the sciences, the arts, entertainment, athletics, public service, or some other field. Specifically, they were curious about: (1) the amount of sleep highly prolific individuals need to function optimally, (2) whether they supplement their nightly sleep with naps—or would like to, and (3) whether they manage to get the sleep they need. A diverse group of creative people—who keep long working hours and have demanding schedules—responded to their questions.

Brian Smith—Outline

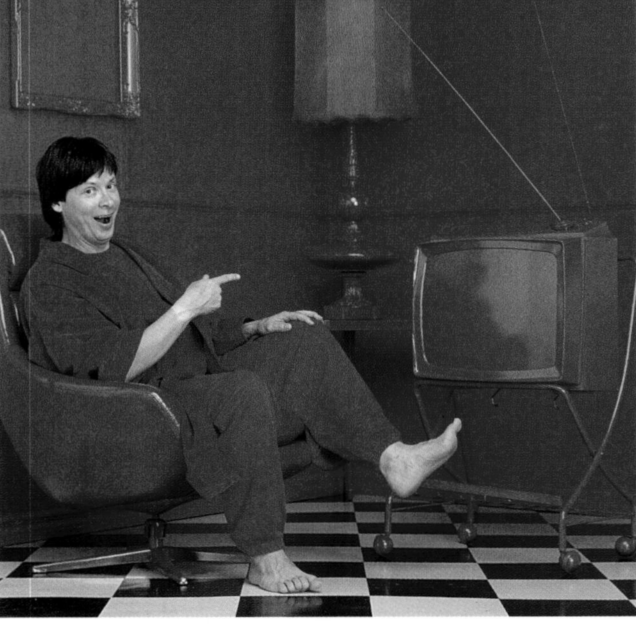

Not-yet-a-Nobelist Dave Barry in his favorite nightclothes

Nobel Prize-winning virologist David Baltimore—pondering a nap?

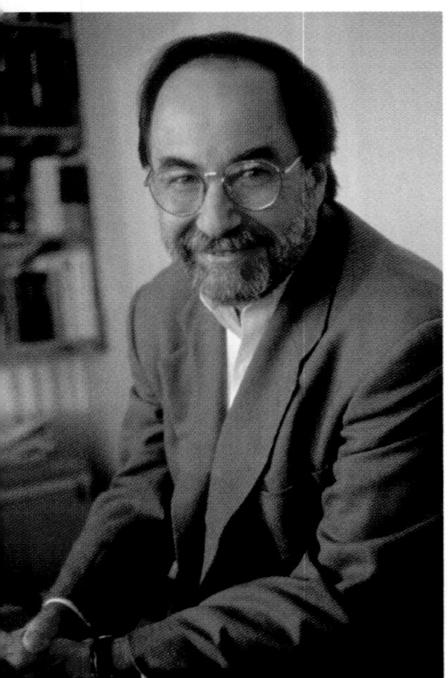

MIT/Associated Press

• • •

In 1975, at the age of 37, **David Baltimore** became one of the youngest recipients of the Nobel Prize for Physiology or Medicine. Today he is an internationally recognized virologist and spokesperson on key scientific issues. His research into cancer-inducing viruses helped make possible the identification of the AIDS virus. Baltimore was director of the Whitehead Institute for Biomedical Research at the Massachusetts Institute of Technology from 1982 to 1990 and in 1990–91 served as president of Rockefeller University, New York City. In 1996 he was named to head a National Institutes of Health committee working to develop a vaccine against AIDS, and in the fall of 1997 he assumed the post of president of the California Institute of Technology.

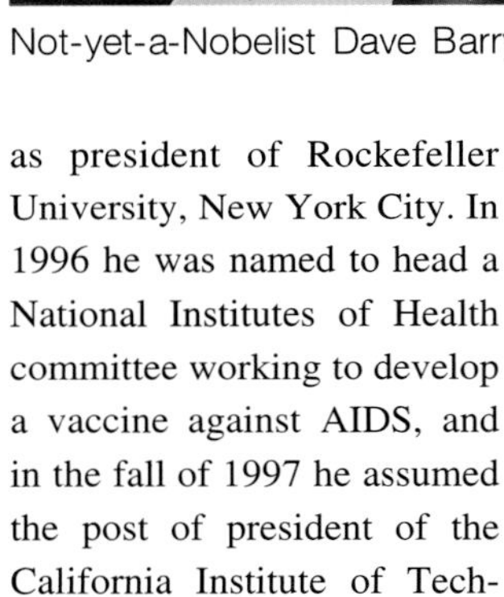

I seem to need seven-plus hours of sleep. It's a shame because I'd love to have those hours for some more productive activity. A nap on a weekend is a special indulgence. As I get older, it is more attractive. Coming awake afterward, though, is so difficult that I must ration my naps and savor the few I can arrange. I get most of the sleep that I need. The rest I make up for in seminars and meetings in Washington.

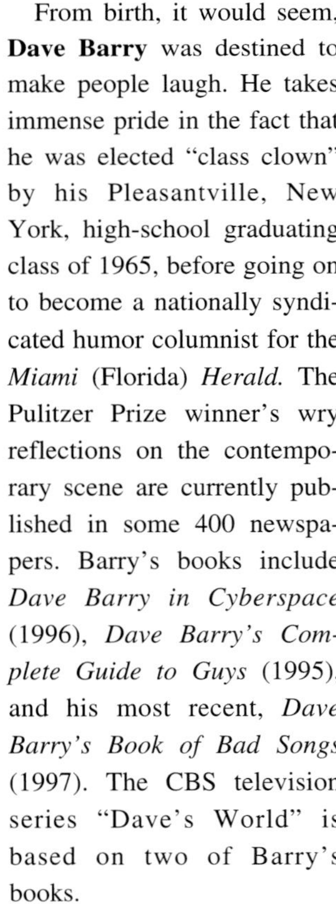

From birth, it would seem, **Dave Barry** was destined to make people laugh. He takes immense pride in the fact that he was elected "class clown" by his Pleasantville, New York, high-school graduating class of 1965, before going on to become a nationally syndicated humor columnist for the *Miami* (Florida) *Herald.* The Pulitzer Prize winner's wry reflections on the contemporary scene are currently published in some 400 newspapers. Barry's books include *Dave Barry in Cyberspace* (1996), *Dave Barry's Complete Guide to Guys* (1995), and his most recent, *Dave Barry's Book of Bad Songs* (1997). The CBS television series "Dave's World" is based on two of Barry's books.

To function optimally, I need roughly 22 hours of sleep a night, supplemented with naps. Unfortunately, I rarely get that much sleep, so I generally am not functioning optimally, which I believe is the reason why I have not yet won the Nobel Prize for Literature.

Country music singer **Clint Black** reached the top of the record charts with his first album, *Killin' Time* (1989). His success as a singer and songwriter has earned him four Grammy award nominations and the 1990 Country Music Association's Male Vocalist of the Year award. In December 1996 he was honored with his own star on Hollywood's Walk of Fame, only the fourth country music artist to receive such recognition.

When I'm on a concert tour, I need at least 8 hours of sleep, sometimes 10 or 11. When I'm not traveling, singing, etc., I can go on 6 easily for a while. Rarely will I nap, although I would like to. If I'm flying, I will always nap a little on the flight. I have managed to be only slightly awakened upon landing and can "go back out" until it's time to disembark. If I am not getting the sleep I need, inevitably, I will sleep for 12 hours and catch up all in one night. When I have things to do that I'm really excited about, I cannot sleep more than about 5 hours. (I'm napping right now.)

(Below) Deborah Feingold—Outline; (bottom) courtesy of Jane Brody

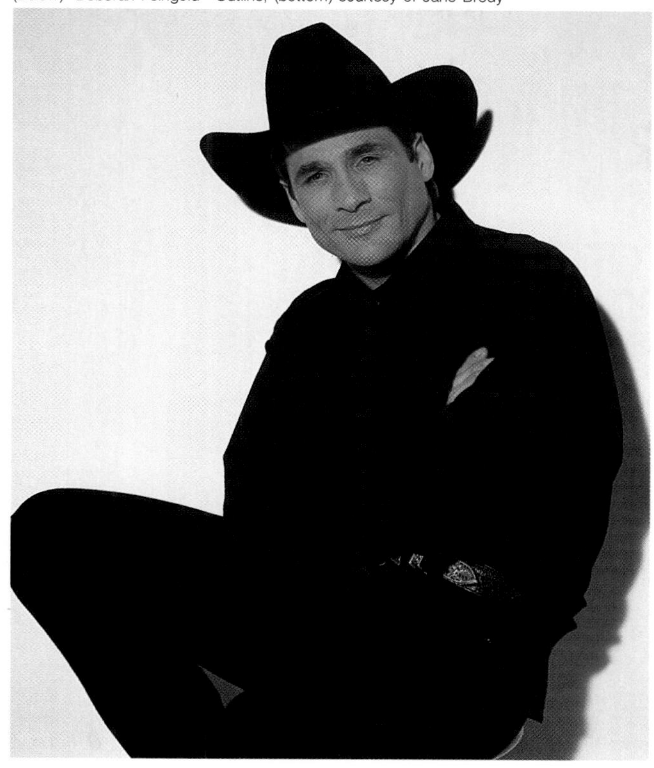

(Above) Clint Black, voluntarily awake; (right) short sleeper Jane E. Brody

Jane E. Brody is a nationally known health columnist for the *New York Times* with a background in medicine and biology. She is the author of nine books, which include *Jane Brody's Nutrition Book* (1981) and her latest, *Jane Brody's Allergy Fighter* (1997). Brody also writes regularly for magazines and lectures frequently on health and nutrition.

I get about five and a half to six hours of sleep a night. I come from a long line of "short sleepers." No matter when I go to sleep, I wake up early in the morning, often well before dawn. If I go to bed really early, I just awaken earlier. I definitely nap—what I call "involuntary naps." If I lie down purposely, I almost never fall asleep. Instead, I doze off while reading in the late morning or early afternoon. I find naps thoroughly restoring and invigorating—as long as they are short, say no more than 20 minutes. I don't always get the sleep I need. Sometimes I have very short nights—three and a half hours when I fly back to New York from the West Coast on the "red eye," four and a half when I stay up very late for a social event. I think I'd be best off retiring at 11 PM instead of 11:30, but I rarely make it.

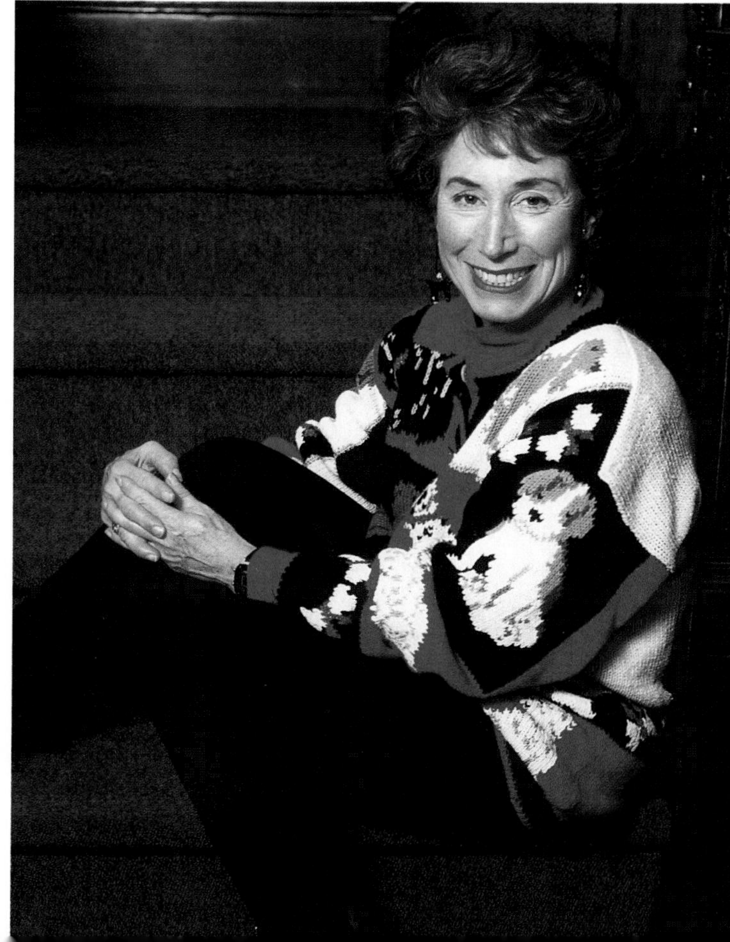

Jimmy Carter, the 39th U.S. president (1977–81), is founder of The Carter Center, Atlanta, Georgia, a nongovernmental, nonprofit organization that promotes peace and human rights, resolves conflicts, fosters democracy and development, and fights hunger, poverty, and disease throughout the world. He is the author of *Keeping Faith: Memoirs of a President* (1982) and of the children's book *The Little Baby Snoogle-Fleejer* (1996; illustrated by his daughter, Amy).

I like to get six hours of sleep a night, which seems to be enough. I rarely supplement my nightly sleep with naps. I think I get the sleep I need.

Former first lady, mother of four, and grandmother of seven, **Rosalynn Carter** is cofounder of The Carter Center and is an advocate for international human rights. She works actively to promote early childhood immunization, nonviolent conflict resolution, and the empowerment of urban communities. By sponsoring the annual Rosalynn Carter Symposium on Mental Health Policy, she hopes to help eliminate the stigma of mental illness and bring attention to the unmet needs of the mentally ill. Every year she and her husband join a crew of over 2,400 volunteers for Habitat for Humanity International, building simple, decent, and affordable housing for the disadvantaged. The Carters chronicled their home-building experiences in *Everything to Gain: Making the Most of the Rest of Your Life* (1987). Rosalynn Carter's most recent book, *Helping Yourself Help Others: A Book for Caregivers,* with coauthor Susan K. Golant, was published in 1994.

I need eight hours of sleep a night to function optimally. Although I would like to supplement my nightly sleep with naps, I don't have a chance very often. I don't think I get the sleep I need.

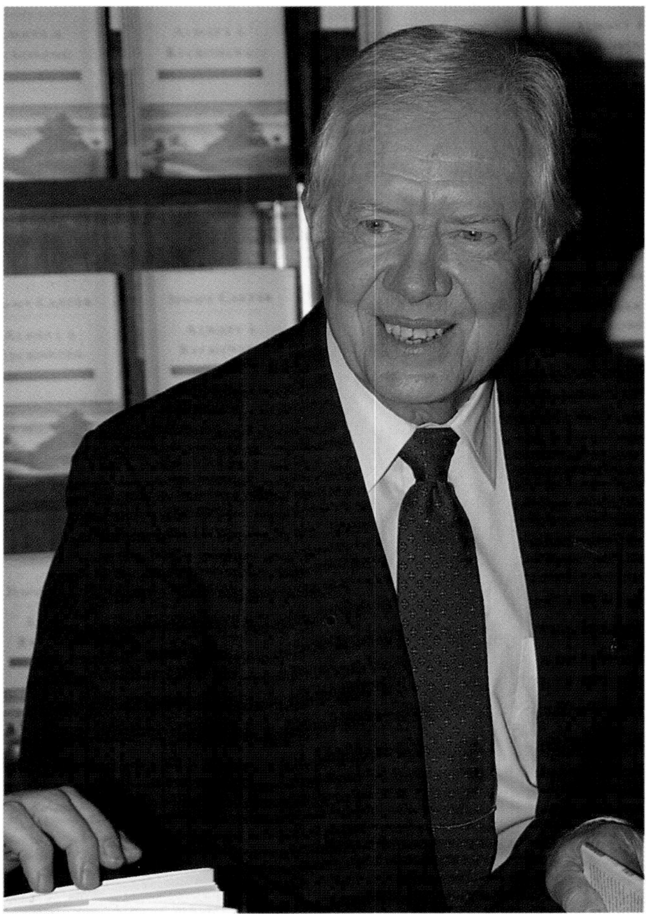

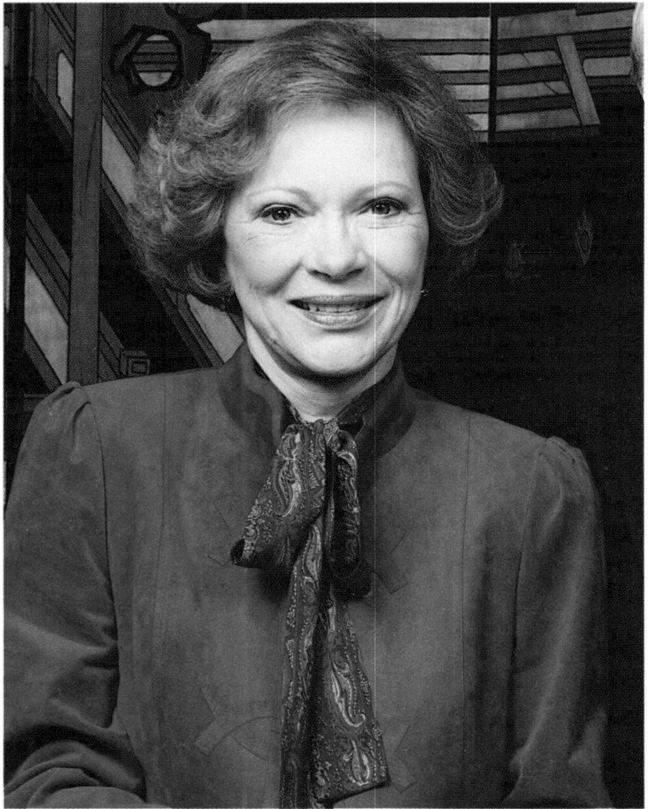

(Top) Porter Gifford—Gamma Liaison; (above) courtesy of The Carter Center

(Left, top and bottom) Jimmy and Rosalynn Carter, who formerly slept in the White House

Italian-born **Mihaly Csikszentmihalyi,** professor of psychology at the University of Chicago, has spent the last 25 years studying creativity and states of "optimal experience." He has written extensively on these subjects, including the national bestseller *Flow: The Psychology of Optimal Experience* (1990), *Creativity: Flow and the Psychology of Discovery and Invention* (1996), and his most recent book, *Finding Flow: The Psychology of Engagement with Everyday Life,* published in 1997. Csikszentmihalyi has written short stories for *The New Yorker;* he also lectures internationally and makes appearances on overseas broadcasting networks, including the BBC and RAI (Italy).

It is hard to know how much sleep I need, but I seem to do best with at least eight hours (although I would

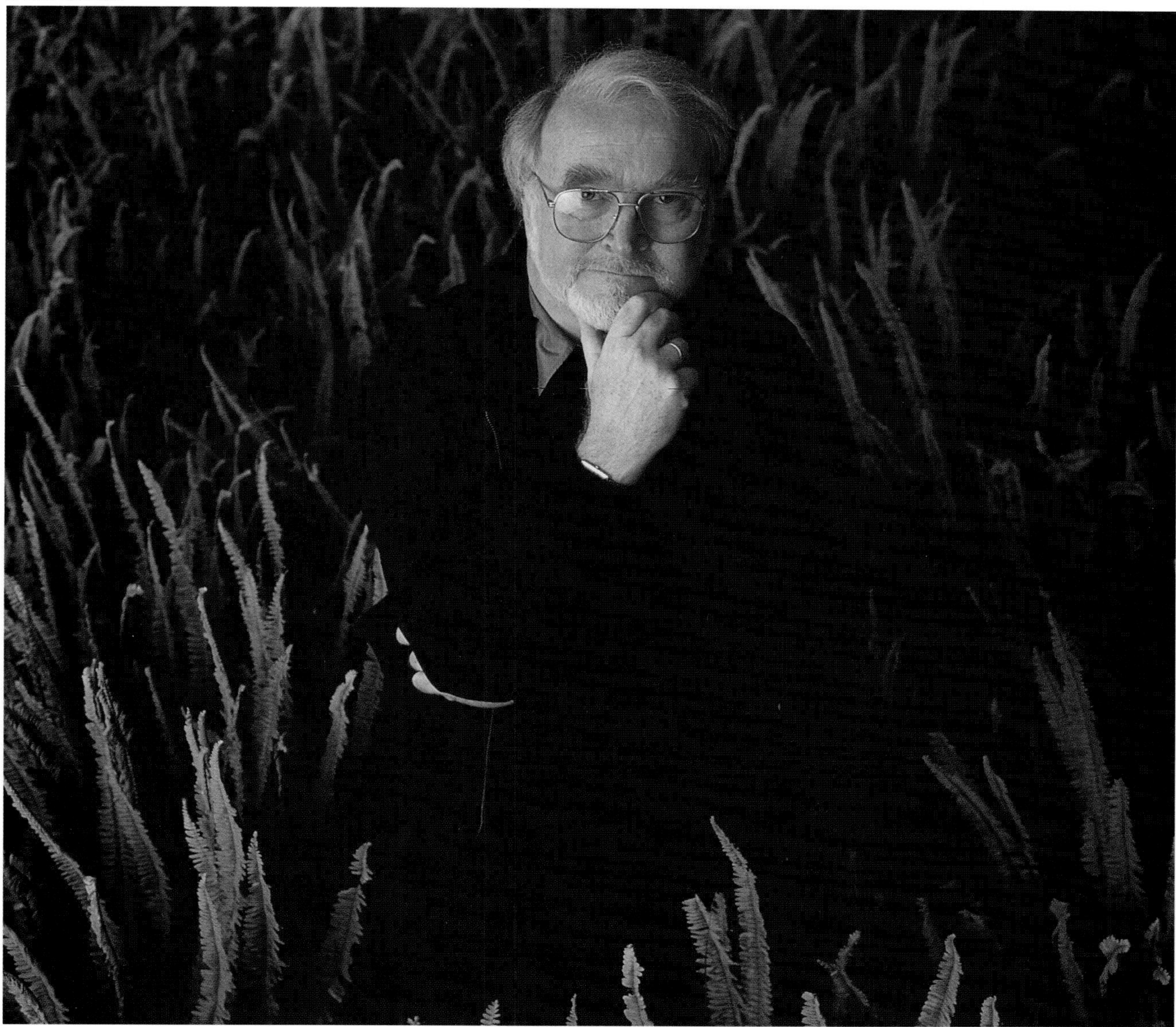

Mihaly Csikszentmihalyi, an eight-hour man

gladly sleep more, but if I try I get woozy). Occasionally, a nap between 2 and 3 PM *feels just right. I honestly would like to have a chance to sleep more, but if I do it's not that satisfying.*

In my work with exceptionally creative individuals, I have found that they tend to sleep quite a lot and often use sleep to resolve problems that were intractable when they were awake.

Michael E. DeBakey is an internationally recognized surgeon, teacher, and innovator who is currently chancellor emeritus and distinguished service professor of surgery at Baylor College of Medicine and director of the DeBakey Heart Center, Houston, Texas. A pioneer in lifesaving surgery, DeBakey in 1964 was the first to perform a successful coronary artery bypass operation. For half a century he has served as adviser to almost every U.S. president and to many heads of state throughout the world. In his role as international medical statesman, he was chief consultant to Renat S. Akchurin, who performed coronary artery bypass surgery on Russian Pres. Boris N. Yeltsin in the fall of 1996. DeBakey is the coauthor of *The Living Heart* (1977), *The Living Heart Diet* (1984), *The Living Heart Brand Name Shopper's Guide* (1992), *The Living Heart Guide to Eating Out* (1993), and *The New Living Heart Diet* (1996).

Sleep is essential for human health, but the amount of time required for sleeping varies considerably from one person to another. I am fortunate in being able to function adequately on about five hours or less daily. I have never found it necessary to take a sleeping pill. Nor have I ever had the need or the urge to nap during the day. I have found that reading classical literature, including poetry, for a short time before retiring is mentally relaxing and pleasantly induces sleep. A day of adequate physical and interesting

Dima Sokolov—Reuters

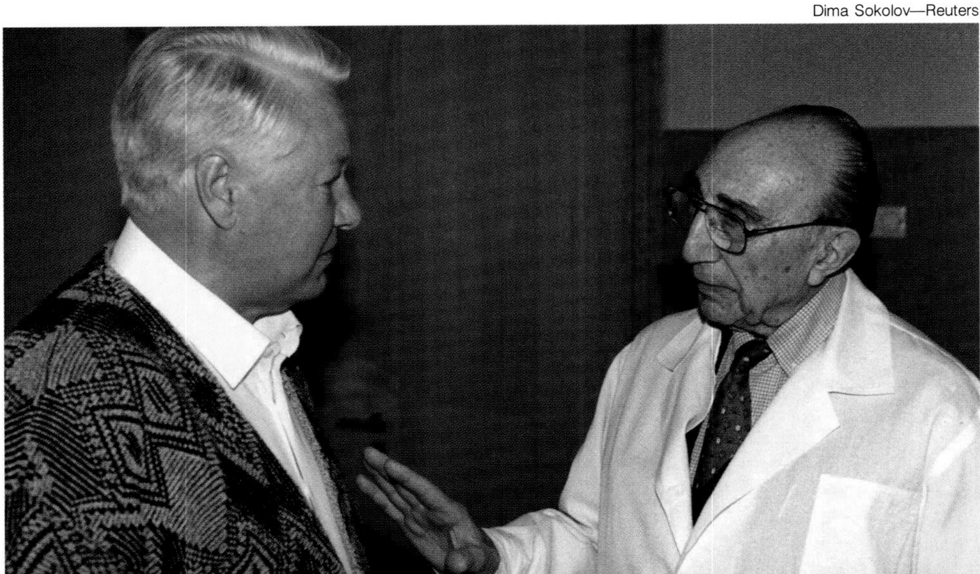

Apparently not suffering from jet lag, heart surgeon Michael E. DeBakey (right) visits Russian Pres. Boris Yeltsin in Moscow's Central Clinical Hospital.

mental activity, a positive attitude, a wholesome diet, and avoidance of late-evening meals and stimulants will help ensure a good night's rest.

Unable to study dentistry because of limited means, **John DeJoria** sold encyclopedias, copy machines, and insurance, then landed a top sales position at Time, Inc. He found his true niche, however, in 1980 when he joined forces with his friend the hairstylist Paul Mitchell to establish a professional hair care products company. Today DeJoria is chairman of the board of John Paul Mitchell Professional Systems, manufacturer of Paul Mitchell Professional Salon Products. A concerned philanthropist and committed environmentalist, he has served as special emissary to the UN Environmental Programme and is adviser to Global Green, the American division of Environmental Green Cross. He has contributed to and worked for the AIDS Relief Fund for Beauty Professionals, Rescue Missions for the homeless, the Big Mountain Weaving Projects, and the Rainforest Foundation, among others. In 1995 DeJoria received the Spirit of Life award from the City of Hope National Medical Center, Duarte, California, where, thanks to his efforts, the $180,000 John Paul Mitchell Research Fellowship in AIDS was established.

A busy person cannot afford to be too busy to get sufficient sleep. The key is to make sure that your waking hours are endowed with maximum energy and acuity. I find I require seven to eight hours of sleep every night to be in tip-top shape. I sleep during the day, but it expands rather than diminishes my working time. I've trained myself to take a five-minute "power nap." The results are amazing! Other than that, I breathe deeply and drink a lot of water when I feel sleepiness coming on. I find I get the sleep I require about 70% of the time. So 3 days out of 10, I do an inordinate amount of deep breathing and I ingest a substantial amount of water, both of which are conducive to health.

Sir Richard Doll, the world's leading cancer epidemiologist, is best known for his discovery in 1950 that smoking causes lung cancer. After his early research established this connection, he undertook further studies on the health effects of smoking, which linked the habit to other serious illnesses, including heart attacks. Doll was the

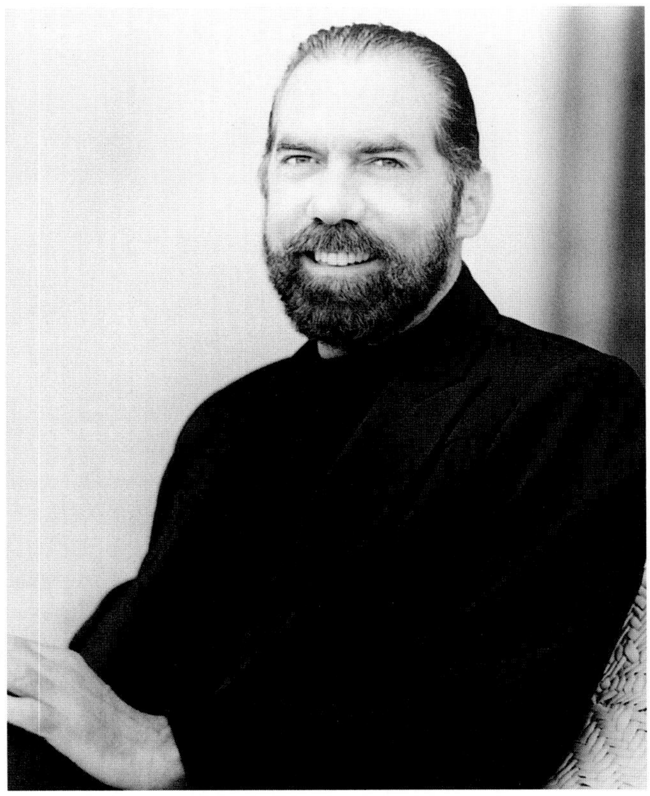

(Right) John DeJoria; (opposite page) Sir Richard Doll

(Above) Courtesy of John Paul Mitchell Systems; (opposite page) © Nick Sinclair

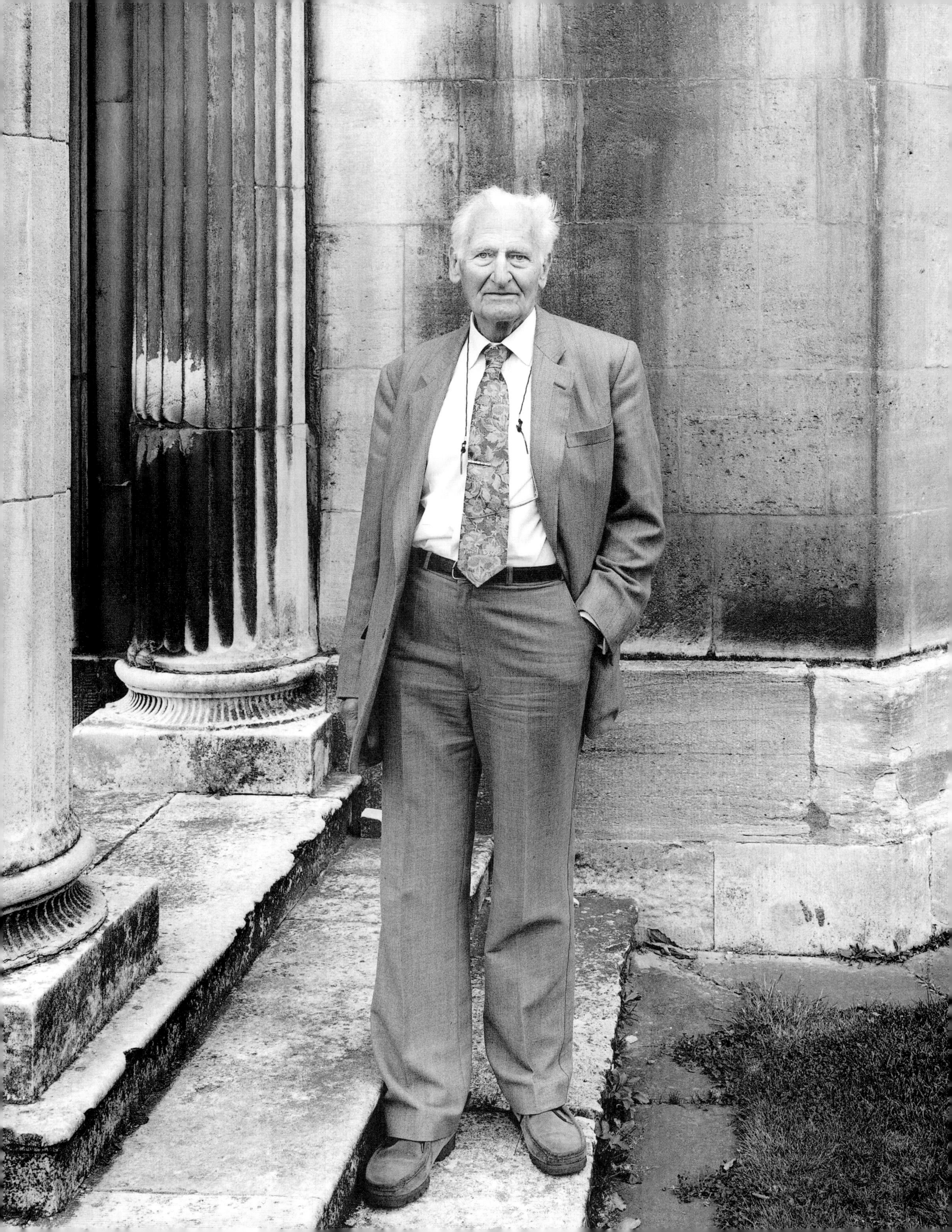

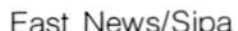
East News/Sipa

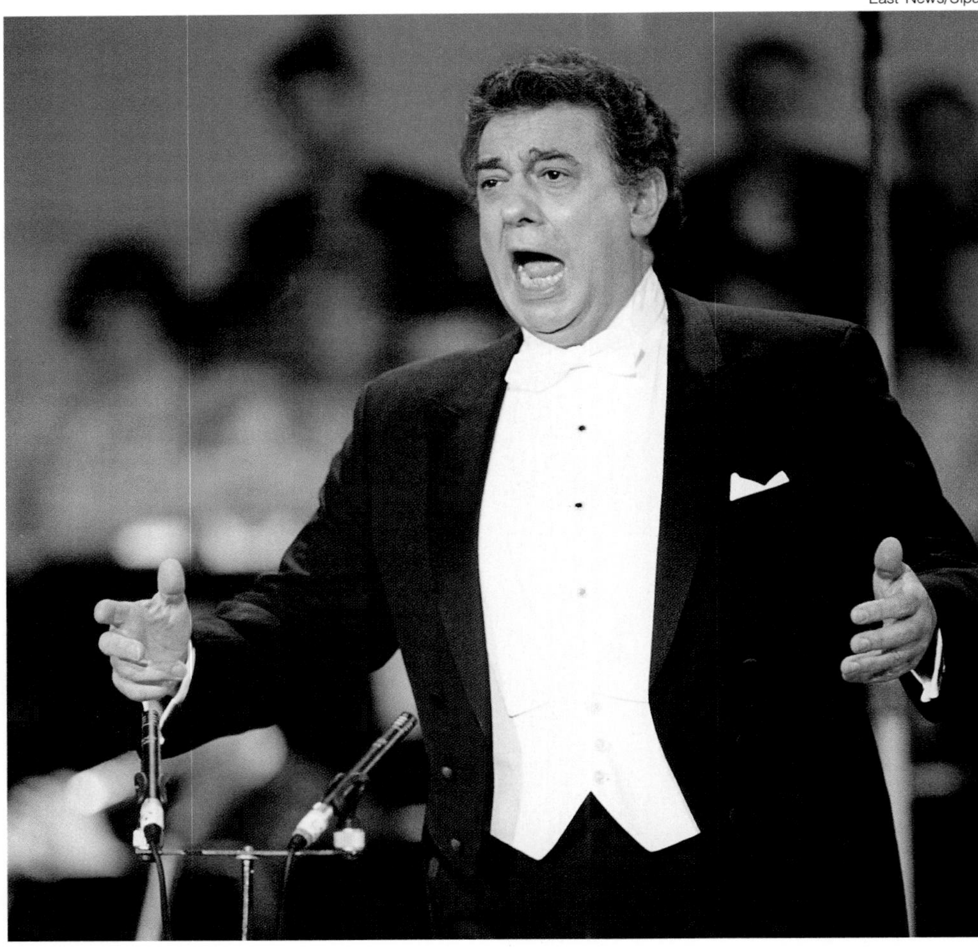

Plácido Domingo, not yawning

first to demonstrate that asbestos causes lung cancer, that exposure to radiation increases the risk of leukemia, and that oral contraceptives slightly increase a woman's risk of blood clots. Though officially retired, he is an honorary member of the Imperial Cancer Research Fund's Cancer Studies Unit in Oxford, England, where he is investigating the causes of childhood cancers, the health effects of electromagnetic fields, and the links between diet and heart disease. He was knighted in 1971 and made a Companion of Honour in 1996. Among the many other honors Sir Richard has received are the United Nations Award for Cancer Research and honorary degrees from 12 universities.

Shortly after I qualified in medicine, I did an experiment to see how much sleep I needed, going to bed a quarter of an hour later every two or three days and always getting up at the same time. I got down to five and a half hours without trouble, but with less than that I found I had no reserve and if, for some reason, I was kept up late or had to get up in the night to see a patient, I felt exhausted the next day. Now I aim for six and a half hours, turning the light out at 1 AM and getting up with the alarm at 7:30 AM. An unbroken night's sleep is a rare luxury, and if I have difficulty in getting to sleep after waking at, say, 4 AM, I take five milligrams diazepam, as I do on the rare occasions when I don't get to sleep quickly upon turning out the light. I don't need naps in the daytime but must admit that I tend to go to sleep in lectures, especially if they are just after lunch and, almost invariably, if I have had a glass of wine with lunch. When I say lectures, I mean, of course, lectures given by other people; I very seldom go to sleep when lecturing myself. On the whole, I think I get about as much sleep as I need. I certainly wouldn't want more if it meant going to bed earlier or missing the half hour's read of a novel before turning out the light.

Spanish-born **Plácido Domingo** has appeared in 109 different operatic roles—more than any other tenor—and regularly performs in the world's leading opera houses. The eight-time Grammy award winner is featured on over 100 recordings, has made scores of videos, and has appeared in three internationally acclaimed films. Domingo is a founder of the Los Angeles Music Center Opera and currently presides as its music adviser and principal guest conductor, as well as being the artistic director of the Washington (D.C.) Opera. He is also the entrepreneur behind the biggest international vocal competition, Operalia, which in 1997 enjoyed its fourth season, and in November 1996 he opened a Spanish restaurant, Domingo, in New York City. In March 1997 he was reunited with his fellow legendary tenors, José Carreras and Luciano Pavarotti, in Melbourne, Australia, for the fifth in a series of "megaconcerts" bringing opera to the "masses."

I need eight hours of sleep to function optimally. I will nap in the afternoon on a performance day. Most of the time I do manage to get the sleep I need.

NIAID, National Institutes of Health

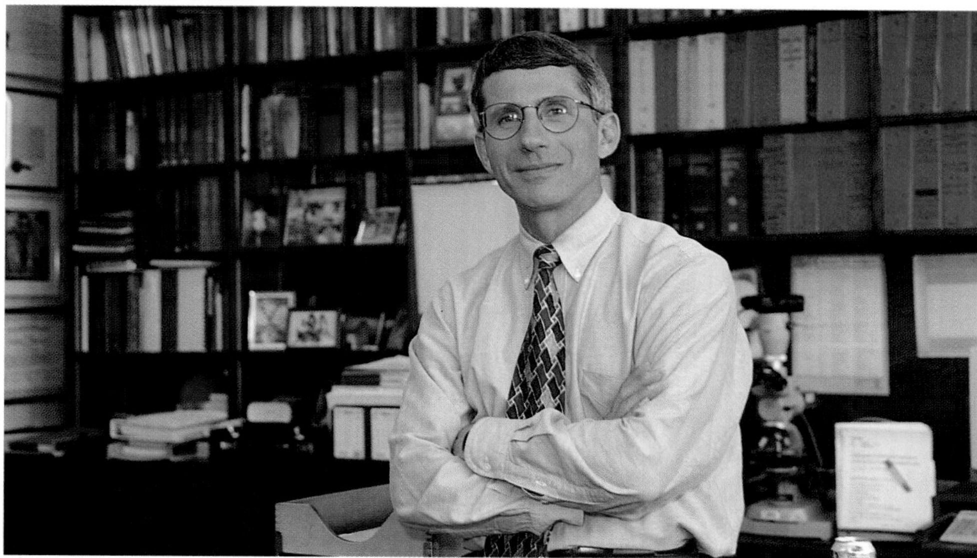

Anthony S. Fauci, up at 5:15

Anthony S. Fauci is a pioneer in the study of the human immune system. In 1980 he became chief of the laboratory of immunoregulation at the National Institute of Allergy and Infectious Diseases, and he was appointed director of the institute in 1984. His work led to the development of a multitude of effective treatments for once-fatal diseases and provided insight into how HIV does its damage to the immune system. Fauci continues to study the repercussions of HIV infection on the body's defense mechanisms.

When I started my medical residency 31 years ago, I quickly learned that sleep is a rare commodity for a young physician. For a house officer in a teaching hospital, late nights and predawn risings come with the territory, and learning to function optimally on minimal sleep is an important lesson in one's training. More than three decades later, I find that my sleeping patterns have changed very little—indeed old habits die hard. As a physician, scientist, research administrator, husband, and father of three young daughters, I find that my days are extraordinarily full, and I am up each morning at 5:15 AM. *Six days a week, I am in the office by 6:45; Sundays, my wife and I "sleep in," which generally means that we are awakened at 7 by one of our daughters. I try to get to bed by midnight unless a good movie or a late basketball game happens to keep me up. I've never been able to nap during the day—it takes too long to clear the cobwebs. Rather, a cup of coffee in the morning and a lunchtime run of four to six miles help to sustain my energy level. When I retire I'll no doubt get the seven hours of nightly sleep my body probably needs, but for now, like many busy people, five and a half hours will have to do.*

Al Franken, writer and performer on NBC's "Saturday Night Live" since 1975, is best known for the creation of the character Stuart Smalley, host of the tongue-in-cheek self-help program "Daily Affirmation." Franken is the author of *I'm Good Enough, I'm Smart Enough, and Doggone It, People Like Me* (1992)—Stuart's words of wisdom—and was the star of the 1995 movie *Stuart Saves His Family.* His most recent book, *Rush Limbaugh is a Big Fat Idiot and Other Observations* (1996), hit the top of the *New York Times* best-seller list.

I can get by on four to five hours of sleep if I'm involved in something really exciting. I can do this for about 10 days, and then I crash. As I get older, I find it gets harder and harder to recover from sleep deprivation. So I've learned to pace myself depending on the nature and duration of the project I'm working on. If I'm working on something over a long period of time—say, a book or screenplay—I like to establish a routine and get about seven to eight hours a night.

Lately, I've been traveling a lot, and I am now able to sleep on airplanes, which is a very efficient use of time. Sometimes I'm the only passenger on the plane who's disappointed when it's announced that we're landing. I'd rather we circle for an hour or two so I can sleep.

Sue Grafton is the author of 18 novels, including the best-selling "alphabet mysteries," which debuted in 1982 with *"A" Is for Alibi.* Her latest installment, *"M" Is for Malice,* was published in 1996, and at her current rate of productivity, she will have completed the internationally popular series by the year

Al Franken, who likes to sleep in the clouds

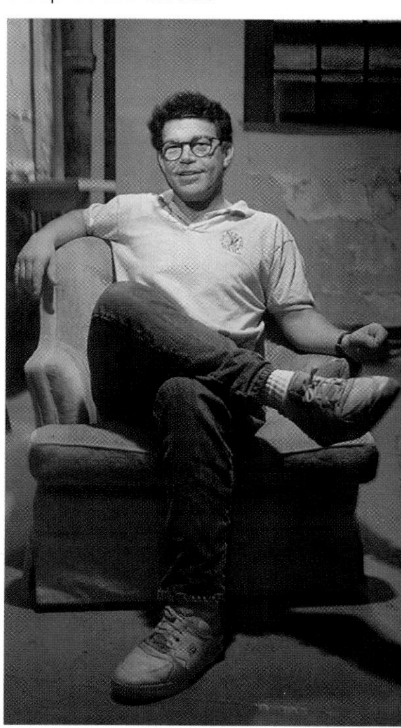

Andrew Brusso—Outline

2015. The crime-solving capers of Grafton's protagonist, private investigator Kinsey Millhone, have been published in 22 languages. In addition to book writing, Grafton spent 15 years as a screenwriter in Hollywood, where she adapted two Agatha Christie novels with her husband, Stephen Humphrey.

Since I rise five mornings a week at 5:38 AM *for my three-mile walk, I find myself generally abed not much later than 9* PM *(sometimes earlier), as I retire there to read and often fall asleep, drooling on myself, my book open on my chest. I used to feel sheepish about this, but I read an article in the Jan. 5, 1997, issue of the* New York Times Magazine *about the hazards of sleep deprivation, and now I feel quite virtuous. I'm happiest with a full eight hours of rest. I used to be a quite talented napper when my children were young. Afternoon naps for preschoolers should be required by law, and I was always ready to set a good example. These days, however, I seem to have lost the knack for napping unless I'm suffering from flu or an old-fashioned head cold.*

One of the reasons I've learned to value sleep is that so much of my creative work is done when my Left Brain is down and Right Brain is playing quietly all by herself in my head. When I'm hard at work on a book, Right Brain presents me with an idea almost nightly, like a rose on my pillow waiting for me when I open my eyes.

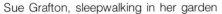

Sue Grafton, sleepwalking in her garden

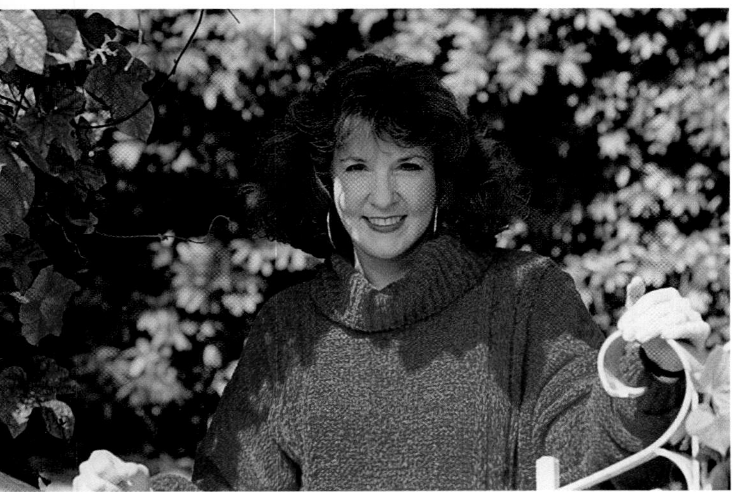

Steven Humphrey

Cardiologist and health policy expert **Bernadine Healy** is dean of the College of Medicine at Ohio State University, where she is also professor of medicine. From 1991 to 1994 she was director of the National Institutes of Health, Bethesda, Maryland, where she established the Shannon Awards, grants designed to foster creative, innovative biomedical research, and launched the Women's Health Initiative, a $625 million program to study the causes, prevention, and cures of diseases that affect women. As president of the American Heart Association (1988–89), she inaugurated a women-and-minorities leadership task force and a program on women and heart disease. She is editor in chief of the *Journal of Women's Health* and author of *A New Prescription for Women's Health* (1996).

Terry Ashe—Gamma Liaison

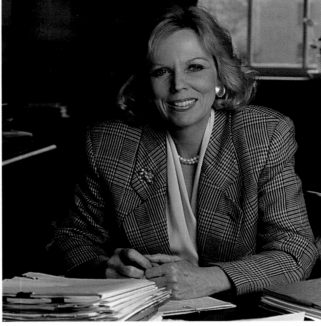

Dean Bernadine Healy, looking forward to the weekend

I generally get six to seven hours of sleep a night and try to take a nap on weekends if I can. Most of the time, I think I get the sleep I need.

The world's foremost advocate of yoga, **B.K.S. Iyengar** has dedicated his life to the study and practice of this ancient art, philosophy, science, and therapy. He began teaching in 1936 and over the years developed the school of yoga that bears his name. He heads the Shrimati Ramamani Iyengar Memorial Yoga Institute in Pune, India; through the hundreds of Iyengar institutes all over the world, he continues to inspire and educate several million students. His classic *Light on Yoga* (1966) has become the "bible" for yoga practitioners the world over. As his student violinist Yehudi Menuhin wrote in the introduction: "[Yoga] is a technique ideally suited to prevent physical and mental illness and to protect the body generally....This book will serve to spread the basic art and will ensure that it is practiced at the highest level." Iyengar has modified many of the basic yoga postures for the benefit of people with physical impairments and is recognized by medical professionals around the world for his expertise in treating complex medical problems.

Sleep is a state of deep rest where activities of the body and mind are abated and thoughts cease. According to Yoga and Ayurveda (ancient Indian medicine), it is a state where consciousness remains dormant, whereas waking and dreaming are active states of consciousness. Sleep is a rejuvenating experience that charges the neurons and electrons of the brain. It is a state of awareness without self-consciousness.

*Sleep has its qualities: light and joyous (*sattvic *in Sanskrit), disturbed and unpleasant (*rajasic*), and dull and confused (*tamasic*), which are known only after one wakes up.*

I get three hours of sound sleep, which is sufficient for me to function optimally. When deprived of this much sleep, I do Niralamba Sarvangasana *(the most difficult of the "shoulder-stand" poses) and* Halasana *(the "plough"), which make up for the sleep deficit, but I do not take naps.*

B.K.S. Iyengar, who needs a mere three hours of sleep a night, in *Kandasana,* a pose that most people would *not* find restful

With six Olympic medals, three of them gold, and five individual records in the heptathlon, long jump, and 50- and 60-meter hurdles, **Jacqueline ("Jackie") Joyner-Kersee** has been called the "world's greatest female athlete." Despite her glory on the track, she is proudest of her off-the-track endeavors. A lifelong asthma sufferer, Joyner-Kersee is a spokesperson for the Asthma Control Program, a patient-education campaign sponsored by the pharmaceutical company Glaxo Wellcome Inc. She established the JJK Youth Center Foundation in her hometown of East St. Louis, Illinois, and is an active participant in numerous other urban leadership programs. She has frequent speaking engagements and often tells her audiences: "The only person who can stop you from reaching your goals is you!"

I get about six and a half hours of sleep a night and take naps occasionally, perhaps once a week. I think I get the sleep I need.

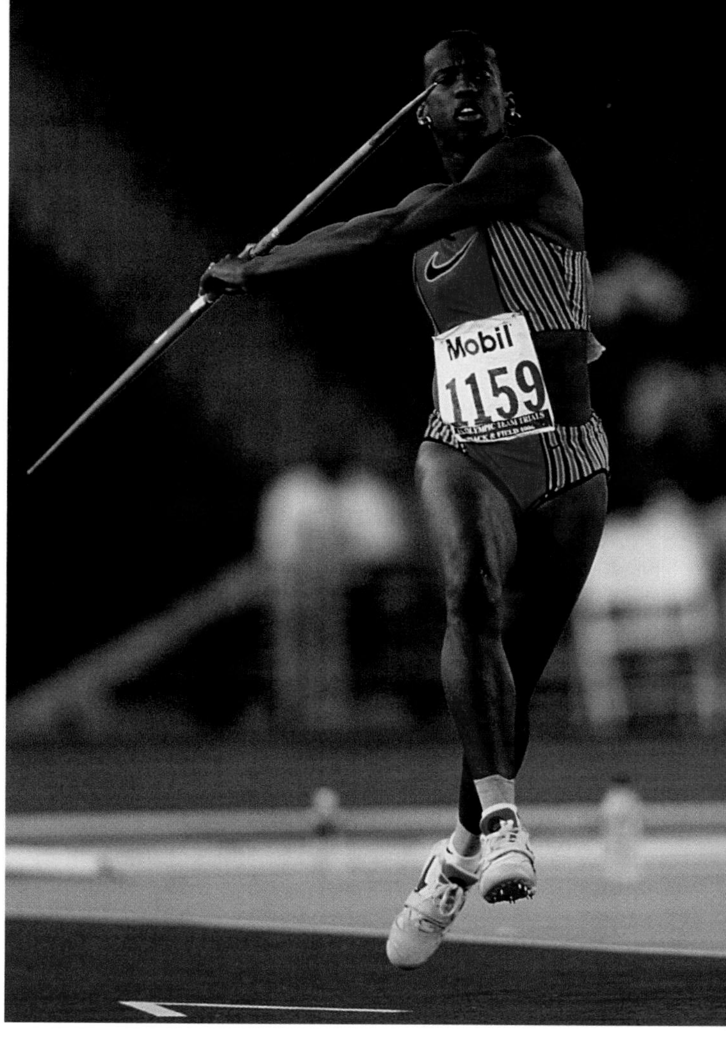

Tireless athlete and educator Jackie Joyner-Kersee

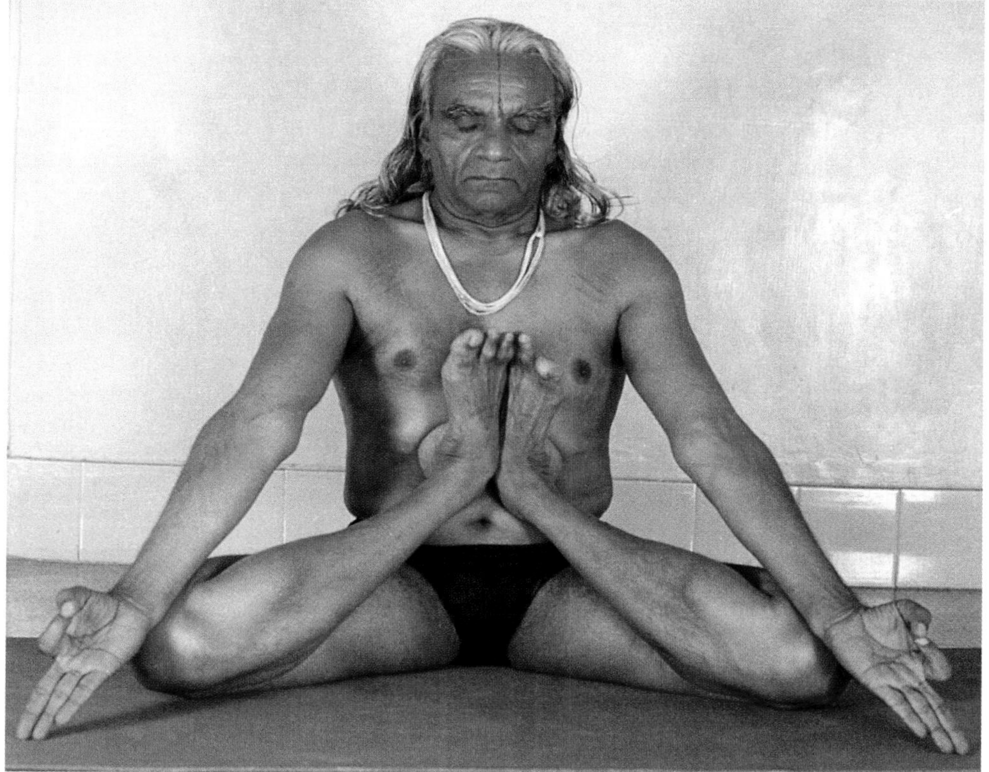

(Top) Steven E. Sutton—Duomo; (above) photograph courtesy of The Yoga Circle and by permission of B.K.S. Iyengar

Dirck Halstead—Gamma Liaison

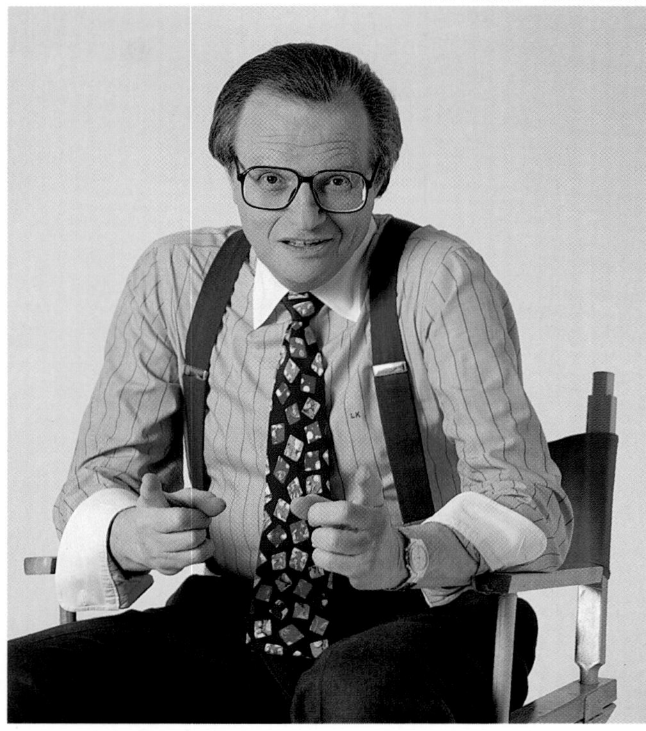

Larry King, live and awake

As host of "Larry King Live," the only live international phone-in TV talk show and one of CNN's consistently highest-rated programs, **Larry King** has conducted over 30,000 interviews with individuals as disparate as Marlon Brando, Barbara Bush, and Yasir Arafat. His nightly show has become a forum for aspiring political candidates and a venue for political debates. King also serves as the host of special programs on the TNT network, writes a weekly column for *USA Today,* and chairs the Larry King Cardiac Foundation, which provides grants to help heart disease patients pay for lifesaving treatment.

I manage to get the sleep I need: six hours a night and a nap once a day for half an hour.

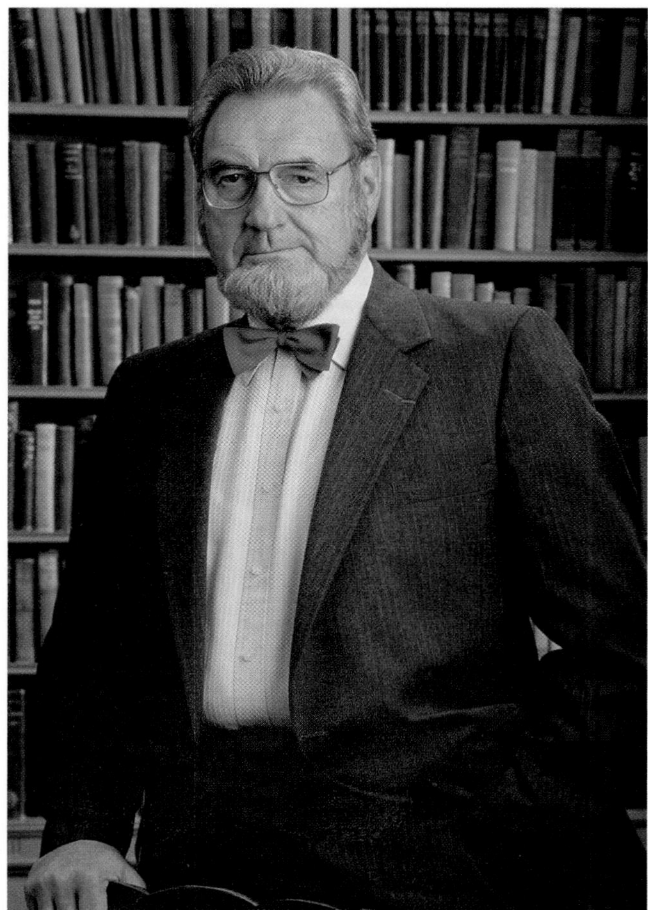

(Above) Thomas Ames; (opposite page) Dana Fineman—Sygma

An internationally known pediatric surgeon, **C. Everett Koop** was surgeon in chief of Children's Hospital of Philadelphia for 33 years, serving in that capacity until 1981, when he was appointed U.S. surgeon general by Pres. Ronald Reagan. Koop resigned from that post in 1989 but is remembered as one of the most forthright and independent individuals ever to have held the office, campaigning tirelessly against smoking and raising public consciousness about AIDS. Koop continues to educate the public about health issues through his frequent speaking engagements, books and articles, and appearances on TV and radio. In 1992 he established the C. Everett Koop Institute at Dartmouth College, Hanover, New Hampshire, with the mission of reshaping medical education and improving U.S. health care delivery. In 1995 he was awarded the Presidential Medal of Freedom.

I need a minimum of six hours' sleep to function optimally. I seldom sleep longer than that, and eight hours is a rarity. I do better if I can have an afternoon nap, usually 30–40 minutes. If I am to give an evening lecture or to function in an earlier time zone, such a nap is a necessity. I do not really feel sleep-deprived at any time.

Surgeon **Susan Love** is an adjunct associate professor of clinical surgery at the University of California, Los Angeles, and director of the Santa Barbara Breast Cancer Institute. She is one of the founders of the National Breast Cancer Coalition and served on the medical advisory committee of the Women's Health Initiative, the largest U.S. study to date of the health of postmenopausal women. Her books (cowritten with Karen Lindsey) *Dr. Susan Love's Breast Book* and *Dr. Susan Love's Hor-*

(Left) Indefatigable antismoking crusader C. Everett Koop; (opposite page) Susan Love, who avoids naps "like the plague," with a favorite companion

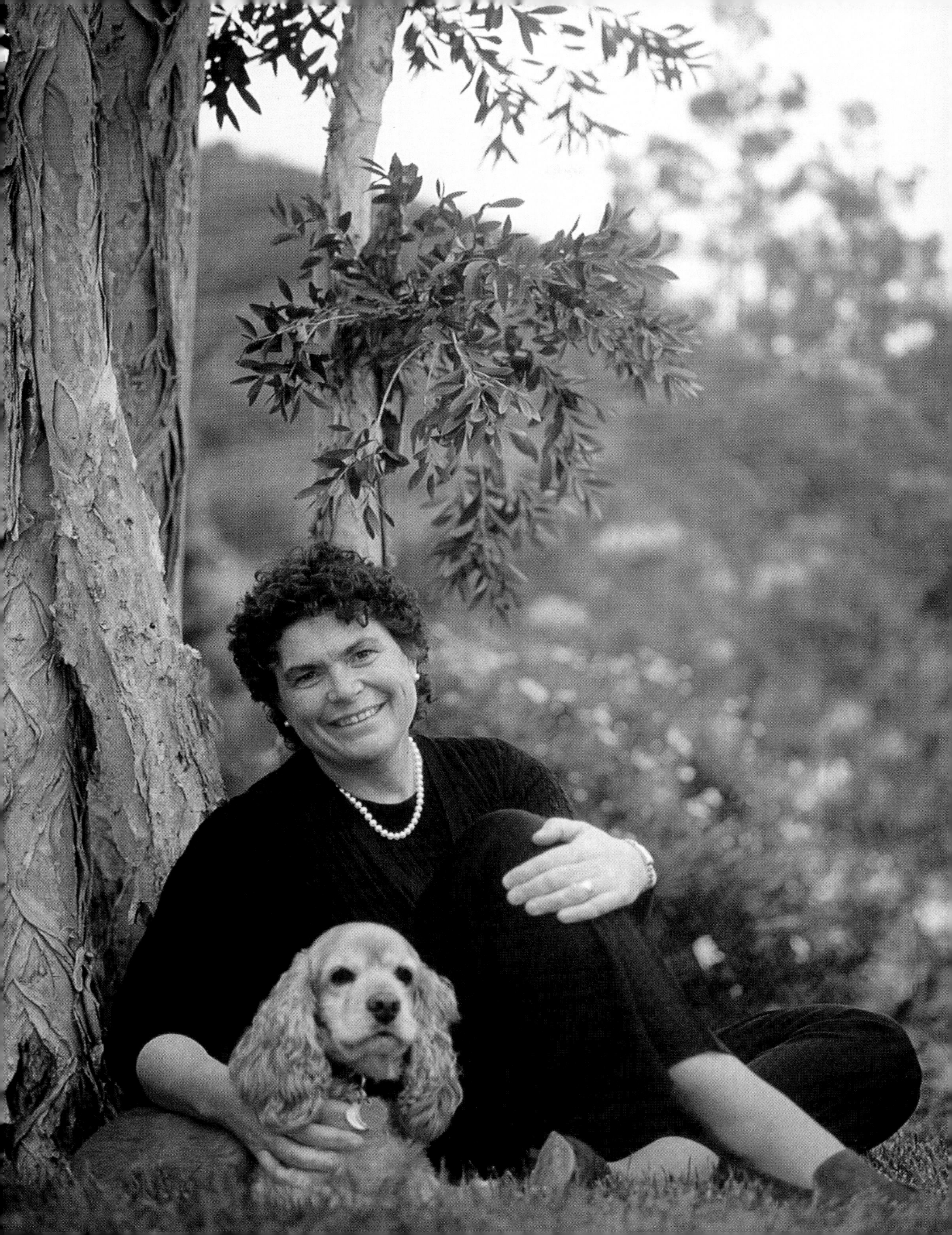

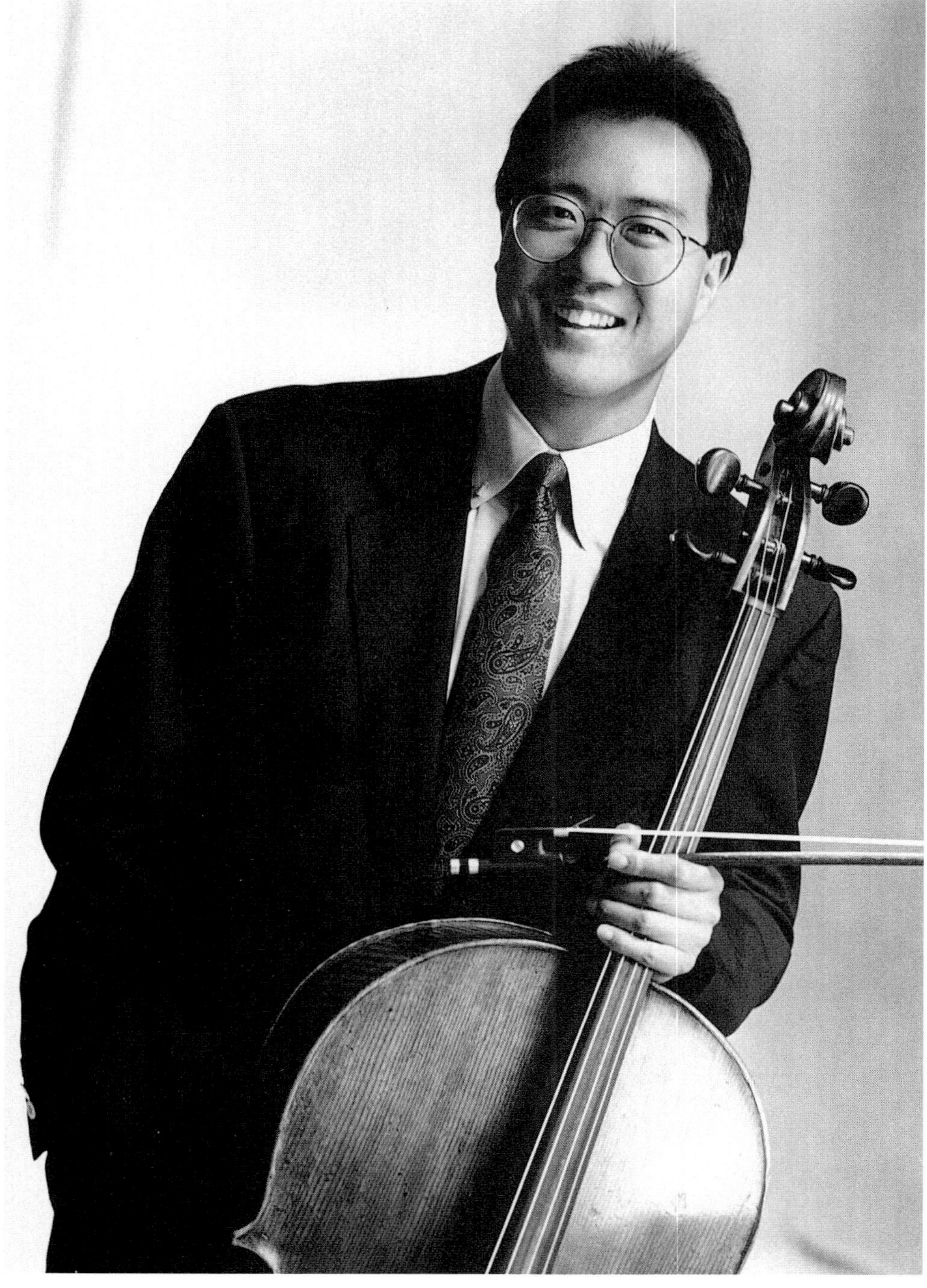

ICM Artists, Ltd.; photograph, J. Henry Fair

Yo-Yo Ma, somewhat sleep-deprived

mone Book were published in 1990 and 1997, respectively.

In order to function optimally, I usually sleep about seven hours. I fall asleep shortly after putting my daughter to bed and get up around 6 AM. *Not only do I not supplement my nightly sleep with naps, but I avoid naps like the plague, since they were a practice that deserved derision in my family. I think I do get the sleep that I need, but most commonly I sleep five to six hours a night and then have to do a couple of catch-up nights. Luckily, as a surgeon and a mother, I have developed the skill to wake up in the middle of the night, attend some life-threatening crisis, and then immediately fall back asleep. This skill has served me in good stead and may be my greatest talent.*

Cellist **Yo-Yo Ma** gave his first public recital at the age of 5; by 19 he was being compared to the great masters of the instrument. He has performed solo and with symphony orchestras around the globe and earned a reputation as an ambassador of classical music. In an effort to learn and demonstrate the vital role music plays in cross-cultural communication, Ma has immersed himself in native Chinese music and the music of the Kalahari bush people of Africa, learning to play the instruments of both. Because he believes music enriches children's lives and stimulates their creativity, he regularly takes time out of his busy schedule to work with and perform for youngsters. Ma has released more than 45 albums, 10 of which have won Grammy awards.

To function optimally, I need seven to nine hours of sleep a night while at home and four to six hours while on the road performing. I supplement my nightly sleep with naps, but overall I feel that I do not get the sleep I need.

In 1990 the National Institutes of Health (NIH) established the Office of Research on Women's Health, and since November 1991 **Vivian W. Pinn** has been its first full-time director. She is also the NIH's associate director for

Office of Research on Women's Health, National Institutes of Health

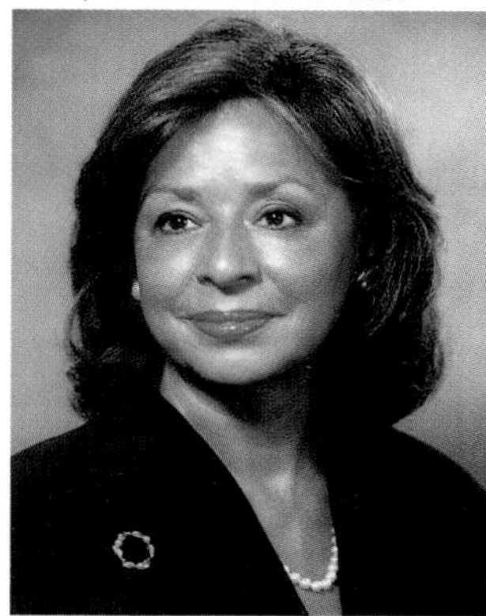

Night person Vivian W. Pinn

research on women's health. Before going to work for the U.S. government, she was professor and chair of the department of pathology at Howard University College of Medicine, Washington, D.C. At the time she received her M.D. in 1967, Pinn was the only woman in her University of Virginia School of Medicine graduating class, as well as the only minority member. Her efforts to improve the health status of and career opportunities for women and minorities have won her many awards and honors, including five honorary degrees of law and science. In 1995 she was elected to the Institute of Medicine of the National Research Council. That same year the *Ladies Home Journal* named her one of the "Ten Most Important Women in Medicine."

As a medical student and resident, I learned to function on very little sleep. I need at least five hours of sleep each night, but because I am a "night person"—with my best creative energies expressive in late-night hours—and yet must be up early, I often get as little as four hours of sleep, and naps are out of the question. Because of demands on my time during the week, and often also on the weekend, I try to get seven hours of sleep at least one night during the weekend. Another legacy from my medical training is that while I can sleep through ringing alarm clocks, a ringing telephone always wakes me up!

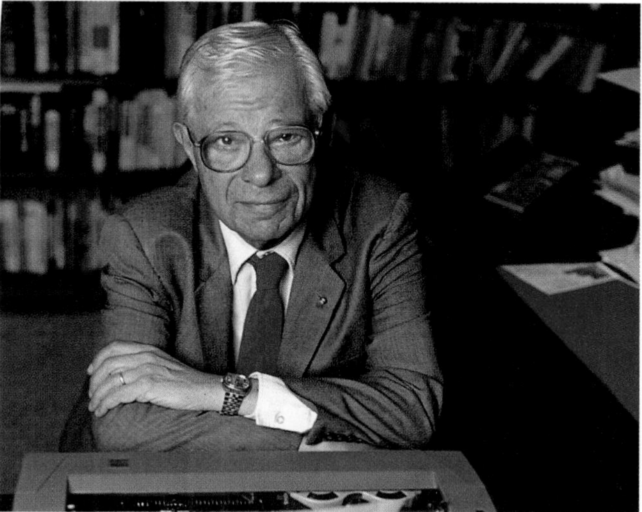

Daniel Schorr, senior news analyst for National Public Radio, began his journalistic career in 1946 as a foreign correspondent writing from Western Europe on post-World War II reconstruction for *The Christian Science Monitor* and later the *New York Times.* In 1953 he entered broadcasting as a correspondent for CBS-TV News, where he remained until 1976. During his prodigious career Schorr has witnessed and reported on some of the most monumental historical events of the last half century, including the anticommunist hearings headed by Sen. Joseph J. McCarthy, the Eisenhower-Khrushchev meeting in Geneva in 1955, and the Reagan-Gorbachev meeting in Moscow in 1988. Schorr was the first reporter ever to conduct a formal interview with the Soviet leader Nikita Khrushchev in his Kremlin office (1957). His exclusive coverage of the Senate Watergate hearings in 1972 earned him three Emmy awards. Schorr is the author of *Don't Get Sick in America* (1970) and *Clearing the Air* (1977).

I need eight hours of sleep a night. Badly, sometimes desperately, I need an afternoon nap but never seem to get enough sleep. My problem is I am recovering from a case of the shingles, which still disrupts my sleep, so even after nine hours I wake up unrefreshed. You had to ask!

Humorist **David Sedaris**—who describes his occupation as "typist"—is a playwright, fiction and nonfiction writer, regular commentator on National Public Radio, and con-

(Left) Serious napper Daniel Schorr; (below) David Sedaris, unemployed, who sleeps as long as he likes

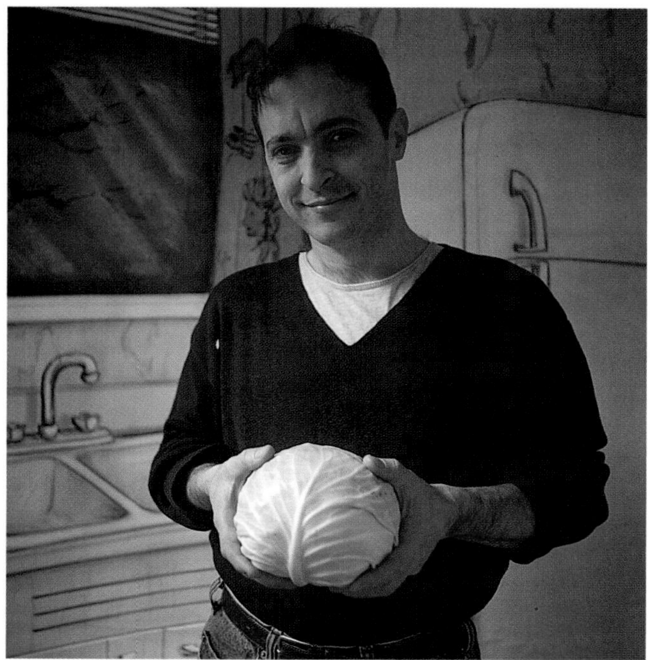

(Center) ©Paula Darte; (above) Karen Kuehn—Matrix

tributor to *The New Yorker.* He is the author of two collections of essays, short stories, and personal reminiscences, *Barrel Fever* (1994) and *Naked* (1997). Sedaris and his sister Amy have written three plays, *Stitches, One Woman Shoe,* and *The Little Freida Mysteries.* Sedaris was recently described in the *Washington Post Book World* as "one of America's most prickly, and delicious, young comic talents."

The numbers change. In my 20s and early 30s, I did best on six hours of sleep. Now I favor eight or nine. I don't know if this is due to a change in my metabolism or a change in my drinking habits. I love a nap in the late afternoon, usually no longer than 15 minutes, and I never take it in bed, as that tends to give me a headache. I nap on the sofa or on the floor. Seeing as I have no job, I'm allowed to sleep as long as I want. This being the case, I think I get the sleep I need.

None of this is particularly interesting. I wish I could say I slept in a coffin and took 14-hour naps, but I don't.

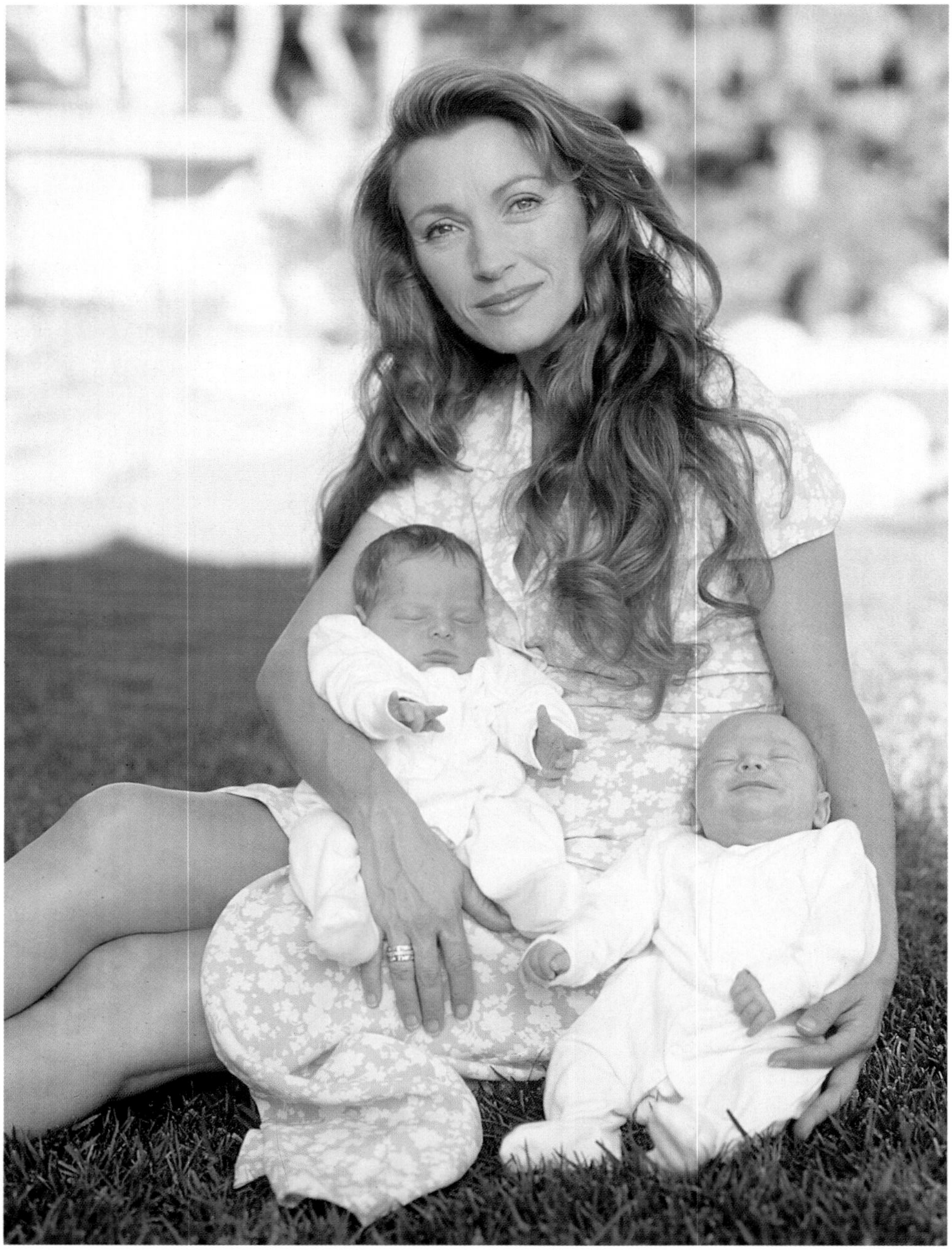

While she is not a doctor, actress **Jane Seymour** plays a very competent and compassionate one on television. She is the star of the Emmy award-winning weekly series "Dr. Quinn, Medicine Woman." Seymour has numerous other leading roles, including mother of twins, artist, and active fund-raiser for several charitable organizations.

I need seven hours of sleep to function at optimum harmony. With my work schedule and infant twins, not to mention the "mom agenda" of having two older active children, good luck! I have to schedule my sleep and then try to hold to the schedule.

I do not take naps. I find that by focusing my attention and energy on the challenge at hand, I can fend off sleepiness. I always try to be wide awake during active hours and fast asleep during resting hours.

I rarely get the sleep I need. I always think I will catch up during vacation breaks, but they seem to be even more packed with things to do. R&R can be hard work if you do it right.

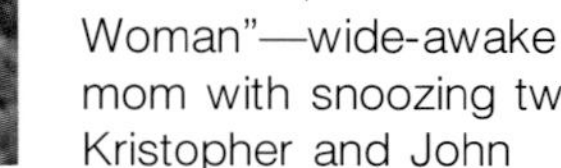

Jane Seymour, television's "Dr. Quinn, Medicine Woman"—wide-awake mom with snoozing twins, Kristopher and John

George Lange—Outline

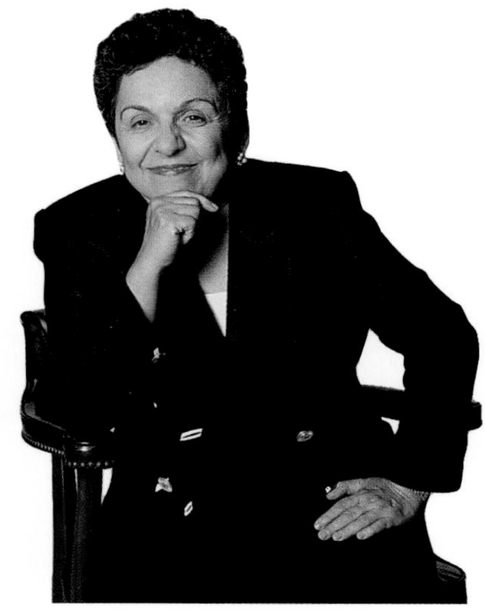

Always-alert Donna E. Shalala

Prior to being appointed U.S. secretary of health and human services by Pres. Bill Clinton, **Donna E. Shalala** served as chancellor of the University of Wisconsin for six years. For more than a decade, she was a member of the board of the Children's Defense Fund, and she became its chairperson in 1992, the same year that *Business Week* magazine named her one of the top five managers in U.S. higher education.

I need eight hours of sleep a night and generally take naps only on the weekends. I think I get the sleep I need.

Most people probably have never heard of **Walter C. Willett,** but chances are that their diets have been influenced by the findings of the landmark studies he and his colleagues have conducted. Willett is professor of epidemiology and nutrition at the Harvard School of Public Health, chairman of the school's nutrition department, and professor of medicine at Harvard Medical School. He directs two huge ongoing epidemiological investigations: the Health Professionals Follow-Up Study, involving about 52,000 men, and the Nurses' Health Study (of over 121,000 older and 116,000 younger female nurses). Among other things, Willett's research has shown that margarine may not be as heart-healthy as nutrition authorities once assumed. A leader in the development of nutritional epidemiology—a discipline that focuses on the roles played by dietary and lifestyle factors in the development of disease—he is the author of more than 400 scientific papers and one of the classic textbooks in his field.

I need six to seven hours of sleep a night. Sometimes I take a short early-evening nap to be able to think and write full steam until midnight. Medical training was excellent for developing the skill to reenergize with a quick nap. Overall, the amount of sleep I get is sufficient.

Energized from a nap, Walter C. Willett at work

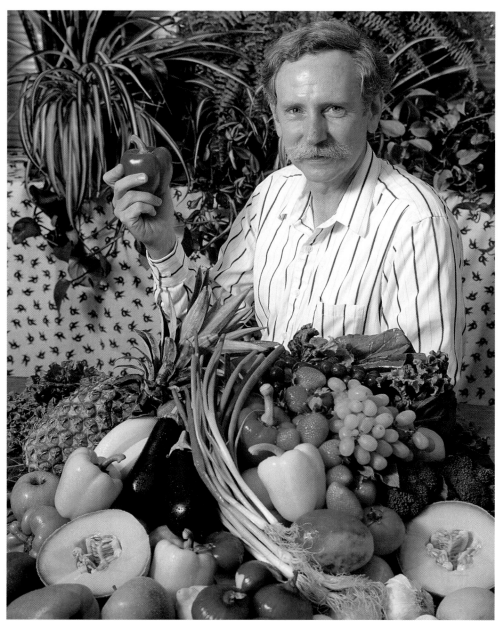

(Top) Janette Beckman—Outline; (above) ©Paula Lerner

Reinventing the Wheelchair

by Ralf D. Hotchkiss

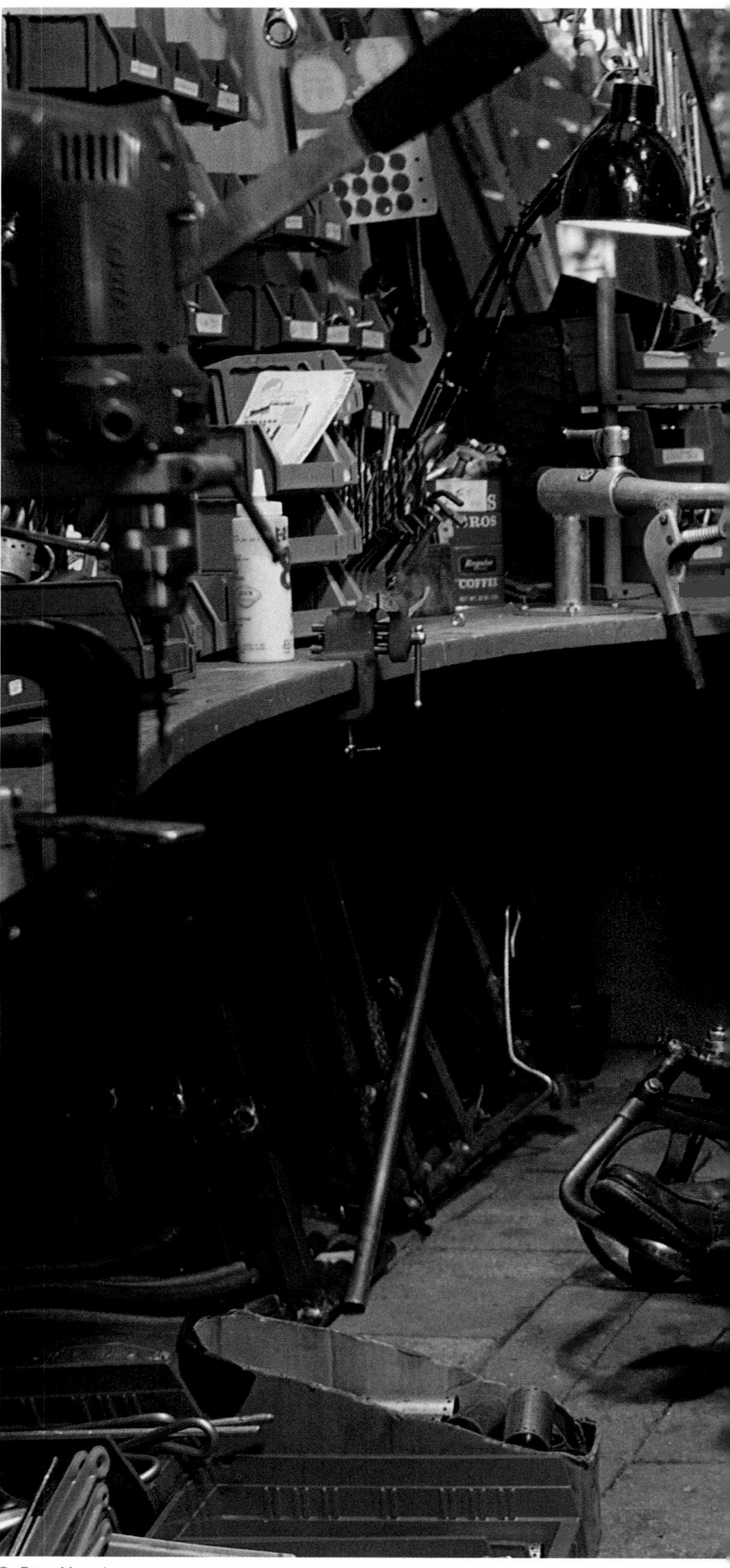

© Peter Menzel

High in the Sierra Madre Occidental, in Sinaloa, Mexico, a young boy named Polo Leva caught polio in the early 1970s. In time Polo recovered, regaining his vigor and his generally robust health. But he needed a new way to get around because his legs could no longer carry his weight. Going to school was out of the question—he had no way to get there. He spent the next decade sitting on the dirt floor of his family's home, helping to care for his younger brother and sister.

In his Oakland, California, home workshop, the author reinvents the wheelchair. For more than 25 years, he has been designing wheelchairs of exceptional durability and low cost to meet the needs of people with physical disabilities living in less-developed countries.

Ralf D. Hotchkiss *is Technical Director of Whirlwind Wheelchair International, based at the School of Engineering, San Francisco State University. He was the recipient of a MacArthur Foundation fellowship in 1989, an Honorary Doctor of Science degree from Oberlin (Ohio) College in 1991, the Henry B. Betts Award for work in disability rights and rehabilitation medicine in 1994, and the Chrysler Innovation in Design Award in 1995. Hotchkiss travels regularly to Third World countries as an advocate for people with disabilities and a leader of workshops on building wheelchairs that work.*

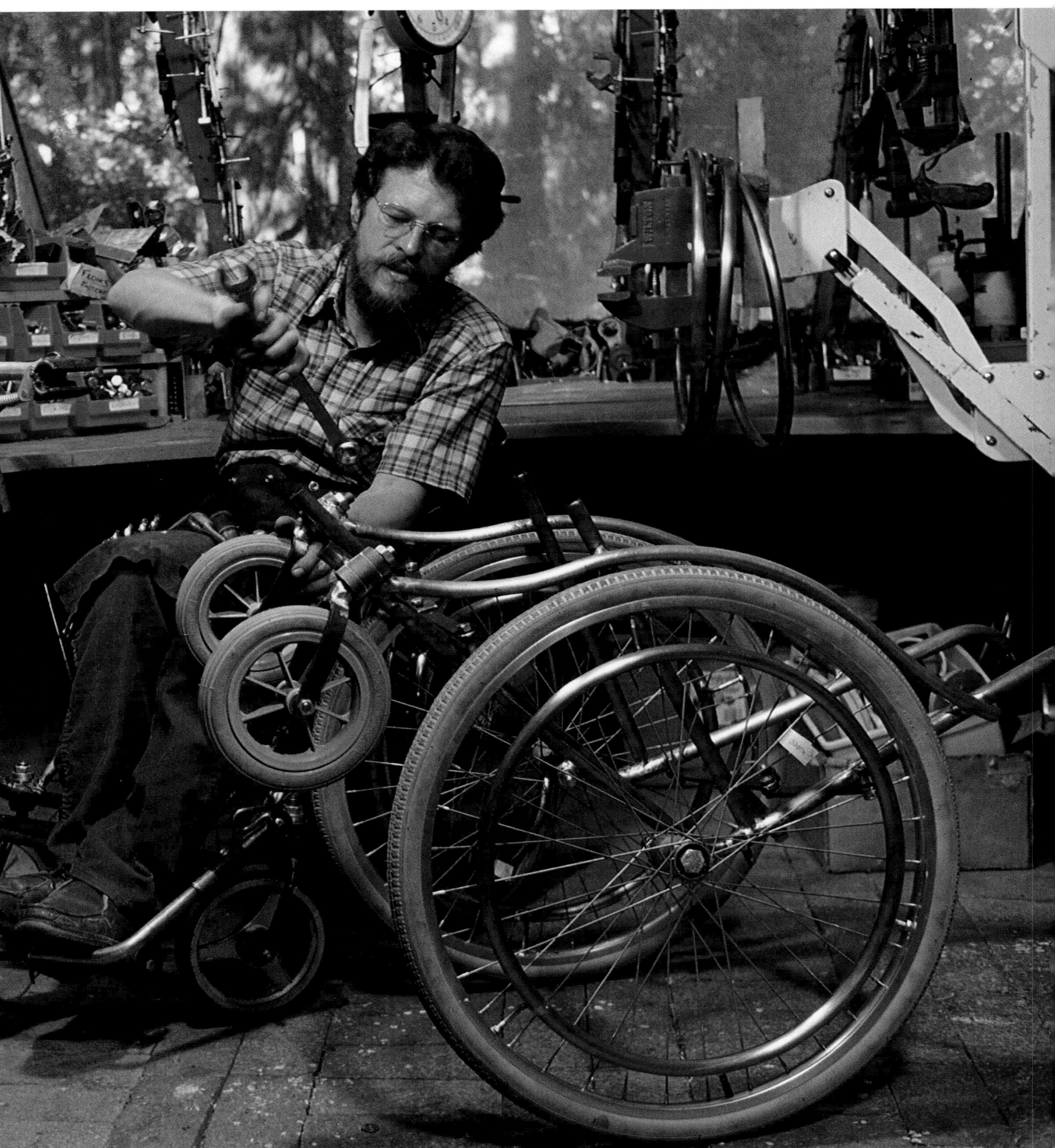

Then, when Polo was 16, he heard about a small rehabilitation center in Ajoya, a several-days' walk away across the mountains. Polo's older brother dragged him there on a wooden board pulled by a rope. At the clinic Polo was given a clumsy American hospital-type wheelchair. For the first time in his life, he could take himself where he wanted to go, though it was a struggle to maneuver on Ajoya's unpaved streets. After just a few days, the front caster wheel of his chair fractured. But Polo had tasted freedom and refused to be held back. By the time he finished repairing his front wheel at the clinic workshop, everyone had seen how handy he was—and the job of wheelchair repair for the entire clinic was bestowed upon him.

A short time later, a wheelchair of a new design was sent to the Ajoya clinic by a small group of disabled people working in Managua, Nicaragua. This chair, the first "Whirlwind," was designed to be made entirely out of parts and materials available in small towns like Ajoya. Polo quickly mastered the skills of building wheelchairs from scratch and constructed a full-featured, lightweight, folding Whirlwind for himself; now he could race around town despite the challenging terrain. Over the next few years, he helped to make hundreds of wheelchairs for other disabled people. Polo's chairs had the best features of the expensive imports, yet they cost only

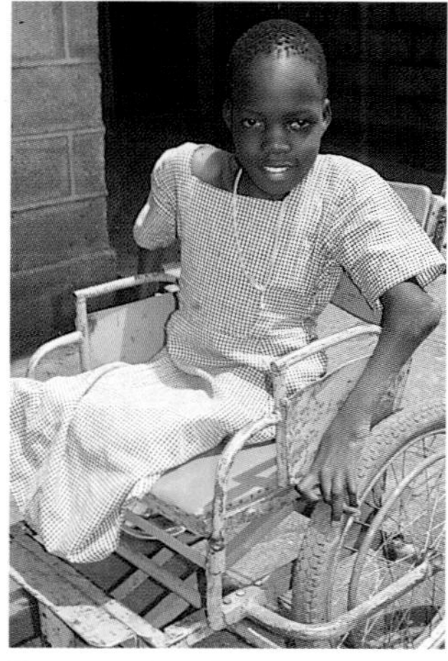

(Left) Courtesy of Ralf D. Hotchkiss; (below) Peter Turnley—Newsweek/Black Star

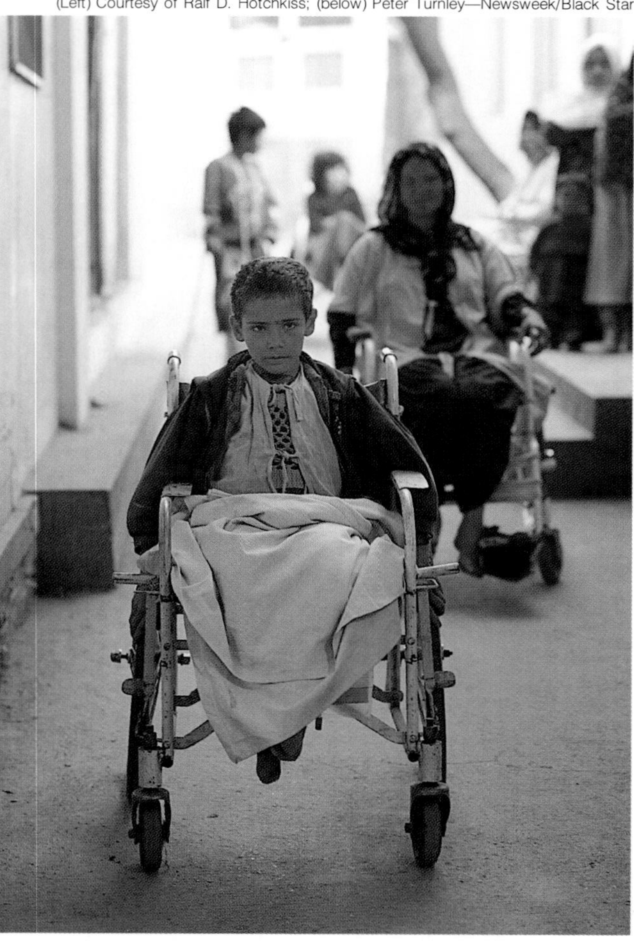

For people who cannot get around on foot, a wheelchair can mean freedom and self-sufficiency. A young girl in Nyabondo, Kenya (above), and land mine victims in Kabul, Afghanistan (right), unfortunately, must make do with antiquated "clunkers" donated from the West.

one-fifth as much, and, most important, they held up even on the roughest of roads.

As Polo's skills increased, he swelled with pride; before long his own chair was upholstered with black leather and decorated with brass studs. With his new earnings, Polo was able to save enough money to move away from Ajoya and enter an even more lucrative profession.

Different spokes for different folks

Throughout history people with disabilities have had distinct disadvantages—one of which is low social status. In some cultures disabled people are in a category akin to India's untouchables. More often than not, people with mobility impairments have been confined and forgotten—"out of sight, out of mind." For anyone who lacks the ability to get around on foot, a wheelchair has the potential to bring about a social transformation; mobility means that people with disabilities can overcome the long-held expectation that they have no future. In order to gain self-sufficiency, people in the world's poorer places need the strongest-possible, highest-quality wheelchairs—as Polo's situation so clearly demonstrates. To offer any chance of success, Third World wheelchairs must do several things very well:

- travel over difficult terrain—*e.g.,* through mud and rain

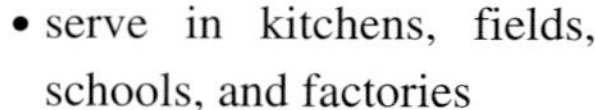

- serve in kitchens, fields, schools, and factories
- fold to fit on a bus, usually the only available and affordable form of transportation from village to town
- go long distances on unpaved pathways with a minimum of assistance
- never miss a day because of a broken part

Needless to say, getting around is easier for most wheelchair riders in Western industrialized countries than for those in the Third World. City streets in the former are usually paved, and many public buildings have ramps. Private cars and vans are widely available, and public transportation is rapidly becoming accessible to wheelchair riders. Moreover, replacement parts for broken wheelchairs are usually available (if the rider can pay the price).

The poorer people are, the less they can pay to replace broken wheelchair parts and the less access they are likely to have to other forms of transport. When a wheelchair fails in a Third World country, the rider cannot get from place to place, cannot earn a living, cannot raise a family. Quite obviously, the people with the greatest need for strong, dependable wheelchairs are not those living in the well-endowed industrialized countries of the West; rather, they are the four out of five people with disabilities who live in less-developed countries.

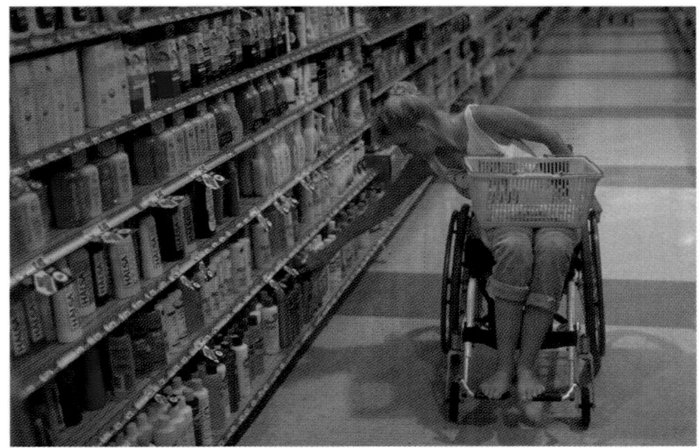

A revolution in wheelchair technology has made it possible for people with disabilities living in wealthy countries to go almost anywhere and do almost anything. Selecting items in a supermarket and boarding a public bus are everyday activities.

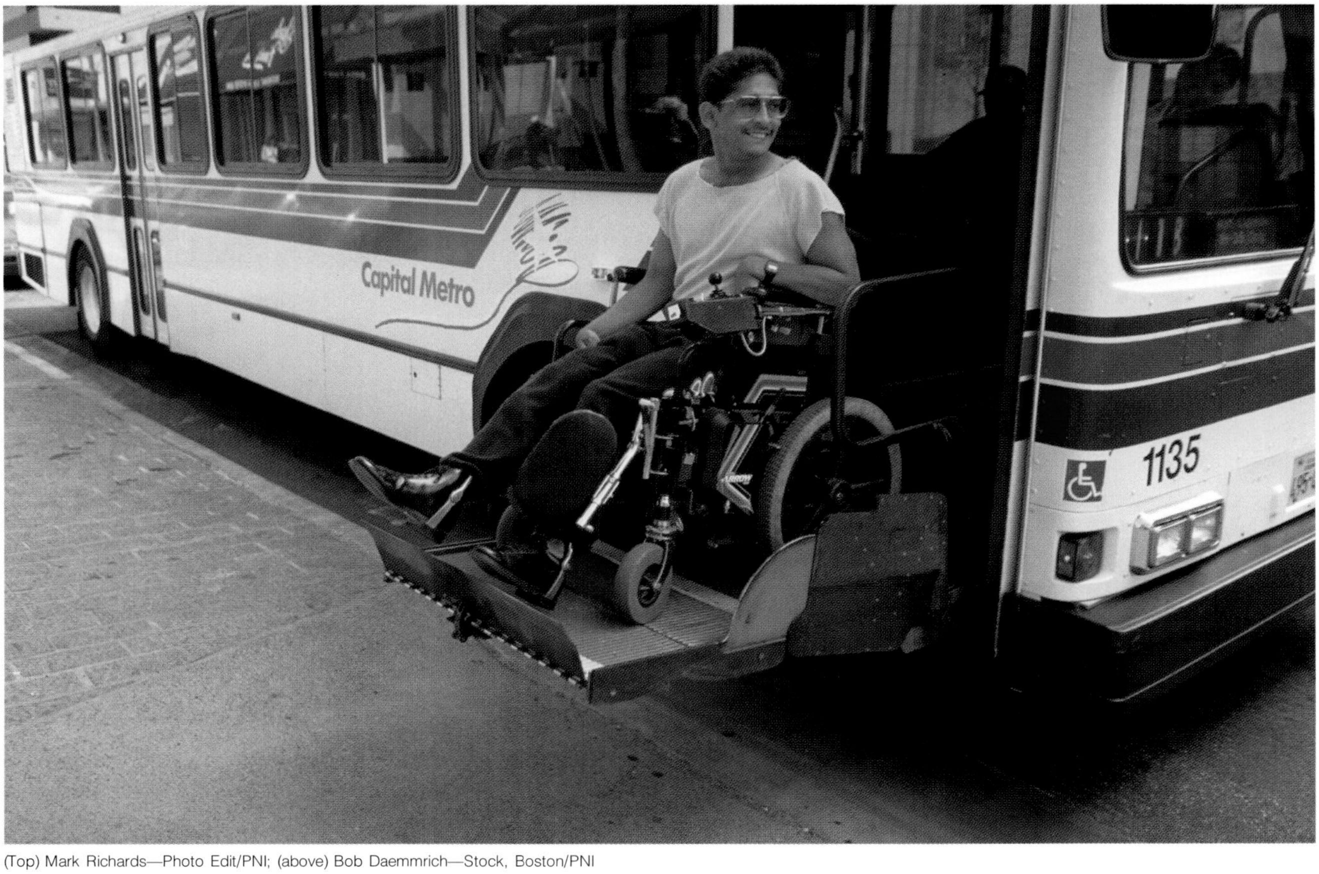

(Top) Mark Richards—Photo Edit/PNI; (above) Bob Daemmrich—Stock, Boston/PNI

A typical Western hospital chair is designed for gentle use on smooth floors. Its short-lived components must be regularly replaced with expensive parts from a factory. If a hospital chair is imported into a Third World community, it can quickly become useless because replacement parts are not available. Not only are Western hospital wheelchairs the least appropriate for people in less-developed countries; they are also the most expensive per year of use.

Over the past 20 years, there has been a true revolution in the design of higher-priced wheelchairs in the West. The heavy, unreliable, poorly engineered wheelchairs of the past—hospital "clunkers"—have been replaced by chairs that are much lighter and stronger. Older-model chairs were made in only one or two widths and were intended to fit nearly everybody; instead, they fit almost nobody well. The newer chairs are made in a multitude of sizes. They provide a snug fit by bringing the wheels in close to the rider's hips. This streamlined design gives the rider better leverage for pushing on the wheels and narrows the overall width of the chair, which makes it possible for the chair to fit through tighter passageways.

Unfortunately, the light weight of most of these new chairs requires the use of sophisticated aluminum alloys that cannot be welded or repaired in most Third World facilities. Moreover, replacement parts for these new models, like the parts for the hospital chairs, are impossible to get. When active use results in damage to a high-tech imported chair, there is often no alternative but to throw it away.

Well-meant but worthless

Why, then, are well-meaning charities in the wealthier countries still donating secondhand Western wheelchairs to less-developed parts of the world? Many donors believe there are no better options, so they continue to export wheelchairs that serve their users poorly, if at all. It is easy to understand how this happens; to a donor any wheelchair seems better than nothing. But to disabled people struggling to pull themselves out of dire poverty—seeking education, employment, and social integration—the physical and economic setbacks that come with each wheelchair failure can be too great to bear.

One reason Western wheelchairs are sent to Third World countries is that these donations are supported by U.S. and European income-tax deductions. When a wheelchair is no longer needed in the United States, because it is either outmoded or in need of repair, it often has no value on the U.S. market. Yet a tax deduction worth hundreds of dollars can be claimed if this otherwise worthless chair is donated to an organization working in the Third World. Shortly after that chair is delivered to a less-developed country, it is likely to be beyond repair. Dumped chairs can be seen rusting by the hundreds behind hospitals. In fact, the same effort and expense (for collecting, warehousing, replacing missing parts, shipping, and distributing Western wheelchairs—plus the value of the deductions) would have considerably greater impact over the long term if, instead, they were invested in the local manufacture of state-of-the-art wheelchairs.

Third World: full of inventors

People with disabilities in less-developed countries have not been sitting idly by waiting for better wheelchairs to come their way. For more than two decades, active groups of disabled people have been searching for "appropriate technology"—a concept for which these grassroots engineers have developed their own rigorous definition: *the very best methods that can be employed, using available materials at an affordable cost.* They have improved on the design of imported wheelchairs and are manufacturing their own new models at much lower cost. Moreover, when wheelchairs are built by the very people who have been freed by them, pride ripples outward, spreading throughout the community.

It is not just the self-made chairs that have long and useful lives; so do the users. Consider Rafael Muturi, a 15-

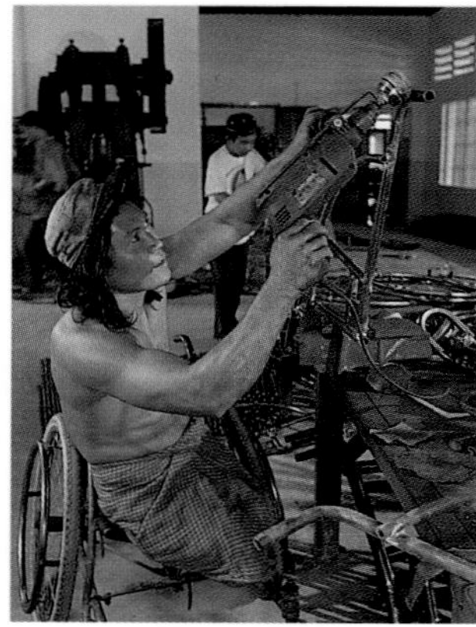

People with disabilities in less-developed countries have not been sitting around waiting for suitable wheelchairs to come their way. A war vet (right) works in a wheelchair factory in Cambodia; a Kenyan woman (below) perfects her spoking skills.

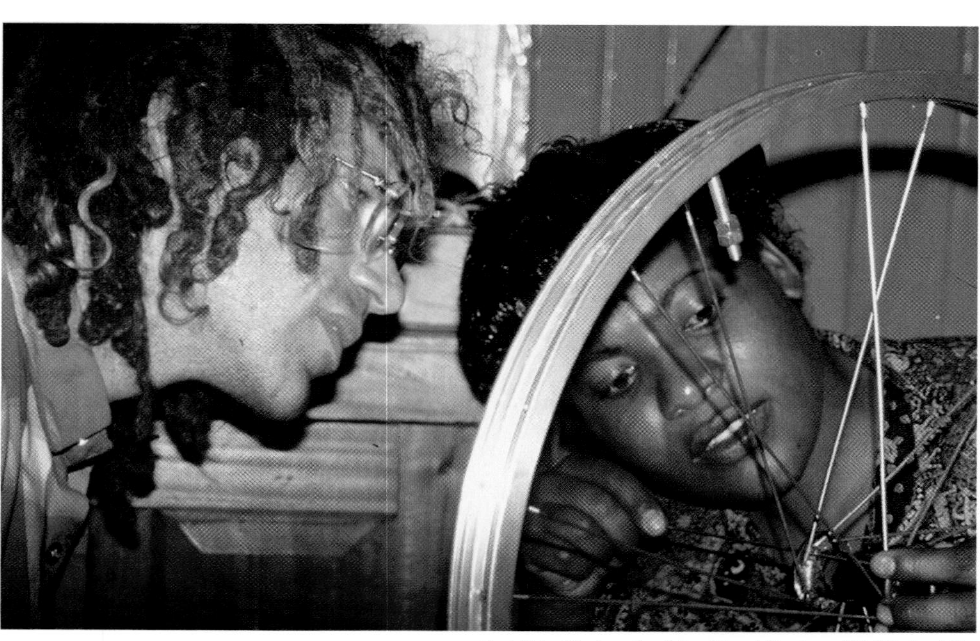

(Top) Peter Charleworth—Saba; (above) Courtesy of Ralf D. Hotchkiss

Courtesy of Ralf D. Hotchkiss

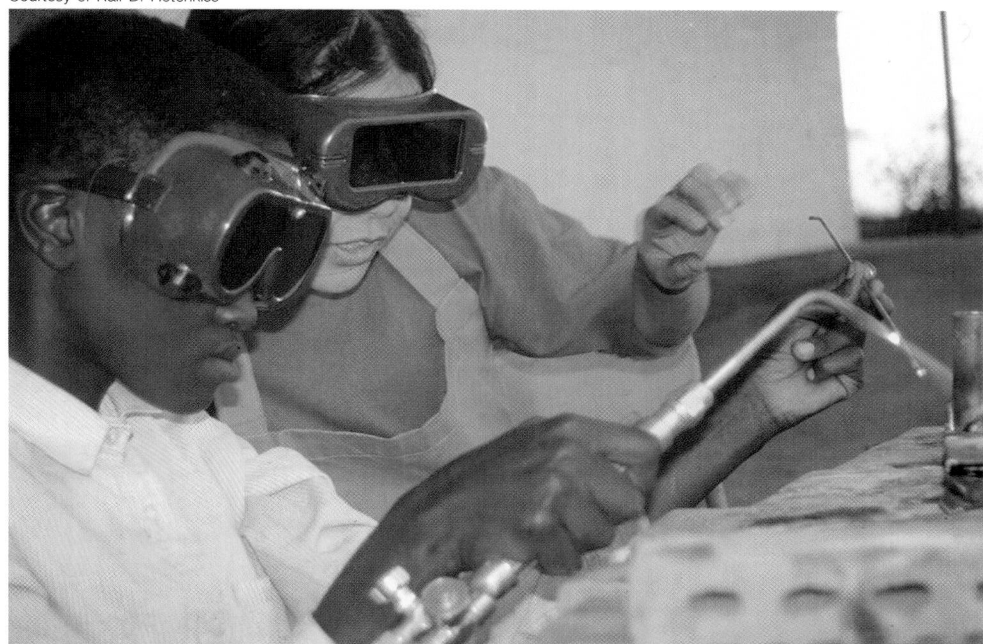

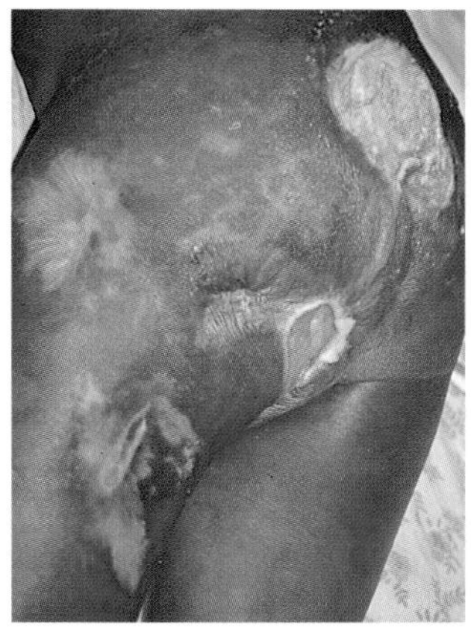

Rafael Muturi of Kenya (in the foreground above) developed life-threatening pressure sores (left) from his old wheelchair. Before he had fully recovered, he had the chance to build himself a new chair specially designed to fit *his* body.

year-old youth in Maua, Kenya, who had sustained a major spinal-cord injury. For eight years he had relied upon a dilapidated German wheelchair that pressed so severely into his bones he had developed life-threatening pressure sores (discussed in greater detail below). Simply put, his chair was killing him. Despite a high fever caused by a serious infection that resulted from his sores, Rafael was determined to take advantage of a special workshop that would enable him to build his own Whirlwind wheelchair. At one point during the construction process, he went into convulsions for over an hour and stopped breathing. Doctors expected him to remain in a coma, if he lived at all. But youth, strength, and extremely good fortune were with him, and a few days later Rafael was back at work.

Now that he has his own custom-built chair, his pressure sores are starting to heal. He also understands what caused them and how he can prevent them in the future. Because the chair is his own creation, he is keeping it in tip-top shape. Furthermore, his improved health and increased determination helped persuade the local primary school's headmaster to admit him after having refused to do so for eight years. No one in his town doubts that Rafael has embarked on a rich new life full of opportunity, which could never have happened had he not gained the freedom that his new wheelchair provided.

Birth of the Whirlwind Network

In the 1970s the first wheelchair-building collective comprising a large group of people with disabilities began work in the Philippines. Known as Tahanan Walang Hagdanan ("House with No Steps"), the group designed chairs that were a vast improvement over the imported chairs upon which Filipinos with disabilities had previously depended. Instead of having expensive, hard-to-repair, and impossible-to-replace parts, they had low-cost components available in the local marketplace. What had been the weakest points on the imported chairs—those that typically fractured on unpaved roads—were reinforced, tested, and then reinforced again until failures were few. Indeed, Tahanan's chairs were as heavy, sturdy, and dynamic as the imports that they were modeled after, but unlike the imports, they withstood rough usage.

In 1980 the Whirlwind Network of Third World wheelchair builders officially began in Managua. Four teenagers sharing one wheelchair made a plea for the materials to build three more chairs. The U.S. Agency for International Development provided support, and Nicaragua's first independent living center and wheelchair shop were established. Consumers were at first wary of the chairs made locally by disabled people. That changed when Nicaragua held the first wheelchair marathon, and disabled builders in sturdy self-designed chairs competed against riders in expensive chrome-plated imported chairs. To the astonishment of the community, a young woman in her self-made Whirlwind pulled ahead of the pack; by the time she reached the finish line, winning the race, the new local enterprise had received its first orders for custom-built chairs.

The wheelchair rider-builders in the Philippines were ea-

Courtesy of Ralf D. Hotchkiss

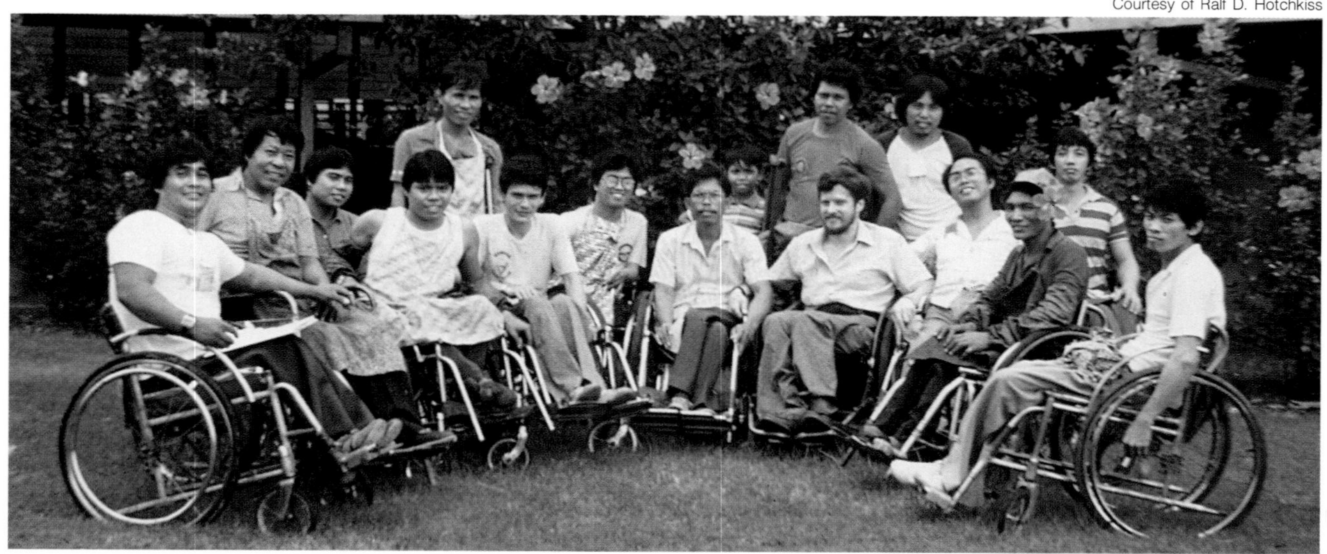

(Above) In the 1970s disabled people in the Philippines became pioneer wheelchair builders and formed the collective known as "House with No Steps."

ger to share their technology and join forces with the Nicaraguans in search of still-better, still-more-appropriate designs. The first achievements of the new network were the reduction of the weight of chairs to three-quarters that of the imports—from about 21 kilograms (46 pounds) to about 16 kilograms (35 pounds)—and also reduction of the time it took to build each chair from 21 person-days to 5.

Capitalizing on creativity. During its evolution some remarkable innovations have percolated up through the Whirlwind Network. For example, what became the "Zimbabwe Wheel" was first observed by a member of the network on a pushcart in Harare, Zimbabwe's capital, in 1988. The pushcart wheel was wide and flexible, and it rolled easily over dirt paths. Just as important, the wheel could be easily molded in a local rubber shop. It showed promise of being the best design yet for a flexible, long-lived wheelchair caster wheel. It took a lot of experimentation, however, to refine and adapt the wheel to replace the standard casters on the front of a wheelchair. Prototypes were made in India, Thailand, Mexico, and Fiji; in each case the design improved upon the one before it. The Zimbabwe Wheel was produced first in Siberia, then in Cambodia, Vietnam, and Kenya; then, in 1997, the wheel finally returned to its country of origin—wider, longer-lasting, cheaper, and more mobile over soft ground than any wheel that had previously been used on a lightweight wheelchair.

(Below) An early version of the Whirlwind—the Land Rover of wheelchairs—was designed for very rugged use, yet it can be repaired by anyone who can fix a bicycle.

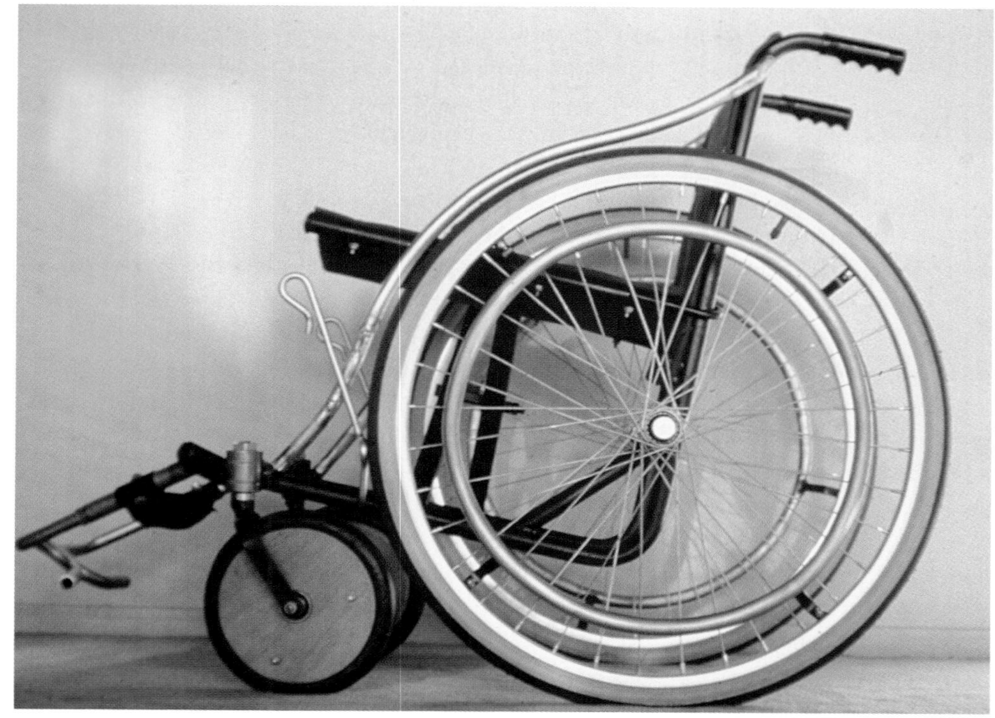

Courtesy of Ralf D. Hotchkiss

The current folding frame of the Whirlwind Wheelchair was even slower to evolve and did so through a considerably more tangled web. In Nicaragua in the early 1980s, pioneer builders adapted the triangular frame of a bicycle to the wheelchair. The design had the same effect upon the wheelchair as it does upon a bicycle—it provided strength but was lightweight. Furthermore, it was cheaper than the standard "box" design to manufacture; getting rid of the cumbersome box shape allowed further simplifications that eventually eliminated about half of the original parts. The new frame was an immediate success in Nicaragua and is widely appreciated by riders in the dozen or more countries where it is now used.

Despite its many advantages and wide acceptance, this new frame too had its problems. The folding mechanism required very precise alignment in order to operate smoothly. The wheelchair's upholstery had to be fastened to the chair with screws; lacing the fabric to the chair would have been cheaper and easier. These problems were solved in 1996 by a combination of a new welding fixture invented by a blacksmith in western Kenya and an ingenious improvement to the folding frame devised by architect Jan Sing, one of the founders of "Whirlwind Women."

Courtesy of Ralf D. Hotchkiss

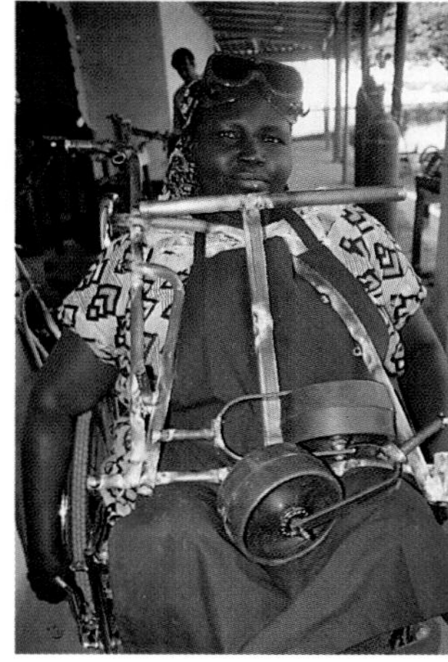

Achan Fatuma of Arua, Uganda, carries the folding frame and front caster wheels of the Whirlwind II that she is constructing from scratch.

Women whirl into action. Disabled women have particular responsibilities and needs that determine what kind of wheelchairs will accommodate them best. It is easier to care for a child, for example, if the mother can easily maneuver in and out of her wheelchair—say, to the floor or a bed. Peninah Mutinda of Kenya wanted to be able to care for her young daughter more effectively, so she helped design a "jump seat," a second seat between the floor and seat of a wheelchair. That innovation is helping wheelchair users around the world care for their youngsters easily.

Women with and without disabilities from various countries have worked as designers, inventors, mechanics, trainers, and testers of the Whirlwind Wheelchair since the network began. Despite their many contributions, they have been discouraged from participation in some of the workshops by male mechanics, who dominate the metalworking trades. Recognizing the need to resist such paternalistic attitudes and to promote the managerial and wheelchair-building talents of women, three enterprising women affiliated with the Wheeled Mobility Center (now Whirlwind Wheelchair International) at San Francisco State University formed Whirlwind Women. The mission of this grass-roots collaboration is to make practical improvements in their own and their "sisters'" lives and to address the double discrimination disabled women face daily.

Where have the Whirlwind Women been, and what have they achieved?

- In September 1995 three of the original Whirlwind Women attended the UN Fourth World Conference on Women in Beijing, where they provided techni-

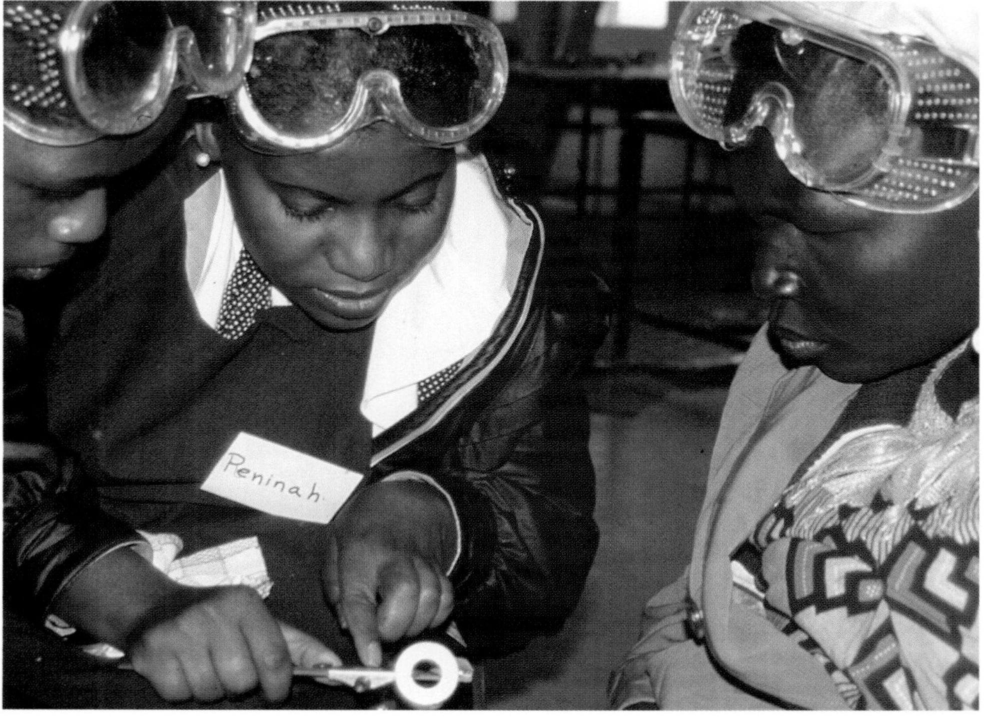

At a wheelchair-building workshop in Limuru, Kenya, Peninah Mutinda teaches other women how to use a vernier caliper to make very precise linear measurements.

Courtesy of Ralf D. Hotchkiss

cal support to women with disabilities and conducted training workshops in wheelchair building. Many disabled women attending the conference participated in the workshops, and representatives from several countries then expressed a keen interest in studying wheelchair fabrication further. The Disabled Women's Association of Uganda went on from that conference to attend a training course in Kenya in 1997; members of that group are now working hard to become the first female-run production shop in the Whirlwind Network.

- In January 1997 in Limuru, Kenya, Whirlwind Women conducted an intensive one-week course to teach six women from Kenya and Uganda basic metal-working techniques. The course gave the women the head start they needed to work side by side with men during a subsequent three-week training course. Most of the women had not worked with metal in a workshop setting previously, although all had experience with other crafts. During their initial training, the women built the side frame of a durable, lightweight, folding Whirlwind. After that, using their newly acquired skills—of measuring, welding, grinding, drilling, and bending thin-walled tubing—the women went on to construct entire Whirlwinds from raw hardware.
- In June 1997 members of this dynamic group demonstrated wheelchair production to participants at conferences on the two U.S. coasts: the International Leadership Forum for Women with Disabilities in Washington, D.C., and the International Leadership Institute for Women with Disabilities in Eugene, Oregon. At both meetings women seeking better wheelchairs joined in the fabrication exercises. They also realized that they could establish similar wheelchair-building projects at home.

Whirlwind growth. The Whirlwind (or Torbellino in Spanish) of the early 1980s, so-named by builders in Peru, was a resounding success. Light and strong, the wheelchair was state-of-the-art. Still, that was not enough. Many problems remained to be solved. The cost of the bearings and front wheels, for example, had added substantially to the total materials cost of the chairs. To find new solutions, the tiny network clearly needed to grow.

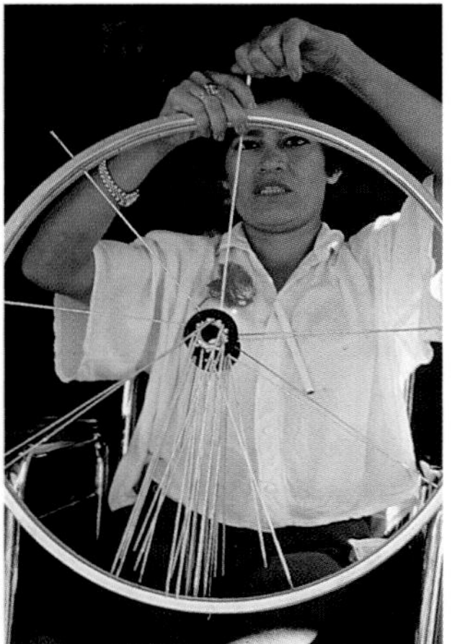

Courtesy of Ralf D. Hotchkiss

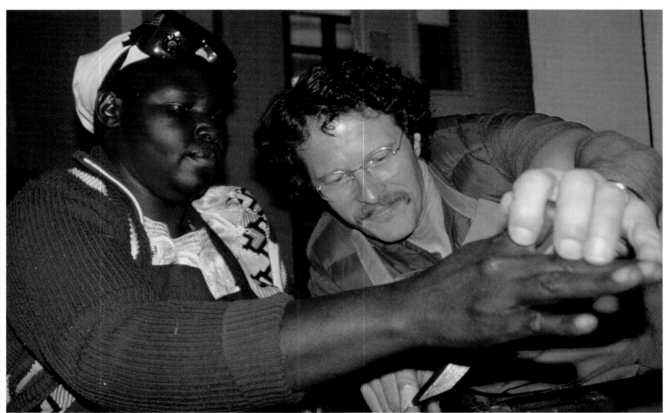

And grow it did. Over the past 17 years, Whirlwind's members have been working together in an informal, persistent network that presently spans much of the globe and includes some 35 shops in 25 countries. Members from every country in the network traveled to find and train new wheelchair rider-builders and bring them into the collaborative effort. The book *Independence Through Mobility,* published in 1985, disseminated the technology for building Whirlwind Wheelchairs around the world and enabled many aspiring builders to get started. Coordinated by attorney and wheelchair builder Jenny Kern, Whirldwind Women are collaborating with the emerging International Network of Women with Disabilities to involve more women in every aspect of wheelchair design, production, and marketing. Attorney and wheelchair builder Marc Krizack took the Whirlwind technology to Siberia, where he and other network members picked up some of the tricks of higher technology. Engineering professor Peter Pfaelzer at San Francisco State University brought the network into his academic setting, where the Wheeled Mobility Center was established, and network members found an endless stream of new inventors and a foundation of core support. One of those inventors, physical therapist Patty Ruppelt, got the network involved in consideration of appropriate designs of wheelchairs for very young children. She is developing a family of wheelchair designs that will provide a better foundation for custom-seating inserts (discussed below). Another inventor, engineer Dwight Johnson, established a testing program for Whirlwind designs with standards more exacting than those of some of the top commercial wheelchair manufacturers. Dozens of partners, ranging from local Rotary and Lions Clubs to the UN, have supported the growth of the Whirlwind Network in many different but complementary ways.

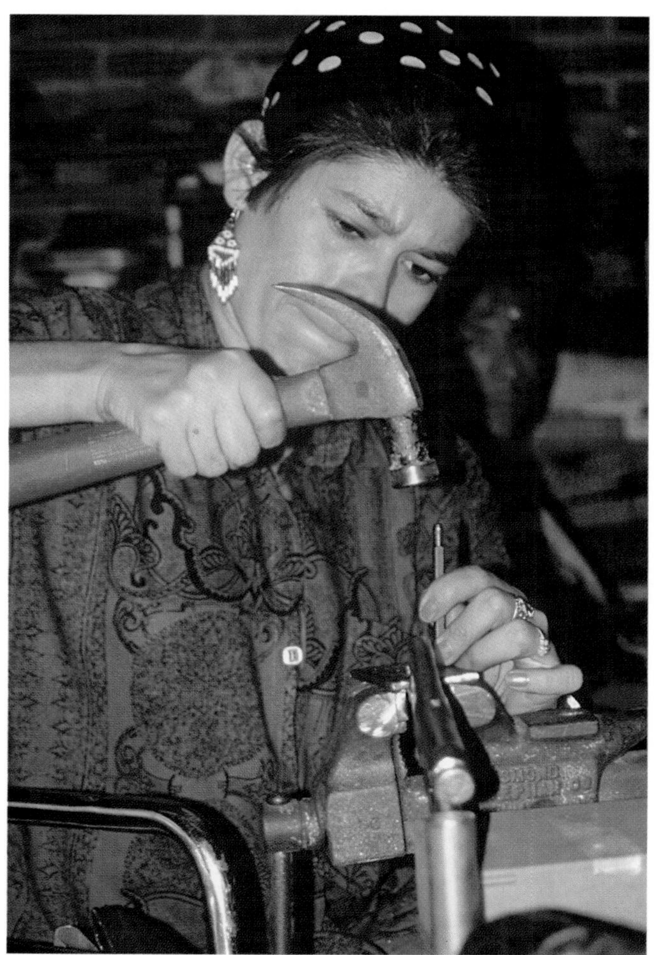

Around the world, women with disabilities are getting involved in every aspect of wheelchair design and construction. (Opposite page, bottom) Achan Fatuma of Uganda gets some tips from the author. (Opposite page, top, and below) Enterprising wheelchair builders in Ajoya, Mexico.

Courtesy of Ralf D. Hotchkiss

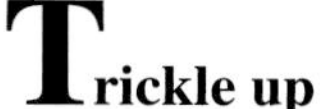

Trickle up

Historically, much of the new technology that is used for rehabilitation of people with mobility impairments has been based on the "trickle up" of new approaches and new technology from the consumer. Most breakthroughs in wheelchair design, for example, have come directly from active users. The same is true of other rehabilitation practices. The best rehabilitation professionals gain experience by working with people with disabilities, by respecting the firsthand information that only the latter can provide.

In the recent book *Nothing About Us Without Us* (1997), David Werner describes hundreds of technical developments that have come from people with disabilities. When equipped with workable tools and resources, disabled people often find highly inventive solutions to their own problems. Some of these people have formed teams with rehabilitation professionals and expert technicians. The result has been a profusion of new devices. Some have been highly effective, some total failures, but each one has underscored the value of working with the most legitimate experts on the needs of people who have mobility impairments and live in difficult environments: the disabled people themselves.

All aspects of rehabilitation need workers who understand disability firsthand. If such experience is lacking, the equipment or treatments that are likely to be imposed will not meet the real-life needs of the person with the disability. At best, this top-down approach results in a lost opportunity. At worst, injury and lasting physical harm can result. The latter often occurs when people with postpolio disabilities are discouraged from using wheelchairs, even though overdependence on walking may be causing dam-

David Constantine—Panos Pictures

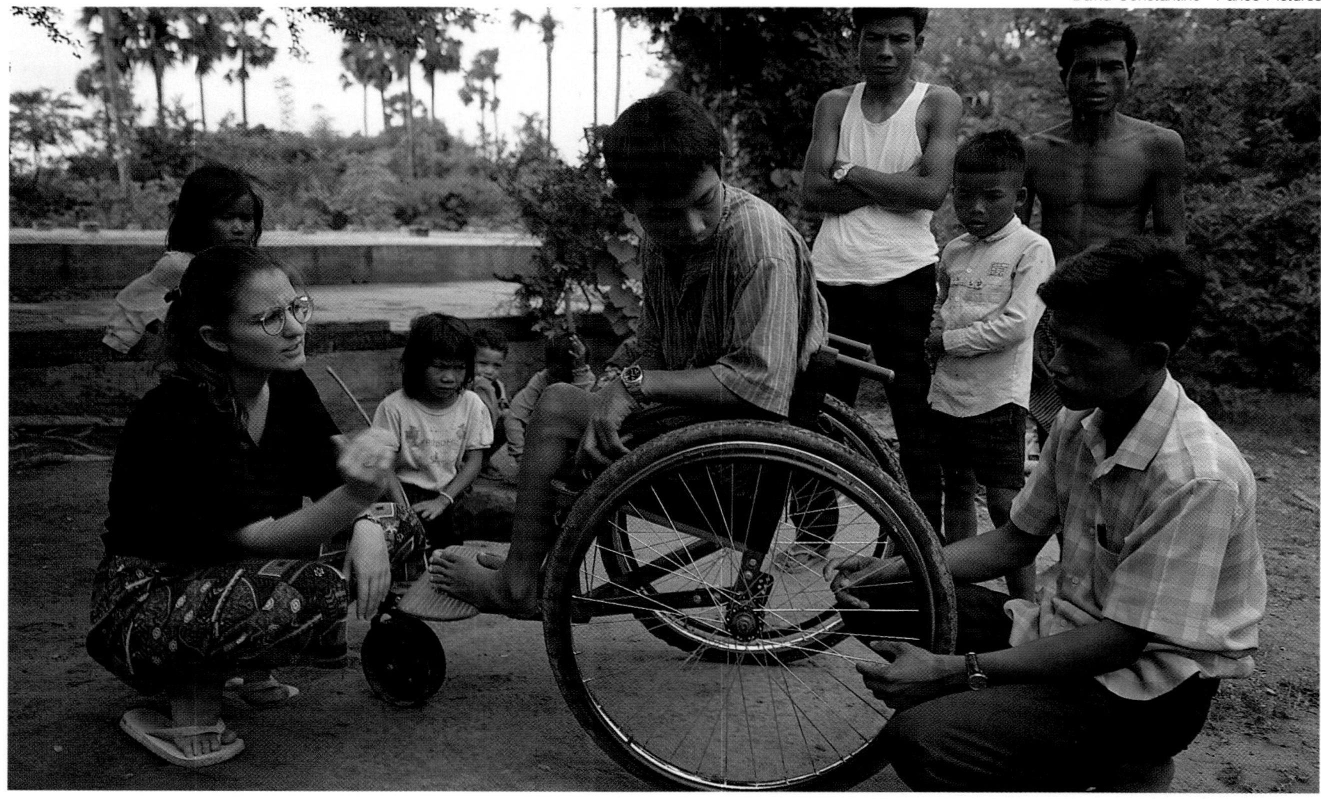

A member of Motivation Charitable Trust discusses the mobility needs of a young Cambodian. The U.K.-based organization—closely allied with Whirlwind Wheelchair International—helps make suitable wheelchairs available to people in the Third World.

age to their muscles and joints. Some symptoms of postpolio syndrome can be delayed or partially prevented by the part-time use of a wheelchair. Nonetheless, it is not uncommon for rehabilitation professionals to persuade their clients not to "give in" and use a wheelchair. This stigma associated with wheelchairs, ironically, has sentenced many people with postpolio syndrome and other mobility impairments to struggle with crutches until their bodies are so worn out that they must abandon walking forever.

Sitting: a life-or-death matter

Project Sore Butts is an example of a successful collaboration in which rehabilitation specialists truly listened to the needs of wheelchair riders. Pressure sores are a life-threatening but often overlooked problem for those who spend long periods sitting. Their primary cause is sustained pressure over the bony prominences of the buttocks—*i.e.,* the ischial tuberosities on the posterior of the pelvis, or the tailbone, that bear the weight of the seated body. Although the skin and underlying tissue can withstand very high pressure over short periods, irreversible damage can begin within two hours if the pressure is not relieved. Even fairly low pressure, if unrelieved, can cause tissue breakdown. Prolonged pressure stretches and compresses blood and lymphatic vessels, preventing tissue from receiving oxygen and hampering the skin's ability to rid itself of waste products. Underlying muscle, fat, tissue, and bone are eventually affected. Factors such as moisture and friction can easily exacerbate the problem.

Until the pressure sores on his buttocks heal, this wheelchair builder in Ajoya, Mexico, must ride prone on a scooter board mounted on the back of his wheelchair.

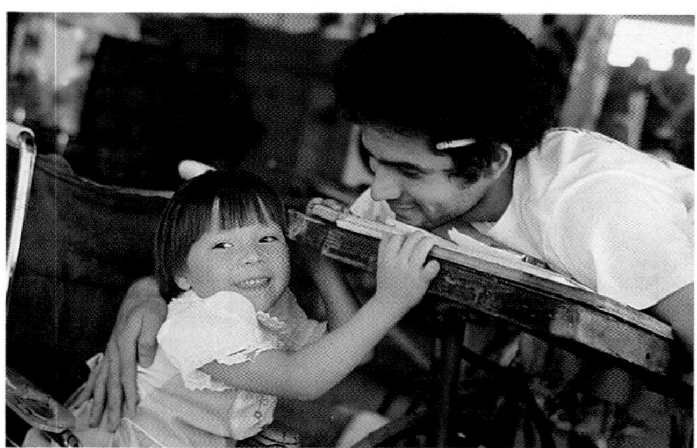

Courtesy of Ralf D. Hotchkiss

Beans, cardboard, and comfort. For the last five years, an international special-interest group within the Rehabilitation Engineering and Assistive Technology Society of North America (RESNA) has enlisted the help of rehabilitation technicians, engineers, and therapists to develop new approaches to preventing pressure sores with pressure-relief cushions and education. The first steps were listening to consumers and taking a close look at all the existing solutions to the problem of wheelchair-induced pressure sores. In 1992, during preliminary discussions of this group, an easily constructed pressure gauge was conceived by rehabilitation engineer Michael Heinrich in Chicago. The device enables users to test the effectiveness of pressure-relief cushions anytime and anywhere. (A problem that some wheelchair riders face is a lessening of sensation in the buttocks, resulting in a lack of awareness of pressure and consequent tissue damage.)

In 1996 at RESNA's annual conference, Project Sore Butts sponsored a pressure-relief-cushion design contest. A number of winning designs using unique materials resulted. The three top-ranked cushions included one made from dried beans and rice, one made from seven bicycle inner tubes, and the Whirlwind cushion, made from many layers of corrugated cardboard, molded to the shape of the individual rider, with a layer of foam on top. All three showed excellent pressure distribution. The first two had the advantage of fitting any rider, while the latter had to be custom fit. The Whirlwind provided the best posture control but required more skill to make. Time will tell how well the first two cushions will accommodate riders; the Whirlwind cushion has had the chance to prove itself over the last 15 years. RESNA will hold repeated contests over the next several years until a selection of suitable cushions for different situations has been found.

At a workshop in Mexico, Sara Hotchkiss, the author's sister, cuts layers of corrugated cardboard to help fabricate the custom-fitted base of a Whirlwind seat cushion.

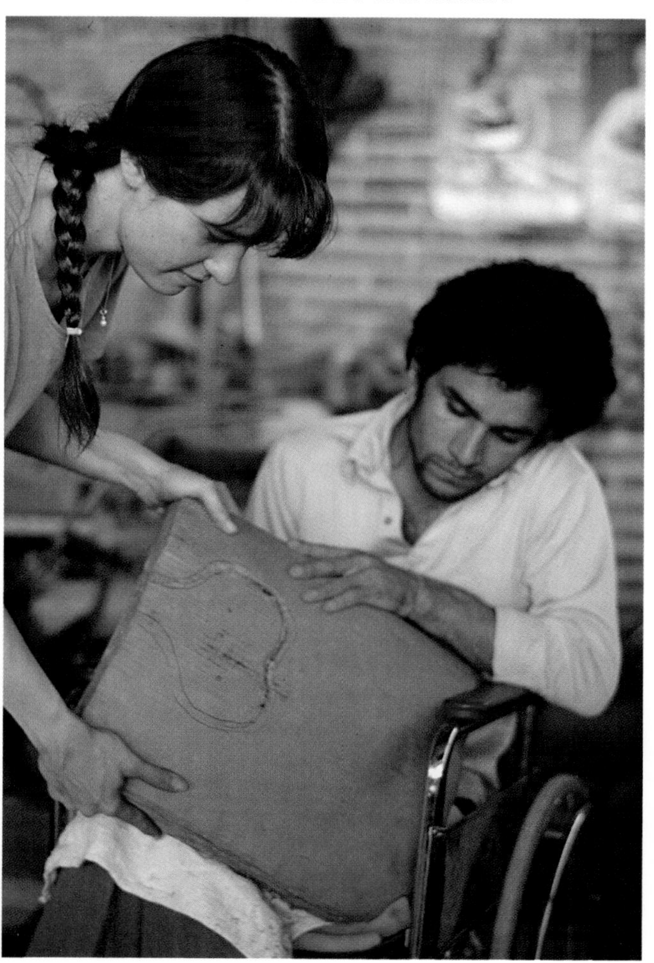

Courtesy of Ralf D. Hotchkiss

Focus on Third-World children. For the past 10 years, the focus of physical therapist Jean Anne Zollars's work has been on seating needs of wheelchair riders—especially of children—in Third World countries. In 1995, when Zollars was scheduled to lead a workshop in El Salvador, the expected funding did not come through. She taught the class anyway. Along with other physical therapists and some very motivated parents of kids with disabilities, she was able to gather all the needed materials (*e.g.,* Styrofoam, wood, glue, tape, tools) to assemble individually designed seat inserts that include back and sides for each child who needed one. No one had preconceived notions about how a child "should" be supported. Each child's unique needs were reflected in his or her custom-made seat insert. Once basic insert prototypes had been devised, building techniques were taught to the parents and therapists by local carpenters. Moreover, since the parents, children, and local therapists were involved from the start, designs could be modified and adapted as the children grew and their needs changed. (All this is the subject of a recently published book by Zollars, *Special Seating: An Illustrated Guide.*)

The big question of cost

The cost of labor and materials for a high-quality wheelchair is between $100 and $300, depending on the country. But people who require wheeled mobility because of physical disabilities are typically among the poorest of the poor. So how can they possibly afford one? The answer, at present, is that most cannot and probably will never have a wheelchair. But this situation can be turned around. Many disabled people, even in the poorest countries, can raise enough money to buy and maintain a wheelchair—if the price is low and the durability high. People too poor to buy their own are nonetheless beginning to get them through innovative combinations of international aid and local advocacy. Such resources include:

- **Consumer credit programs.** Over 10 years ago, a consumer fund was established in Colombia to help hundreds of people buy their first wheelchairs. A similar consumer credit fund is being established in Siberia.
- **Wheelchair rental.** Without the large initial outlay required for purchasing a wheelchair, more people could afford one. In such a scenario, outside donors would underwrite the construction of a wheelchair fleet; the wheelchair manufacturer then would retain ownership of chairs, charging customers a nominal rental fee. The manufacturer would have a considerable incentive to make durable wheelchairs that would work well over a long period. This approach, though not yet in practice, is under discussion in Russia and Kenya.
- **Partial subsidies.** Consumers who pay for their own wheelchairs will often insist on high quality. By contrast, people who receive free wheelchairs usually do not complain when the wheelchairs break. For one thing, it is not clear to whom they should complain, and experience has shown that complaining generally does not help. With partial subsidies from outside sources, wheelchairs can be made affordable to those who need them. In addition, this strategy leaves the critical consumer-manufacturer feedback loop intact.

Newer types of wheelchairs, designed specifically to meet the daily challenges of life in poorer rural areas, are needed. Though wheelchair riders in the Third World have developed chairs with the kinds of features needed for mobility in a rough urban or rural setting, there are still considerable limits to where they can go. While Westerners can usually avoid obsta-

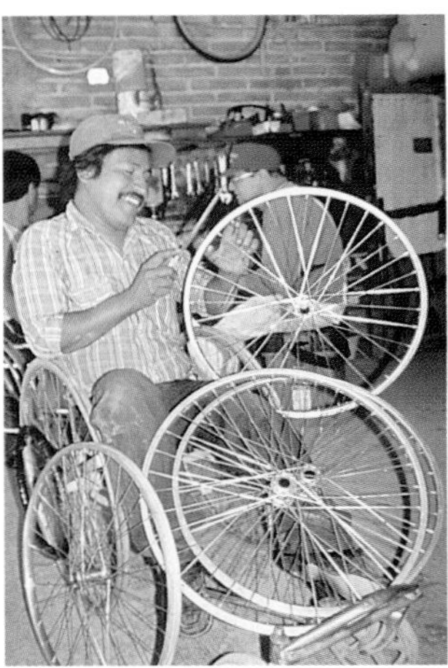

Wheelchair rider-builders in some of the world's poorest countries are meeting their own real-life mobility needs, fashioning chairs that meet meticulous design standards out of locally available and affordable materials.

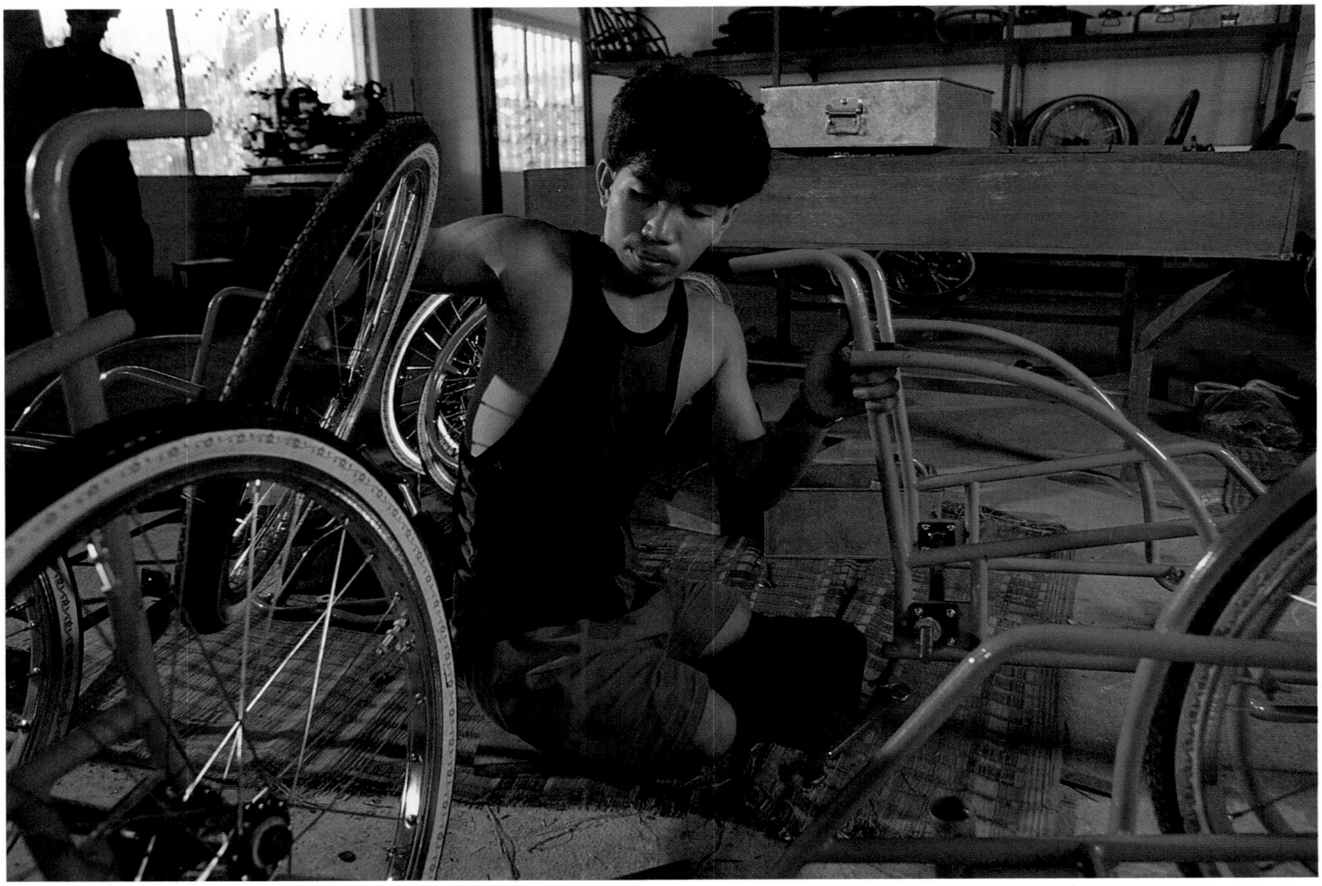

(Top and opposite page) Courtesy of Ralf D. Hotchkiss; (above) Peter Charleworth—Saba

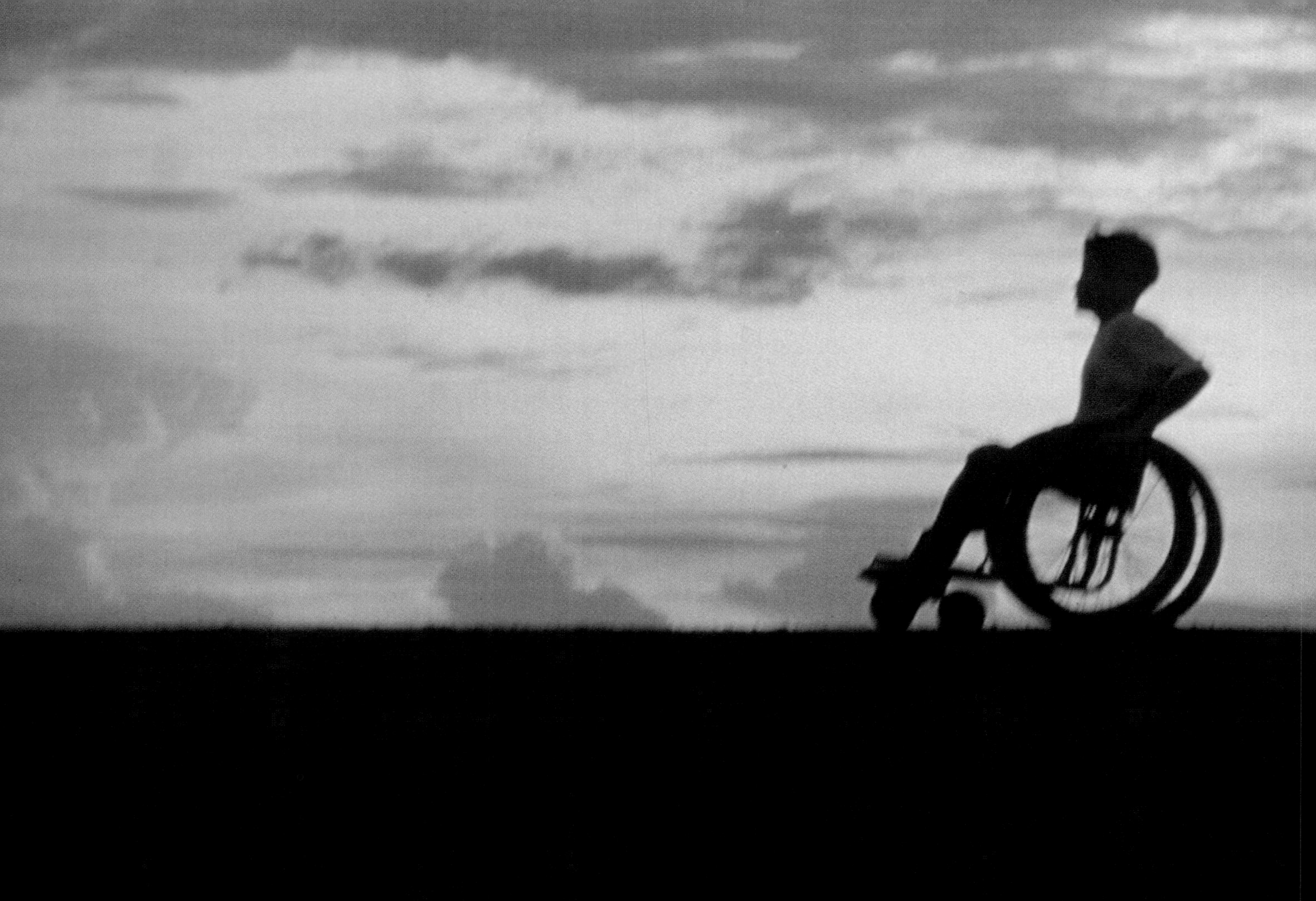

A dream come true for a Cambodian: riding into the Phnom Penh sunset in a self-built wheelchair.

cles and still get where they need to be, riders in less-developed countries are reminded many times a day that they need to invent chairs that are even more capable of negotiating rough terrain than the ones they have. Among the limitations of current wheelchair design are:

- the inability to ascend or descend a steep slope or traverse a side slope
- the inability to traverse a path that is any narrower than 61 centimeters (2 feet)
- the limited ability to cross challenging terrain such as soft sand, mud, loose gravel, and rocky paths
- a limited curb-climbing ability (of 5 to 18 centimeters [2 to 7 inches], depending on the rider)
- the inability to get across town at a sustained swift speed

New tools, new rules

When consumers in industrialized countries must solve technological problems, they generally (1) look for ready-made solutions, (2) rely on "experts," or (3) seek a newer, more advanced model of an appliance or tool that will do the job. In contrast, in less-developed countries, where there are generally no such options and people can rarely afford manufactured goods, they must show exceptional persistence and ingenuity to solve everyday problems. In the process, grass-roots inventors have come up with novel means of improving the lives of people with disabilities.

Around the world, people with mobility impairments are developing a "survival culture." Just getting out of their houses and going about the routines of daily living are acts of determination, creativity, and adaptation. Physical and cultural barriers force disabled people to be continually inventive—as well as politically active. The need to bend society's "rules" in order to live productively will surely lead to the creation of ever more innovative and useful tools in the future.

FOR FURTHER INFORMATION

- Burns, August; Lovich, Ronnie; Maxwell, Jane; and Shapiro, Katherine. *Where Women Have No Doctor* (1977). Hesperian Foundation, PO Box 11577, Berkeley CA 94712-2577.
- Werner, David. *Where There Is No Doctor* (1977; rev. ed., 1992). Hesperian Foundation.
- Werner, David. *Disabled Village Children* (1987). Hesperian Foundation.
- Werner, David. *Nothing About Us Without Us* (1997). HealthWrights, 964 Hamilton Ave, Palo Alto CA 94301.
- Zollars, Jean Anne. *Special Seating: An Illustrated Guide* (1996). Otto Bock Inc., 3000 Xenium Ln, Minneapolis MN 55441. MHA

THE BOOKSHELF

Because the editors of the *Medical and Health Annual* suspect that its readers are people who appreciate a good book, they have selected and reviewed 26 recent medicine- and health-related volumes from among the hundreds that have been published in the past year or so—books that they think should appeal to people with a lively curiosity about medicine, health, and/or the biological and psychological sciences. The list is a broad one and includes some titles that have received wide acclaim and others that have been less well noted. There are personal accounts of living with and triumphing over illness, books that offer practical advice, others that grapple with pressing bioethical and legal questions, and fascinating histories. There are even a novel about psychoanalysis by a practicing psychiatrist and a collection of essays about the neurophysiology of celebrated athletes from Michael Jordan to the late golf legend Ben Hogan. An excerpt from the text precedes each review.

The Broken Mirror: Understanding and Treating Body Dysmorphic Disorder
KATHARINE A. PHILLIPS, M.D.
New York City: Oxford University Press, 1996.
357 pp., appendixes, glossary, index.
$25.00

> *"I don't like talking about my problem," [Jennifer] said. "You'll probably think I'm silly or vain. But I'm not," she said with tears in her eyes. " This is a very serious problem. I can't even tell you how bad it is." She sat silently for a minute, looking down anxiously, as if trying to decide what to say and how to express it.... "I think I'm really ugly. In fact, I think I'm one of the ugliest people in the whole world."*

While most people would agree that vanity is not a characteristic that should intentionally be cultivated, they would also acknowledge that appearances are important. Studies show that attractive individuals have advantages over those whose appearance is less pleasing to the eye. Moreover, the public is bombarded daily by images of "supermodels" and movie stars who represent standards of physical beauty that—for most people—are unachievable. It is no wonder, then, that many people spend a considerable amount of time worrying about how they look.

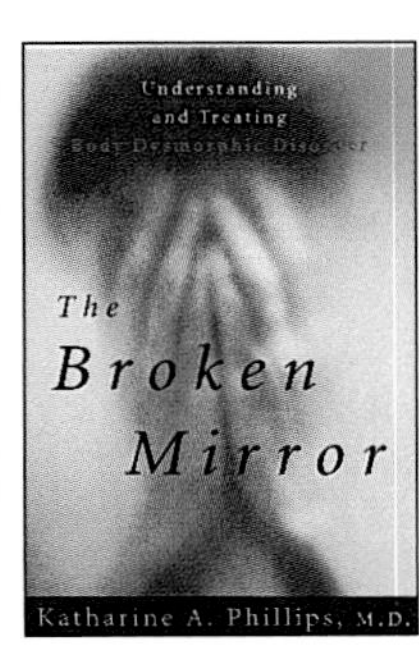

For some, a preoccupation with physical appearance—and physical imperfections—becomes an obsession that rules, and in many cases ruins, their lives. Like Jennifer, these people have a psychiatric condition called body dysmorphic disorder (BDD). Although they may be unremarkable looking—or sometimes even very attractive—the image they see in the mirror is distorted.

Not only are those with BDD haunted by physical defects that do not exist; the defects are perceived as huge, monstrous, alien-like. So overwhelmed are they by this imagined ugliness that they may not be able to look in a mirror, leave the house, or think of anything except their defect, be it "blotchy" skin or a "hideous" nose. Many people would be tempted to dismiss such concerns as silly, but the consequences of BDD are no laughing matter. Patients may drop out of school, avoid friends, become reclusive; some will commit suicide.

Katharine A. Phillips, chief of outpatient services and director of the Body Dysmorphic Disorder and Body Image Program at Butler Hospital in Providence, R.I., is a pioneer in the study of BDD and has written widely about the subject for professional journals. *The Broken Mirror* is the first book on BDD written for a nonspecialist audience.

Phillips defines BDD as a preoccupation with an imagined or slight defect that causes clinically significant emotional distress or impairs normal social functioning. Although the disorder is not uncommon—it affects an estimated 2% of the population—it often goes undiagnosed or is misdiagnosed because patients are ashamed to discuss the problem for fear of seeming vain and superficial. Another common fear is that, like their friends and families, the physician or therapist will attempt to reassure them that there is nothing wrong with them, which makes them feel that their distress is not being taken seriously. Ironically, when given reassurance that they look perfectly fine, they assume it is a lie—of course, no one would be cruel enough to tell them the truth: that they are grotesquely ugly.

Symptomatic behaviors of BDD include excessive grooming (*e.g.*, tweezing, combing, teasing), persistent picking at the skin, camouflaging (*e.g.*, swathing the face with bandages), repeatedly seeking and sometimes undergoing plastic surgery, requesting reassurance ("Does my nose look okay?"), and making comparisons ("My hair is so much thinner than his"). Affected individuals may go to great lengths to avoid mirrors or, in some cases, to check their appearance in virtually every reflective surface they pass. Some refuse to leave home for fear of ridicule.

Phillips suspects that BDD is caused by a combination of three factors: (1) a shortage of the neurotransmitter serotonin in the brain; (2) psychological problems such as low self-esteem or a history of emotional abuse; and (3) sociocultural influences such as the impossibly high standards of physical attractiveness promoted by the fashion, advertising, and other industries. Of all the treatments that have been tried for BDD, a relatively new class of drugs called selective serotonin reuptake inhibitors, of which the best known is Prozac (fluoxetine), has been the most successful. These drugs increase the amount of serotonin available to nerve cells in the brain. Many patients treated with Prozac and related compounds not only cease to be preoccupied with their defects but actually perceive a physical change. Thus, it has been reported by patients that skin blemishes have cleared up, thin hair has become thicker, or a "lopsided" face has suddenly become symmetrical. Discontinuing the medication or reducing the dosage has caused the defect to return. On the basis of these observations, Phillips has concluded that BDD is primarily a biological rather than a psychiatric condition.

In *The Broken Mirror* Phillips's patients describe their tortured existences in their own words. The author provides guidelines for distinguishing BDD from normal concerns about appearance and explores other mental disorders—such as obsessive-compulsive disorder, anorexia nervosa, depression, and social phobia—that have features in common with BDD and may overlap or coexist with it. She hopes that this book and her research will lead more BDD sufferers and their families to seek help.

—*Katherine I. Gordon*

The Cambridge Illustrated History of Medicine
ROY PORTER, ed.
Cambridge, Eng.: Cambridge University Press, 1996.
400 pp., reference guide, index of medical personalities, bibliography, index. $39.95

> *Perceptions of sickness have varied greatly over time and place, shaped by diverse circumstances.... In Shakespeare's time, melancholy was called the 'courtier's coat of arms' and regarded as an eligible, fashionable disorder of the elite; but a poor person suffering similar symptoms—what we might call depression—was considered 'mopish' and rebuked for being sullen. Gender has counted too: the condition that in 1800 would have been called 'hysteria' in a woman might have been diagnosed as 'hypochondria' in a man.*

In reading a history of an unfamiliar subject, the nonexpert tends to be most satisfied if the authority dispensing the information can discern some sort of authentic pattern. The six contributors to this volume do just that. Thus, readers of this excellent history will learn a great deal about what has made people sick through the ages. The first infectious diseases occurred more than 2,000 years ago when hunter-gatherers settled down to farm. Proximity to domesticated animals and residence in permanent dwellings promoted the transmission of infectious disease, as did such basic agricultural activities as breaking the sod, clearing the land, and flooding fields for irrigation. When, eventually, agriculture succeeded in producing food surpluses, cities were able to grow, though at first they were so unhealthy that more inhabitants died than were born, and the population size was maintained only through constant migration from the countryside. Ill health was fueled in the 18th and 19th centuries by the Industrial Revolution and in the present century by drastic changes in lifestyle.

History, by its very nature, is replete with fascinating "stories." Medical history is no exception. In one of the 10 chapters into which the book is divided, "The Rise of Medicine," the reader learns that the crusaders in the 11th and 12th centuries were so impressed by Byzantine medicine—and especially hospital care—that they copied many of its features back home in feudal western Europe. A chapter that traces the evolution of medical science shows how certain of its heroes, like the pioneering 17th-century physiologist William Harvey (who discovered the circulation of the blood), helped launch the "New Science," which was then popularized during the Enlightenment. The rise of science as it is known today (*e.g.,* the germ theory of disease), however, had to wait until the 19th century. At that time doctors from the United States and Great Britain flocked to study in France and, particularly, in Germany and Austria. A chapter on the history of primary care concludes with observations on the ironic "flip side" of today's miracle drugs and technological innovation: growing dissatisfaction among patients, who, perceiving doctors as "remote and arrogant," respond not with gratitude but with malpractice suits.

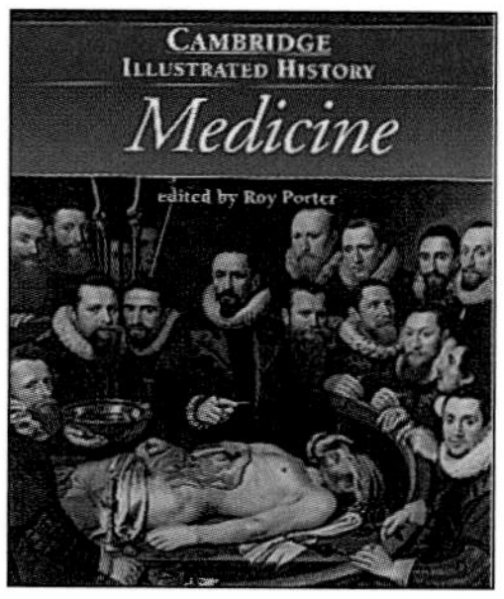

This carefully researched, splendidly illustrated history concludes with a chapter that peers into medicine's future, considering, among other things, computers in medicine, robots in surgery, the development of new drugs and new drug-resistant pathogens, global warming, reproductive dilemmas, and future ways of death. The text throughout this volume is enlivened with quotations from diverse sources. Extracts from doctors' memoirs and diaries provide some particularly illuminating glimpses into medical practice in earlier times: "In some cases I knew, even in the beginning, that my efforts would be futile.... Of course, one left [the patient] some medicine.... It was just about as important as the deacon's 'Amen' during the preacher's sermons—it did no harm and it was an evidence of good faith."

If there is any one topic that is slighted in this superb volume, it is pediatrics—pity! Although its history is relatively short, the discipline of caring for children makes up as much as a quarter of today's medical practice.

While the contributors approach their subjects from a distinctly British point of view, the book is international in its scope. Editor Roy Porter, a respected scholar at the Wellcome Institute for the History of Medicine, London, contributes four of the chapters, along the way dispelling some common myths and coming to some unsettling conclusions. The reader learns, for example, that the accepted stereotype of the 17th- or 18th-century surgeon as "Dr. Sawbones"—a blundering and bloody operator—is unjustified. The surgeon's main business, Porter shows, was in fact taking care of minor repairs: pulling teeth, trussing ruptures, and managing the occasional inflamed finger or toe.

In the chapter on mental illness, Porter offers some depressing observations about the state of contemporary psychiatric practice, concluding that the once-hailed "drug revolution"—which was supposed to enable the release of institutionalized mental patients—has been only partially successful. Has society in effect gone "back to square one," he wonders, with so-called community care replacing institutionalization as a new form of heartlessness? Is psychiatry perhaps the exception to the rule that, as the other contributors to this well-written, well-organized book show, medical disciplines improve over time? In themselves, those questions are reason enough for readers to take this particular history of medicine seriously.

—*Stephen Lock, M.D.*

Cheating Time: Science, Sex, and Aging
ROGER GOSDEN.
New York: W.H. Freeman and Co., 1996.
427 pp., illustrations, glossary, bibliography, index. $23.95

> *Trade-offs between longevity and reproduction help to explain why some species live much longer than others. The balance of advantages is influenced by the circumstances of life.... Species that live in risky environments would be well advised to invest heavily—and soon—in reproduction, even if it threatens their very existence. When the food supply fluctuates wildly or where predators and parasites are abundant, those that are more fecund early on will be the winners in the struggle for genetic survival.*

The search for the fountain of youth is probably as old as the human species itself. Explorers, mystics, mountebanks, and scientists all have looked for an elixir, a regimen, an incantation, or some other marvel that would either maintain or restore vitality. In *Cheating Time,* Roger Gosden offers a brief but wide-ranging history of rejuvenation therapies, along with a summary of current knowledge of the intricate biochemistry of the reproductive and aging processes in many organisms. The author also describes the ongoing scientific search for a way to arrest, or at least retard, the inexorable process of human aging. A professor of reproductive biology at the University of Leeds, Eng., Gosden began his long career in the field under the tutelage of the pioneering infertility specialist Robert Edwards (who, with his coworker Patrick Steptoe, was responsible for the birth in 1978 of the world's first test-tube baby).

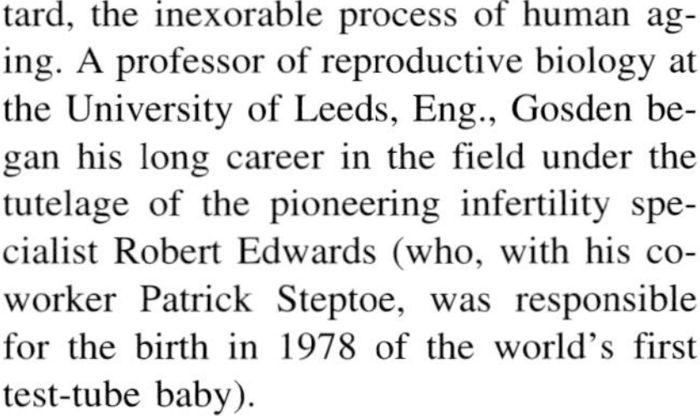

Gosden's observations on the reproductive strategies of nonhuman organisms are instructive and memorable. These strategies range from the ceaseless division of so-called immortal cell lines to the procreative frenzy of the male brown marsupial mouse, which dies, aged and desiccated, at the end of a single mating season. This precipitous descent into old age and death wipes out all of the species' adult males, which thereby reduces competition for food and ensures a fresh supply of vigorous adolescent male impregnators for the next year's mating season.

Because, at least from an evolutionary perspective, individuals need survive only until they have reproduced, scientists speculate that some advantages must accrue to creatures that mature more slowly. Not the least of these advantages is that longer-lived species have more opportunities than their short-lived counterparts to mate and produce offspring. But, as Gosden notes, a longer period of reproductive vigor is an advantage only as long as the genes that are transmitted are healthy. In the case of many animals, humans among them, there comes a time when a sort of genetic law of diminishing returns sets in, possibly influenced by the built-in mechanism known as the "biological clock." Given that human life expectancy in some developed countries has nearly doubled in the past century—while the average age of menopause is unchanged—Gosden predicts that hormone replacement and similar strategies will continue to expand the opportunities for postmenopausal pregnancy.

Citing the high rate of miscarriage in human pregnancies and the purported negative effect of environmental pollution on sperm counts, Gosden suggests that recent increases in life expectancy have done little more for humankind than add extra years of disease and disability at the end of life. Nonetheless, he is optimistic about the future of antiaging research. While he believes that replacement of male and female hormones is currently the most effective bulwark against aging, he predicts that gene therapy and other, as-yet-undiscovered molecular genetic interventions will eventually surpass hormones as a means of delaying, if not preventing, the whole spectrum of age-related deficits.

As is clear from the title, the author views time as an adversary, a force to be not only reckoned with but countered and resisted. Even in evolutionary terms, however, time can be a positive factor in the shaping of outcomes. Gosden's penetrating look backward and ahead might have been at least as well served if he had called his book *Keeping Time, Using Time,* or even *Saving Time.*

—*Jean S. Gottlieb, Ph.D.*

The Diving Bell and the Butterfly
JEAN-DOMINIQUE BAUBY
(translated by Jeremy Leggatt).
New York: Alfred A. Knopf, 1997.
132 pp. $20.00

> *Once, I was a master at recycling leftovers. Now I cultivate the art of simmering memories. You can sit down to a meal at any hour, with no fuss or ceremony.... If I do the cooking it is always a success. The* **bœuf bourguignon** *is tender, the* **bœuf en gelée** *translucent, the apricot pie possesses just the requisite tartness. Depending on my mood, I treat myself to a dozen snails, a plate of Alsatian sausage with sauerkraut, and a bottle of late-vintage golden Gewürztraminer; or else I savor a simple soft-boiled egg with fingers of toast and lightly salted butter. What a banquet! The yolk flows warmly over my palate and down my throat. And indigestion is never a problem.*

On Dec. 8, 1995, Jean-Dominique Bauby, then the 43-year-old editor in chief of the French fashion magazine Elle and the divorced father of two, suffered a massive stroke that left him paralyzed, speechless, and unable to breathe or swallow on his own. Amazingly, he emerged from this catastrophe mentally intact and fully conscious—a victim of a rare condition known as "locked-in syndrome." Not until the final pages of this moving memoir does Bauby describe the cataclysmic stroke itself and the events that transpired during his last minutes as "a perfectly functioning earthling." Most of his poignant story oscillates between descriptions of the rich interior life he created for himself and the strange existence locked-in syndrome thrust upon him.

Awakening from a coma in a hospital in Berck-sur-Mer, France, 20 days after the stroke, Bauby found that capricious Nature had left him a single gift: the ability to blink his left eye. With this minute gesture, he was able to reestablish communication with the rest of the world. The system was ingeniously simple; the alphabet was rearranged so that the

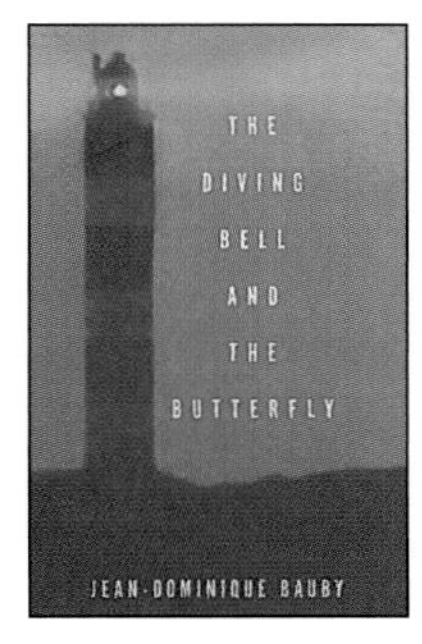

most frequently used letters in French (E, S, and A) were first in order. Bauby's visitors would read the list of letters aloud. By blinking his eye when a reader got to the letter he sought, Bauby could spell out, letter by letter and word by word, his end of the conversation with anyone who had the patience and instinct to master the "code," as he called it. With the assistance of a faithful transcriber, he used this painstaking system to write *The Diving Bell and the Butterfly,* his remarkable meditation on being alive.

Although an ineffable sadness pervades his narrative—so much is irretrievably lost—it is still radiant with a love of life in all its beauty and perversity. Bauby marvels at the things he once took for granted—getting out of bed in the morning, shaving himself, drinking a cup of hot chocolate. He loves to be taken in his wheelchair to the beach near the hospital, where his greatest pleasure is in the redolent aroma of potatoes deep-frying at a waterfront food concession. He spends hours watching and smelling the sea from a hospital balcony.

His children bring heart-wrenching sweetness to his solitary life—their innocence, their solicitude, their drawings, their youth. Spending Father's Day in their company, he longs to ruffle his son's hair and is overcome with the enormity of his physical isolation: "There are no words to express it. My condition is monstrous, iniquitous, revolting horrible. Suddenly I can take no more. Tears well...."

Yet Bauby wastes few words feeling sorry for himself or railing against his fate. His vibrant imagination can spirit him out of the prison of his immobile body and take him anywhere he wishes: to the market, where he assembles the ingredients for a luscious meal; to scenes from his childhood; to exotic far-off places; or home to his Paris apartment to sleep beside his beloved. It is almost as if, having been robbed of most physical manifestations of being alive, Bauby has liberated his sense of aliveness from the confines of his body, setting it free with even greater intensity in his mind and imagination. The strength he draws from his interior life is a form of grace through which he manages to transcend his own grief and suffering. In a tragic ending to an already heartbreaking story, Bauby died in March 1997, two days after the French publication of his book.

—*Jean S. Gottlieb, Ph.D.*

Do We Still Need Doctors?
JOHN D. LANTOS, M.D.
New York: Routledge, 1997.
214 pp., notes, index. $24.95

> ***I've made quite a few mistakes in my time. They come back to haunt me late at night. Missing a diagnosis, prescribing the wrong drug, botching a procedure. Sometimes, patients have died as a result of my mistakes. Other times, my mistakes have increased their suffering. When they come back to me, late at night, I hold court in my mind, replaying events, wondering whether they were honest mistakes, forgivable mistakes, or if not, how I can go on.***

In this book John D. Lantos, a pediatrician and bioethicist at the University of Chicago, reflects on the state of his profession and wonders in what form it—and he—will survive the radical changes that are engulfing doctors, patients, and the health care system itself. "Do we still need doctors?" he wonders. With this question he challenges himself and his readers to think analytically about the state of health care in the United States. Concerns about patient autonomy, assisted suicide, and burgeoning technology and skyrocketing costs are transforming the way doctors view their profession, the way patients see their doctors, and the way both perceive hospitals and other health care institutions. Doctors, in Lantos's view, must continue to listen, advise, support, and comfort—rather than allowing themselves to be turned into medical administrators or merely the interpreters of test results.

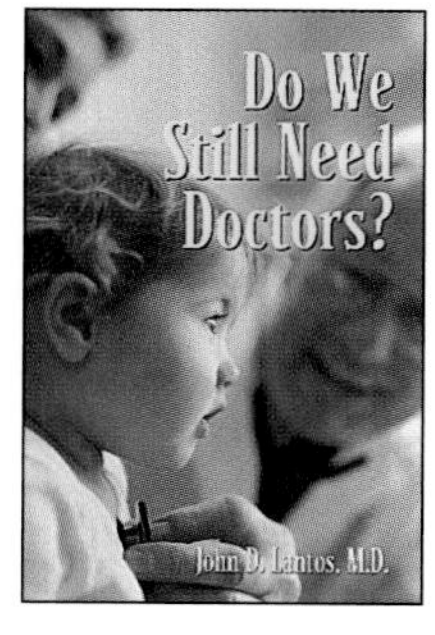

Lantos is, first and foremost, a compassionate human being who is keenly aware of his own fallibility. These qualities emerge clearly in his accounts of many real-life situations that he has faced over many years as a practicing physician and ethics consultant at a major urban medical center. He is also a person of a thoughtful and philosophical nature who has read widely. His reading has not been confined to discourses on health care policy but includes major works of fiction by such disparate writers as Leo Tolstoy and the late Canadian novelist Robertson Davies. Quotations from several of these sources enrich his text.

Lantos examines aspects of contemporary medicine such as "doctor productivity" and "delivery of health care services," suggesting that they exemplify the move toward an impersonal, economics-driven style of medical care that inserts services into patients, assembly-line style. He looks at economic concepts such as "opportunity costs" (*i.e.,* a dollar spent on health care is a dollar that could be spent for something else) used to evaluate the relative merits of health care compared with other public health and safety needs like safe water, crime reduction, and care of the homeless. He imagines future generations looking back on the late 20th century and asking why certain inequalities were tolerated and choices made: "How could we have devoted so many resources to medical care for a few people with rare diseases and failed to provide prenatal care for pregnant women, immunizations or lead-free housing for our children?"

Developments in research and technology—from the decoding of the human genome to the development of sophisticated diagnostic imaging devices—are landing doctors and their patients on terrain as unexplored as outer space. Ethical and moral concerns are prominent features of this new landscape, and Lantos speculates on how they will be integrated into future medical practice. Many of the ethical dilemmas that trouble doctors today are as old as humankind itself: What and how much should a physician tell a dying patient about his or her condition and prognosis? How should the doctor balance a patient's "right" to know against another patient's unspoken but nonetheless ardent wish not to?

Lantos describes how virtuoso technologies keep a critically ill baby alive—at staggering cost—and he agonizes over the question of "best interest." Whose interest comes first? The infant's? The parents'? Those of the medical institution? Economic considerations must be factored in; if hospitals are to profit, they must promote the use of income-producing technologies such as those of the neonatal intensive care unit. Yet every dollar spent to keep a doomed child alive is a dollar taken away from the funding of public health programs that would benefit enormous numbers of children.

Clinical trials in which patients are randomly assigned to either a treatment or a control group for the purpose of testing a drug or procedure and "informed consent" are two concepts that bear directly on another issue of great concern to Lantos: "truth telling." The author has the philosopher's curiosity about the nature of truth and the scientist's respect for it as a pillar of scientific method.

Lantos's humanism radiates throughout this book. While he maintains a sense of optimism about the future of medicine, he is also wistful about the passing of the family doctor who made house calls and listened compassionately not only to patients' lungs but also to their litany of small complaints.

—Jean S. Gottlieb, Ph.D.

In the Shadow of Polio: A Personal and Social History
KATHRYN BLACK.
Reading, Mass.: Addison-Wesley Publishing Co., 1996.
307 pp., appendix, notes, bibliography, index. $23.00

> *The summer passed, and then the fall, the measure kept by the whooshing of the chest respirator and the mesmerizing creaks of the rocking bed; from anywhere in our small house, one could hear the humming, mechanical sounds of Mother being breathed. These were reassuring, lulling sounds. We became unaccustomed to silence, which was a signal for alarm. A fear of death, which no one spoke of, shadowed those months.... Mother was like a bubble we tiptoed around, fearing the worst. Often enough, something would happen to remind us of how fragile her existence was.*

Although polio was described as long ago as 1500 BC, the disease was not identified until the end of the 18th century, and the first epidemic—44 cases in Stockholm—was not recorded until 1887. In earlier centuries the majority of the population developed immunity to polio by contracting mild cases of the disease in infancy. Ironically, the development of modern sanitation systems reduced the public's exposure to the poliovirus and, consequently, the opportunity to acquire immunity. Accordingly, during the 20th century polio epidemics increased in severity, at first sporadically and only in certain places.

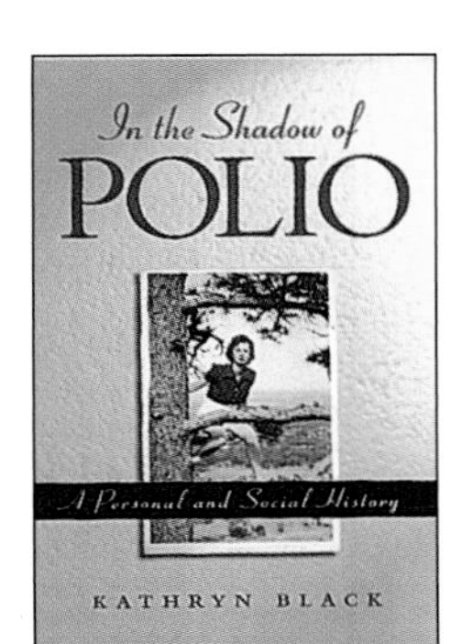

In the 1940s and early '50s, the annual number of cases in the U.S. mushroomed. A climate of fear came to prevail during the summer, the "polio season." Anxious parents refused to let their children engage in any activities that had been linked to the onset of symptoms—overexertion, swimming at public beaches or pools, going to the movies or other crowded venues. Where the next outbreak would occur or which year would be the worst could not be predicted. Seemingly, luck alone determined who would get the disease.

Today the fear and superstition that surrounded polio seem almost medieval. Author Kathryn Black lived "in the shadow of polio" virtually all her life. In 1954, when she was four years old—and the first polio vaccine was being tested—her mother, Virginia, was hospitalized with a severe form of the disease known as bulbospinal polio, which rendered her quadriplegic and unable to breathe, cough, or swallow. After nearly a year of treatment, Virginia Black returned home, still completely paralyzed, suffering from kidney trouble, and breathing only with the aid of a rocking bed. A little less than a year later, she died. The family coped by burying the painful past along with Virginia. The father's ties to the family—never strong—dissolved, and Kathryn's memories of her mother gradually faded.

More than 30 years later, a series of events convinced her that she could no longer repress this important part of her past. With the help of relatives and family friends, she set out to search for the real, vibrant person her mother had been. She became reacquainted with her father, combed through newspaper accounts of polio outbreaks, and was able to track down some of her mother's doctors, therapists, and even fellow patients. At the same time, she set out to learn as much as she could about the disease itself and to examine its profound impact on other patients, their families, and society at large. Her book is a result of this quest. In it, Black skillfully interweaves the story of her mother's struggle, the history of polio, and accounts of polio patients' and the public's reactions to the disease. Particularly intriguing is her exploration of how, in the face of society's emphasis on triumphing over polio—the pervasive attitude that any adversity could be overcome or, at the very least, heroically and cheerfully borne—those left disabled were forced to deny feelings of loss and grief.

Although paralytic poliomyelitis has largely faded from the public consciousness—the disease has been vanquished in the Western Hemisphere and is on the brink of worldwide eradication—it has also made an unexpected reappearance in many former patients who are now experiencing a condition called postpolio syndrome. As well as dealing with a recurrence of physical symptoms and effects they thought they had left far behind, these individuals are now having to confront long-buried emotions about their childhood ordeal. In her account of how she came to grips with her own loss, Black has given a voice to those who experienced polio firsthand; perhaps equally important, she has also created a work that will enlighten a generation for whom the word *polio* figures as just one more in a list of routine immunizations.

—Barbara Whitney

Inside the Brain: Revolutionary Discoveries of How the Mind Works
RONALD KOTULAK.
Kansas City, Mo.: Andrews and McMeel, 1996.
194 pp., index. $21.95

> *Pushing the right biological buttons in the brain, scientists are finding they can make the future brighter for many children whose development otherwise would have been stunted. Based on preliminary results, they can boost IQ levels by ten to twenty points, reduce mental retardation by 50 percent, and cut school failure rates by much more.*
>
> *That there are biological buttons, and that they work to physically reshape the brain by engaging its genetic gears and hormonal levers, is only now being understood. How the buttons work is perhaps the most amazing thing of all. The buttons are the senses—vision, taste, smell, touch, sound—and they can be pushed by experiences from the outside world.*

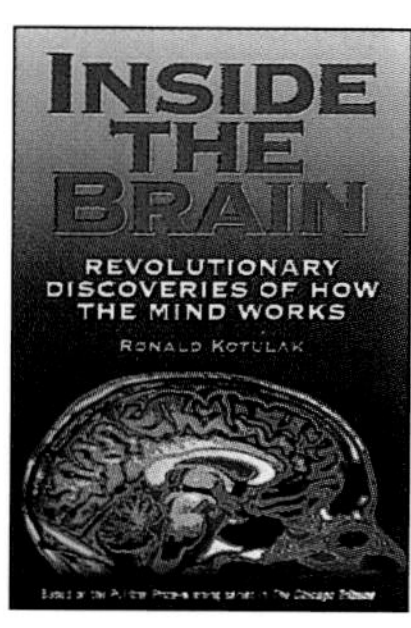

Key developments of the eventful past decade in neuroscientific research are distilled in this volume by Pulitzer Prize-winning *Chicago Tribune* science reporter Ronald Kotulak. The book represents two years of work during which Kotulak interviewed more than 300 neuroscientists, psychologists, and other authorities from around the world. His purpose is not simply to summarize the research data but rather to explore the broader implications of these findings for society as a whole. A better understanding of how the brain develops, he suggests, could point the way to solutions for many of today's most pressing societal problems, including violence, mental illness, and substance abuse.

Despite occasional lapses into oversimplification, Kotulak is adept at illuminating scientific concepts, such as the interrelationship of nature and nurture, with metaphors and similes: "[the] genes, the chemical blueprints of life, establish the framework of the brain, but then the environment takes over and provides the customized finishing touches....The genes provide the building blocks, and the environment acts like an on-the-job foreman, providing instructions for final construction." Because the brain is the product of genetic endowment in combination with life experience, Kotulak explains, it is constantly changing in response to experience. Just as experiences may be positive or negative, so may be their effects on the brain.

Kotulak examines the negative influences of childhood neglect and abuse on brain biochemistry and, ultimately, individual behavior. He also cites recent research indicating that IQ is *not* static and immutable; rather, with education, intelligence level can actually rise. Moreover, it appears that learning is constantly enhancing the brain, forging new connections between neurons. As Bruce McEwen, a neuroscientist at Rockefeller University, New York City, explains, "The brain...feeds on stimulation and it is never too late to feed it."

Neuroscientists have been aware for many years that the brain is most receptive to certain kinds of learning at certain times. The classic example is the mastering of a new language, which is most easily accomplished before the age of 12. As Kotulak points out, the educational establishment has paid little heed to this finding, and this has resulted in funding cuts for foreign-language programs in the early grades—the very time at which children's brains are most receptive.

Inside the Brain is fascinating reading for all who wish to learn about the current state of research in neuroscience. Readers should be aware, however, that it is too early to draw any definite conclusions about the practical applications of this knowledge—to improve public education, for example, or solve such pervasive social problems as crime and violence. The field of neuroscience, like the weather, can change in a minute. Depending on one's point of view, this state of affairs may be either frustrating or exciting. For Kotulak, clearly, it is the latter.

—Andrea Gellin Shindler, M.A.

The Island of the Colorblind, and Cycad Island
OLIVER SACKS.
New York: Alfred A. Knopf, 1997.
298 pp., notes, bibliography, index. $24.00

> *There are no powered vehicles on [the island of] Pingelap, no paved roads, only trodden-earth or gravelled paths through the woods, all connecting, directly or indirectly...with a broader tract with houses to either side, some tin-roofed, and some thatched with leaves. It was on this main path that we were now being taken, escorted by dozens of excited children and young adults....There was a lovely festive quality to this spontaneous procession, which had no order, no program, no leader, no precedence, just a raggle-taggle of wondering, gaping people (they at us, we at them and everything around us), making our way, with many stops and diversions and detours, through the forest-village of Pingelap. Little black-and-white piglets darted across our path....We were struck by the fact that the pigs were black and white and wondered, half seriously, if they had been specially bred for, or by, an achromatopic [colorblind] population.*

Any new book by Oliver Sacks, the eminent British-born U.S. neurologist, is likely to be greeted enthusiastically—especially by readers familiar with *Awakenings* (1973), his classic work on the survivors of the early-20th-century global encephalitis epidemic, or one of his more recent volumes, such as *The Man Who Mistook His Wife for a Hat* (1985) and *An Anthropologist on Mars* (1995). The son of a distinguished physician, Sacks grew up in a comfortable London suburb, fascinated at once by the worlds of nature and literature. The prospect of a research expedition to a tropical atoll stirs in him fond memories of a lifetime of reading—Herman Melville and Robert Louis Stevenson when he was a child and later Charles Darwin, Alfred Russel Wallace, and the other great naturalists. Confronting the "trackless vastness of the Pacific," where sky and ocean fuse into "a single blue bowl," Sacks readily calls to mind the philosopher Immanuel Kant's description: "the terrifying Sublime."

In the 1980s, having treated a patient (an artist, incidentally) who lost his color vision following an automobile accident, Sacks began to wonder about those born with the condition of achromatopsia; would they be compensated by, say, an excessive curiosity or an especially sharp memory? He then discovered that there was a large community of congenitally colorblind individuals on two Micronesian islands, Pingelap and Pohnpei, and set out for a few weeks' research with an ophthalmologist colleague and a Norwegian physiologist, the latter also totally colorblind from birth.

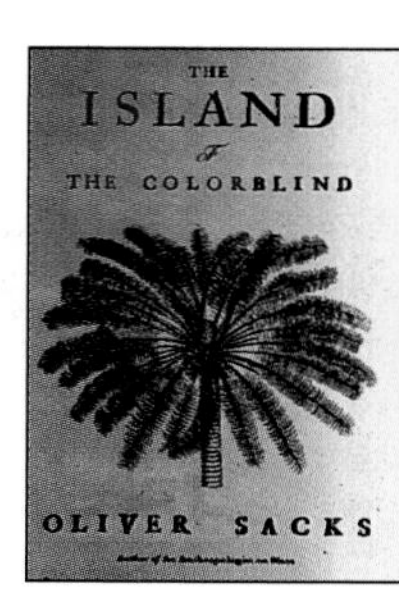

Maskun (literally, "not-see"), the local name for the condition, affects one out of every 12 of the islanders (elsewhere in the world, the prevalence of hereditary colorblindness is one in 30,000), and a third of the population carries the gene for the condition. Sacks found that colorblindness was already well established on Pingelap by 1820, almost 50 years after the island was devastated by a typhoon that reduced the population of nearly 1,000 persons to a mere 20. Following this disaster, the population grew again through extensive inbreeding; among the survivors were the hereditary ruler of the island, who apparently carried the *maskun* gene. Today many of those affected are disadvantaged—often, for instance, they have never learned to read because their poor eyesight meant that they could not see the teacher's handwriting on the blackboard. They are also less likely than other islanders to marry. Nonetheless, sufferers have developed compensatory mechanisms that enable them to cope with daily life, such as exceptionally acute hearing and the habit of working at dusk and dawn when it is easier for them to see than in the bright midday light.

Sacks's narrative is much more than just a clinical or an epidemiological report. It offers the excitement of travel to an exotic destination, together with scintillating accounts of the jungle, the coral reefs, and the amiable society of the local people. As a counterpoint, Sacks also provides descriptions of what 20th-century civilization can do at its worst. The islands have been used for the testing of atomic bombs; the U.S. military maintains a repressive atmosphere in areas where missiles are still being tested (even in the post-Cold War era); and as many as 15,000 low-paid laborers are crowded onto an island about 1.6 kilometers (one mile) long and 185 meters (200 yards) wide (people in these parts will do anything to get work).

Fortunately for the reader, most of this section of the book is occupied by his accounts of *maskun* and the Micronesian environment. He visits a deserted city in its way as impressive as the pyramids or the Colosseum but virtually unknown to the outside world. He gets mildly "stoned" on *sakau,* a potent local brew. He describes life in the tropics in such attractive terms that many readers will be tempted to follow him, if not all the way then at least to some similarly remote and tropical part of the world for their next vacation. And his conclusion about congenital color blindness is mildly encouraging; though geographically separated, much of the world's colorblind community is now united by modern communications. There is even a Web site on the Internet. "Perhaps this new network," Sacks concludes, "this island in cyberspace, is the true Island of the Colorblind."

Cycad Island, the second part of this book, should in theory be equally compelling reading. It concerns another of Sacks's quests to study a strange neurological condition—"lytico-bodig," a cross between amyotrophic lateral sclerosis (ALS, also known as Lou Gehrig's disease and motor neuron disease) and a Parkinson's-like disorder—seen only among the Chamorro people, the inhabitants of the island of Guam. To be sure, there are some captivating descriptions of local fauna and flora, with a special emphasis on the primitive plants called cycads, the seeds of which furnish a source of food for the Chamorros and may be implicated in the disease. On the whole, however, this part of the book is devoted to an exhaustive analysis of the clinical features of the illness and the reasons why none of the competing theories about causation has ever been confirmed. This account is hard going even for somebody accustomed to reading medical texts. And in any case, lytico-bodig is dying out, and the disease may quite possibly disappear altogether before medical science can determine its true cause.

As a literary endeavor, the second section of the book clearly takes a subordinate position. This reviewer got the feeling that the volume started off with the brilliant section on *maskun*—which by itself would not have been commercially viable as a full book—and *Cycad Island* was added to make up the length. Significantly, while Sacks's trip to Guam took place before that to Pingelap, its description is relegated to second place. Nevertheless, there are passages of prose that this reader would not want to have missed, such as this description of a stroll on the beach: "The sand itself, broader with the tide's retreat, was still wet with the phosphorescent sea, and now, as we walked upon it, our footsteps left a luminous spoor."

—*Stephen Lock, M.D.*

Joycelyn Elders, M.D.: From Sharecropper's Daughter to Surgeon General of the United States of America
DR. JOYCELYN ELDERS AND DAVID CHANOFF.
New York: William Morrow and Co., Inc., 1996.
355 pp., illustrations, index. $25.95

> ***One of my points of contention with the religious right is that they are massively engaged on the abortion issue, yet you never see them out there fighting to provide adequate housing or to fund early-childhood education or to improve medical coverage for poor families. In my view, that does not show a will to protect our society's helpless and hopeless. On the contrary...I challenge the Christian Coalition to put its resources into finding ways to care for children in need. If it did that, it would at least have the standing to argue about abortion. There are those in the antiabortion movement whose stand is part of a philosophy that includes opposition to the death penalty and a commitment to the poor. Those groups deserve respect, no matter how deeply I disagree with them about a woman's right to choose. But there are others whose moralizing is hollow because it is not accompanied by charity of the heart.***

This remarkably frank memoir documents the journey of Joycelyn Elders from her birth in a small town in rural Arkansas to her appointment to a series of offices that brought her to the forefront of public health policy making for her state and then for her country. Elders has never been one to mince words. Her views on such highly charged issues as sex education, abortion, and the legalization of drugs were both groundbreaking and politically dangerous. Her candid public response to a question about sex education ultimately caused the firestorm of criticism that led to her resignation from her post as U.S. surgeon general only 15 months after taking office.

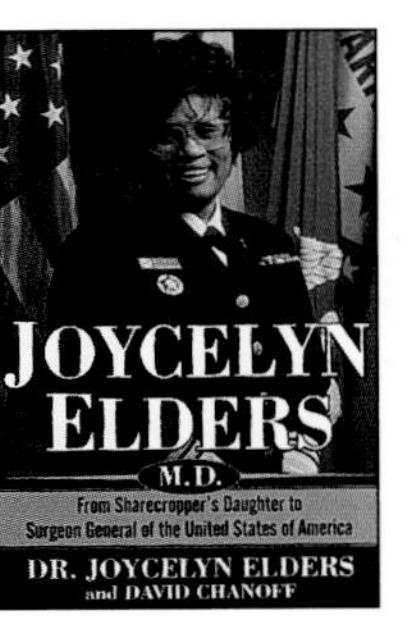

With a few exceptions, Elders tends in this account to downplay the poverty and deprivation of her early days. While it is perfectly clear that her family lacked money and basic necessities such as health care—as a young child her brother Bernard nearly died of a ruptured appendix because, as she puts it, "there were no hospitals around there for any black children"—it is also apparent that Elders was never deprived of love and family support. As the eldest of eight children, she naturally took on the role of caregiver to her siblings. She excelled in school and, as valedictorian of her high-school class at the age of 16, secured for herself one of the few college scholarships to be had at that time.

Throughout Elders's life, opportunities seem to have had a way of presenting themselves, something she modestly chalks up simply to having been in the right place at the right time. That she chooses to portray herself as one who was often privileged rather than underprivileged is perhaps as revealing as any of the personal and professional anecdotes in the book.

She writes openly of her struggle to cope while her husband battled depression; of the stillbirth of their third child, who, had he lived, would have been severely disabled; of the deaths by violence of her foster child and her well-loved brother Bernard; and of the substance-abuse problems of one of her sons. The same determination that enabled her to ignore racial slights and overcome career obstacles seems also to have sustained her through these private trials.

Elders embarked on a career in medicine at a time when women—and especially poor black women—were just beginning to enter this hitherto white-male-dominated profession. Later, as a member of a hospital staff, a university medical school faculty, and state and federal government administrations, she became intimately acquainted with politicking in all its forms, although, as she emphasizes, she herself never set out to be a "politician." Instead, she grew into the role out of necessity, in order to provide her patients with what she felt they needed. Regardless of her office or those who appointed her, she has always been critical of incompetence and bad management wherever she has encountered them.

In addition to learning about the life of an extraordinary woman, readers of this book will also learn—as Elders did in the course of her career—of the distinctions between clinical medical practice and public health administration. As she explains, the health problems of groups require different strategies from the health problems of individuals. It was as health director of the state of Arkansas that she first became acutely aware of the issues about which she is now most passionate—poverty, ignorance, child abuse and neglect, and teen pregnancy—and it is when she writes of these subjects that Elders is most persuasive.

—Sara Brant

Level 4: Virus Hunters of the CDC
JOSEPH B. MCCORMICK, M.D., AND SUSAN FISHER-HOCH, M.D., WITH LESLIE ALAN HORVITZ.
Atlanta, Ga.: Turner Publishing, 1996.
379 pp., maps, illustrations, appendixes, index. $22.95 ($29.95, Canada)

> *The majority of people in the area around Nzara and Yambio [on the Sudan-Zaire border] lived in family compounds, which could be reached only by following tortuous footpaths through the bush consisting mainly of elephant grass nine feet tall. There were, of course, no local maps, so we had to find someone to show us the way.... Then we had to cope with the challenge of figuring out who was related to whom, and who was not. A man might have more than one wife. A woman might identify someone as her brother, and you would write this down. Then she would point to a second man and say, "Yes, that is my brother."... Pretty soon we would have all these brothers listed—maybe nine or ten.... Even with very large families, that was a lot of brothers. It took us some time to realize that her idea of a brother and ours were completely different. In many cultures, calling a man a brother... is only another way of saying that someone was important enough to be accorded all the love and respect due a blood relation. While this practice... might be endearing, it certainly wasn't of much help when it came to defining a group—or "cohort"—in an epidemiological study.*

In 1989 research monkeys in a Reston, Va., laboratory began to die from a mysterious illness that was suspected of being transmissible—and possibly fatal—to humans who came into contact with the animals or their body tissues. Virologist Joseph McCormick was one of the scientists who identified the agent as a new form of the feared Ebola virus. That episode, the subject of the 1994 best-seller *The Hot Zone,* pales beside some other experiences McCormick describes in this suspense-filled story of his 30 years as a virological sleuth.

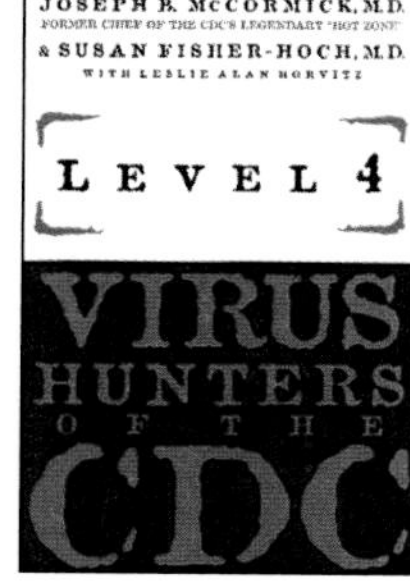

McCormick and his colleague (and later, wife) Susan Fisher-Hoch have lived and worked in some of the world's most inaccessible and impoverished regions. Their mission: to ferret out the sources of a group of virulent diseases, known as viral hemorrhagic fevers, that have periodically erupted into devastating epidemics, principally in Africa. Ebola and Lassa fever, two of the deadliest of these illnesses, have become familiar names in the West now that air travel and international tourism have given the viruses new opportunities to spread. The authors have traveled across continents and cultures pursuing these "Level 4" viruses (as the U.S. Centers for Disease Control and Prevention, or CDC, designates the most lethal and treatment-resistant agents of infection), as well as searching for clues to the epidemiological puzzles posed by AIDS, meningitis, hepatitis C, Legionnaires' disease, the hantaviruses (one of which was responsible for an outbreak and a number of deaths in the southwestern United States in 1993), and others.

Accompanying the virus hunters from one disease and locale to the next, readers of this book learn, among other things, of the ingenuity needed to conduct an epidemiological investigation in the Third World without violating local customs. While investigating an outbreak of Crimean Congo hemorrhagic fever (CCHF) among nomads in the southern Sahara, for example, McCormick and his colleagues were told that a large percentage of the tribe's sheep were infected with the CCHF virus. The question was, how many animals were there? The people refused to count the sheep because of their belief that "only Allah should know how many animals you own, lest He take them away." A resourceful researcher developed a method for estimating the sheep population: he counted freshly deposited droppings in the overnight holding pen and extrapolated the size of the herd from that number. In another situation Muslim strictures against the appearance of unchaperoned women in public resulted in a potentially disastrous (for the research program) confrontation between Fisher-Hoch and the local authorities. It took intervention at a high political level for her to be permitted to register at a hotel or dine in a restaurant as a single woman.

The authors vividly describe what they have seen: the terrible wasting diseases, the agonizing deaths, the overworked and often poorly trained Third World nurses and doctors, and the rudimentary medical facilities utterly lacking in such essentials as clean water, electricity, and basic supplies. They are equally forthcoming about the vicissitudes of epidemiological fieldwork—the squalid quarters, less-than-appetizing meals, and constant perils of close contact with lethal infectious agents. McCormick's own experience of waiting to see if he would become ill after accidentally sticking himself with a contaminated needle makes for breath-stoppingly suspenseful reading.

While McCormick and Fisher-Hoch obviously admire the courage of the health workers who combat these deadly outbreaks and feel great sympathy for the victims, their training compels them to place the issue of emerging infections into a broader public health context. They declare, in fact, that viruses rarely "emerge" but are forced into the open when humans, under pressure from overpopulation, venture into previously uninhabited areas. At the same time, migration from the countryside into the fetid slums of overcrowded cities creates an ever-expanding pool of rootless poor who are highly vulnerable to these already-endemic agents of disease. While acknowledging that scientific and technological advances have the potential to improve health care worldwide, the authors contend that a tragic failure of conscience and responsibility on the part of wealthy nations has sown disruption, disease, and death. They do not mince words about the grisly consequences of this failure for future generations or the role they believe the developed world should assume in the face of this threat.

—Jean S. Gottlieb, Ph.D.

Life After Medical School: Thirty-Two Doctors Describe How They Shaped Their Medical Careers
LEONARD LASTER, M.D.
New York: W.W. Norton & Co., Inc., 1996.
344 pp. $27.50

> *When it comes to medicine, I'm an idealist. I think things should be done more for the good of the patient and less for the "good of society." When I helped arrange for a bone marrow transplant on a illegal alien, who paid for it? For my patient faced with a life-threatening disease, it was the best treatment since he had an identical twin. But you and I paid for the transplant and he isn't a citizen. Was it right or wrong? I don't know....I try to do good and not to do harm.*

Life After Medical School is addressed primarily to medical students facing the challenge of negotiating a career path through the increasingly complex labyrinth of modern medicine. The fact that the book is directed at students should not, however, discourage other potential readers, including the families and advisers of students—who are likely to find it informative, illuminating, and reassuring by turns—and physicians considering a change of direction in their own careers. In fact, anyone who has ever been a patient—and especially a skeptical, suspicious, or dissatisfied patient—will find this book enlightening. As these first-person accounts make clear, dedicated physicians carry heavy responsibilities and make many sacrifices. Apparently, most have no regrets.

Leonard Laster, a professor of medicine and health policy at the University of Massachusetts Medical Center, talked to physicians representing virtually every aspect of medicine. Their stories are presented here in the form of monologues, each preceded by a brief introduction describing the subject's present clinical work and academic appointments. The interviews follow roughly the same format. After some remarks about family background and education, interviewees elaborate on the factors that influenced the crucial decisions of their careers—why *this* school or city, why *that* area of concentration or institutional affiliation. They tell what it is like to work with specific patient populations: the homeless, people with AIDS, cancer patients, individuals seeking care in the emergency room. Their fears and frustrations are discussed with as much candor as their joys and satisfactions. These insights produce some surprises for the uninitiated: "People don't realize how much agony a pathologist goes through in rendering a diagnosis....Many of us feel there's a clock ticking and that if we haven't made an error yet it's going to happen one day."

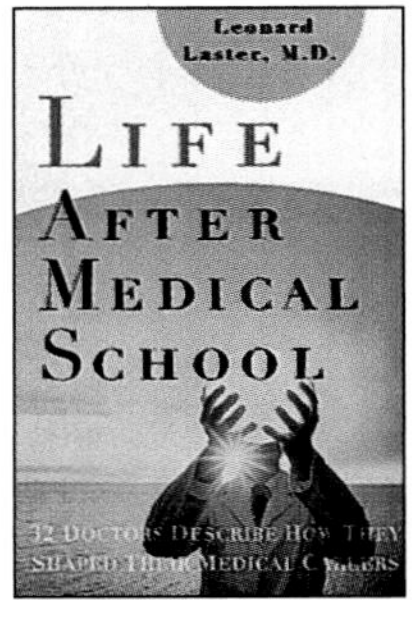

The book is organized around five basic career paths: medicine; surgery; psychiatry and related pursuits; specialties such as pathology, anesthesiology, and radiology that do not require a sustained relationship with patients; and careers in corporate life or politics that have only a tangential relationship to medicine. A section on national health policy includes interviews with Howard Dean, an internist who became governor of Vermont; Joycelyn Elders, the outspoken pediatric endocrinologist from Arkansas who captured national attention as surgeon general of the United States; and Arnold S. Relman, a specialist in kidney diseases who served for many years as editor in chief of *The New England Journal of Medicine.* The book concludes with a section on physicians who faced racial prejudice, had physical disabilities, or were the subjects of malpractice suits. Several interviewees comment on the obstacles faced by women in medicine, and many make reference to the struggle of paying for a medical education.

A common thread is the intensely individual nature of the decision about which path to follow. The very same qualities that drew some medical students into a field repelled others. Some relished the opportunity to form long-term relationships with patients; others shrank from the emotional commitment it implied. Some loved the bold, immediate solutions of surgery; others were attracted to the thoughtful, puzzle-solving approach of internal medicine.

Despite the vast disparities in the physicians' ethnic and socioeconomic backgrounds, their stories have recurrent themes: the importance of mentors and role models, the need to know oneself, the necessity of remaining flexible and open to chance and change, the role of temperament and personality type in choosing a career path, and the demands and rewards of a life in medicine. Many of those interviewed offer observations about the evolution of medical education over time and the changes in medical practice that have accompanied the trend toward managed care. Their predictions about the future of health care and the medical profession range from apprehensive to optimistic. The concluding comments of the interviewees are telling:

"Despite the problems, I'm happy to be a doctor."

"I don't have reservations about advocating a career in medicine."

"I have never once regretted my choice."

"After all these years, I'm still having a wonderful time."

"Medicine today is exciting to me. I love what I do and can't think of any path that I might have taken instead."

"Being a physician is a wonderful adventure."

—Anita Wolff

Living Downstream: An Ecologist Looks at Cancer and the Environment
SANDRA STEINGRABER.
New York: Addison-Wesley Publishing Co., Inc., 1997.
357 pp., notes, index. $24.00

> *There are individuals who claim, as a form of dismissal, that links between cancer and environmental contamination are unproven and unprovable. There are others who believe that placing people in harm's way is wrong—whether the exact mechanisms by which this harm is inflicted can be precisely deciphered or not. At the very least, they argue, we are obliged to investigate, however imperfect our scientific tools: with the right to know comes the duty to inquire.*
>
> *Happily, the latter perspective is gaining esteem as many leading cancer researchers acknowledge the need for an "upstream" focus. As explained at a recent international conference, this image comes from a fable about a village along a river. The residents who live here, according to parable, began noticing increasing numbers of drowning people caught in the river's swift current and so went to work inventing ever more elaborate technologies to resuscitate them. So preoccupied were these heroic villagers with rescue and treatment that they never thought to look upstream to see who was pushing the victims in.*
>
> *This book is a walk up that river.*

In 1960, while U.S. biologist Rachel Carson was researching and writing her prophetic *Silent Spring* (1962), the classic work on the deadly fallout of post-World War II chemical use, she was diagnosed with breast cancer. Carson spoke little about cancer's effect on her life—the devastating surgery and radiation treatments, the spread of the disease throughout her body, which eventually numbed even her writing hand. So worried was she that the details of her condition would be used by her detractors to discredit the scientific authority of the book's message that she instructed even her closest friend to avoid speaking about her medical condition.

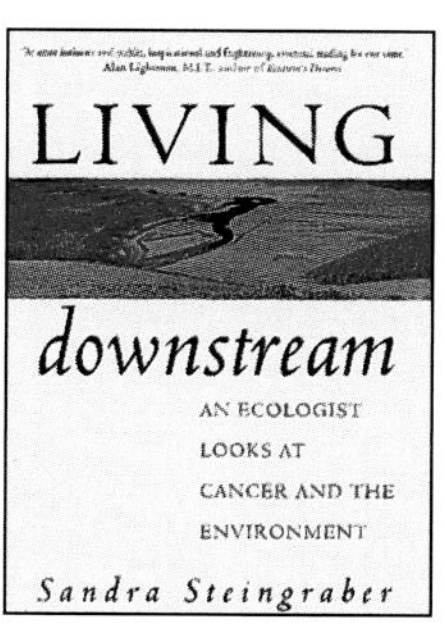

In *Living Downstream,* Sandra Steingraber, who is also a biologist and has herself been diagnosed with cancer, has broken Carson's silence by assigning a human face to an ecological nightmare. What could be more personal, she asks, than to be exposed without one's knowledge or consent to some of the deadliest substances ever created, poisons that insinuate themselves into the most hidden recesses of the body, where they blossom into agony one cell at a time?

Steingraber received her Ph.D. in biology from the University of Michigan and has taught at Columbia College, Chicago, and held fellowships at several other institutions. The book interweaves her own personal narrative with a larger discussion of the relationship between environmental pollutants and cancer. Recovered from a bout with bladder cancer diagnosed when she was 18, Steingraber returns to her hometown in central Illinois to track the industrial and agricultural contaminants she was exposed to as a child. Her own illness is part of what she describes as a family history of cancer: a mother who contracted breast cancer, an aunt and an uncle who died of colon cancer, another aunt who succumbed to bladder cancer. Steingraber says this familial legacy makes it easy for people to dismiss her own brush with cancer, attributing it to a genetic susceptibility to the disease. Except for one hitch: Steingraber is adopted. When she reveals this fact, she says, the typical responses "remind me how unfamiliar many of us are with the notion that families share environments as well as chromosomes or with the concept that our genes work in communion with substances streaming in from the larger, ecological world."

The connection between these substances and cancer has begun to receive renewed attention, particularly in the aftermath of recent research that suggests how, by mimicking sex hormones, certain chemicals may have the potential to disrupt some of the most basic bodily functions. Readers could not ask for a more competent, articulate guide into this new territory than Steingraber, whether she is exploring the history of the wartime conversion of new and deadly chemicals for civilian uses, providing clear explanations for the ways in which environmental toxins can become ticking time bombs in the body, or expressing anger over a national cancer prevention strategy that emphasizes personal behavior (*e.g.,* diet and exercise) but ignores the part played by exposure to known toxins. In the end, readers are sure to share Steingraber's moral outrage; allowing "untested chemicals free access to our bodies," she says, is a "form of homicide."

—Adelheid Fischer

Lying on the Couch: A Novel
IRVIN D. YALOM, M.D.
New York: Basic Books, 1996.
369 pp. $25.00

> *Perhaps priestly consolation was exactly what he should be offering. Surely there was something to be learned from the church's two thousand years in the therapy business. Ernest had always wondered about priests' training. How good were they really at providing consolation? Where did they learn their technique? Courses in consolation? Courses in confession-booth counseling? Ernest's curiosity had once led him to do a literature search at the library on Catholic confession counseling. He had come up with nothing. Another time he had inquired at a local seminary and learned that the curricula offered no explicit psychological training. Once, while visiting a deserted cathedral in Shanghai, Ernest sneaked into the confessional booth and, for thirty minutes, sat in the priest's seat, inhaling the Catholic air and murmuring, again and again, "You are forgiven. My child, you are forgiven!" He emerged from the booth full of envy. What powerful Jovian weapons against despair the priests wielded; in contrast, his own secular armamentarium of interpretations and creature comforts seemed puny indeed.*

The protagonist of Irvin D. Yalom's second novel is Ernest Lash, a former psychopharmacologist (specialist in the treatment of mental disorders with psychoactive medications) who has converted to the practice of "talk therapy." Although he has taken part in the censure of a distinguished colleague for flouting the dictates of the profession, Lash himself has come to believe that a therapist should be creative and flexible, tailoring treatment so as to create an "existential," or "authentic," situation between doctor and patient. His ideas are put to the test, however, when he accepts as a new patient a woman who is out for revenge.

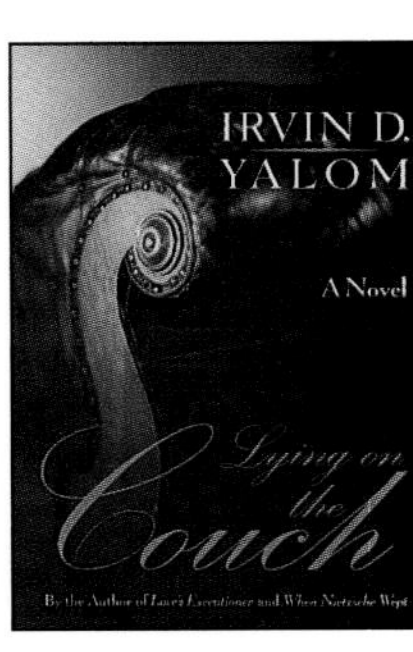

Lash's supervisor, Marshal Streider, who also plays a role in the censure of a colleague for straying from orthodoxy, practices more traditional psychoanalysis, but he is motivated as much by political ambition and greed as by his commitment to the profession. Streider too tests the boundaries of professional relationships—one former patient offers him what seems like a fabulous investment opportunity, while another in effect blackmails him, threatening to sue the analytic institute where he practices.

Yalom, professor emeritus of psychiatry at Stanford University, has written several works on psychotherapy. These include textbooks as well as *Love's Executioner* (1989), a collection of fictionalized case histories, and the award-winning novel *When Nietzsche Wept* (1992). In *Lying on the Couch,* set in San Francisco, Yalom shows how therapists sometimes have matters other than the treatment of patients uppermost in their minds; patients sometimes conceal things from their therapists and sometimes lie (hence, one suspects, the title is intended to be read as a double entendre). The book is an entertaining thriller, but one in which the suspense is largely internal and psychological. Filled with talk by doctors and patients about therapy, its techniques, and its effects (is it science or art?), the novel takes a number of surprising turns. Unbeknownst to the characters Lash and Streider, their worlds become intertwined in unexpected and even shocking ways, and the book ends with stunning role reversals.

In the end the novel makes a forceful case for the psychoanalytic process—for the power of self-knowledge to transform behavior and life. Once an individual is launched on the road to understanding, there may be no turning back. Anyone practicing, undergoing, or interested in psychotherapy ought to find this book a compelling read.

—Robert Rauch

Making PCR: A Story of Biotechnology
PAUL RABINOW.
Chicago: The University of Chicago Press, 1996.
190 pp., notes, bibliography. $22.50

> ***It has become a commonplace that during the 1970s there was a blurring of the once supposedly distinct line between "applied" and "pure" research in the biosciences. Often this story is constructed as a corruption tale: how molecular biology became a handmaiden (to use a dated metaphor) to an industry relentlessly—and, by definition, unscrupulously—in search of profit. For example, one prominent historian of modern biology writes: "Prior to the emergence of recombinant DNA technology, the practice of molecular biology was guided largely by the traditional ethos of academic research and its commitment to the development of knowledge through an essentially cooperative and communal effort." Anyone the least bit familiar with the history of science...could hardly describe it as an "essentially cooperative and communal effort." This view...is historically and anthropologically inadequate.***

Like many other students of the history of science, Paul Rabinow, an anthropologist at the University of California, Berkeley, sees science as a deeply social enterprise whose progress depends more on the routine day-to-day work of technicians than on the occasional imaginative leaps of the lone genius. It is not surprising, then, that the story of PCR (polymerase chain reaction) and the man credited with discovering it, biochemist Kary B. Mullis, appealed to him.

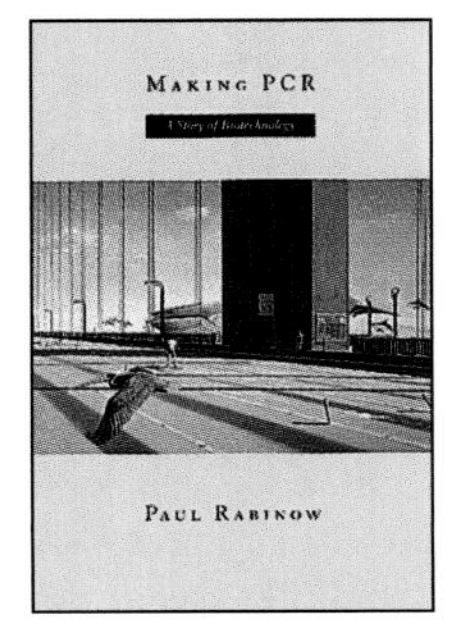

Rabinow spent several years interviewing researchers at the California biotechnology firm Cetus Corp. (Mullis's former employer), reconstructing the discovery and development of PCR, a revolutionary technique for copying specific genes or other discrete segments of DNA. In PCR these segments, called target sequences, are isolated, and the two helically wound complementary strands of the segment are separated from each other by heating. Then, in a process that involves the application of polymerase, an enzyme essential to the synthesis and repair of DNA, a complementary sequence is created for each of the individual strands. The result is two copies of the target sequence where originally there was only one.

This process, which takes only a few minutes, is then repeated. With each repetition the DNA sample doubles in size; after 30 repetitions and a few hours, the original DNA sample has been copied a billion times. Previous methods for copying DNA were both expensive and extremely time-consuming; PCR virtually mass-produces DNA, quickly, reliably, and at low cost.

As Rabinow observes, the technique has "profoundly transformed the practices and potential of molecular biology" by making "abundant what was once scarce." It has found uses in a variety of fields, from molecular biology to criminology to clinical medicine. In fact, versatility is one of PCR's hallmarks. As a Cetus technician told Rabinow, "Once [PCR] existed, problems began to emerge to which it could be applied....PCR is a tool that has the power to create new situations for its use and new subjects to use it."

PCR was originally conceived by Mullis in 1983; 10 years later he was awarded the Nobel Prize for Chemistry for this pathbreaking discovery. Rabinow makes the case, however, that a number of other scientists, technicians, and managers at Cetus were instrumental in turning Mullis's basic idea into a useful tool. Without their work in refining the technique, ensuring its reliability, and demonstrating its practical utility outside the field of synthetic chemistry (Mullis's own specialty), he argues, PCR might never have become "the exemplary biotechnological invention to date," and Mullis would almost certainly never have become a Nobel laureate.

Not only does Rabinow show how important these other figures were in "making PCR," he also provides a revealing look at the world of corporate biotechnology research. He suggests that because corporate biotechnology is less hierarchical than its academic counterpart, as well as more informal and faster to reward achievement and support innovative research, corporate scientists actually have *more* freedom to pursue their goals than their colleagues in academia.

—Alex Soojung-Kim Pang, Ph.D.

The Medicine of ER: Or, How We Almost Die
ALAN DUNCAN ROSS AND HARLAN GIBBS, M.D.
New York: Basic Books, 1996.
232 pp., index. $18.00

> *Major trauma is a big deal in any ER, and it seems that almost every week at [the fictional] County General's ER at least one major trauma case is presented. They've got to get the television viewers' blood pressures and pulses soaring as the staff pulls out all the stops in an attempt to cheat death! In real life as much as in a television drama, major trauma will get an ER staff rocking, and the procedures you see employed [on the TV show] every week are for the most part the kind of livesaving maneuvers used in emergency rooms around the country.*

A 20-year-old male comes to the emergency room by ambulance complaining of spreading muscle weakness.... Harry, a 60-year-old man, has a heart attack.... Jody, an apparently healthy pregnant woman, shows up in the emergency room complaining of urinary frequency.... In the course of recounting these and other everyday emergency room scenarios, Alan Ross and Harlan Gibbs compare what transpires in an *actual* hospital emergency department with the dramatic goings on in "ER," the television series that has mesmerized a substantial portion of the American viewing public on Thursday nights for the past three seasons.

The authors' credentials make them well-suited to their task. Gibbs is a practicing emergency room physician, and Ross is a movie and television scriptwriter who has had some experience in hospital administration.

In some respects the authors find "ER" to be an accurate representation of what transpires behind the trauma suite's swinging doors—as, for example, in the show's portrayal of a territorial dispute between the head nurse and a physicians' assistant. At the same time, they do not hesitate to acknowledge the script's many departures from reality. A case in point is the Emmy award-winning episode "Love's Labor Lost," in which a medical resident's misjudgments are responsible for the death of a woman in childbirth. Ross and Gibbs also examine the personality quirks, medical training, and level of professionalism of the TV drama's "staff"—senior attending physician Mark Greene, surgical resident Peter Benton, department chairman David Morgenstern, and others—finding some aspects of these fictional characters to be compatible with reality and others utterly far-fetched. In contrast, the chairman of one major hospital emergency department interviewed by Ross and Gibbs was unreservedly critical of the series, calling it "an inaccurate portrayal of what goes on in an ER, both in its extreme positives and its extreme negatives."

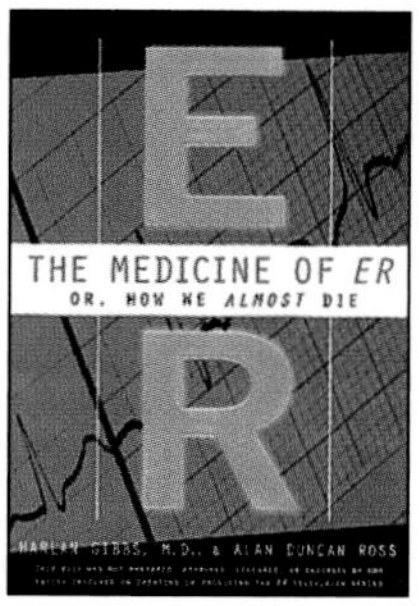

Accurate or not, the show has a devoted following, and "ER" fans are likely to enjoy this book. Terms such as "pulse ox" (short for pulse oximetry), "V-fib" (ventricular fibrillation), and "lytes" (electrolytes), heard in virtually every episode of "ER," are defined in detail, as are such common emergency room procedures as intubation and peritoneal lavage. The terms are set in bold-faced type, and the authors seem to think that readers will refer to them while watching the show. Probably, however, a glossary would have been more helpful for reference purposes.

Anyone who is not an "ER" watcher but is nonetheless fascinated by the subject of emergency medicine (if such a person exists) will find the book informative. Ross and Gibbs explain the physical layout of the ER, the work of the physicians and other staff, and the roles played by pharmaceuticals and machines. There is even a section on the history of emergency medicine, as well as a useful comparison of the training and capabilities of emergency medical technicians and paramedics. (The authors would want the latter in *their* ambulances.)

Although they frequently accuse the "ER" scriptwriters of histrionics, the authors are clearly fascinated with the dramatic aspects of emergency room medicine. The subtitle *How We Almost Die* is at once a parody of the title of surgeon Sherwin B. Nuland's acclaimed 1994 book *How We Die* and a clue to the authors' personal view of the emergency department as a place that pulsates with the grand excitement of saving lives. Even more than the television show, the book is resolutely upbeat about emergency room outcomes; few of the anecdotes Ross and Gibbs recount end in death.

In keeping with this optimistic emphasis, the authors accord little attention to some of the more contentious issues in contemporary emergency room medicine. The health hazards that physicians and other ER staff members increasingly face, such as exposure to tuberculosis, hepatitis, and HIV, are referred to only briefly and toward the end. The book justifies the ER's high costs, but it ignores the struggles these have engendered between some hospitals and managed-care organizations. In general, there is hardly any discussion of the U.S. health care system as a whole or the changing relationship of the emergency department to it. In short, *The Medicine of ER* is an engaging companion to the TV show and a source of basic information for people who are curious about what goes on in the ER. If it encourages readers to delve into more serious sociomedical issues, so much the better.

—Joseph Turow, Ph.D.

One Blood: The Death and Resurrection of Charles R. Drew
SPENCIE LOVE.
Chapel Hill: The University of North Carolina Press, 1996.
373 pp., notes, bibliography, index. $29.95

> *It is hard to overstate the archetypal familiarity of the theme of a black man bleeding to death at white hands. Even the most cursory investigation of black history or literature summons up such images, and each era has offered its*

twists on the theme. The theme of the shedding of blood runs like a dark stream through the history of blacks in America. One of the first major African American historians, George Washington Williams, described his lifework in 1882: "I have tracked my bleeding countrymen through the widely scattered documents of American history; I have listened to their groans, their clanking chains, and melting prayers, until the woes of a race and the agonies of centuries seem to crowd upon my soul as a bitter reality."

On April 1, 1950, Charles Drew, a pioneering researcher in the science of blood banking and one of the few African-American surgeons in the U.S., was critically hurt in an automobile accident and subsequently died of his injuries. Whether Drew received appropriate medical care at the small segregated Southern hospital to which he was taken or, as another popular version of the story insists, was refused treatment because of his race is the question that forms the core of this well-researched book by Spencie Love, a graduate student in American history at Duke University, Durham, N.C.

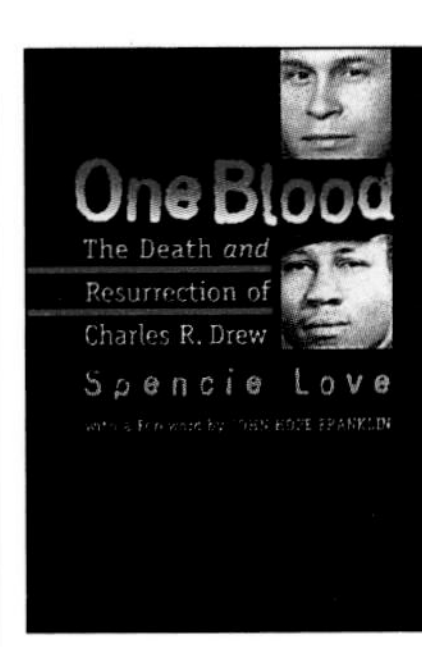

Drew was born in 1904 to a well-educated Washington, D.C., family. He struggled financially to attend medical school and then struggled to be admitted to a program that would permit a black candidate to qualify as a surgeon at a time when African-American physicians faced many barriers; they were not welcome in Southern affiliates of the American Medical Association, and none had yet been admitted to the American College of Surgeons. While he worked to develop a method for the storage of human blood and plasma, Drew also campaigned tirelessly to open his profession to others of his race. In 1940 he was instrumental in the establishment of a groundbreaking wartime program for blood banking known as Blood for Britain. It must, then, have been a bitter blow to him when the U.S. Army announced that black donors would be excluded from the American Red Cross blood banks then being established. Subsequently, the Red Cross adopted a policy that the race of donors would be identified along with their blood type—the U.S. blood supply was thus "segregated" and remained so until 1950.

Drew went on to become a professor of medicine at Howard University Medical School, Washington, D.C., one of the two institutions in the country training black physicians. On the morning of his death, he and three colleagues were traveling to a medical conference in Tuskegee, Ala. The truth of Drew's story, according to Love, who interviewed an eyewitness and members of Drew's family, is that the white doctors at Alamance General Hospital in Burlington, N.C., did everything possible to save his life.

But, as Love points out, there is also a larger truth: that of hundreds of years of mistreatment of American blacks, from the indignities of segregation to the Tuskegee syphilis study (in which black men were used unknowingly as subjects of medical research). The refusal of hospitals to treat black patients, a common practice in Drew's day, formed the core of experience that allowed his legend to flourish despite attempts by those who knew the truth to correct the record. Love provides a detailed history of the prejudicial treatment—or, in some cases, nontreatment—blacks regularly received from the medical community in the U.S.

The closing section of the book is an account of the demise of Maltheus Reeves Avery, a black man who *was* refused medical treatment and *did* die, the same year as Drew and at a nearby location. Severely injured in a car crash, Avery was transferred from Alamance (because the hospital had no neurosurgeon) to Duke University Hospital, where he was refused treatment because no beds were available for black patients that night. He was transferred to yet another hospital but arrived there near death and died soon after. Love's purpose in telling Avery's story is not simply to account for the origin of the Drew legend, although it is easy to see how the two events may have become conflated in people's minds. In fact, rumors of Drew's being denied admission to the hospital—or, in another version, of the refusal of white doctors to give him a lifesaving blood transfusion—had begun to surface even before Avery's death. (Indeed, a similar story, also untrue, is told about the death of the singer Bessie Smith.) Instead, as Love sees it, Avery's treatment on that night in 1950 is the ultimate reason for the necessity of the legend in which Charles Drew, hero and martyr, dies before his time owing to bigotry and negligence. In Love's analysis, the legendary account of Drew's death is, in the end, a mythic or poetic truth that "points the way to historical realities even more tragic than the one it specifically describes." Readers of all races will be enlightened by this book.

—Christine Sullivan

The Practical Pediatrician: The A to Z Guide to Your Child's Health, Behavior, and Safety

HOWARD MARKEL, M.D., PH.D., F.A.A.P., AND FRANK A. OSKI, M.D., F.A.A.P.

New York: W.H. Freeman and Co., 1996. 346 pp., illustrations, index. $16.95

In short, focus on the many do's of parenting. Remember that raising an infant and child should be a positive, pleasurable experience. You can do it, and do it well.

The attitude reflected in the above quotation is, in large part, what makes this advice book for parents a really good one. The authors acknowledge that pediatricians have the valuable perspective that comes from seeing scores of children every week, but, they emphasize, parents have a different although equally important advantage—that of knowing one child, *their* child, really well. The subtext of this practical-advice book is that parents should have a little confidence in their own judgment; this attitude is refreshing and a much-needed change from the approach usually taken by books of this type.

The Practical Pediatrician, written by Howard Markel of the University of Michigan and Frank Oski (who died in December 1996) of the Johns Hopkins Children's Center, Baltimore, Md., is satisfactory in a number of ways. On the mundane level, its alphabetical organization enables the panicked parent to locate information quickly, without having to resort to the index. Thus, information on head injury is found under "Head and neck injuries," not under "Concussion, *see* subdural hematoma" or the like. (A search for advice about temper tantrums, on the other hand, *does* require a glance at the index. The topic, it turns out, is covered in an extensive entry entitled "Discipline.") On a broader level, the information provided is worth knowing once it has been found.

Many of the entries are unusually helpful for a book of this type. This reviewer was particularly impressed by the 14 pages devoted to breast-feeding. Oski was strongly committed to encouraging American mothers to breast-feed, and the level of information and support provided in this section reflects that commitment. Another outstanding entry, entitled "Negotiating with your child," takes pains to distinguish between rewards for accomplishment and "bribes" and thus settles a question that leaves many parents feeling confused and, sometimes, slightly guilty. The authors explain that rewards, when given properly, not only motivate children to behave but can also reinforce the learning of responsibility and help to build self-esteem.

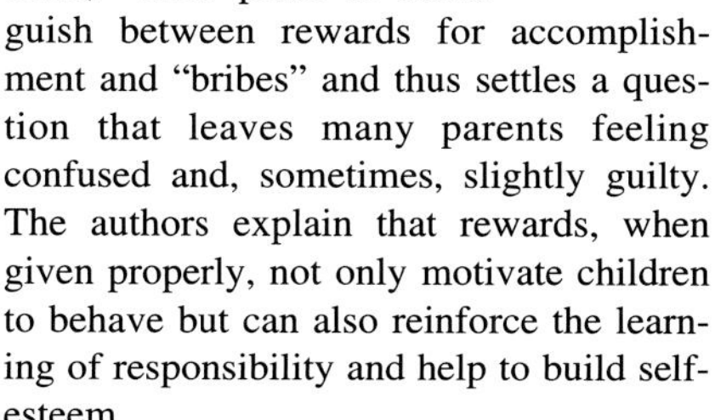

The extensive section on bites (16 pages, covering human, pet, wild animal, and insect bites) shows that the authors have a clear understanding of the most common reason parents consult a book like this: they want to know (1) Do I need to call the doctor? and (2) If I need to call the doctor, can I wait until the office opens at 8 AM? One page into the entry is a section headed "Bites that require immediate medical attention"—just the ticket for the worried parent trying to decide what to do about a spider bite that seems to be swelling pretty fast. Practical advice of this nature is also found in the sections on fevers and croup, two common problems that cause a lot of middle-of-the-night agonizing over just exactly what course of action to take. Also noteworthy are the many helpful charts on, among other things, well-child pediatric visits, immunizations, and developmental milestones in speech and hearing. New parents in particular will find these useful. A few entries end with a section headed "Okay, doctor, none of these worked." Here parents will find out what to do about really desperate diaper rash, stubborn constipation, etc. (Curiously, or maybe not, all of these sections seem to involve bathroom issues.)

Not all of the entries are equally illuminating. In the entry on sudden infant death syndrome (SIDS), for example, the authors discuss recommended sleep positions, the link between secondhand smoke and SIDS deaths, and how to avoid smothering by bedding. In a separate entry on sleep and sleep problems, a section devoted to the issue of bed sharing by parents and babies mentions accidental suffocation and cross-refers the reader to SIDS. It would have been much more enlightening if the entry on SIDS provided a thorough explanation of the connection between SIDS, smothering, and suffocation by "overlaying." Another entry this reviewer took exception to is the one entitled "Computers and the Internet," which, at half a page, is too brief to do justice to the subject and takes a narrowly negative approach, comparing computers to passive forms of entertainment like television and videos and ignoring their enormous educational potential.

One last criticism: the book is marred by numerous typographical errors. Most are obvious enough that they do not obscure the meaning, but one in particular could lead to misunderstanding. On page 20, parents of children with attention deficit disorder are urged to "learn their cures to prevent social embarrassment or battles." Since the heading above this statement reads "Know your child's behaviors and cues," surely, it is *cues,* not *cures,* that the authors feel parents should learn.

—Christine Sullivan

Science on Trial: The Clash of Medical Evidence and the Law in the Breast Implant Case
MARCIA ANGELL, M.D.
New York: W.W. Norton & Co., 1996.
256 pp., notes, index. $27.50

> *Science plays a hugely important role in our daily lives, and not just because we are dependent on its technological fruits. In addition, we base many of our habits and activities on the results of research studies, as interpreted for us by the media. Medical research, in particular, increasingly informs our lives. We are subject to an almost incessant barrage of warnings and recommendations based on new medical information. Yet, despite the practical importance of science in our lives, most Americans find the nature of scientific research a complete mystery. To many of them, the conclusion is all that matters. It's as though Americans said to medical researchers, "Tell us what we should and shouldn't eat, which vitamins to take, and how much to exercise, and don't bother us with how you found the answers or how sure you are." But in science, the conclusions cannot be separated from the process of reaching them.*

Science on Trial is a detailed examination of the U.S. breast implant controversy. The author, Marcia Angell, executive editor of *The New England Journal of Medicine,* was involved in the controversy from its early stages. In June 1992 she wrote an editorial ("Breast Implants—Protection or Paternalism?") critical of the decision by David Kessler, then commissioner of the U.S. Food and Drug Administration (FDA), to order sharp restrictions in the use of silicone-gel-filled implants. (An estimated 80% of the devices are implanted for cosmetic reasons and 20% for reconstruction following mastectomy or for other deforming breast conditions.)

Two years later she wrote another editorial on the occasion of the journal's publication of the first epidemiological study exploring a possible connection between implants and systemic diseases, primarily connective tissue disorders such as systemic lupus erythematosus and scleroderma. While no studies have found a definite cause-effect relationship between implants and these diseases (although other problems—like leakage and rupture of implants—are well known), there have been widespread reports of such links in the media. A class-action settlement of $4,250,000,000 was reached in 1994, and a number of women who sued manufacturers individually won huge awards. (The class-action settlement dissolved in 1995 when Dow-Corning, the company that had sold half of all implants, declared bankruptcy.) How, the author asks, could the issue have

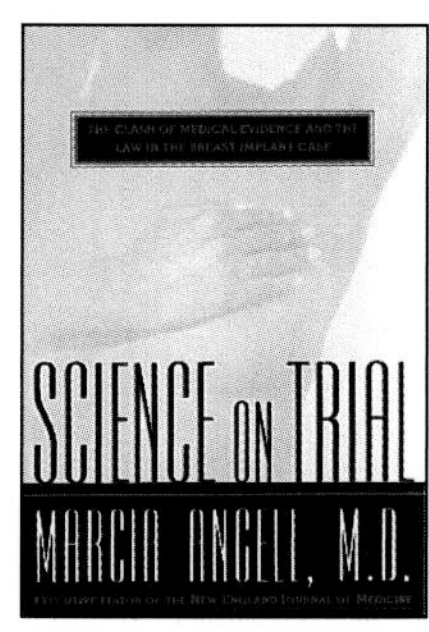

worked itself out in this way in the absence of any firm scientific evidence that breast implants do, in fact, cause systemic disease?

One by one, Angell examines the institutions and processes that shaped the controversy: the regulation of drugs and medical devices, the U.S. tort law system, the scientific method in medical, and specifically, epidemiological research, the use—and abuse—of scientific data in the courtroom, and the media as disseminator and interpreter of scientific findings. Her account of the regulatory process makes it clear that the FDA, although an independent governmental agency, is nonetheless subject to political and other influences. Indeed, it was the actions of public-interest groups that helped bring about the FDA's virtual ban on implants. The ban, which was instituted not because the implants had been demonstrated to be harmful but because manufacturers had not proved them *not* to be harmful, led to an explosion of lawsuits against manufacturers. Most of this litigation, Angell emphasizes, was brought by a relatively small but, in this age of electronic communications, closely connected network of lawyers. Moreover, the U.S. tort system—which operates on the principle of contingency fees (*i.e.,* the lawyer's fee is contingent on the client's winning the case) and which, unlike many other systems, allows jury trials—encourages the filing of such suits.

Meanwhile, the media fueled the public's fears with dramatic stories of women who claimed that their implants had made them sick. Given the general public's inability to understand many scientific issues and the tendency of groups as disparate as humanists, feminists, and religious fundamentalists to reject science, perhaps, the author concludes, it should not be surprising that events developed as they did.

Although Angell's immediate subject is the indictment of silicone breast implants in the absence of solid scientific evidence against them, her larger concern is the way in which the government, courts, media, and public deal with questions involving science and medicine. When citizens do not understand the difference between scientific and legal evidence, when a legal system encourages the filing of suits and allows paid experts to use "junk science" to influence juries, and when the news media give more coverage to bad news than to good, herald initial scientific discoveries but ignore later caveats or retractions, and neglect to explain the implications of the information they present, science and medicine may well lose out to the forces of fear and greed. Any person interested in the breast implant case or the larger medicolegal issues it raised should find this book compelling reading.

—*Robert Rauch*

Signs of Life: A Memoir of Dying and Discovery
TIM BROOKES.
New York: Times Books, 1997.
271 pp. $23.00

> *It's the last thing you want to think about, of course, and even now you can barely bring yourself to say the word. You've successfully kept the subject at bay for a remarkably long time, despite the loss of pets, of school friends who tried to take the curve at eighty with a blood alcohol level of 2.5, of a distant relative or two. Yet sooner or later the perpetual youthfulness you've been taking for granted is nibbled away in small injuries and disappointments, and you think, half joking, half with your heart sinking, that immortality doesn't seem to be an option after all. Or perhaps someone close to you is gravely ill and you don't know how to help, knowing nothing except your own queasy aversion. One way or another, death gets to you, stealing your willful blindness, and you find yourself wondering what it is like to die.*

As this opening paragraph of Tim Brookes's beautifully written memoir, *Signs of Life,* suggests, the most difficult thing about this book for many people will be to pick it up in the first place. The second most difficult, however, may be to put it down.

The British-born Brookes teaches writing and media criticism at the University of Vermont and serves as a regular commentator on National Public Radio. He is also the author of an earlier book, *Catching My Breath,* about his own asthmatic condition. *Signs of Life* began as a reportorial project, an investigation into the hospice movement. Shortly after starting his research, however, Brookes learned that his mother had been diagnosed with terminal pancreatic cancer. Thus, as he puts it, "the cerebral, journalistic part of my education, fascinating but largely theoretical," came to an abrupt end. What followed was Brookes's personal odyssey.

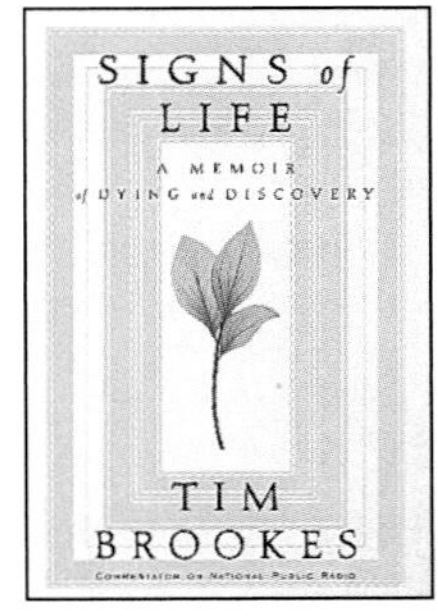

His approach is nothing if not thorough; he examines from every possible viewpoint the issues raised at each stage in his mother's dying and compares her experience with the quite different death of his father—also from cancer—some years earlier. Because his mother and siblings resided in England, Brookes gets an insider's view of British health care practices; from his vantage point as a resident of the U.S., he is able to make perceptive comparisons between the two countries' approaches to the dying process.

The American medical establishment comes in for harsh treatment. Brookes is highly critical of a system that promotes belief in miracle cures and, as he sees it, feeds off false hope. Physicians and surgeons, he writes, are often judged (by patients and even by themselves) by the number of patients they save from death. No doctor wants to lose a patient, and when death becomes inevitable, one by one, beginning with the specialists at the top of the hospital hierarchy, the medical personnel withdraw. The dying person, feeling confused and abandoned, is left in the care of nurses—the only ones who cannot leave. As Brookes notes, palliative care, long a subspecialty in Britain, Australia, and New Zealand, is not given similar status in the U.S.

This book is clearly an endorsement for "hospice," as both the movement and the form of care are often called, but Brookes is measured in his assessment of the successes of the individual facilities he visited. He points out a number of specific problems with the hospice care he has observed and is critical of some branches of the movement. Not surprisingly, he finds that despite problems with community funding and support, good hospice care still depends principally on good staff members.

One cavil: in the final chapter, following an examination of grief counseling (in which Brookes points out that the U.S. Medicare system does not reimburse hospices for time spent on bereavement counseling), the author calls at one port beyond where this reviewer wanted to stop. "My research into death...demanded one last effort," he writes. This effort took him to visit a psychic, to whom, according to Brookes's account, his mother appeared and through whom she spoke to him. While he acknowledges that he never actually saw his mother in spirit form, he presents her descriptions of the afterlife in the same even-handed, matter-of-fact reportorial style as he recounts his conversations with physicians, nurses, and hospice workers. Despite this rather startling—and to this reviewer, disturbing—turn of affairs, *Signs of Life* remains an educational, personal, and intensely moving memoir. Few readers will be able to remain dry-eyed to the end.

—*Charles P. Trumbull, Ph.D.*

The Trouble with Testosterone: And Other Essays on the Biology of the Human Predicament
ROBERT M. SAPOLSKY.
New York: Scribner, 1997.
288 pp., illus. $23.00

> ***This is what many people fear, that scientists, as they learn more and more about less and less, will inadvertently go and explain everything, will turn us with their knowledge into sterile assemblages of molecules and networks and equations, and that with each new fact accrued, another light in the heavens will be extinguished.***
>
> ***I do not worry about this. This is not because I am an unemotional scientist just intent on reaching that holy grail of turning dancing flames into equations. I am a reasonably emotional person and that is central to the science that I do. Yet I am not worried if the scientists inadvertently go and explain everything. This is for a very simple reason: an impala sprinting across the savannah can be reduced to biomechanics, and Bach can be reduced to counterpoint, yet that does not decrease one iota our ability to shiver as we experience impalas leaping or Bach thundering. We can only gain and grow with each discovery that there is structure underlying the most accessible levels of things that fill us with awe.... The purpose of science is not to cure us of our sense of mystery and wonder, but to constantly reinvent and reinvigorate it.***

A fascination for the living world drives the study of biology, but all too often the dull, dry prose in which biologists present their research obscures their sense of wonder. How refreshing then to read the lively and engaging pieces in this collection by behavioral neuroendocrinologist Robert Sapolsky. The wit, enthusiasm, and insight he brings to this work leave no doubt about the excitement to be found in a career in biology.

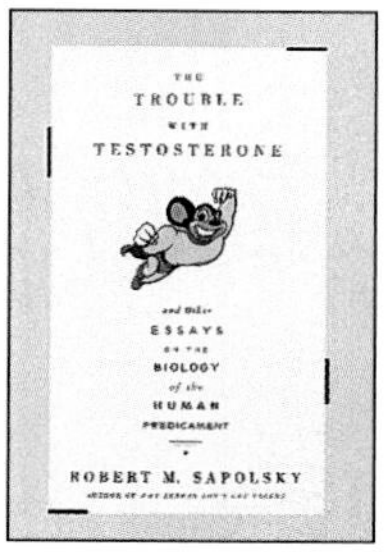

Sapolsky, a professor of biology and neuroscience at Stanford University, studies the effects of stress in primates. He spends summers in East Africa observing baboon behavior, then returns to his laboratory during the school year to study how hormones secreted during times of stress affect the brain.

In these essays, many of which were published previously in the magazines *Discover* and *The Sciences,* to which Sapolsky is a regular contributor, he discusses both his own research and a wide assortment of other topics in behavioral biology. In the title essay, for example, he examines the link between testosterone levels and aggressive behavior, addressing the question of whether the hormone regulates the behavior or, as might seem less likely, the behavior the hormone. The point he makes at the end of this piece, that "behavioral biology is usually meaningless outside the context of the social factors and environment in which it occurs," is a common theme throughout the book. Other topics addressed include the influence of family stability on the time of onset of puberty in girls, the physiological mechanisms of fever and other flulike symptoms, and the part "friendship" plays in determining whether an aging male baboon remains with his troop.

In the essay entitled "Curious George's Pharmacy," which was first published (under a different title) in *The Sciences,* Sapolsky questions the belief of some scientists that certain animals intentionally ingest medicinal plants to treat their own illnesses. As an epilogue to this chapter, he offers an irate letter *The Sciences* received from the investigators whose data he had criticized, along with his own reply. Lest the reader misinterpret this confrontation of rival theorists, the author sums up the seemingly contentious dispute this way: "In other words, we were being a bunch of academics having a fine time arguing with each other over something." Clearly, Sapolsky and his fellow scientists revel in the spirited debate that characterizes scientific inquiry.

No matter the subject, the author provides a lucid, jargon-free explanation of the relevant research, often enlivened by perceptive comments pertaining to the social and political implications of the particular finding in question. For the reader whose curiosity has been piqued, at the end of each piece is an annotated list of suggested further reading materials.

In his introduction to the volume Sapolsky observes that from time to time everyone is called upon to act as a "behavioral biologist," analyzing and interpreting the behavior of others. Often, as when one is called to serve on a jury or appraise an employee's job performance, there may be a great deal at stake. Since these situations are inevitable, Sapolsky contends, people might as well develop the skills to handle them competently. It is his hope that these essays may help readers become more thoughtful and insightful interpreters of human behavior.

—*M.J. Friedrich*

Typhoid Mary: Captive to the Public's Health
JUDITH WALZER LEAVITT.
Boston: Beacon Press, 1996.
331 pp., illustrations, notes, index. $25.00

> ***When [investigator] George Soper walked up the steps of the Park Avenue brownstone in which Mary Mallon was working in March, 1907, and accused her (albeit, in his terms, diplomatically) of making people sick with her cooking, he initiated a new public health encounter. Investigators previously had looked into other home- and community-based typhoid epidemics. They had come to examine the water supply, the food, and the disease histories of the people in the household. But never before, in Mallon's experience or anyone else's, had an epidemic investigation led to an accusation that a specific healthy individual was causing typhoid in others. Soper himself admitted that "such a thing had never been heard of."***

There really was a Typhoid Mary. Her name was Mary Mallon, and she apparently was the first person to be identified as a healthy carrier of the bacillus that causes typhoid fever. She was born in 1869 in Ireland and in 1883 immigrated to the United States, where she found employment as a cook for several prosperous families in the New York City area. After being linked to a number of outbreaks of typhoid fever in the households where she worked, Mallon was apprehended by the city health department in 1907 and detained until 1910.

She spent most of that time in isolation on North Brother Island, in the East River just off the Bronx, which was then the site of the Willard Parker Hospital. She was released on the condition that she not work as a cook again, but four and a half years later she took a job in the kitchen of a maternity hospital. When another cluster of typhoid fever cases was linked to her, she was taken into custody again in 1915 and returned to North Brother Island, where she lived until her death in 1938.

Judith Walzer Leavitt, a professor of the history of medicine and of women's studies and dean of faculty at the University of Wisconsin Medical School, examines Mallon's life in exhaustive detail. She tells the Typhoid Mary story from many different perspectives, among them that of the emerging science of bacteriology, which provided the tools needed for investigating disease outbreaks; that of public policy makers of the day, who were establishing the limits of the powers and duties of public health departments; and that of the law and the legal issues raised by the detention of persons said to pose a threat to the public health. Leavitt also examines the influence of what she calls the "social expectations and prejudices" of the period, the role of newspapers and journals in publicizing and sensationalizing the case, and the subject's own feelings about who she was and how she had been treated. She reviews the many writings on Mallon, fiction and nonfiction, sympathetic and hostile, published in the nearly 60 years since her death. The results of Leavitt's research should appeal to readers with a strong interest in the history and issues of public health, as well as those interested in the social history of the U.S. in the early 20th century.

Typhoid Mary

Captive to the Public's Health

Judith Walzer Leavitt

As the author's account makes clear, the "truth" about Typhoid Mary varies, depending on one's viewpoint and personal prejudices; moreover, many questions about the case remain unanswered to this day. One of these is the degree of Mallon's culpability. It is not clear if she understood the concept of a healthy carrier of disease (few people at the time did) or the fact that she posed a danger to others.

Another issue subject to varying interpretations is her treatment by the authorities—she was punished much more harshly than other known carriers, including some who, like her, broke their promises to authorities not to work with food and some who infected more people than she did. Nor is it apparent why the press seized on Mallon in particular as a symbol of the threat of disease. The author believes that bias against gender, class, nationality, and even religion played a part, but it also seems possible that Mallon was simply in the unfortunate position of having been the first healthy carrier to be so identified. Although Leavitt devotes the final chapter to a discussion of lessons to be drawn from Mallon's story, she does not examine contemporary issues—for example, mandatory HIV testing or laws barring people with certain communicable diseases from entering the U.S. Nor does she make detailed proposals for addressing the balance between the rights of individuals and the need to protect the public health.

—Robert Rauch

Vitamania: Vitamins in American Culture

RIMA D. APPLE.

New Brunswick, N.J.: Rutgers University Press, 1996.

245 pp., illustrations, notes, index. $18.95 (paper)

Science has often been regarded as a secular religion in the modern U.S.; its pronouncements are taken as akin to gospel. Each participant in [the vitamin] controversy exploited this view of science. From one perspective, faithful vitamin takers have been brainwashed by vitamin companies, which continue to hammer home their science of vitamins. Yet this book shows us that the U.S. consumer rejects such a dogmatic view of science. It is significant that when scientists rancorously disagree, many Americans remain passionately committed to vitamins and to science. Scientific experts and expertise are not rejected unilaterally. It is only that consumers demand the right to decide for themselves, once a day, every day.

Rima Apple holds appointments in both consumer science and women's studies at the University of Wisconsin—appropriate credentials for the author of a book whose cover pictures a gingham-aproned Mom administering a dose of vitamins to a reluctant tyke. Apple is also author of *Mothers and Medicine: A Social History of Infant Feeding, 1890–1950* (1987). Her stated intention in *Vitamania,* published as part of the Rutgers University Press series *Health and Medicine in American Society,* is to explore why people buy vitamins and, specifically, why individuals who have no serious vitamin deficiencies feel the need to take vitamin supplements. Along the way, however, she becomes fascinated by the development and regulation of the vitamin-supplement industry—the book's true topic. The history of vitamins in the United States intertwines with the histories of academic research, advertising, mass marketing, government regulation, nutrition science, and consumer rights. At the center of the controversy over regulation is the U.S. Food and Drug Administration (FDA), the agency charged with overseeing, among others, the food, drug, and cosmetics industries.

Are vitamins a food or a drug? Do they pose a danger to consumers? Who should control the development, manufacture, marketing, and sales of vitamin supplements? These questions recur throughout *Vitamania.* Apple cites publications from as early as 1914 in which it was asserted that poor soil and agricultural practices, overprocessing of foods, and bad eating habits were combining to make the American diet inadequate in many essential micronutrients. The proponents of vitamin supplements claimed that these products could provide "insurance" against the subclinical nutritional deficiencies that were thought to be pervasive and a barrier to optimum health. They argued that consumers should be allowed to choose for themselves which vitamins to take and in what quantity.

Nonsense, countered opponents; for the average person, a balanced diet is enough to provide all needed nutrients. Money spent on supplements is mostly wasted, this group asserted, and they demanded that the public be protected from snake-oil salesmen and their extravagant claims. "Science" was cited as an authority by both sides, but, as Apple takes pains to point out, the findings of nutritionists, doctors, and researchers were often contradictory, and many scientific studies raised more questions than they answered.

Nonetheless, for the public, vitamins seem to possess an enduring mystique. How else to explain why, in 1994, when Congress was debating a bill to protect the vitamin industry from proposed FDA restrictions, legislators received more than 100,000 calls and letters in support of the law? Not since the Vietnam War and Watergate had a public policy issue provoked such a passionate outpouring.

Apple's cultural history of vitamins explores, among other things, the cod-liver-oil industry, the transition of vitamin sales from pharmacy to grocery store, Linus Pauling's advocacy of large doses of vitamin C, and endless congressional hearings on the regulation of vitamins. In one chapter she recounts the efforts during the 1920s of University of Wisconsin biochemist Harry Steenbock to reconcile the values of science and commerce as he sought to patent his process of enriching foods with vitamin D by irradiation. In another she describes the legal battle waged in the early 1960s to prevent the sale of a specious vitamin remedy for acne.

Although she repeatedly restates her central question ("Why do Americans take vitamins?"), Apple avoids giving obvious answers. American vitamin takers—typically middle-class, well-fed, and fairly healthy—apparently seek something more than relief from disease; they want insurance against it. They look to vitamins to supply them with vigor, vitality, stamina, and zest for life—an essentially American point of view that identifies the pursuit of optimum health as a personal right with which legislators tamper at their peril.

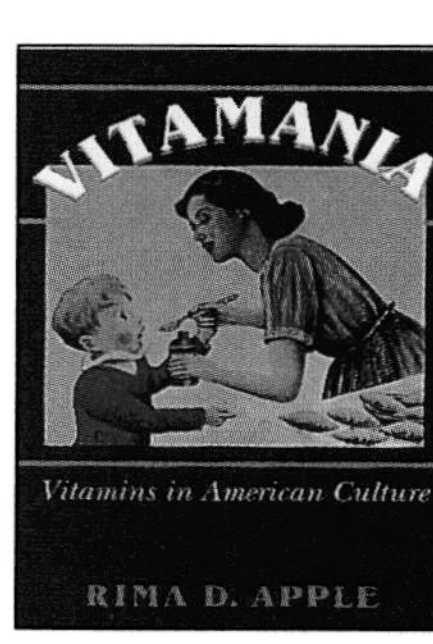

—*Anita Wolff*

Why Michael Couldn't Hit and Other Tales of the Neurology of Sports
HAROLD L. KLAWANS, M.D.
New York: W.H. Freeman and Co., 1996.
308 pp., bibliography, index. $22.95

> *Each hard blow to the head of a boxer causes a sudden movement of the brain, a displacement. Each time the head is snapped back, the brain is sent sailing back and forth within the spinal fluid. ...Each displacement, each acceleration and deceleration, leaves its trace in the axons that cross from the brain stem to the brain.... But is boxing designed to injure these axons? Make no mistake about it: the answer is yes. Grass grows, fish swim, and boxers attack each other's brains and especially the wires of the brain that travel from the brain stem to the brain proper. The damaged axons of the substantia nigra are not the prime target, they are a form of what we call collateral damage—quite a euphemism for death and destruction.... And it's all part of the game.*

In 1994, at age 31, one of the world's greatest basketball players, Chicago Bulls superstar Michael Jordan, attempted to begin a new career—in professional baseball. Despite training earnestly, Jordan was able to become only a mediocre minor league player, an outcome that neurologist Harold L. Klawans believes had less to do with Jordan's abilities as an athlete than with some fundamental realities about the development of the human brain. According to Klawans, most professional athletes and accomplished performers in other fields begin to acquire their specific skills during critical developmental periods, or "windows of opportunity," that occur in childhood and the early teens. It is at this time that the brain is most susceptible to new experiences and stimuli. As Jordan discovered, acquiring such complex skills later in life is an exceedingly difficult, if not impossible, task.

In this highly instructive and entertaining collection of essays, Klawans, a professor of neurology and pharmacology at Rush Medical College in Chicago and author of several books of clinical tales, including *Toscanini's Fumble* (1989) and *Newton's Madness* (1990), combines his passion for neurological discovery with his lifelong enthusiasm for sports. Though Klawans never personally treated any of the famed athletes whose stories he tells, he has observed them all from the unique perspective of a practicing neurologist, has read their biographies and autobiographies, and in some cases has had access to their medical reports, X-rays, and other revealing documents.

In *Why Michael Couldn't Hit* Klawans demonstrates how both the accomplishments and failures of many great athletes may ultimately be traced to the activities of the brain. The success of Italian boxer Primo Carnera, for example, was due in large part to a pituitary tumor that caused him to grow to an enormous size, though his strength and coordination were limited. The compulsive perfectionism associated with Tourette's syndrome resulted in Denver Nuggets star Mahmoud Abdul-Rauf becoming one of basketball's most accurate shooters. The dystonia suffered by golfing legend Ben Hogan, on the other hand, ended his career prematurely when the involuntary jerks caused by this muscle disease interferred with his ability to putt. Klawans also explains in detail how Muhammad Ali's boxing style and genetic endowment resulted in his developing a form of Parkinson's disease; in the course of this narrative, Klawans presents a convincing argument for banning boxing as a sport.

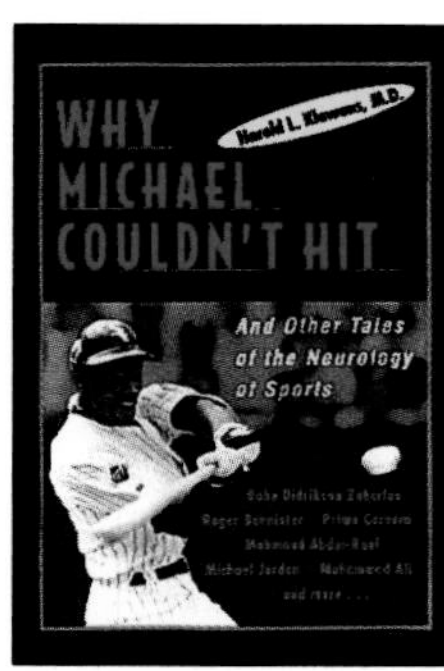

Although Klawans discusses the neurological problems encountered by other sports figures such as baseball great Lou Gehrig and Olympic sprinter Wilma Rudolph, the focus of these essays is not simply on the brains of athletes but on the *human* brain and its ability to learn and adapt itself to the environment. In one fascinating essay that compares the early musical training of Mozart with the training undertaken by current golf prodigy Tiger Woods, Klawans shows why early exposure to learning experiences is the factor that makes acquisition and development of skills during later periods of life possible. As Klawans points out, windows of opportunity exist for every activity, from learning to hit a baseball to learning to read. If skills are to be learned well, it is imperative that these critical periods be exploited.

—Sherman Hollar

The Wisdom of the Body
SHERWIN B. NULAND.
New York: Alfred A. Knopf, 1997.
395 pp., glossary. $26.95

> *Suppressed, repressed, regressed, cathexed, sublimated, symbolized, inhibited, fixated, displaced, transferred—these are some of the names given to the maneuvers of our minds as they attempt to avoid direct confrontation with the reproductive cell's essentially simple desire to meet its mate. It should be so easy, and among animals whose cerebral limitations prevent the manufacture of a psychological maelstrom like our own, it* is *easy. But to let it remain easy is not the human way. The human way is that the simplest stimuli are sufficient to send all manner of signals along all manner of pathways, and to make something vastly complex of what was biologically meant to be quite clear. Sexual reproduction is apparently too direct for us—we have taken on this enormous bundle of baggage we call sexuality.*

Having engagingly explained the physiological catastrophes that precede the cessation of life in his award-winning *How We Die* (1994), Sherwin B. Nuland undertakes in his latest book the daunting task of explicating how we live. Nuland is a practicing surgeon and clinical professor of surgery at Yale University, as well as being a prolific writer. His superior gifts as expositor and story-teller find ample scope in *The Wisdom of the Body,* a work that endeavors to describe and make plain for nonhealth professionals how the body functions in health and disease.

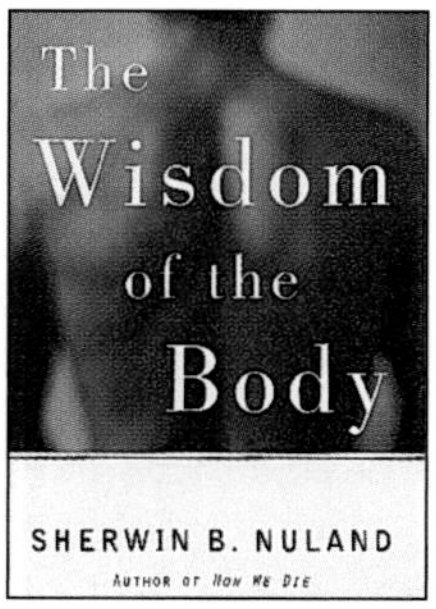

The title, as Nuland points out in the introduction, is not new but has graced volumes by illustrious scientists of past eras, among them the physiologists Ernest Starling and Walter B. Cannon. Nor is it difficult to see why the appellation has enjoyed such favor. In the reactions of the body—the delicate equilibrium of its complex chemistry and the uniquely fitting responses and finely tuned adaptations of each one of its component parts—it is impossible for the scientist not to detect something like a portentous organizing principle, a purposeful, astonishingly efficient ruling order. This is what, for lack of a better word, Nuland, like so many authorities before him, feels compelled to call "wisdom."

In 12 chapters and an epilogue, Nuland canvasses the extraordinary mechanism of the human body. His approach, insofar as the narrative is concerned, is more effective than that of writers of previous books by the same name. He draws from his own clinical experience to illustrate the perturbations wrought by disease upon the harmonious whole. Thus, in order to introduce concepts of circulatory function, Nuland recounts the dramatic case of a woman suffering a massive episode of intra-abdominal bleeding and the heroic efforts of the surgical team to rescue her from irreversible circulatory collapse.

Similarly, a disquisition on the lymphatic and venous systems leads to a discussion of the dissemination of cancer cells via lymphatic routes and then to an engrossing anecdote: "Years ago, I took care of a woman who...." Again, the disease acquires a human face, and the interest of the reader is captured. Other chapters deal in a similar manner with various aspects of human physiology, among them the functioning of the nervous system, the digestive tract, and the organs of reproduction.

The sense of immediacy is enhanced by the inclusion of patients' own subjective perceptions of their disease and treatment, quoted at length in italics to distinguish them from the rest of the text. Thanks to Nuland's clinical experience, he succeeds in lending to these utterances an air of authenticity. And since writers are notorious for using their own lives as grist for the mill, readers will not be surprised to find that the chapter on childbirth includes the author's own experience with paternity; here the italicized "patient's" comments are those of his second wife, Sarah, pregnant with their son, Will. Of the overwhelming sentiments he experienced in the delivery room, Nuland writes, "We are told there are no atheists in foxholes—let it be known that there are no cynics at the birth of their own children." The hallmarks of Nuland's writing—a touch of light humor, a physician's compassionate outlook, and an unassuming, lucid style—which have already earned his books wide acclaim, are fully in evidence in his latest effort.

—F. González-Crussi, M.D.

The Yale Guide to Children's Nutrition
WILLIAM V. TAMBORLANE, M.D., ed.
New Haven: Yale University Press, 1997.
415 pp., appendix, index. $18.00 (paper), $40.00 (cloth)

> *Some children love food and eat many foods with enthusiasm, whereas others are much choosier about what they put into their mouths. Most children vary in what they like: one day they love peas and the next day they spit them into their napkin. One day they love canned ravioli, but as soon as the parent buys a case to have on hand, the passion for ravioli has abated. Normal childhood eating habits provide challenges for responsible adults; picky eaters provide the consummate challenge....*
>
> *Children who recognize the family cook's tremendous investment in providing appetizing meals can garner attention by refusing to eat what has been prepared. This often heralds the introduction of the short-order cook, the person who leaps to the stove when the child rejects what is on the table.*

Often, books on children's nutrition can be downright scary for parents. Some contain a lot of frightening statistics about the health hazards of food additives and pesticide residues; others make the idea of properly nourishing a child seem so overwhelmingly difficult that the average parent feels defeated before she or he starts. This book is different. The contributors are people who have practical experience and thus understand that it is one thing to recommend that parents serve homemade muesli instead of "Choco-munchie-crunchies" and another thing to get kids to *eat* the muesli. As these experts know well, in order for kids to benefit from nutritious foods, they must actually consume them. Thus, for example, their sample lunch-box menus include such child-pleasing foods as bologna (albeit *turkey* bologna).

William V. Tamborlane is chief of pediatric endocrinology at the Yale University School of Medicine and director of the medical school's Children's Clinical Research Center at Yale-New Haven Children's Hospital. The contributors to the volume include more than 75 physicians, dietitians, nurses, and social workers from both the school and the hospital. The book is divided into major parts that cover (1) developmental nutrition from birth to adolescence, (2) common concerns about children's eating habits (including chapters on vegetarianism and feeding the young athlete), (3) children with special nutritional needs, (4) the building blocks of good nutrition, and (5) shopping for food, packing school lunches, and eating out. A sixth part includes nearly 100 pages of recipes—from squash and apple puree for infants to sweet corn ravioli—some from well-known chefs.

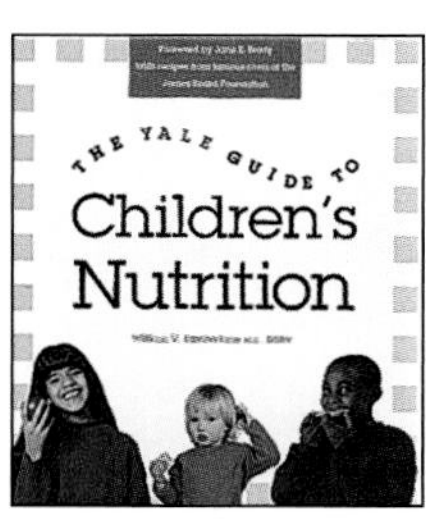

Each chapter is impressive for its breadth of coverage. Part three, for example, entitled "Beyond the Basics: Special Challenges in Nutrition," contains separate chapters on a broad range of problems that can affect children's eating habits and nutritional needs, including, among others, eating disorders, allergies, elevated cholesterol levels, diabetes, chronic gastrointestinal disorders, and cleft lip or palate. Part four is a crash course in the fundamentals of nutrition, covering the functions of calories, fat, protein, carbohydrate, and fiber. Many chapters end with a "Resources" section, which lists organizations that might be helpful (the American Celiac Society, for example, is cited in the chapter on childhood gastrointestinal disorders) or suggests books for further reading.

Some fairly complex subjects—how the body digests food, what functions vitamins perform, how tastes are perceived—are explained so simply and lucidly that one could probably read them aloud to a small child who is curious about these processes. The chapter on "Taste, Smell, and Food Preferences" is a fine example of this book at its best, explaining why much of what people associate with their sense of taste really depends on their sense of smell. The authors even provide a simple experiment involving a Lifesaver candy to help readers demonstrate for themselves the different parts played by these two senses. A discussion of genetic differences in taste perception contains the amazing fact that the number of taste buds on the human tongue can range from as few as 11 per square centimeter to more than 1,000. Again, an experiment is suggested for those who want to estimate the number of their own taste buds.

At the beginning of each chapter a common myth or misconception is dispelled. Is fish really "brain food"? (No. While it is an excellent source of protein and other nutrients, fish has not been shown to have any particular benefits for neurological development.) Should parents "starve a fever, feed a cold"? (No. Sick kids need to eat—and get adequate amounts of fluids—regardless of the illness.) Does diet play a part in acne or attention deficit disorder? (No to both.)

Some of the recipes in the last section come from celebrated chef-restaurateurs, among them Alice Waters of Chez Panisse in Berkeley, Calif., and Odessa Piper of L'Etoile in Madison, Wis. Many require minimal preparation and call for only a handful of ingredients. This reviewer has not yet tried any of them but would be willing to bet that Piper's cantaloupe soup would be a hit with her four-year-old.

—*Christine Sullivan*

Yellow Fever, Black Goddess: The Coevolution of People and Plagues
CHRISTOPHER WILLS.
Reading, Mass.: Addison-Wesley Publishing Co., 1996.
324 pp., glossary, notes, index. $24.00

The plague changed the face of Europe in many ways, both physically and intellectually. In 1348 the city of Siena was about to triple the size of its cathedral, intending that its grandeur would exceed that of St. Peter's in Rome. This immense project was stillborn when Siena's population was decimated by the plague. Petrarch's Laura perished, as did many members of the intellectual and artistic elite. And while there was no great upsurge in disbelief in the efficacy of organized religion, like that which would be sparked by the earthquake in Lisbon in 1755, the obvious helplessness of the Church in the face of this apparent act of God began to raise questions that would help to sow the seeds of the Reformation a century and a half later.

From Exodus in the Old Testament to Boccaccio's *Decameron,* accounts of plagues have always held a peculiar fascination. Given the current vogue for "doomsday" books about lethal microbes, prospective readers might easily make the mistake of assuming Christopher Wills's book to be yet another in the same vein. Wills, however, does not regard epidemic diseases as a sort of Malthusian revenge on modern civilization but rather considers them a natural and, in some sense, even beneficial phenomenon.

Wills, a biology professor at the University of California, San Diego, rejects the popular argument that unsustainable population growth is, in itself, responsible for the emergence of more numerous and more virulent pathogens. Rather, he suggests, the existence of larger numbers of human "hosts" has quite naturally resulted in larger populations of bacteria and viruses and, consequently, an increased likelihood that new, more lethal infectious agents will evolve.

He points out that population growth inevitably results in the movement of people into previously uninhabited or sparsely inhabited lands, where they encounter new strains of pathogens. Moreover, human populations tend to "simplify" the ecosystem they inhabit—clearing land, for example, and replacing a highly varied indigenous flora with a single agricultural crop. This process enables disease-spreading animals such as rats and cockroaches to colonize freely where once they might have been restrained by native predators. The human inhabitants of these modified ecosystems encounter fewer species of animals on a regular basis, which may lower their resistance to many pathogens.

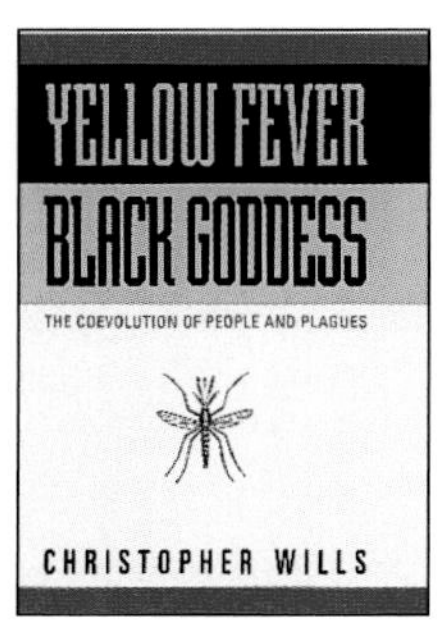

On the other hand, Wills suggests, exposure to a genetically diverse world may actually be health-promoting. His explanation of these interactions is central to his basic premise: that disease has fueled humankind's genetic evolution and diversity and that human evolution has, in a similar manner, shaped the development of pathogens.

Having laid this groundwork, Wills then gives a lucid account of bubonic plague—the notorious Black Death—examining the human suffering and social havoc wrought by plague; the process by which the pathogen effects its changes in rats, fleas, and humans; the genetic modifications that have occurred in the disease-causing bacillus, *Yersinia pestis,* to make it so deadly; and the rivalry between the scientists who searched for *Yersinia.* Wills shifts from scientific explanation to personal history with astonishing facility. The story of his British grandmother's near-fatal encounter with typhoid fever acquired in colonial India serves as a preface to his discussion of that disease. He is also able to explain in readily understandable terms the complex biological mechanisms of disease—*e.g.,* why there are more plague bacilli in warm areas than cold and how the pathogens that inhabit colder regions manage to be more lethal than their temperate-zone counterparts.

The writer is particularly adept at using metaphors and similes: "Fleas, of course, are nothing more than mobile hypodermic needles." Of the broad array of virulence genes that bacteria have at their disposal, he says, "It is as if assault weapons were to grow on the trees of Central Park, available for anyone to pluck down."

Wills's coverage of infectious scourges from antiquity to the present includes—in addition to plague—cholera, typhoid, syphilis, and AIDS. Curiously, the yellow fever of the title is referred to only in passing. The "black goddess" is apparently Kali, the Hindu goddess of death and destruction—called the Black One—who, Wills suspects, may have been connected to cholera.

Despite its confusing name, this book will be enjoyed by anyone who is interested in the biology or history of infectious diseases. Unfortunately, a number of errors of fact somewhat diminish its reliability as a reference source. Latex, for instance, is indeed a product of the tree *Hevea brasiliensis,* but it is not a form of tree sap, as the author states on page 281.

—*Christine Sullivan*

BOOK REVIEW CONTRIBUTORS

Sara Brant
Assistant Editor, Encyclopædia Britannica, Inc., Chicago

Adelheid Fischer
Associate Editor, Encyclopædia Britannica, Inc., Chicago

M.J. Friedrich
Associate Editor, Encyclopædia Britannica, Inc., Chicago

F. González-Crussi, M.D.
Professor of Pathology, Northwestern University Medical School, and Head of Laboratories, Children's Memorial Hospital, Chicago

Katherine I. Gordon
Editorial Coordinator, Encyclopædia Britannica, Inc., Chicago

Jean S. Gottlieb, Ph.D.
Freelance writer and editor and historian of science, Chicago. Author of *A Checklist of the Newberry Library's Printed Books in Science, Medicine, Technology, and the Pseudosciences ca. 1460–1750*

Sherman Hollar
Assistant Editor, Encyclopædia Britannica, Inc., Chicago

Stephen Lock, M.D.
Research Associate, Wellcome Institute for the History of Medicine, London

Alex Soojung-Kim Pang, Ph.D.
Deputy Editor, Encyclopædia Britannica, Inc., Chicago

Robert Rauch
Freelance editor and writer, Chicago

Andrea Gellin Shindler, M.A.
Executive Director and Founder of the Foundation for Human Potential, Wilmette, Ill.

Christine Sullivan
Copy Editor, Encyclopædia Britannica, Inc., Chicago

Charles P. Trumbull, Ph.D.
Director of Yearbooks, Encyclopædia Britannica, Inc., Chicago

Joseph Turow, Ph.D.
Professor of Communication, Annenberg School for Communication, University of Pennsylvania, Philadelphia. Author of *Playing Doctor: Television, Storytelling, and Medical Power* and *Breaking Up America: Advertisers and the New Media World*

Barbara Whitney
Copy Supervisor, Encyclopædia Britannica, Inc., Chicago

Anita Wolff
Managing Editor and Director of Research, Encyclopædia Britannica, Inc., Chicago

Recent Developments from the World of Medicine

AIDS/HIV Update

The level of optimism about many aspects of AIDS was higher in 1996–97 than perhaps at any other time since the disease was first described in 1981. Years of intensive research into the basic biology of HIV and the process by which it causes disease have yielded many of the virus's secrets. The development of effective treatments and methods for assessing response to treatment has prolonged the lives of patients. As a result of these advances, there is now hope that for many patients HIV/AIDS may become a manageable chronic disease—a disease that people "live with" rather than inevitably die from.

The HIV/AIDS epidemic is by no means over, however. The new treatments are complex, costly, and not uniformly effective. HIV transmission continues worldwide, and the limited availability of life-prolonging therapy in less-developed countries further accentuates the disparities between the world's "haves" and "have-nots."

The state of the epidemic

Given that many AIDS patients are living longer and that new cases continue to occur, it was no surprise that the prevalence of AIDS in the U.S. increased in 1996. (Prevalence is the proportion of the population affected by a given disease.) The cumulative number of reported cases from 1981 through 1996 was more than 580,000.

For the first time in the history of the epidemic, however, the Centers for Disease Control and Prevention reported a decline in AIDS-related deaths in 1996. The rate was 19% lower in January–September 1996 than in the same period in 1995. In some areas where data for the full year were available, the numbers were even more impressive. In New York City, for example, AIDS deaths dropped by 30% in 1996 compared with 1995. Similarly, Washington state reported a 35% decline in AIDS mortality. The trends showing a decline in death rates coincided with the introduction of a potent new class of anti-HIV drugs called protease inhibitors. Most experts believe these therapies are an important factor in the improved survival of people with AIDS. Preliminary data suggest, however, that not all those affected have benefited equally; persons of color and women have not experienced the same decline in death rates as the patient population at large, possibly because of differential access to the newer, more effective therapies.

In recent years African-Americans, Hispanics, and women have accounted for an increasing proportion of U.S. AIDS cases. In 1996 African-Americans accounted for 41% of adult cases, outnumbering whites for the first time. The relative proportion of women with AIDS also continued to rise, with women accounting for 20% of new cases in 1996—an all-time high. Most women become infected via heterosexual sex; a smaller proportion acquire HIV through intravenous drug use.

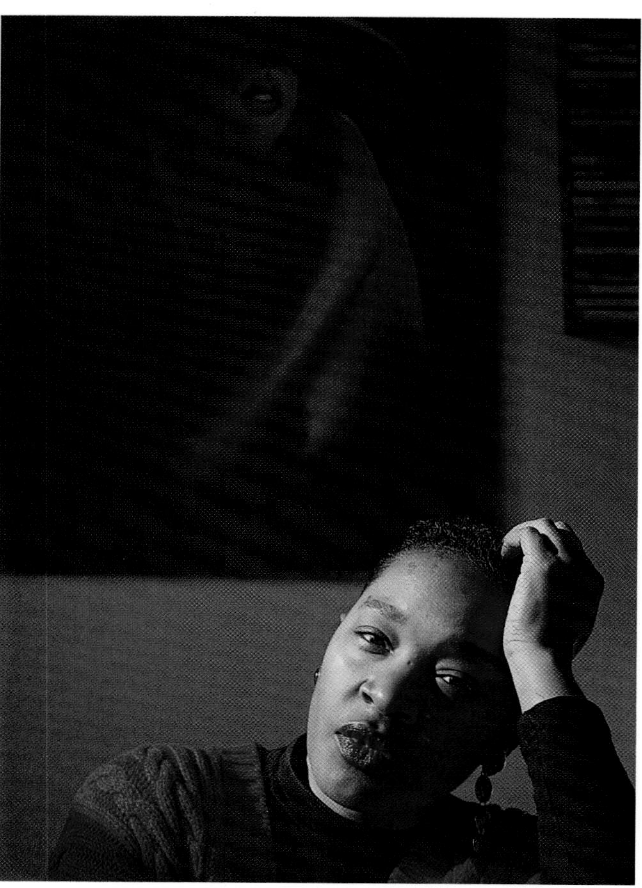

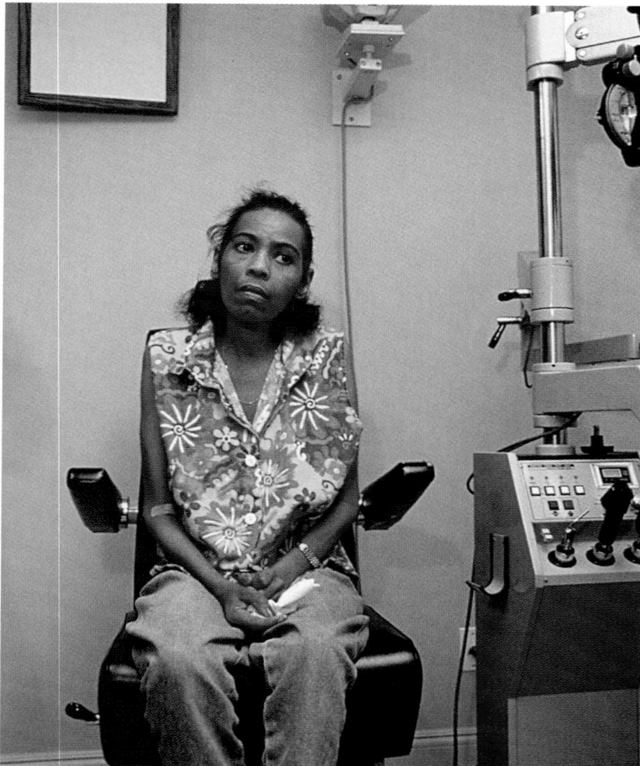

In the U.S. women and members of minority groups continue to account for the fastest-growing groups of AIDS patients. (Right) A Puerto Rican woman who fled her native country and an abusive husband is treated for AIDS in New York City. (Top right) This HIV-positive California woman acquired the infection from a former boyfriend who was an injecting drug user.

(Top) Lynn Johnson—Aurora; (above) Meryl Levin—Impact Visuals

(Below) Leah Melnick—Impact Visuals; (bottom) Pablo Bartholomew—Gamma Liaison

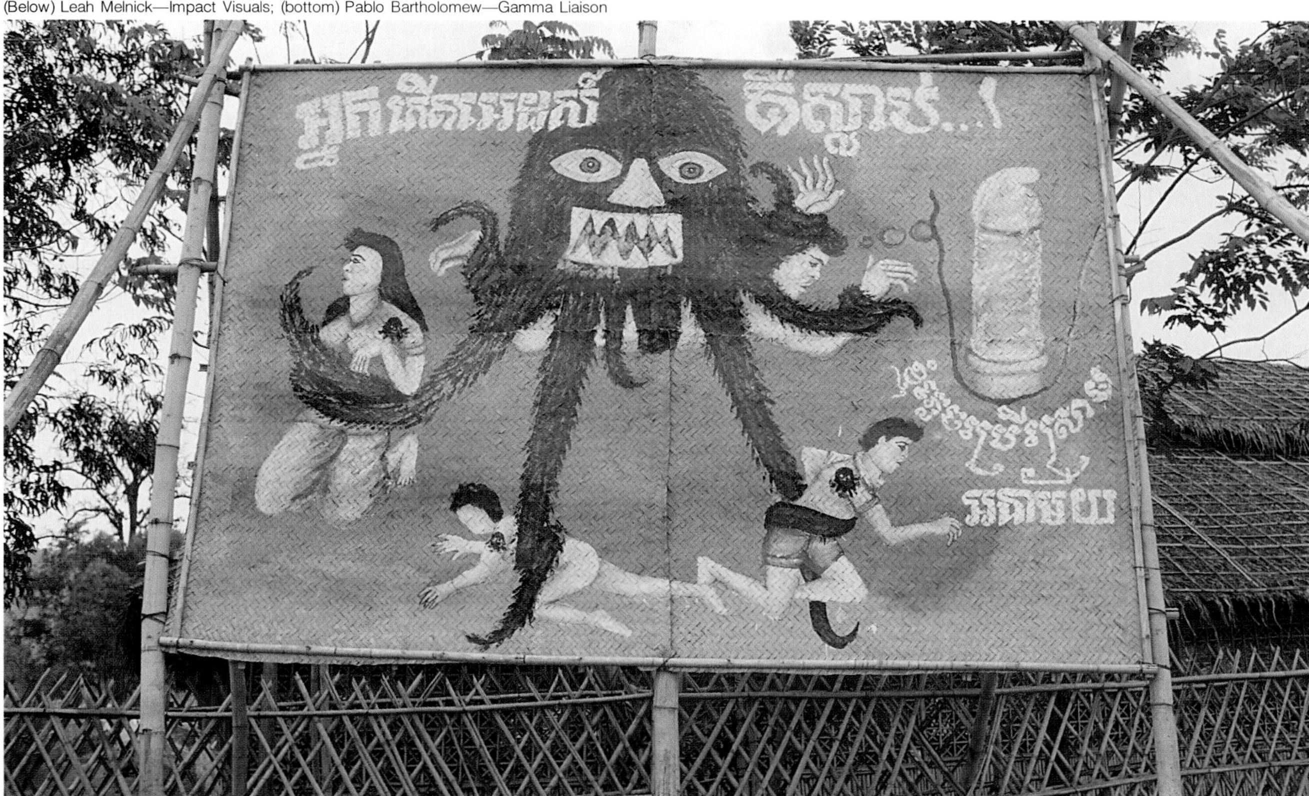

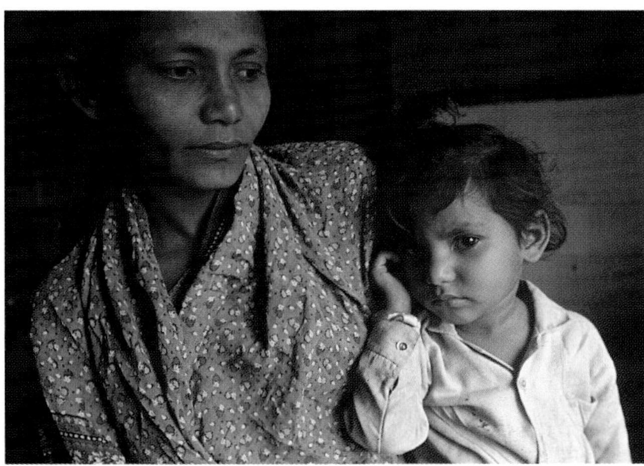

The AIDS epidemic continues to rage in Asia. (Above) In Thailand a hard-hitting AIDS-awareness campaign has slowed the explosive increase in the number of new HIV infections. (Right) India has been less successful in curbing the spread of the disease. This woman and her young daughter are both HIV-positive.

Although the growth of the HIV epidemic has stabilized in many developed countries, a number of less-developed countries continue to see increases—some steady and some explosive—in the number of persons infected with HIV. Three regions of the world show the most alarming increases: sub-Saharan Africa, Asia (particularly India), and Latin America. In mid-1997 the World Health Organization estimated that 14 million persons were living with HIV in sub-Saharan Africa, 4.8 million in South and Southeast Asia, and 1.3 million in Latin America; by comparison, there were an estimated 780,000 HIV-infected individuals in North America and 470,000 in Western Europe. As a result of an aggressive public health campaign promoting the use of condoms, Thailand has managed to significantly reduce the rate of new HIV infections and thereby has provided a ray of hope for other nations committed to prevention.

The infection process: new insights

New models of the dynamics of HIV infection continue to dramatically alter the basic understanding of how the virus acts in the body. According to one recently developed and widely accepted model, more than 10 billion HIV virions, or virus particles, are produced per day in a single HIV-infected individual—a number substantially higher than previous estimates. Moreover, this model estimates that more than 99% of HIV replication occurs in the immune system cells known as CD4+ T lymphocytes. CD4+ T lymphocytes, also commonly called CD4+ cells (as well as T-helper cells), play an important role in coordinating the actions of the other cells of the immune system. They decrease in number in persons with HIV infection and are a widely used measure of the integrity of the immune system.

Once CD4+ cells have been entered by the virus and have begun to actively produce new HIV virions, they live only about two days. In the terminology of the new model, these infected cells are the primary "compartment," or site, of HIV replication in the body. Most of this replication takes place in the lymphoid tissues (*i.e.,* lymph nodes, ducts, and vessels). In the primary compartment the average HIV cycle time—that is, the period from

The Dynamics of HIV Infection: One Model

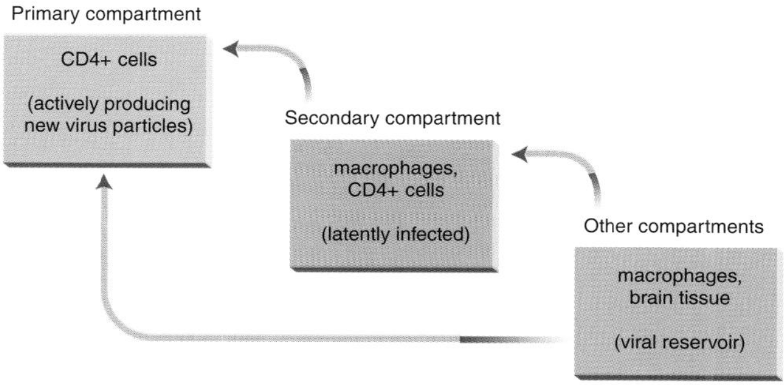

Source: Information from A.S. Perelson *et al.*, presented at the XI International Conference on AIDS, 1996.

the time HIV is released from one cell, infects another, and that cell releases a new progeny virion—is between two and three days; this corresponds to about 140 viral replication cycles per year. Replication of HIV at this rate is thought to begin at the time of infection and to continue throughout the course of the infection.

Preliminary studies indicate that several weeks of treatment with a combination of potent anti-HIV drugs can almost completely suppress viral replication, reducing the amount of virus in the patient's blood to undetectable levels. Soon after drug therapy is discontinued, however, viral levels rebound, which suggests that virus particles sequestered somewhere in the body remain unaffected by drug treatment. The new model proposes that a small but significant amount of active HIV replication occurs in the so-called secondary compartment—populations of cells that are not as instrumental to HIV replication as the CD4+ cells in the primary compartment and that may have a completely different timetable for reproducing. This category includes cells in which the virus is latent (*i.e.,* not actively reproducing) and cells with life spans much longer than that of CD4+ cells.

Even though less than 1% of virus production takes place in the secondary compartment, it apparently functions as a reservoir, harboring virus particles capable of reinfecting cells in the primary compartment. Moreover, eradicating HIV from the secondary compartment is problematic, if it is indeed possible at all. And because of the longer life span of the cells that constitute the secondary compartment, if anti-HIV drugs were capable of eliminating the virus from these sites, a minimum of several years of therapy would be required. To make matters even more complicated, HIV may also be present in still other "compartments," such as in cells of the central nervous system. Again, HIV-infected cells from these compartments could serve as a reservoir of the virus, a source for reinfection of primary or secondary compartments, perhaps years after an individual was thought to be free of HIV. Small-scale experiments are under way to test the feasibility of completely eradicating HIV from the human body.

Unlocking the secrets of coreceptors

When HIV interacts with a cell, it first seeks out and attaches to a protein receptor, known as CD4, on the cell surface. For some time, scientists have generally agreed that in order for HIV to enter into a cell successfully, it must also bind to another receptor. Within the past two years, investigators have shown that HIV utilizes at least two distinct types of "coreceptors," depending on the type of cell being infected and the strain of HIV involved. The major HIV coreceptors are CXCR-4 (also known as fusin, or LESTR) and CCR-5 (also known as CKR-5). Obviously, human cells are not equipped with these receptors simply to facilitate the entry of HIV. Rather, the receptors normally serve as binding sites for hormonelike compounds known as chemokines, which play a role in communication between cells during the processes of inflammation and infection.

Several research groups have shown that some people make a defective form of the CCR-5 receptor protein. In essence, this defective protein does not protrude sufficiently from the cell membrane for HIV to bind to it. Only those individuals who possess two mutant genes for the CCR-5 receptor produce an obviously defective protein. (Nearly all genes exist in pairs, one inherited from the mother and one from the father. The genes encode—carry instructions for the synthesis of—proteins.) Interest in these defective receptors increased in 1996 when researchers from the Aaron Diamond AIDS Research Center in New York City described two individuals who had never become infected despite repeated sexual exposure to HIV; both of these individuals carried a pair of mutant CCR-5 genes. Subsequent work has shown that (1) 1–2% of Caucasians carry two mutant versions of the CCR-5 gene and (2) among HIV-negative homosexual Caucasians at high risk of acquiring HIV, one-third carry two mutant versions of the gene. Moreover, as of summer 1997, among more than 2,700 HIV-infected persons whose CCR-5 receptor genes had been analyzed, only 4 had been found to carry a pair of mutant CCR-5 genes.

Taken together, these findings suggest that the CCR-5 coreceptor plays a key role in the initial entry of HIV into susceptible target cells—at least in sexually transmitted HIV. People who carry two mutant CCR-5 genes have substantive but not absolute protection against sexual acquisition of HIV. Individuals who carry one mutant and one normal CCR-5 gene do not appear to be protected. Preliminary data suggest, however, that these latter individuals, if infected, may progress to AIDS more slowly than persons who possess no mutated CCR-5 genes.

The discoveries regarding HIV coreceptors have important implications. With an improved understanding of where and how HIV enters cells, scientists may be able to develop new anti-HIV therapies; such compounds might act by mimicking the natural chemokines that bind to the receptor and thereby blocking the binding of HIV to the receptor. Another strategy would be to develop antibodies to the receptor. The latter approach could be part of a biological prevention strategy that would work like a vaccine, preventing acquisition of the infection.

Combination therapy: the mainstay

Combination regimens, in which two or more antiretroviral drugs are used concurrently, have become the mainstay of care in the U.S. in past year or two. Eleven anti-HIV agents have been approved by the Food and Drug Administration for use in HIV infection.

Anti-HIV drugs are classified by the part of the virus's life cycle they inhibit. Three different types, or classes, have been developed: nucleoside analogs, nonnucleoside analogs, and pro-

Lacy Atkins—Associated Press

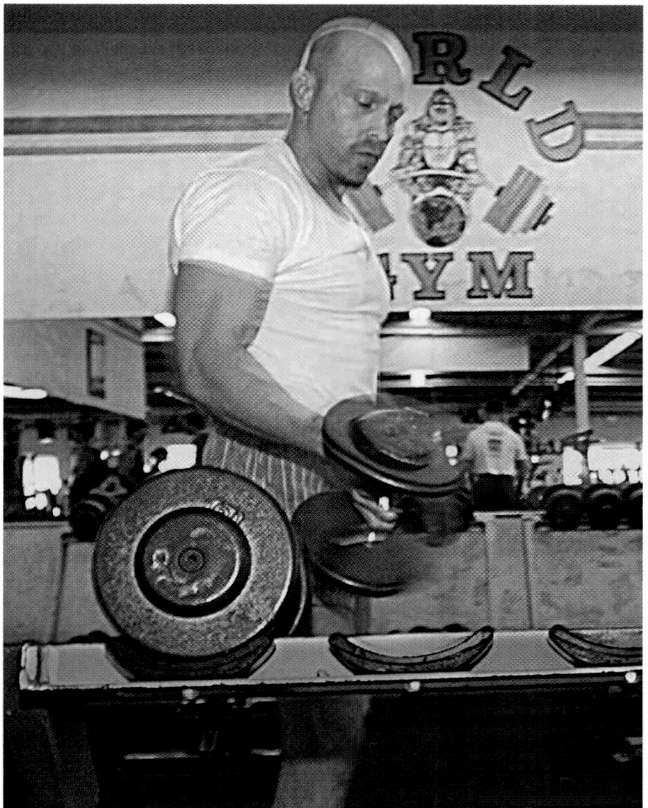

After adding a protease inhibitor to his treatment regimen, this San Francisco AIDS patient, like many others benefiting from this new class of drug, experienced a dramatic improvement in his health.

tease inhibitors. The agents that have been in use the longest, such as zidovudine (AZT), are nucleoside analogs. They inhibit the activity of reverse transcriptase, an enzyme required for the synthesis of DNA from viral RNA, an early step in the events that occur after HIV has entered a cell. Although not very effective in suppressing HIV for long when given as a single agent, the reverse transcriptase inhibitors remain important as components of multidrug regimens. The nonnucleoside analogs also act by inhibiting reverse transcriptase but in a different way from nucleoside analogs.

The most promising addition to the HIV treatment arsenal has been the newest class of compounds, the protease inhibitors. These drugs block the viral enzyme responsible for cutting a "long" protein (*i.e.,* one with a long sequence of amino acids) into the many peptides, or shorter proteins, that are essential for creation of a new infectious virus. Multiple protease inhibitors have been studied, and four (indinavir, nelfinavir, ritonavir, and saquinavir) are now available for use in the U.S. Each of these agents has a different chemical structure, pharmacological characteristics, and side effects. All block the growth of HIV in the laboratory and the living body, and all are costly—$4,500–$8,000 for a year's worth of one drug.

Large studies in which patients have been randomly assigned to receive either a protease inhibitor combined with one or two reverse transcriptase inhibitors or reverse transcriptase inhibitors alone have demonstrated significantly longer survival in patients taking the protease inhibitor. Further, protease inhibitor therapy produces dramatic decreases in the level of virus circulating in the blood, often to a level below that detected in tests used to quantify HIV. Far less is known about the suppressive effects of these drugs in tissues other than blood. Preliminary results from a small number of patients suggest that the amount of HIV in lymph nodes also declines with use of triple-drug regimens that include a protease inhibitor, an important observation if eradication of HIV is ever to be a reality.

Relatively little is known about the effects of protease inhibitors on HIV in genital secretions and, by extension, about their impact on the transmissibility of HIV through sexual intercourse. Another important question is how long the antiviral suppression will last and what the long-term effects of these new regimens will be. Many, but not all, patients treated with these therapies have shown marked increases in the number of CD4+ cells. What is not yet known, but is actively being studied, is whether these cells are functional and whether the immune system can be restored to its original state. The clinical improvements experienced by patients taking protease inhibitors suggest that these drugs must have some immunologic benefits, but many questions remain. Until more data are available, AIDS experts recommend that people with AIDS continue prophylactic (preventive) treatment for opportunistic infections, even if their CD4+ cell counts improve. (Opportunistic infections are those that occur in people whose immune systems are compromised; *see* below.)

The new potent drug combinations pose several practical problems, not the least of which is the complexity of a regimen that may involve taking 10–18 pills per day at two to five different times. Some medications must be taken with food and some on an empty stomach; one treatment requires drinking large amounts of liquid to prevent the development of kidney stones. If a patient does not take the drugs regularly and exactly as prescribed, the virus can develop resistance. The potential side effects range from minor to life-threatening, and, as mentioned above, the costs can be enormous. Treatment guidelines have been developed to aid physicians and HIV-infected persons in using these potent new treatments in the most optimal and cost-effective way.

Ironically, the success of these therapies in improving health

Combination drug therapy is now the mainstay of treatment for HIV infection in the U.S. Although lifesaving, these regimens are not without drawbacks; they are complex and costly and may have serious side effects.

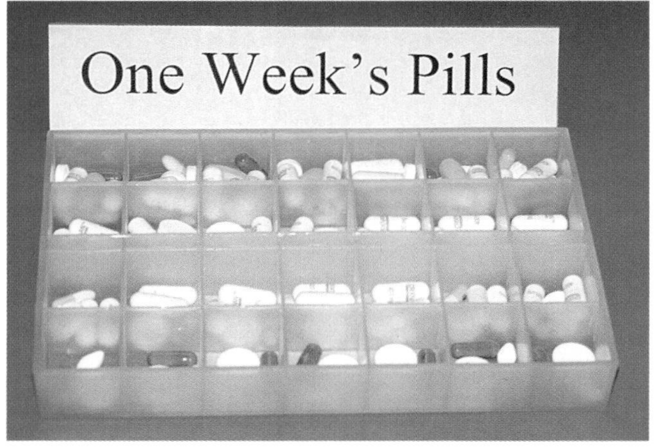

Ann C. Collier

and prolonging life has created some unanticipated social, economic, and psychological complications. What will happen, for example, when a person formerly disabled by AIDS improves enough to return to work but such work disqualifies him or her from receiving the disability benefits that paid for the medications in the first place?

In another innovation in treatment, prophylactic multidrug therapy is now recommended for health care workers who are occupationally exposed to HIV. Data from one study of health care personnel who were exposed to contaminated blood or body fluids suggest that AZT reduces the risk of acquisition of HIV by 79%. Experts believe that the newer combination of drugs may be even more effective. The U.S. Public Health Service has formally recommended use of combinations of antiretrovirals for four weeks after a high-risk occupational exposure to HIV. The prophylactic use of anti-HIV drugs in people exposed through sexual contact is a matter of debate; there are no data on the effectiveness of therapy in this situation.

Another treatment approach

Interest in therapy specifically directed at boosting the immune system has increased in the past year. For several years investigators from the National Institutes of Health have been experimenting with interleukin-2, a natural cytokine (chemical messenger), in HIV-infected individuals. Cytokines normally regulate the growth and development of lymphocytes. In one year-long study, all patients were treated with reverse transcriptase inhibitors, while approximately half also received intermittent injections of interleukin-2. Whereas the patients on anti-HIV drugs alone showed declines in CD4+ cells, those who received interleukin-2 experienced a more than 100% increase in average CD4+ cell counts. On the basis of these encouraging results, further studies with interleukin-2 are in progress, assessing whether the newly created CD4+ cells are functional and whether interleukin-2 will be useful when added to the newer, more potent anti-HIV drug regimens.

Opportunistic infections

Compared with advances in the understanding and treatment of HIV, the past year's developments in the field of opportunistic infections were less dramatic, but they were important nonetheless. In contrast to the late 1980s and early 1990s, when the number of cases of HIV-related tuberculosis (TB) in the United States increased to epidemic proportions, the past two years have witnessed steady and significant declines. This reversal is most likely the result of more effective TB treatments and intensive efforts to identify those needing treatment, both made possible by increased funding for programs to combat the disease.

One of the most significant recent changes in the management of AIDS-related opportunistic infections involved drug treatment for infection with *Mycobacterium avium* and related organisms, a condition known as *M. avium* complex, or MAC. *M. avium* lives in the environment (in water and soil); disseminated infection with this organism develops predominantly in patients with very advanced AIDS. MAC can cause fever, weight loss, anemia, and abdominal pain. Several recent studies have shown that use of azithromycin or clarithromycin in patients with AIDS is effective in preventing MAC infection. These commonly used antibiotics were shown to be more effective than rifabutin, the drug previously recommended for this condition. In addition, azithromycin and clarithromycin offer an advantage over rifabutin in that they have fewer adverse interactions with other important drugs, such as the protease inhibitors. Authorities now recommend the regular use of one of these agents for prevention of MAC in patients with advanced HIV infection.

HIV testing: more options

Until fairly recently, individuals who wished to be tested for HIV had to go to a medical facility to have blood drawn and return in person to receive the test results. A substantial proportion of those who go for testing never go back for their results. In 1996 for the first time, testing for HIV became available via an over-the-counter test kit that enables a person to collect a blood specimen at home, mail it to a laboratory, and obtain the results by telephone; the process is anonymous. Advocates of this method suggest that it will increase access to HIV testing among individuals who are concerned about confidentiality and that it will increase the proportion of those tested who find out the result. On the other side are those who argue that it will be impossible to properly counsel individuals learning over the phone that they are HIV-infected. It is not yet clear what proportion of those at risk will use this method or what the consequences will be.

Alternative methods that do not require a blood specimen have also been developed. One of these is a system for collection and antibody testing of oral secretions. It is intended to be administered only by health professionals, however. Available data suggest that oral secretion HIV testing is highly accurate. Such methods will be of benefit in situations where collection of blood is difficult or problematic, as in young children or where cultural taboos discourage the drawing of blood.

—David H. Spach, M.D.
and Ann C. Collier, M.D.

Spreading the Gospel of AIDS Prevention

> ***Not everything that is faced can be changed, but nothing can be changed until it is faced.***
>
> —James Baldwin

The overrepresentation of black Americans among AIDS cases has been well documented. Blacks constitute 12% of the U.S. population, yet they represented 41% of reported AIDS cases in 1996. Some 55% of women with AIDS are African-American, while 58% of pediatric AIDS cases are among African-American children. Since 1991 AIDS has been the leading cause of death in African-American men aged 25–44, and in 1994 the disease became the number one killer of African-American women of the same age group. In 1995, in states that required confidential HIV testing, African-Americans accounted for 46% of male infections (27,098 cases) and 66% of female infections (12,753 cases). At a time when new HIV infections are declining among white people and new drug therapies are extending the lives of many patients with AIDS, blacks are dying from the disease at an alarming rate. The question is, "Why?"

Lynn Johnson—Aurora

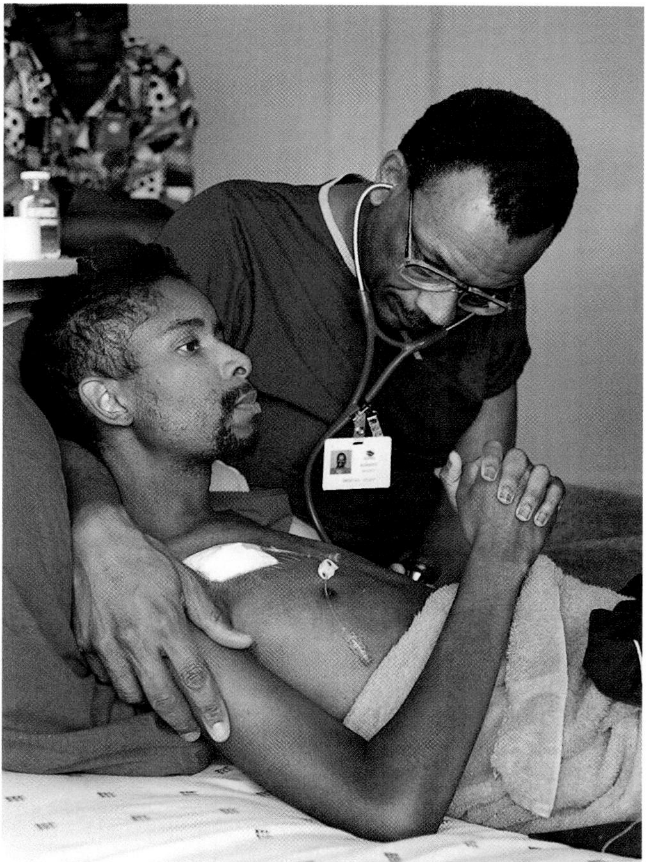

An AIDS patient is attended by his doctor. African-Americans as a group have been disproportionately hard hit by HIV/AIDS. While prevention messages may have helped curb the growth of the epidemic among whites, they have had significantly less impact in the black community.

A matter of trust

African-Americans on the whole have not heeded public health messages aimed at halting the spread of HIV/AIDS. Explanations that have emerged for this lack of response are that blacks have a blanket distrust of government reports on AIDS, that they harbor suspicions about the origins of HIV, and even that many African-Americans believe AIDS is a form of genocide that has been unleashed upon the black race. While some professionals may dismiss such notions as inconsequential or even ridiculous, there is plenty of evidence not only that they exist but that they are widely held. A survey done by the Southern Christian Leadership Conference in the early 1990s found that 35% of respondents thought AIDS was a form of genocide directed at black people, and another 30% thought it might be. In September 1994 the U.S. Public Health Service cosponsored a conference entitled "Breaking Barriers, Building Bridges: National Congress on the State of HIV/AIDS in Racial and Ethnic Communities." One of the questions addressed at the conference was "Is AIDS medical genocide?" The speaker, physician Abdul Alim Muhammad, minister of health for the Nation of Islam and director of the Abundant Life Clinic in Washington, D.C., stated quite directly, "Genocide is the policy of the U.S. government."

In order to fully appreciate the position of Muhammad and the social construction of AIDS in the black community today, it is necessary to know something about the legacy of mistrust toward the U.S. medical establishment that has grown up among black people. In the 1970s, well before the first cases of HIV/AIDS had been diagnosed, Castellano Turner and William Darity at the University of Massachusetts at Amherst surveyed 1,890 black Americans in three cities to assess their attitudes toward family planning. Fear of genocide was a prominent feeling expressed about programs that promoted birth control. Medical historian and physician Vanessa N. Gamble has written about the bitter history of sterilization abuse and coercive birth-control programs aimed at blacks, and she points out that such forced family-planning practices were indeed perceived by the black community at large as genocidal. But by far the most notorious example of medical abuse of black people in the U.S. is the "Tuskegee Study of Untreated Syphilis in the Negro Male."

Tuskegee's dark shadow

The Tuskegee study, the longest-running nontherapeutic experiment on human beings in the history of medicine and public health, has become a metaphor for the violation of human rights in the name of biomedical research. The government-sponsored research project began in 1932 and continued for four decades. In the guise of offering treatment, the U.S. Public Health Service allowed 399 syphilis-infected black male sharecroppers in rural Alabama to go untreated so that the effects of a devastating disease could be monitored. (There was an assumption at the time that the course of syphilis in blacks differed from that in whites.) The subjects were not told that they had syphilis, only that they had "bad blood." Long after penicillin was established as a safe and effective cure for syphilis in the 1940s, the men in the Tuskegee study continued to receive placebos (tonics of no therapeutic value). To ensure that the participants' bodies would be available for autopsy, the government promised free burials and paid the men's families somewhere between $35 and $50; this "burial insurance" was not an insignificant sum for rural blacks born and raised in poverty.

It cannot be emphasized strongly enough that to this day there remains a legacy of distrust and suspicion in the African-American community that hampers most medical research that involves blacks and also minimizes the success of all public health efforts to prevent illness in that community. In *Bad Blood* (1981), the definitive history of the Tuskegee syphilis study, medical historian James Jones specifically linked Tuskegee to the mistrust that now clouds AIDS education, prevention, and treatment efforts. Such a sentiment was also expressed in testimony before the National Commission on AIDS in 1990 by Alpha Thomas, a health educator with the Dallas (Texas) Urban League: "So many African-American people that I work with do not trust hospitals or any of the other community health care service providers because of that Tuskegee experiment. It is like...if they did it then, they will do it again." Indeed, because the researchers who conducted the Tuskegee study patently withheld information about syphilis from participants, black people today may believe that they are not being told the full truth about AIDS.

In February 1997, during Black History Month, Americans who knew little or nothing of the Tuskegee study learned about it when Home Box Office (HBO) aired *Miss Evers' Boys,* a made-for-television movie based on a play of the same name. The movie focused on a fictional black public health nurse (Eunice Evers,

(Below) Centers for Disease Control and Prevention; (right) Everett Collection

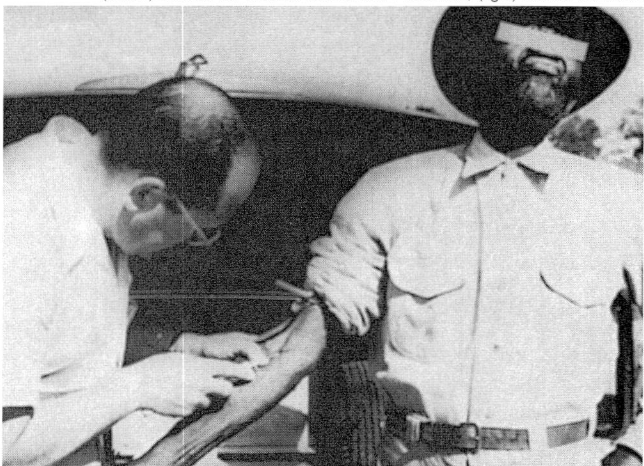

Distrust of the medical establishment runs deep in the black community—in large part because the blatantly unethical Tuskegee syphilis study (above) was allowed to occur. (Right) The events behind the infamous experiment were dramatized in the 1997 cable-television movie Miss Evers' Boys, *starring Alfre Woodard and Laurence Fishburne.*

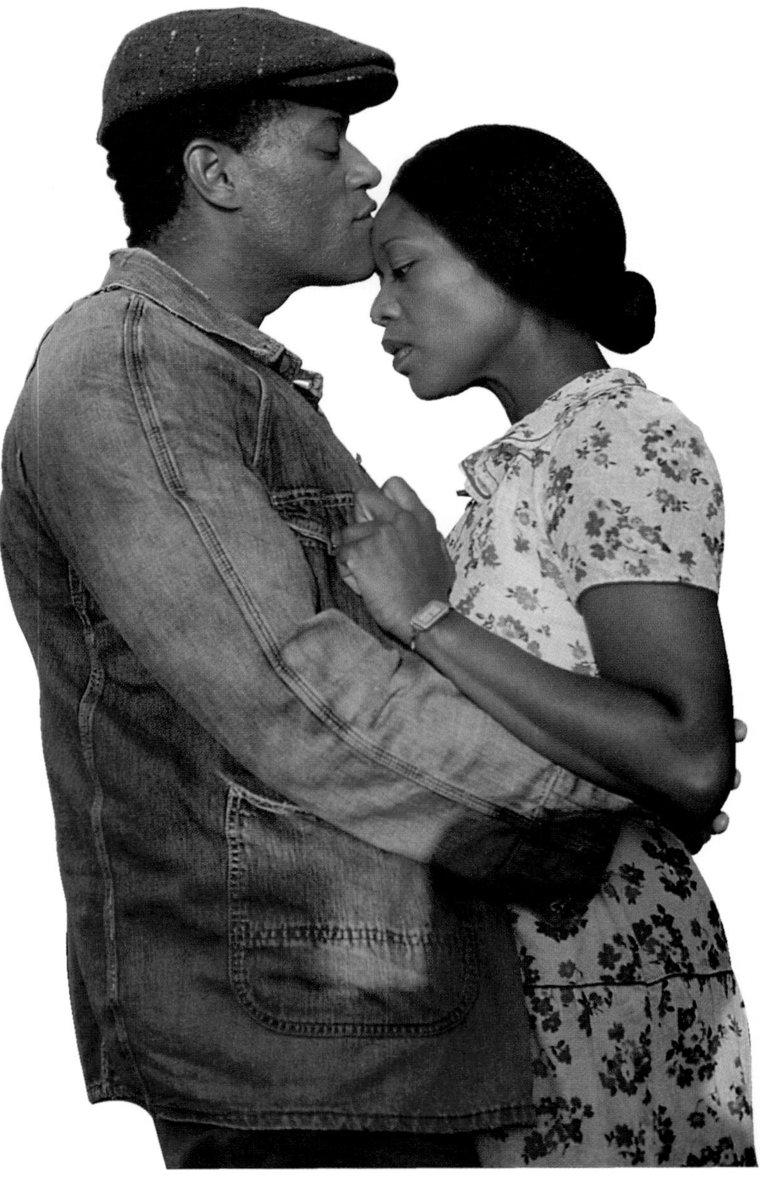

whose character was loosely based on that of Eunice Rivers, the nurse-facilitator who kept the Tuskegee participants involved through the long research project.) For millions of TV viewers, this fictional version of the tragic experiment (which blurred the historical facts in typical Hollywood fashion) will be all they "know." In all likelihood, members of the black community who viewed HBO's blockbuster will only feel further alienated from the medical establishment. It is in this context that African-Americans now confront the worsening AIDS crisis. (On May 16, 1997, Pres. Bill Clinton issued a formal apology for the Tuskegee study in the East Room of the White House.)

When Pernessa Seele saw that churches in her own community (of Harlem, N.Y.) had not responded to the AIDS crisis, she envisioned a "Week of Prayer" for the afflicted. Seele's desire was realized; (below) she joins local clergy in an AIDS prayer march outside Harlem Hospital.

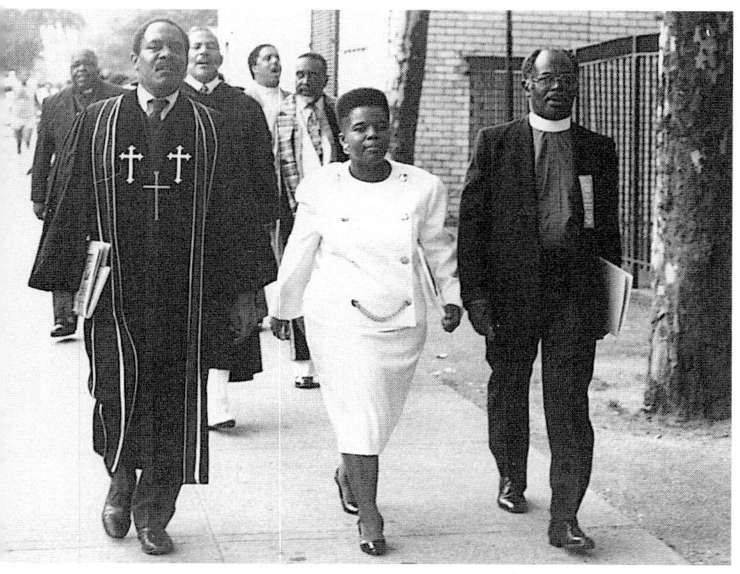

Courtesy of The Balm in Gilead

AIDS response: long overdue

> ***I have found that battling despair does not mean closing my eyes. It means teaching, surviving, and fighting. When I dare to be powerful, to use my strength in the service of my vision, then it becomes less and less important whether I am afraid.***
>
> —Audre Lorde (1934–92), feminist poet and essayist

In 1987 the Centers for Disease Control and Prevention (CDC), Atlanta, Ga., held the first national conference on the prevention of HIV disease in ethnic and racial minority populations. A Black Coalition Caucus that grew out of that gathering issued a report the following year. That report stated:

> ***Blacks in particular demand the truth because some health educators, when asked about the origin of the AIDS virus, answer that Blacks in Africa who were bitten by infected green monkeys running around the villages started the AIDS epidemic and pandemic. As HIV infection continues to increase among black men, women, and children, bringing death to an alarm-***

Photographs, courtesy of The Balm in Gilead

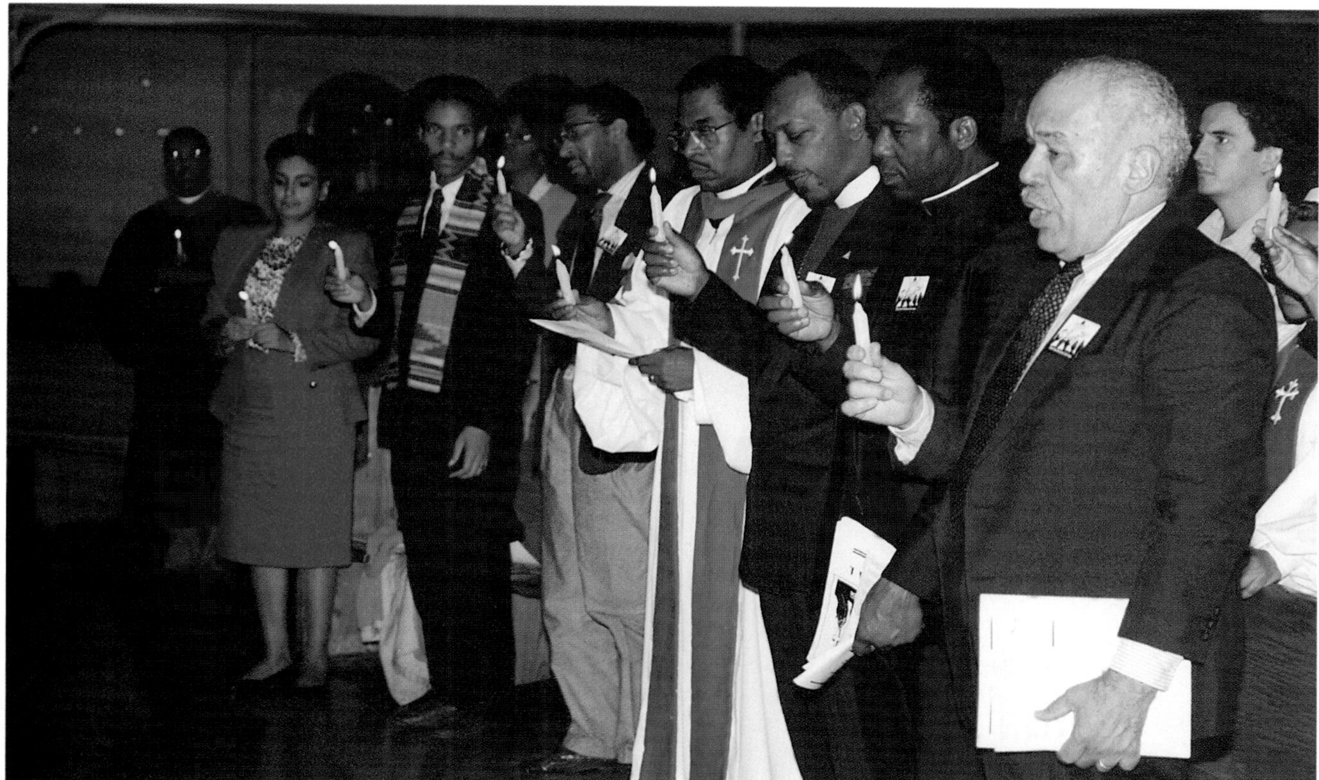

ingly high number of young people, Blacks have come to fear that research scientists have exposed the race to a deadly "Andromeda Strain."

The caucus resolved "to look to our Black clergy and church for absolute assurance that CDC AIDS testing and counseling initiatives are not just another Tuskegee tragedy being perpetrated on the Black race." The caucus articulated the central role that the church can play in combating HIV/AIDS. Indeed, clergy and leaders in the faith community are trusted in ways that health professionals and government officials are not and may never be.

In 1989 Pernessa Seele, a staff member at the Harlem Hospital Center in New York City, daily witnessed African-Americans suffering through the late stages of AIDS, alone and abandoned. She remembers feeling "really devastated by not seeing the kind of spiritual support that I expected" for people who were dying. She was particularly surprised that there did not seem to be any black church response to the human suffering caused by AIDS. Seele had a close friend who was an organist for his church and sang in its choir, but when he was dying from AIDS, his church was silent. Not so long after his death, Seele woke up one morning and said aloud to herself, "We've got to pray on this situation." When she said that, "it was like boom!" she recalls. "That's it, Harlem Day of Prayer. No, this is too much for a *day.* Harlem Week of Prayer! And when I said Harlem Week of Prayer, the whole room just lit up! I knew I had had a cosmic experience." The vision Seele had of a day, then a week, of prayer for AIDS was first realized in Harlem in 1989. It has been repeated annually, and now such prayer weeks are being observed in cities across the nation.

(Above) During the second annual Black Church Week of Prayer for the Healing of AIDS (1990), Harlem's Salem United Methodist Church stages a candlelight prayer vigil for people with AIDS. Communitywide events for the AIDS prayer weeks are coordinated by the not-for-profit organization The Balm in Gilead. (Below) A Sunday-school class at Convent Avenue Baptist Church makes use of materials provided by The Balm in Gilead to learn about HIV/AIDS prevention.

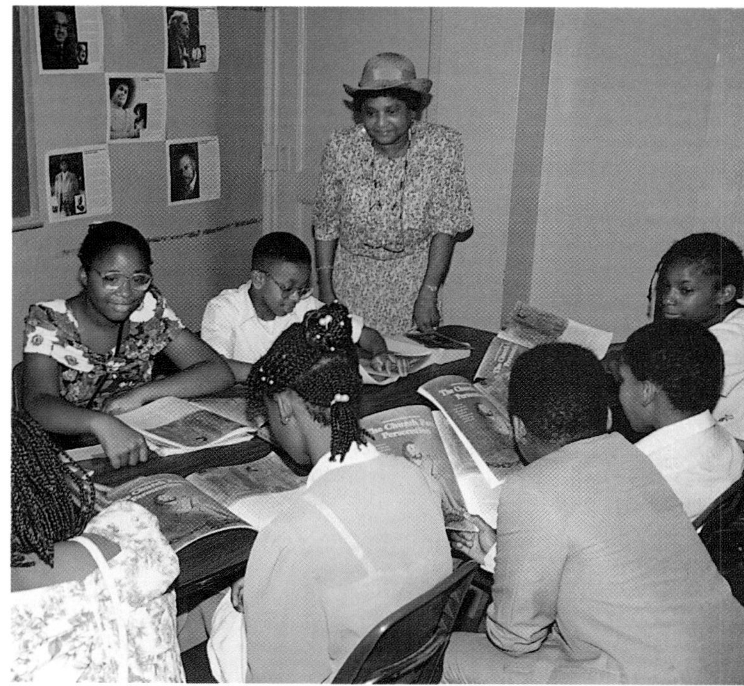

It is the first Sunday in March 1997, and church services are under way in a small, weathered chapel just outside Atlanta. Pastor Yaqar Benowr of Believe and Receive Ministries is delivering a sermon about love and hope for those who live with AIDS. On the same day in the heart of the black community in Durham, N.C., the Rev. Daryl Iverson stands in the pulpit of Orange Grove Missionary Baptist Church and delivers a prayer of compassion; then he calls upon the choir members to lift their voices and sing for the healing of AIDS. Over the next six days, in black churches in Macon, Ga.; Nashville, Tenn.; Cleveland, Ohio; and Kansas City, Mo., choirs sing and ministers preach—all in observance of the Black Church Week of Prayer for the Healing of AIDS.

Since AIDS was first recognized as a new disease in 1981, far too many African-Americans have suffered in silence without the unconditional love and support that is the tradition of black churches throughout the United States. The Rev. Eddie White, pastor of Mount Sinai Baptist Church, Thomasville, N.C., has "seen people who would not sit on the same pew if they knew a person there had AIDS." The Reverend White believes that churches should be "a refuge for people with AIDS. If they can't go to the church, where can they go?" Churches can offer not only messages of compassion for the sick and their loved ones but culturally sensitive HIV/AIDS-prevention messages aimed at the uninfected.

Thanks in large part to the efforts of people like Benowr, Iverson, Seele, and White and many more, the African-American faith community is at long last taking ownership of HIV disease; congregations throughout the nation are celebrating Black Church Week of Prayer for the Healing of AIDS; and more and more ministers are openly conducting funerals for young African-American men and women who die before their time. In the wake of so many AIDS deaths and bearing the burden of loved ones presently suffering from HIV disease, black families are now reaching out to the church for hope and receiving its comfort, compassion, and prayers.

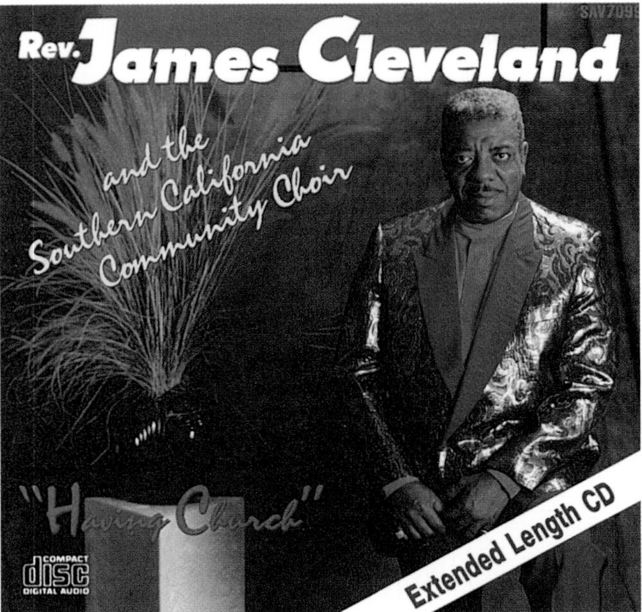

The "king of gospel" died of AIDS in 1991, having suffered alone and in silence. Now the gospel music community is rising up and singing for the healing of the many among its ranks who are ailing and dying.

From the pulpit to the airwaves

AIDS brought forth responses that have tarnished the golden halos of our piety.

—The Rev. James A. Forbes, Jr., pastor, Riverside Church, Harlem, N.Y.

It is in the shadow of suffering and death that black church leaders have broken the silence and cast the light of the gospel on AIDS. Another very credible source of information—one that can reach even more black people than churches and is only starting to be realized as a powerful health communication channel—is gospel radio. Gospel radio is at the core of the African-American cultural experience, with over 150 gospel stations reaching as many as

The Rev. Yvette Flunder (below left) is a nationally known gospel singer, pastor of San Francisco's City of Refuge Community Church, and executive director of the Ark of Refuge, which provides housing and spiritual support for Bay Area residents with HIV/AIDS. Artist Thomas Rohnacher is a member of Flunder's congregation; his painting "Love Your Neighbor as Yourself" (below right) was inspired by her compassionate teachings.

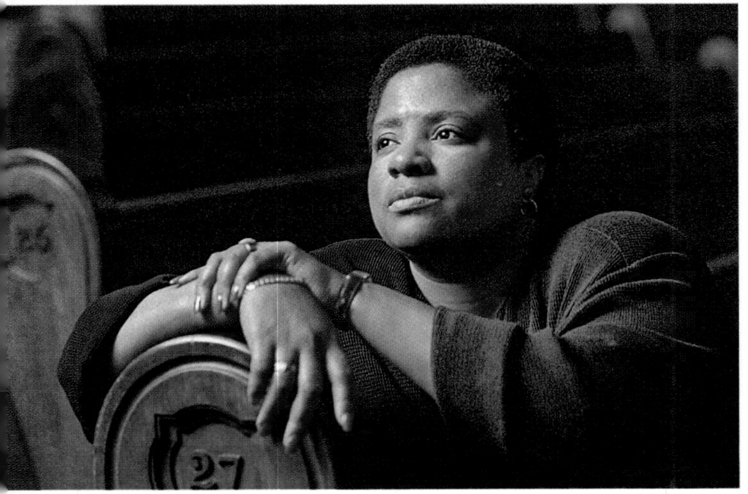

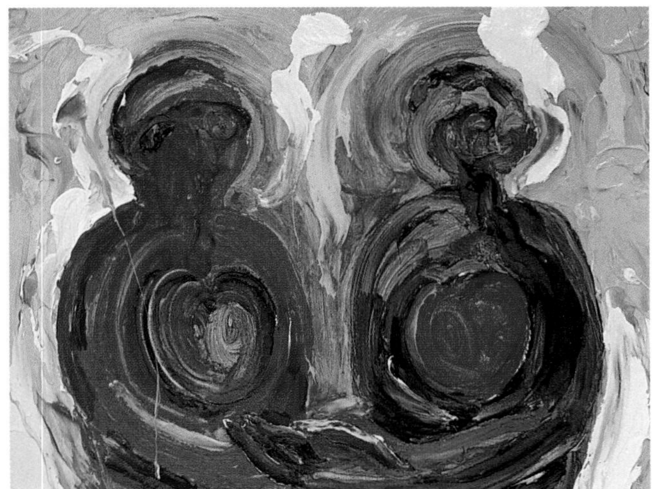

(Left) Katy Raddatz—San Francisco Examiner; (right) painting by Thomas Rohnacher

90% of black households nationwide. Phil Petrie, managing editor of *Gospel Today* magazine, notes: "Once narrowly defined as religious, gospel has transcended those limits to become a profound force in American music and popular culture. As the music moves beyond its incubator—the church...we must hope that the music is building bridges, not walls." Gospel radio is a medium with the potential to break the silence that for so long has shrouded any mention of AIDS in the black community. It can disseminate AIDS-prevention messages aimed at individuals whose behavior places them at high risk of contracting HIV. Gospel radio can air the testimonies of family members and persons living with HIV disease. It can begin to reduce the stigma of the disease and thereby help change social norms. Importantly, gospel radio reaches policy makers and other opinion leaders who can be highly influential in the black community. In short, there is probably no communication channel that has the trustworthiness and reach of gospel radio.

One who knows the power of that medium particularly well is the Rev. Yvette Flunder, a nationally known gospel singer, who has recorded "Oh Happy Day," "Special Gift," and other gospel favorites with the Hawkins Family singers. As pastor of the City of Refuge Community Church in San Francisco, and founder and executive director of Ark of Refuge, an HIV/AIDS support agency and residential facility, Flunder considers it her mission to bring love and acceptance to those who feel that nobody cares, especially African-Americans with AIDS. She is a compassionate pioneer who has lately turned to gospel music to mobilize African-Americans to stop the spread of HIV.

In 1996 Flunder and researchers at the Rollins School of Public Health of Emory University, Atlanta, conducted a survey of gospel music industry leaders. Their research revealed that gospel radio reaches a vast audience; over 75% of 108 gospel radio stations surveyed reached from 10,000 to over one million listeners. The survey also indicated that AIDS is highly relevant to the gospel music community: 75% of 128 respondents knew at least one person connected with gospel music who had HIV disease, and 93% of 172 respondents considered it "very important" for gospel radio to present information about AIDS.

When asked, "Does your gospel radio station deliver information about AIDS?" 59% of 174 respondents answered "yes," 21% said "no," and another 20% "did not know." Flunder and her colleagues in the public health field interpreted the significant gap between what is perceived as "important" and what actual radio stations are doing as challenge and opportunity. Clearly, they saw, gospel radio had been underutilized as a channel for effective dissemination of information about prevention of HIV disease to the African-American community. They also saw that well-devised health education strategies and the application of appropriate behavioral science techniques could go a long way toward remedying that situation.

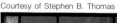

Courtesy of Stephen B. Thomas

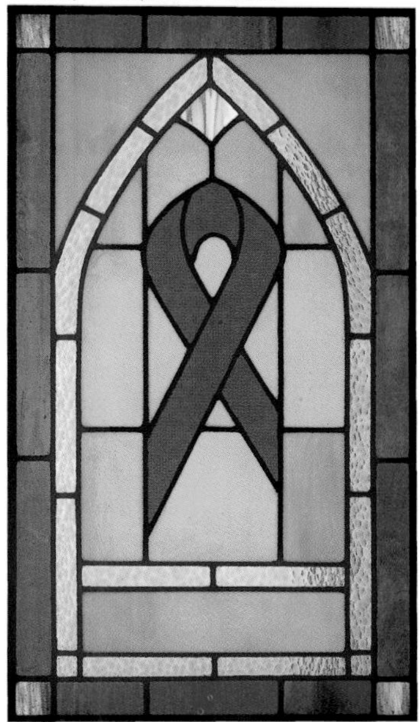

Stephen Thomas, who created this AIDS-awareness window, is leading an effort to bring HIV/AIDS-prevention messages to the gospel radio airwaves.

Lift every voice

> *You know, I remember when I sent every person with AIDS to hell. I remember when I sent every homosexual to hell. But, you know, my nephew died of AIDS, and when my nephew got AIDS, I didn't feel right sending my nephew to hell.*
>
> —Pentecostal minister, Harlem

Just as HIV disease has claimed the lives of thousands of artists from New York to San Francisco, AIDS has devastated the heart and soul of the black gospel music industry. James Cleveland (1931–91), winner of four Grammys—the last awarded posthumously for his album *Having Church*—was considered by many gospel enthusiasts to be the "king of gospel." He mesmerized his audience and brought a high standard of excellence to gospel music through his organization, the Gospel Music Workshop of America. But the Reverend Cleveland, along with other well-known and unknown gospel music singers, died from AIDS and did so in silence.

Kent Brooks, an assistant minister at the Orange Grove Missionary Baptist Church, wrote a song for his church's choir that premiered during the 1997 Black Church Week of Prayer for the Healing of AIDS. That song, "Heal the Land," inspired in part by his compassion and love for a member of his own family living with AIDS, was meant to give "voice to the human spirit...to unite the congregation in lifting the veil of stigma and denial."

The issue of blacks' denial of AIDS was the focus of a conference at Harvard University in October 1996. Henry Louis Gates, chairman of Afro-American studies at the university, chaired the gathering of clergy, health professionals, government officials, media representatives, and academicians. At the conference the Harvard AIDS Institute released frightening figures projecting that by the year 2000 more than 50% of AIDS cases in the U.S. would be among blacks. Gates blamed such an alarmingly high prevalence of disease in the African-American community on "a traditional homophobic tendency in our culture" and "ignorant stereotypes about HIV and AIDS." Calling upon the conference attendees to mount a campaign to stop denying a dreadful situation, Gates said, "This is a human tragedy of monstrous proportions, which could have been and could be avoided."

If one thing is known with certainty about the experience of black people in America, it is that they know how to draw upon an endless reservoir of love and hope in the face of adversity. Churches and gospel radio are wellsprings that are just beginning to be tapped. But many more voices must lift up and sing for the healing of AIDS in the African-American community before anyone can say, "Amen!"

—Stephen B. Thomas, Ph.D.,
and Sandra Crouse Quinn, Ph.D.

One Bold Plan for an AIDS Vaccine

> *A scientist who is also a human being cannot rest while knowledge which might be used to reduce suffering rests on the shelf.*
> —Albert B. Sabin (1906–93)

In the 15 years since the human immunodeficiency virus (HIV) was first identified, more than 6.4 million people worldwide have died from HIV/AIDS. In the United States, AIDS is now the leading killer of adults aged 25–44. Despite massive international public education efforts, HIV continues to take a heavy toll in both developed and less-developed countries, infecting some 10,000 people per day—about one person every nine seconds.

J. Scott Applewhite—Associated Press

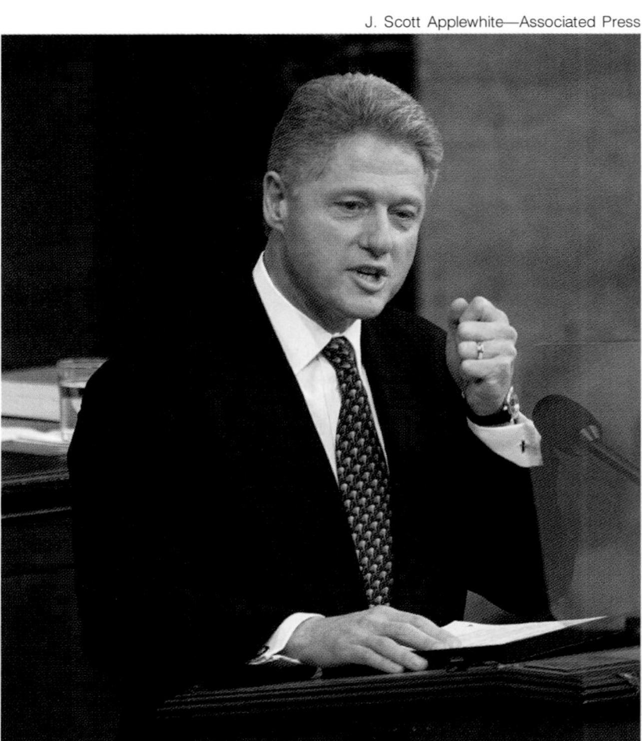

On Feb. 4, 1997, in his state of the union address, Pres. Bill Clinton calls for intensified government-supported HIV/AIDS research and emphasizes the need for an effective AIDS vaccine.

Yet the last two years have offered people living with HIV/AIDS hope for the first time, as several new drugs that truly seem to counter the lethal virus have been approved for use. Clinical trials and broad use of these drugs, known as protease inhibitors, have shown that they greatly reduce patients' levels of HIV ("viral load") when combined with older antiviral agents such as zidovudine (AZT) and didanosine (ddI). Some AIDS authorities have gone so far as to proclaim the beginning of the end for the disease. "No one can call AIDS an inevitably fatal disease anymore," said Peter Piot, executive director of the Joint United Nations Program on HIV/AIDS (UNAIDS).

Others have been more cautious, greeting the clear gains in the clinical management of AIDS with only tempered enthusiasm; they emphasize that infection rates have remained as high as ever and, in fact, have been climbing among certain demographic groups (African-Americans, women, and Latinos in the U.S., for example). Patricia Fleming, chief of the Reporting and Analysis Section, Division of HIV/AIDS Prevention, Centers for Disease Control and Prevention (CDC), Atlanta, Ga., has stressed that as the number of infected individuals who could live effectively with the virus for many years (with few or no symptoms) increases, so will the demand for the limited available resources for treating the disease. Others point out some major pitfalls associated with the newer therapies, including their high cost, the difficulty for the average patient to maintain compliance with the complex regimens, and, for some, the lack of a positive response to the multidrug protocols.

During the first decade of the pandemic, most prevention efforts focused on behavioral interventions. Educational campaigns encouraged people to modify lifestyle practices that placed them at risk of acquiring and transmitting infection. Such public health efforts made a difference but did not solve the problem. Today most experts agree that the best—if not the only—way to prevent future infections is with an immunization against HIV/AIDS.

For many years research into vaccines was held back by some unsubstantiated assumptions. Few scientists believed a vaccine against the AIDS virus was technically feasible. Among other things, researchers thought that HIV became latent (inactive) for many years, that infection with the virus was always rapidly fatal, that continual mutation enabled the virus to evade the immune system successfully, and that HIV/AIDS was drastically different from all other known diseases.

Recent advances in vaccine science and important insights into the virus itself, however, have given scientists new confidence that an AIDS vaccine will be developed. Researchers now appreciate that HIV/AIDS has distinct similarities to other viral diseases and that much can be learned from the expertise of those who developed effective vaccines against them. Furthermore, successful immunizations against other long-lasting viral infections already exist. These include vaccines for hepatitis B, varicella (chicken pox), and a number of HIV-like retroviruses that infect animals, including domestic cats.

The value of vaccines cannot be overstated. They have had a greater impact on the health and well-being of society than any other medical intervention. Vaccination strategies are responsible for the global eradication of the deadly disease smallpox in 1977 and the projected eradication of paralytic poliomyelitis by 2000. Immunizations are also credited with dramatic decreases in the international incidence of many other infectious diseases, including diphtheria, hepatitis B, rubella, measles, and mumps.

In fact, the critical step for the development of an AIDS vaccine—growing the virus in a test tube—was achieved some 14 years ago. Currently, U.S. pharmaceutical companies are testing over 120 new agents for HIV, AIDS, and AIDS-related illnesses, but only a few of these potential new products are preventive. Despite the evident need for a vaccine, many pharmaceutical manufacturers are reluctant to commit resources to a project that until recently was not given much chance for success. Moreover, the incentives for the pharmaceutical industry to invest in a preventive agent are negligible, especially when compared with the incentives for investment in new drugs to treat full-blown AIDS.

Before the new combination therapies were in use, the average lifetime direct medical costs for each HIV-infected patient in the United States were about $119,000. Assuming, conservatively, that costs will increase to at least $200,000 per new case and that an estimated 40,000 to 80,000 Americans a year will become newly infected, every year of delay in developing a preventive vaccine adds $8 billion to $16 billion to future health care costs, which will be borne by all citizens paying health insurance premiums and taxes. Fiscal prudence alone would support the investment of far greater sums than are now being allotted for AIDS vaccine development; such funds would be recouped many times over in future savings in health care costs. Indeed, history has shown that the long-term cost-benefit ratios almost always favor prevention over treatment.

On Feb. 4, 1997, in his state of the union address, U.S. Pres. Bill Clinton underscored the importance of an AIDS vaccine: "Every year we move up the discovery of an AIDS vaccine will save millions of lives around the world. We must reinforce our commitment." At the same time, federal spending on vaccine development was increased to about 10% of the total $1.5 billion earmarked for HIV/AIDS research.

One who agrees with the president and has long stressed the urgency of an immunization against HIV/AIDS is H.R. Shepherd, a disciple of the late Albert B. Sabin, creator of the oral polio vaccine. In 1993 Shepherd established the Albert B. Sabin Vaccine Foundation (now the Albert B. Sabin Vaccine Institute at Georgetown University, Washington, D.C.) to carry out his mentor's mission: *to prevent the suffering caused by debilitating and deadly disease by promoting advances in vaccine development, delivery, and distribution.* Says Shepherd, "It is imperative that our priority should be to facilitate the measures necessary for the development, broad use, and success of an AIDS vaccine to prevent additional infections." An AIDS vaccine not only would halt the epidemic and prevent disease, Shepherd emphasizes, but would do so for a fraction of what it costs to care for the afflicted.

To meet this extraordinarily complex challenge, in 1997 the Sabin Institute launched "Operation BOLD STROKE," an ambitious plan aimed at eradicating AIDS in the U.S. The initiative's goals are threefold: in cooperation with government and industry to establish a timely agenda for the development, testing, production, and delivery of an AIDS vaccine; to engage the financial resources that will be necessary for the vaccine's delivery, in part by setting up an AIDS Vaccine Trust Fund that will provide for those who cannot afford immunization; and, finally, to strengthen and sustain the national commitment to this immense task.

While there are still some formidable scientific and political obstacles to overcome, scientists at major research institutions are collaborating in the international search for an AIDS vaccine.

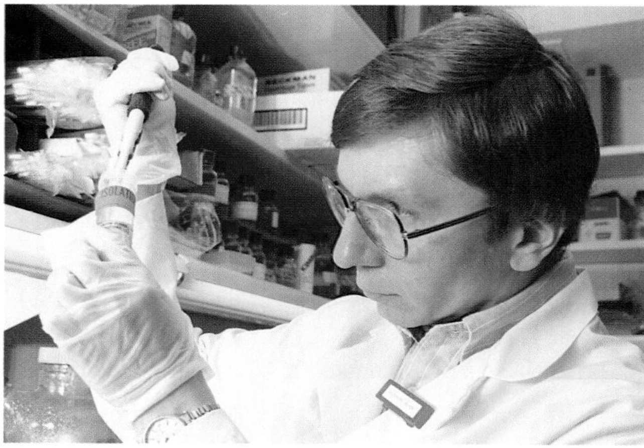

NIAID, National Institutes of Health

Many questions remain to be answered. For example, once an HIV/AIDS vaccine becomes available, who will receive it? Recently, members of the National Vaccine Advisory Committee of the CDC recommended the formation of a national immunization public awareness program for all vaccines. The members expressed the concern that continuing misperceptions of vaccines in general already discourage participation in existing vaccination programs. An AIDS vaccine would be doubly difficult to administer under such adverse circumstances. The Sabin Institute is intensely aware that people will not immediately line up for an AIDS vaccine as they did during the panic days of the polio epidemic when "Sabin Oral Sundays" (SOS) mobilized hundreds of thousands for oral polio vaccination, sometimes delivered in a sugar cube.

The foundation also realizes that simultaneous with scientific efforts to bring forth an AIDS vaccine, there must be an equally heroic planning and public education effort. People must become convinced of the urgency of immunization and the safety and efficacy of any end-product AIDS vaccine. A strategic plan for distribution will be needed to earn the confidence of people worldwide. In this context Operation BOLD STROKE is stressing the importance of delivering a vaccine to the populations of greatest need and least means in the most expeditious manner possible. The actual delivery method—along with many other strategic issues—has yet to be settled.

Operation BOLD STROKE is, of course, just one of many U.S. vaccine-directed efforts. Many government agencies and programs are engaged in the search. The National Institute of Allergy and Infectious Diseases (NIAID) has developed a scientific agenda for the "discovery and development of prophylactic HIV vaccines" despite "formidable scientific obstacles." NIAID's comprehensive program incorporates both basic and applied research and is built on a number of assumptions—among them, that progress toward a vaccine will be made in incremental steps and that multiple vaccine designs will need to be evaluated. At the same time, NIAID is also pursuing various nonvaccine strategies.

On a much broader scale, the Rockefeller Foundation's International AIDS Vaccine Initiative has set the goal of removing all barriers to the development of safe, effective, long-lasting, and affordable AIDS vaccines *for the world.* Some 90% of new infections occur in less-developed countries; therefore, it will be important to ensure that vaccines target strains of HIV that are most prevalent in the world's poorest countries and that they are available to those at highest risk. Africa, for example, currently bears 60% of the world's HIV burden but has the weakest economy of any continent. Among the partners in this global initiative are the World Bank, UNAIDS, Until There's a Cure Foundation, the American Foundation for AIDS Research, the Merieux Foundation, and others. If Sabin were alive today, he would undoubtedly be gratified to know that globally there are many scientists who share his vision of a world in which people do not suffer from preventable diseases.

—*Rick Curran*

Traditional Chinese Medicine Under Scrutiny

While the Chinese are eager to import modern medical technology from the West, increasing numbers of Westerners are equally interested in adopting the traditional medical remedies of China. According to the *China Daily,* annual foreign sales of traditional Chinese medicines are expected to double to more than $2 billion by the year 2000. Helping to fuel interest in traditional Chinese medicine (TCM) is a growing disenchantment in the West with technology-based medicine, which often overlooks the patient's psychological and spiritual needs. Today many Westerners view China's traditional medicine as a more dynamic approach—one that treats the *whole* patient rather than just a patient's disease.

China has one of the world's oldest medical systems. Acupuncture and Chinese herbal remedies date back at least 2,200 years, although the earliest known written record of Chinese medicine is the *Huangdi nei jing* ("The Yellow Emperor's Classic of Internal Medicine") from the 3rd century BC. That opus provided the theoretical concepts for TCM that remain the basis of its practice today. In essence, traditional Chinese healers seek to restore a dynamic balance between two complementary forces, yin (passive) and yang (active), which pervade the human body as they do the universe as a whole. According to TCM, a person is healthy when harmony exists between these two forces; illness, on the other hand, results from a breakdown in the equilibrium of yin and yang.

To restore harmony, the Chinese healer may use any of a staggeringly large array of traditional remedies. The patient may be treated with acupuncture, in which thin needles are inserted into the skin at key points along invisible channels of the body, called meridians. Chinese healers believe that the body's vital energy, or *qi* (also spelled *ch'i;* "divine breath"), flows through these channels. By stimulating the appropriate point with the needle—or with a finger in acupressure—the healer attempts to correct the flow of *qi.* The healer may also perform the method known as moxibustion, or moxa treatment, in which a dried herb, usually wormwood (*Artemisia moxa*), is burned like incense above the skin at the appropriate point. Placing hot glass cups on the patient's skin, a process called cupping, is an ancient practice used to draw blood to the skin. Alternatively or additionally, the Chinese healer may prescribe a brew prepared with one (or some combination) of thousands of medicinal plants or dried animal parts (*e.g.,* snakes, scorpions, insects, worms, bear gall bladders, deer antlers, tiger penises) in the Chinese pharmaceutical armamentarium.

A visit to a traditional Chinese pharmacy is like a visit to a small natural history museum. The hundreds of cabinet drawers, glass cases, and jars in a typical pharmacy hold an enormous variety of desiccated plant and animal material. In 1578 Li Shih-chen published his famous *Pen-ts'ao kang-mu* ("Compendium of Materia Medica"), which lists 1,892 drugs and about 10,000 formal prescriptions for specific ailments. A recent national survey by the Chinese Academy of Medical Sciences in Beijing counted 7,295 species of plants currently used as medicines in China and nearly 200 modern medicines that have been developed either directly or indirectly from those plants. For example, ephedrine, an alkaloid used in treating asthma, was first isolated from the Chinese herb *ma huang*.

A more recently discovered alkaloid, which was isolated from the widely prescribed herbal medicine *qian ceng ta,* may lead to the development of new drugs to treat Alzheimer's disease and other dementias; the compound huperzine A (named for the Chinese moss *Huperzia serrata*) has recently aroused the interest of investigators in the United States. Laboratory and X-ray studies suggest that this agent may compare favorably with tacrine and donepezil, the two drugs now approved in the U.S. for treating Alzheimer's disease.

The meditation exercises *tai qi* and *qigong* are other integral features of traditional Chinese healing. *Tai qi* is characterized by deliberately slow, continuous, circular, well-balanced, and rhythmic movements that were originally practiced as a martial art. *Qigong,* which was known in ancient China as "the method to repel illness and prolong life," contains elements of meditation, relaxation training, martial-arts techniques, and breathing exercises that are intended to cultivate *qi* and transmit it to all the bodily organs. Many Chinese regularly perform these exercises to promote health and may indeed derive health benefits from the exercise and relaxation. Unfortunately, *qigong* is also being promoted as a way to develop superhuman and supernatural powers. *Qigong* "masters"

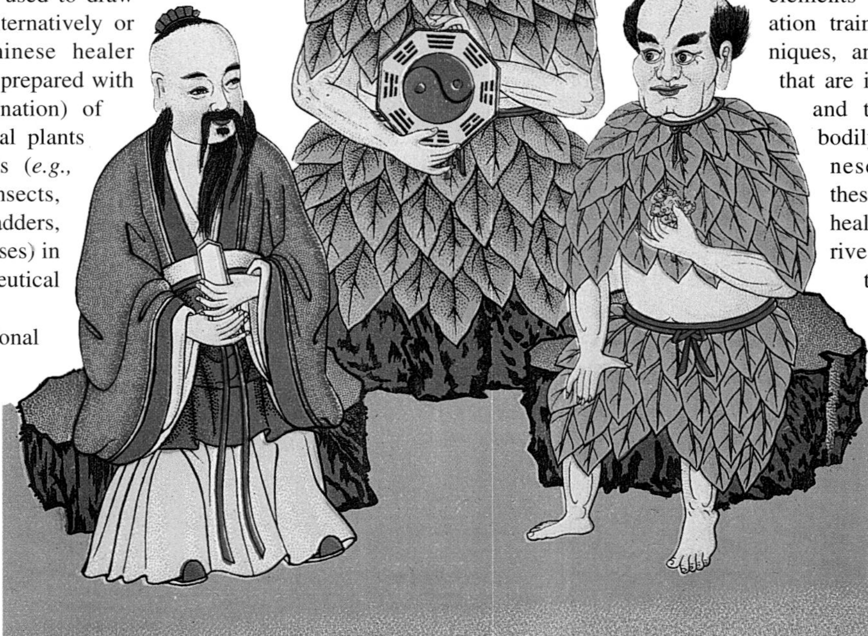

(Left) Gamma Liaison; (right) Charles Walker Collection—Stock Montage, Inc.

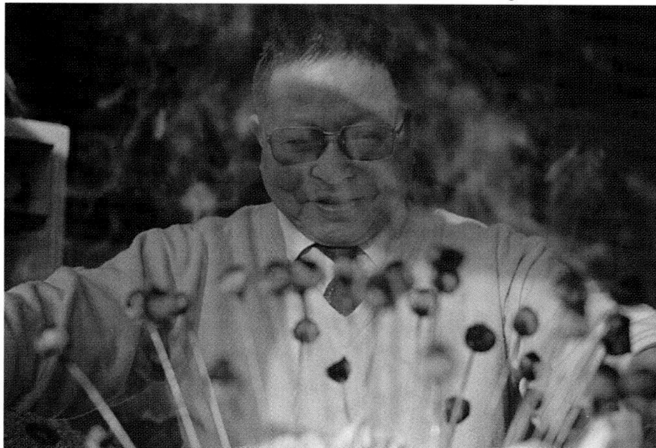

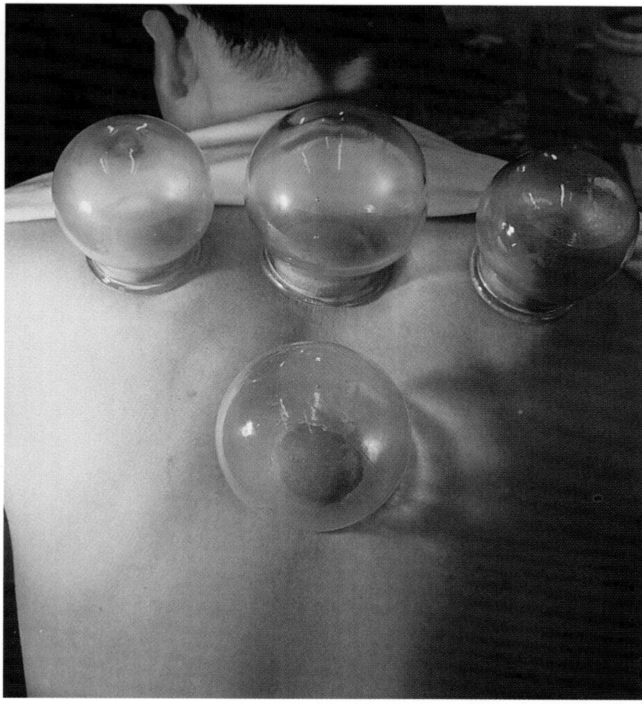

(Left) A Chinese healer ignites herbs in preparation for performing moxibustion, one of a number of traditional treatments aimed at restoring equilibrium between the forces of yin and yang in the human body. (Above) In the ancient practice of cupping, hot glass cups are placed on a patient's back to draw blood to the skin.

have gained followings throughout China using tricks to perform "miracles" that purport to demonstrate the power of the "internal" and "external" *qi* they command. Han Xiaoming, deputy secretary-general of the Chinese Medical Association, points out that while many physicians and scientists in China view the "internal" (meditational) practice of *qigong* as beneficial, they are trying to educate the public about the tricks of practitioners who claim the ability to use "external" *qigong* (control of *qi* outside the body) to heal others.

Acupuncture is probably the best-known traditional Chinese healing technique practiced in the West. In China it is routinely used as an anesthetic during surgery. While acupuncture appears most promising for treating chronic musculoskeletal pain, it is also being promoted as a treatment for other health problems, including asthma, alcoholism, and addiction to nicotine. Han Jishen, director of Beijing Medical University's Neuroscience Research Center and a pioneer in research on the neurochemical basis of acupuncture's analgesic effects, says acupuncture can reduce pain in about 80% of patients who receive it, but he dismisses the more sensational therapeutic claims. According to Han, many of the studies involving acupuncture published in the medical literature are, unfortunately, methodologically flawed.

Challenging superstition and pseudoscience

These are times of great changes and contradictions within Chinese society. While the government promotes modernization and makes strides toward implementing an open-market economy, it is trying to hold on to many Chinese traditions. Although the government is proud of China's traditional medicine and is eager to export it to the West, it is uncomfortable with the superstitions behind some of those traditions and is growing concerned about the medical frauds who exploit those superstitions.

Throughout Beijing, Shanghai, and other cities, women in white smocks sit at tables in front of pharmacies, where they offer passersby free examinations and health advice. Some of these "healers" take a "pulse diagnosis" or run an electrified needle over the prospect's palm and, judging by the way the person reacts to the mild electric shock, make a diagnosis such as "neck trouble," "digestive weakness," or "hot liver"—all of which can be treated with remedies sold at the pharmacy. Elsewhere, *qigong* masters sell jars of water that they "charge" with their *qi* by waving their hands over the jar. Patients are told that by drinking the charged water, they will restore their internal *qi* to a balanced, healthy state.

The effort to "integrate" TCM with modern medicine sometimes leads to dangerous practices. Owing to the one-child-per-family law imposed by the Chinese government, many women are demanding—and receiving—medically unnecessary and risky cesarean sections, performed to ensure that their sole child is born on an astrologically auspicious day.

In 1996 the China Association of Science and Technology announced a national campaign against pseudoscience. In that same year, in order to curb the marketing of products carrying fraudulent health claims, China's Ministry of Public Health ordered manufacturers of medicinal food products to apply for licenses. According to a report in the *Workers' Daily,* the scarcity of qualified physicians in China's rural areas has spawned a plague of "traditional witch doctors," who "parade feudal superstitions under the cloak of science" and threaten the health and lives of the uneducated peasants they prey on. To counter this problem, the association established a forum for organizing public seminars that underscore the importance of "scientific thinking, scientific methods, and scientific spirit."

(Opposite page) Traditional Chinese medicine dates back at least 2,200 years. China's ancestral gods of medicine, Huangdi, Fu Xi, and Shen Nong, are depicted at bottom. (Top) A drawing dating from 1031 shows points of insertion for acupuncture. In China today, acupuncture is used routinely as an anesthetic during surgery.

(Opposite page, bottom) Jean-Loup Charmet; (top) Bettmann-Corbis

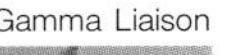

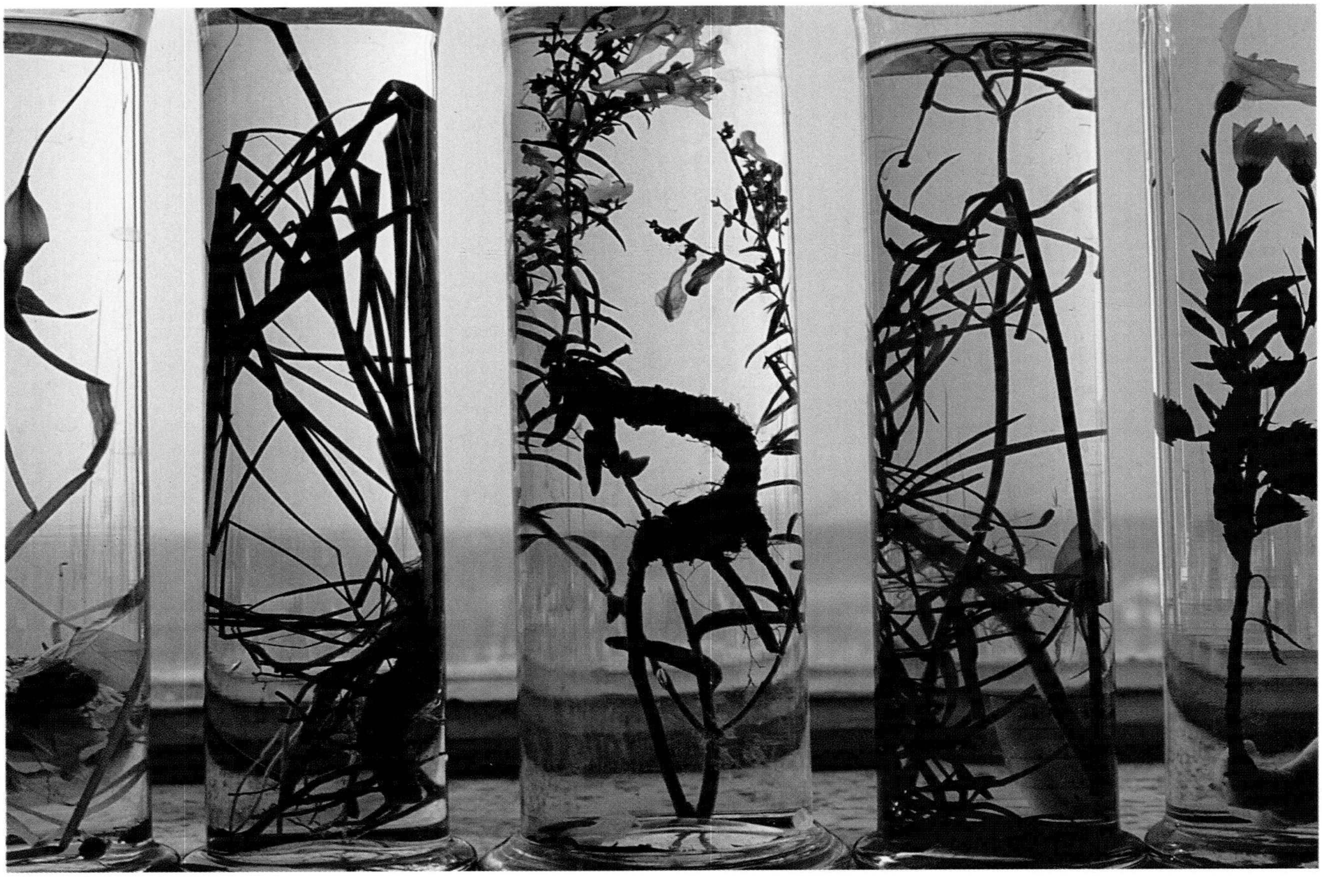

Jars of medicinal plants line the walls of a traditional Chinese pharmacy. A recent survey by the Chinese Academy of Medical Sciences in Beijing counted 7,295 species of plants that are currently being used as medicines in China.

Increasingly, Chinese scientists are beginning to speak out against the more outlandish claims of traditional healers. Lin Zixin, the retired editor of China's largest-circulating scientific publication, *Science and Technology Daily,* considers the unmitigated acceptance of superstition in China "shameful," as well as a threat to China's technological and economic development and to the public health. Lin has been a leading organizer of academic exchanges between Chinese and Western scientists working to promote scientific literacy and combat pseudoscience and quackery. The first of several such exchanges took place in 1988, when Lin invited members of the Amherst, N.Y.-based Committee for the Scientific Investigation of Claims of the Paranormal (CSICOP) to visit China; that was followed by a reciprocal visit by Chinese scientists to CSICOP conferences in the United States. In 1995 Shen Zhenyu, director of research at the China Association for Science and Technology's Office for Academia in Beijing, and colleagues at the State Science and Technology Commission invited two experts from CSICOP and this author to visit leading TCM centers in Beijing and Shanghai and to participate in scientific seminars examining the validity of traditional healers' claims.

Lin, Shen, and other outspoken critics of pseudoscience recognize the many venerable contributions of traditional healers. They also recognize the enormous potential for developing powerful new therapies based on TCM and do not dismiss the important role traditional healers play in caring for and providing comfort to the sick, many of whom have no other access to health care. Whether because of a demonstrable efficacy of the actual remedies used or a placebo effect, many recipients of TCM report a high degree of satisfaction with their treatment.

Integrating East and West, old and new

Medical scientists like Ka Kit Hui, director of the Center for East-West Medicine at the University of California, Los Angeles, School of Medicine, hope to integrate TCM with modern medicine to create a new discipline of "integrative medicine." Hui believes that the clear limitations of modern medicine have heightened the need for a more integrative approach to health care. "We believe that incorporating the systems perspective of TCM and its many time-tested therapeutic methods to make up for the limitations of conventional medicine will enhance the care of our patients," he wrote in a letter published in the *Journal of the American Medical Association* (March 5, 1997). "Traditional Chinese medicine will be the most important contribution to the betterment of humankind by the Chinese civilization in the coming millennium."

Others, however, like Wallace Sampson, a clinical professor of medicine at the Stanford University School of Medicine, and Barry Beyerstein, a biopsychologist at Simon Fraser University,

Andrew A. Skolnick

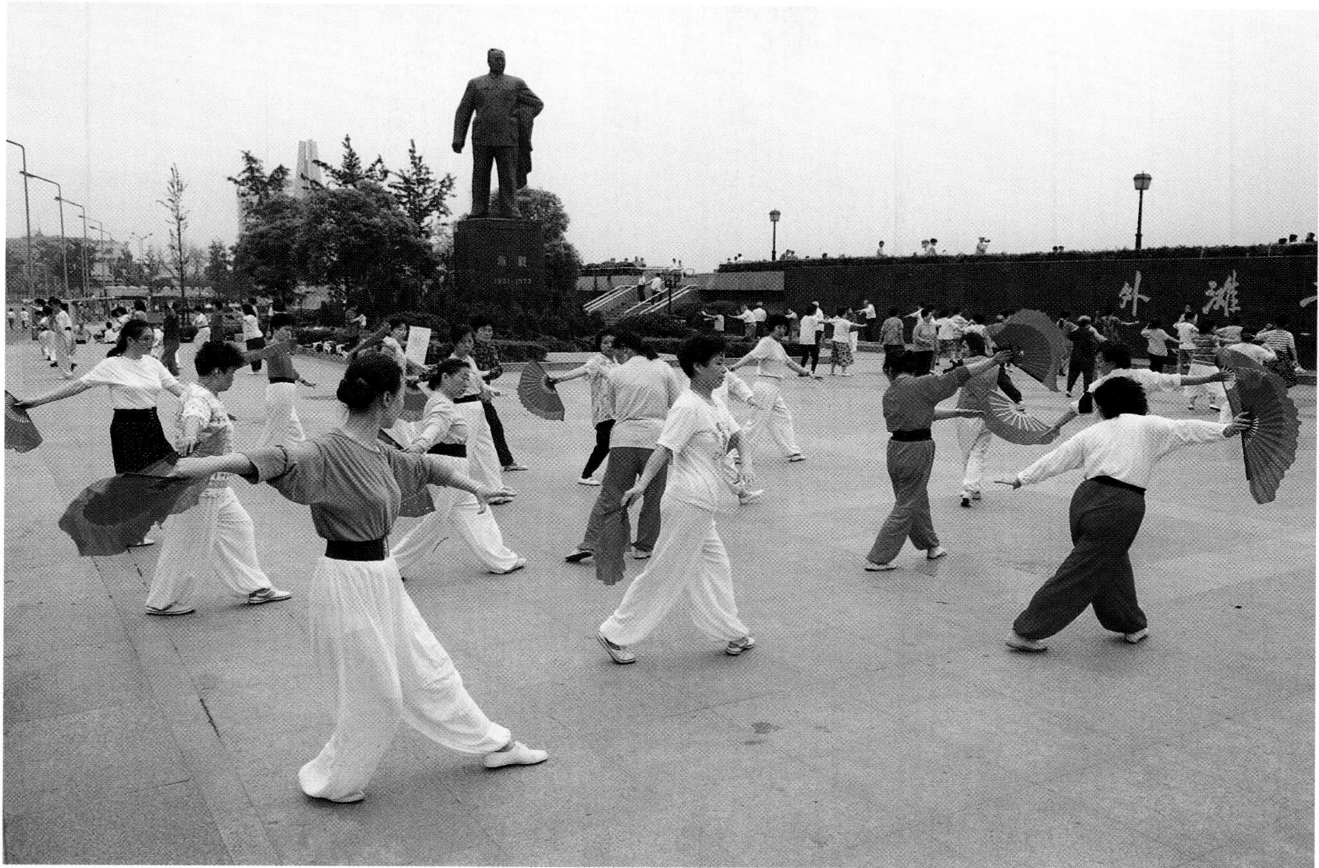

Shanghai residents gather in one of the city's many parks to perform the slow, rhythmic movements of the ancient meditation exercise tai qi. *Though long valued for promoting emotional well-being,* tai qi *can also improve balance and help tone muscles.*

Vancouver, B.C., do not share Hui's optimism. In CSICOP's journal, the *Skeptical Inquirer,* they noted that the health of the world is not going to be improved by the uncritical acceptance of health claims from either the East or the West. The vast majority of traditional Chinese herbs have not yet been adequately tested. According to Sampson and Beyerstein, traditional Chinese herbalism remains a mixture of some safe and effective remedies, some inert placebos, and some dangerous substances. In most instances it is difficult, if not impossible, they believe, to tell which concoctions belong in which of these categories. One encouraging sign is that there are increasing numbers of attempts, particularly in China, to apply scientific methods to separate the effective herbal remedies from the placebos and to isolate the active ingredients in those that have a true pharmacological effect.

Herbal remedies are being widely promoted as "natural," "safe," and "without side effects." Such claims can be dangerously false. *Jin bu huan,* a Chinese patent medicine linked to three recent U.S. cases of liver damage, is one of a number of herbal remedies listed by the U.S. Food and Drug Administration as causing severe side effects. *Hai ge fen* (powdered clamshell) and several other Chinese remedies used in the United States have been associated with cases of lead and other heavy metal poisonings. Eight deaths and hundreds of adverse reactions have been reported in Texas alone from the use of *ma huang* or other health products containing ephedrine alkaloids. Even the practice of *qigong* has been associated with adverse effects. "*Qigong* deviation syndrome" is the name that researchers in China are using to describe the abnormal physiological and psychological effects—including hallucinations—that some *qigong* devotees have experienced. Although rare, serious infections, punctured lungs, and even fatalities have resulted from improperly performed acupuncture.

The ancient texts of TCM were based on observations shaped by supernatural precepts rather than on controlled scientific studies. While much of the knowledge may be more than 2,000 years old, it would be wrong to say that TCM is based on 2,000 years of experience. Unlike modern medicine, which is constantly being challenged and corrected by scientific reports in the medical literature, new observations have had little impact on the basic TCM dogma. Medical advances occur so rapidly that any Western physician today practicing medicine based on the medical literature of even a decade or so ago could probably be charged with malpractice. Traditional Chinese healers, however, are using treatments that have not changed in centuries.

One of the problems is that TCM theories rest upon a foundation of essentially untestable supernatural precepts. *Qi,* for example, is not detectable in any objective way, nor are meridians. Indeed, no two acupuncturists are likely to insert needles in the same spot on the same patient. "It is possible that some of the procedures might still work, but for reasons unrelated to the

Andrew A. Skolnick

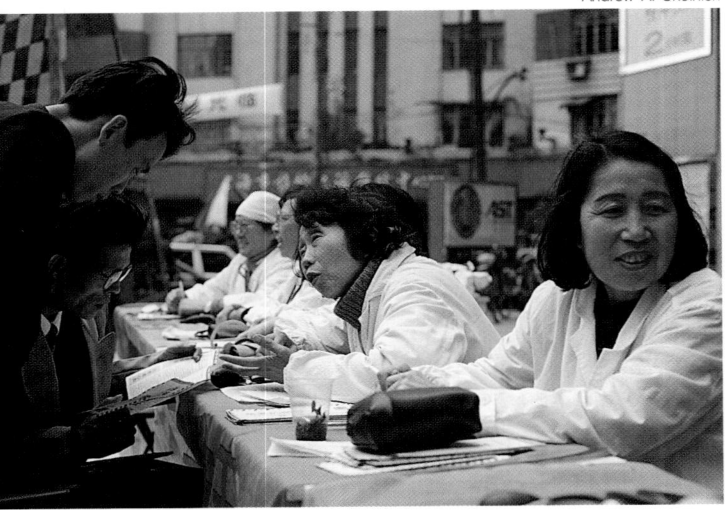

In front of a pharmacy in Shanghai, untrained medical practitioners offer passersby information about purported remedies. Efforts to combat pseudoscience and quackery in China are increasing.

magical belief system that supplied their rationale thousands of years ago," says Paul Kurtz, CSICOP chairman and professor emeritus of philosophy at the State University of New York at Buffalo. As he points out, "Open-minded physicians everywhere would welcome any treatment that could benefit their patients, regardless of its origins, providing it can demonstrate its value in properly controlled clinical trials."

Two studies sponsored by the National Institute on Aging indicate that the practice of *tai qi* can help people aged 70 and over reduce the risk of falls. Currently the National Institutes of Health's Office of Alternative Medicine is studying such questions as how acupuncture compares with the drug methylphenidate (Ritalin) in combatting attention-deficit hyperactivity disorder in children, whether acupuncture is effective in treating severe depression in women, and whether *qigong* is beneficial to patients with late-stage reflex sympathetic dystrophy, a chronic nervous system disorder.

It remains to be seen what the full impact of TCM on health care in the West will be. To compete with the promoters of all kinds of unproven and ancient therapies, however, today's practitioners of scientific-based medicine are being challenged to do what traditional Chinese healers have been doing for centuries—to look not just at the patient's symptoms but at the whole patient and all the factors affecting his or her life. That in itself could be one of China's greatest contributions to world health.

—*Andrew A. Skolnick, M.S.*

Acupuncture in the United States

Acupuncture is a healing method that has been used in China for at least 2,200 years. The practice of acupuncture involves the insertion of fine needles (approximately 0.25 mm [0.01 in] in diameter) into specific points on the surface of the body. Typically, between 4 and 30 needles are inserted in the course of one treatment. The depth of insertion varies with the location being treated and the technique being used.

Acupuncture is often used in conjunction with moxibustion—the local application of heat produced by burning small amounts of an herb (usually *Artemisia moxa*) on or near the skin surface. Collectively, these two practices are termed acumoxatherapy, or *zhen jiu* (meaning "needles and burning") in Chinese. The medical theories guiding the application of these therapies were first described in the ancient Chinese medical treatise *Huangdi nei jing* ("The Yellow Emperor's Classic of Internal Medicine"), which was committed to written form around 200 BC.

The essential theory underlying the practice of acupuncture is that the entire body—surface and interior—is traversed by an extensive network of channels that conduct both *qi* (also spelled *ch'i;* the vital life force) and blood. The unimpeded movement of *qi* and blood through these channels is thought to be integral to health. In some areas of the body, the channels can be reached by holes (*xue*), or what are known in the U.S. as acupuncture points. By inserting needles at these points, the acupuncturist can influence the movement of *qi* and, as a consequence, relieve various symptoms and illnesses. Acupressure, the application of manual pressure to acupuncture points, has long been a part of the practice of Chinese medicine. More recently, electricity, magnetic fields, and lasers have been used to stimulate acupuncture points.

Over the course of many centuries, acupuncture and the theories of Chinese medicine spread to Korea, Japan, and Vietnam and eventually to the West. Today acupuncture is international; its practitioners include professional acupuncturists and a variety of other health care providers, including physicians. It was not until the 1950s, however, that the practice of acupuncture came

The Canadian physician Sir William Osler wrote of the efficacy of acupuncture in treating back pain. For doctors who had no acupuncture needles, Osler advised that "ordinary bonnet-needles...will do."

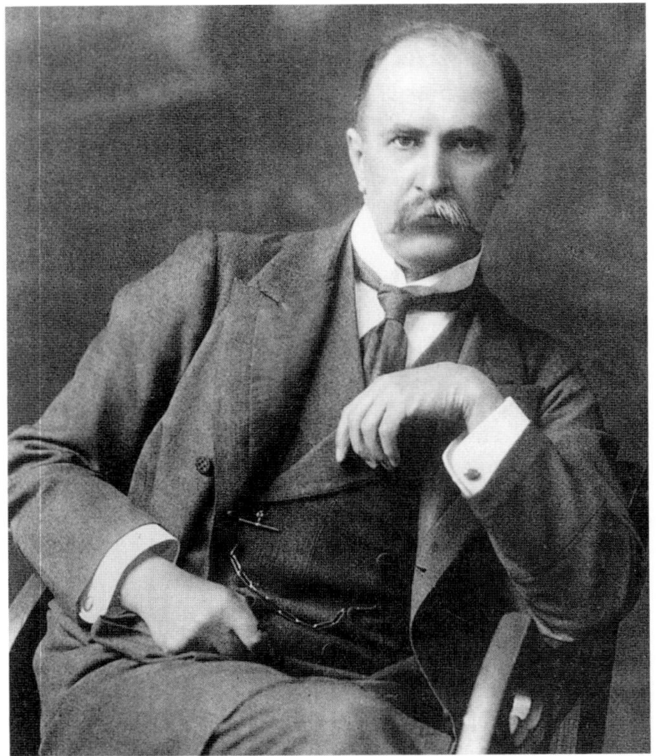

Brown Brothers

under scientific scrutiny, first in Asia and later in Europe and the U.S. Its clinical benefits have been substantiated by much of this research.

Lost and found in America

Knowledge of acupuncture was introduced into Europe in the 17th century by practitioners like Willem Ten Rhyne (1647–90), whose writings on the subject were based on information gathered in Japan during his service as a physician for the Dutch East India Company. As a result of such publications, European and English physicians—and, therefore, colonial American physicians—were often aware of acupuncture. According to the medical historian J.S. Haller, a physician named Bache became one of the first Americans to employ it as a treatment in about 1826. Ten Rhyne's text was a part of the library of the distinguished Canadian physician Sir William Osler, and in the eighth edition (1912) of his classic textbook *The Principles and Practice of Medicine,* Osler prescribes acupuncture for acute lumbago (muscular back pain):

> *For lumbago acupuncture is, in acute cases, the most efficient treatment. Needles of from three to four inches in length (ordinary bonnet-needles, sterilized, will do) are thrust into the lumbar muscles at the seat of pain, and withdrawn after five or ten minutes. In many instances the relief is immediate, and I can corroborate fully...its extraordinary and prompt efficacy in many instances.*

In the U.S. another reservoir of knowledge about acupuncture and other Chinese healing traditions was the Chinese medical practitioners who accompanied the influx of Chinese laborers into the American West in the mid-19th century. A number of these individuals developed substantial reputations among both the Chinese and the non-Chinese communities for their skillful management of many medical conditions. In 1903 Ah Fong Chuck, who had been treating patients in Boise, Idaho, since 1866, became the first of these practitioners to receive a medical license in the U.S., despite a pervasive climate of popular and official racism. Other Asian acupuncturists gained considerable local reputations. In Oregon, for example, Ing Hay was credited with saving many lives during the influenza epidemics of 1915 and 1919.

As the U.S. made the transition from frontier society to industrial nation, the practice of acupuncture and other Asian healing arts gradually retreated into the "Chinatowns" and other ethnic enclaves. It was not until the restoration of diplomatic relations between the U.S. and China in the early 1970s that the technique suddenly burst into the American consciousness. Accounts by travelers who witnessed or underwent acupuncture in China were instrumental in this process. A notable example was journalist James Reston's front-page article "Now, Let Me Tell You About My Appendectomy in Peking..." in the *New York Times* in 1971.

Learning the art

With the surge of American interest in acupuncture in the early 1970s came a demand for educational resources. Motivated individuals sought out teachers anywhere they could be found. By

Jean-Loup Charmet

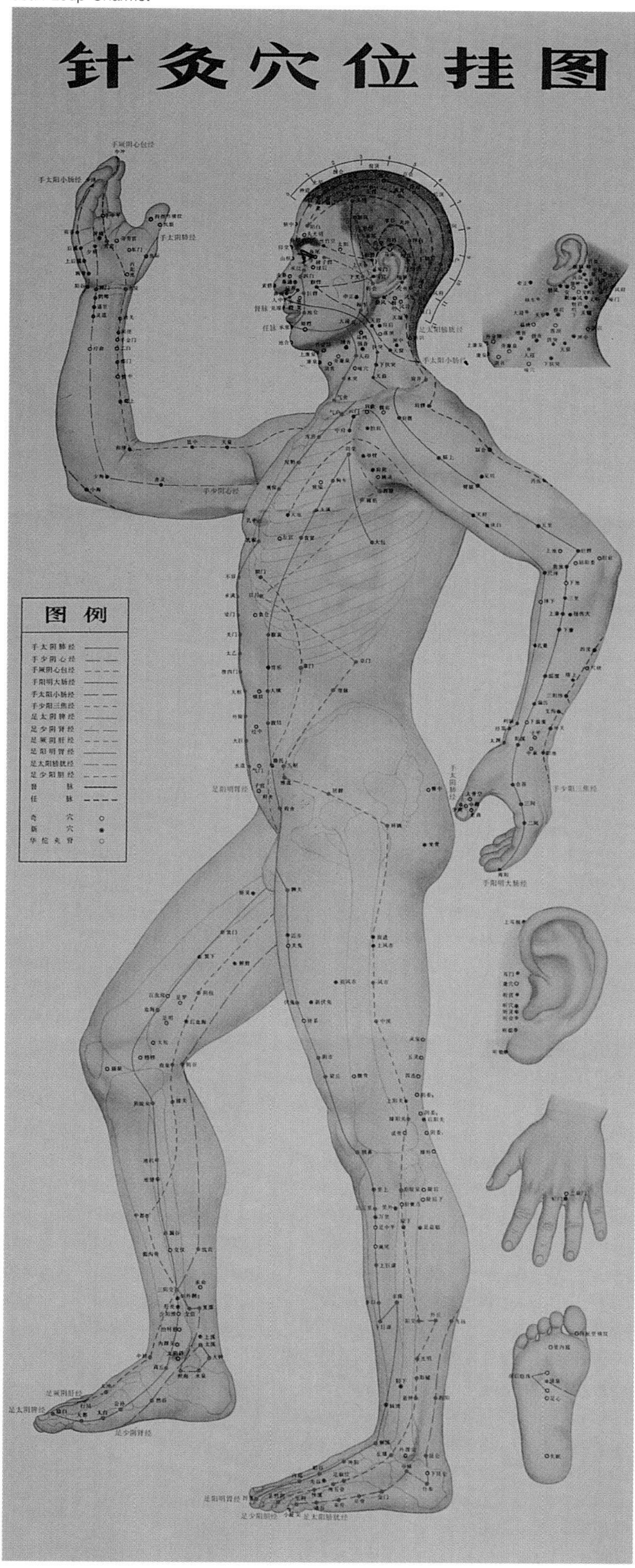

A chart shows the xue, *or acupuncture points, on the human body. Practitioners believe that needles inserted at these locations influence the movement of* qi, *or energy, throughout the body.*

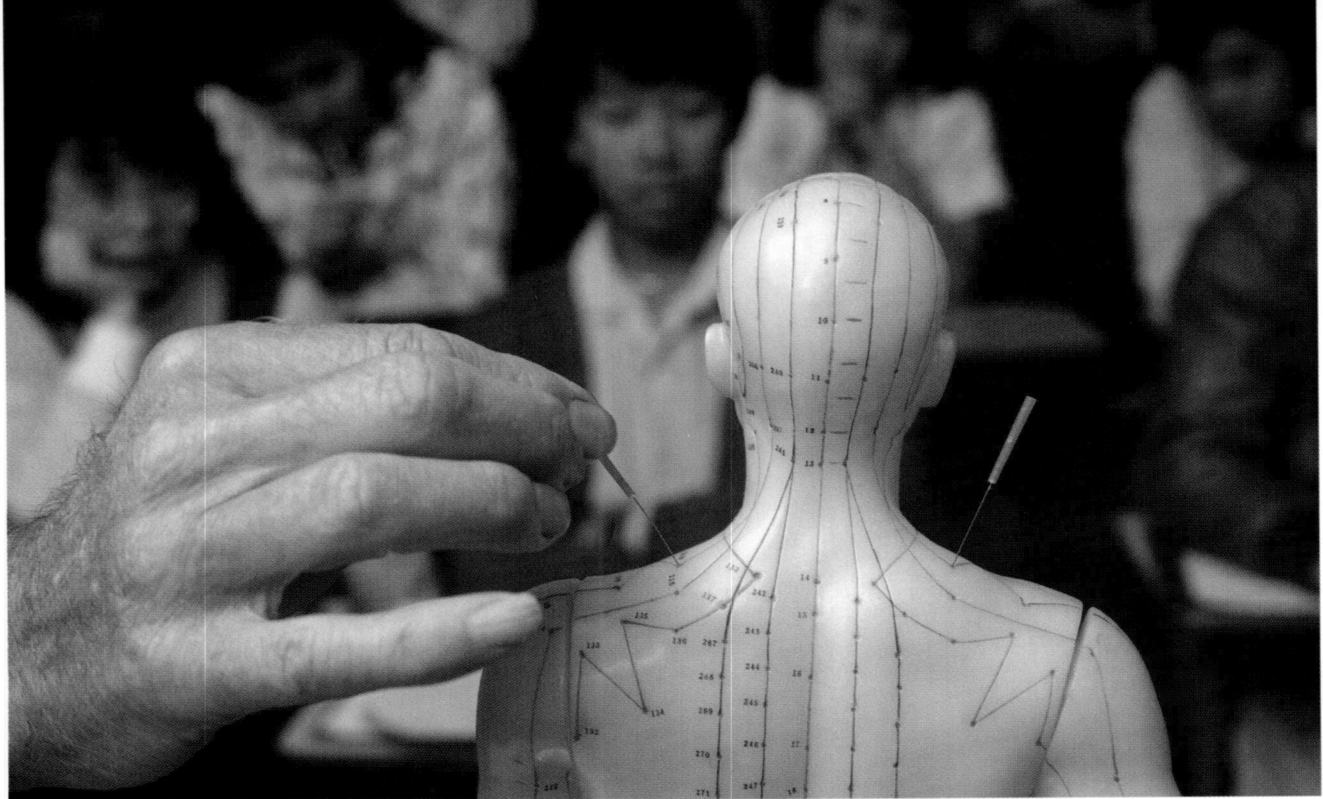

Prior to the 1970s, Americans who wanted to learn the practice of acupuncture had to travel overseas. Today they can enroll at any of the 24 schools around the U.S. whose training programs are accredited by the Department of Education.

1973 students from the U.S. were traveling to England to work with such celebrated practitioners as J.R. Worsley, the developer of the form known as Five Element acupuncture. Renowned instructors like James Tin Yau So of Hong Kong were invited to teach and conduct research in the U.S., and within the U.S. itself Miriam Lee and other experienced practitioners began to share their knowledge with the medical profession and the public.

By the mid-1970s several formal instructional programs had been created. The New England School of Acupuncture was established by So in 1975. Homer Cheng created the Samra University in Los Angeles in 1975, and the California Acupuncture College, also in Los Angeles, was established in 1978. By 1982 there were a sufficient number of schools to warrant the creation of the National Council of Acupuncture Schools and Colleges (known today as the Council of Colleges of Acupuncture and Oriental Medicine). Later that year the group established an independent accreditation commission, the National Accreditation Commission for Schools and Colleges of Acupuncture and Oriental Medicine (later shortened to Accreditation Commission for Acupuncture and Oriental Medicine, or ACAOM). In 1988 the commission established acupuncture education as a legitimate field of study, gaining the recognition of the U.S. Department of Education for its accreditation process. Today 32 programs are within ACAOM's purview, of which 24 are accredited and 8 are candidates for accreditation. A number of training programs that do not yet subscribe to ACAOM standards are also in operation.

Most U.S. schools of acupuncture offer a course of training that complies with—and in many cases exceeds—the minimum ACAOM standards. These include, for programs providing training in acupuncture and Oriental medicine, a minimum of 123

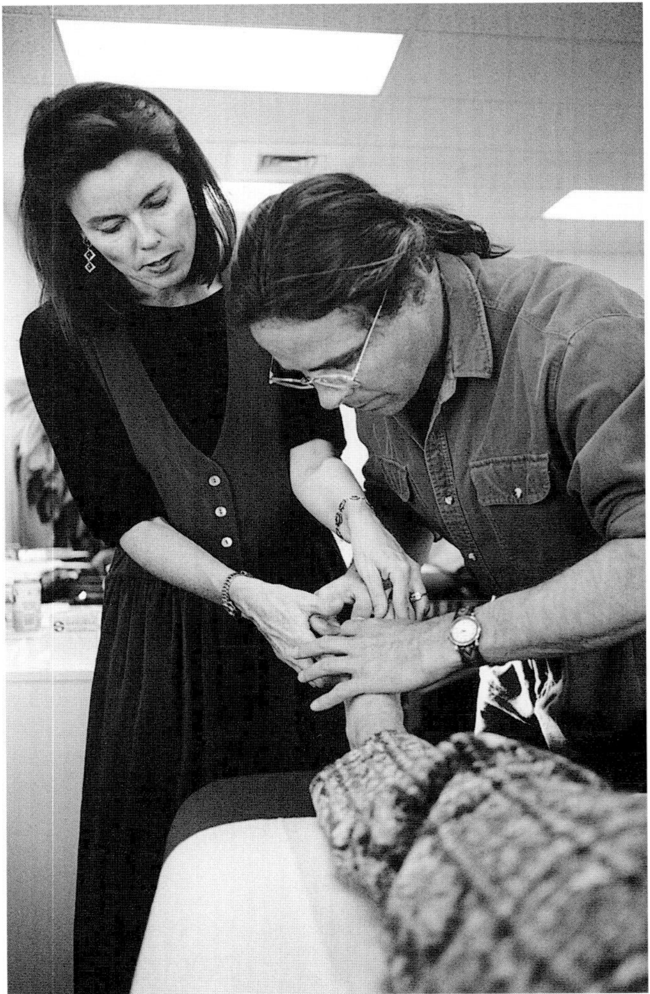

(Top) Phil Schermeister—Corbis; (above) Jill Fineberg

semester credits (2,175 hours), including 47 semester credits (705 hours) in Oriental medical theory and diagnosis and treatment techniques, 30 semester credits (450 hours) in studies related to Oriental herbal medicine, 24 semester credits (360 hours) in biomedical clinical sciences, and 22 semester credits (660 hours) of clinical observation and practice. On average, accredited programs provide more than 30 semester credits (450 hours) of training above and beyond this standard, and the leading programs in the field provide considerably more. Programs typically accept students with a minimum of two years of college course work and award a master's degree or master's-level diploma upon completion of the program. Although the different programs award a variety of titles—master of acupuncture, master of science in traditional Chinese medicine, master of traditional Oriental medicine, diploma of acupuncture—within a given state, all graduates of these programs receive the same type of license.

Training programs in China typically award a medical baccalaureate, or M.B./B.S., which indicates that the graduate has completed four to five years of education after finishing high school. China's system of medical education is similar to that of Great Britain in that it does not award the title M.D. but considers graduates of these programs doctors. Advanced training in the field in China can lead to either an M.S. or a Ph.D. with an emphasis on research.

The title O.M.D. ("Oriental medical doctor"), which gained some currency in the United States in the 1980s, has never been awarded by a state licensing agency or by authorized training programs in China, nor is the title currently conferred by any legally operating and accredited program in the U.S. Often this title indicates that a practitioner has had less comprehensive training than those educated in the master's degree programs.

Licensure

One of the most remarkable aspects of the reawakened interest in acupuncture in the 1970s was the rapidity with which states adopted legislation to permit its practice by individuals who were not medical doctors. In 1972 California passed a law permitting nonphysician acupuncturists to practice with physician supervision for the purpose of research. The first system of licensure for professional acupuncturists was adopted in Nevada in 1973. Oregon followed suit shortly thereafter, and New York adopted standards for licensure in 1975. By 1997, 34 states and the District of Columbia had adopted regulations governing the professional practice of acupuncture.

Acupuncture licensing laws vary from state to state. Typically, they specify the meaning of "acupuncture," outline the scope of the acupuncturist's practice, and set minimal educational qualifications and standards of professional conduct. Many states use the examinations provided by the National Certification Commission for Acupuncture and Oriental Medicine (NCCAOM) to test those applying for licensure. These examinations test for entry-level competency in acupuncture, Oriental medical theory, and Oriental herbal medicine, but they do not assess knowledge in the biomedical sciences. Most states require that candidates for licensure meet a minimum educational standard, usually the standard provided by ACAOM. Some states, such as California, require a higher standard than that used by ACAOM and develop their own tests independently of the NCCAOM.

States have discretion over the title that may be used by the holder of the license. Thus, in the United States a licensed practitioner of acupuncture may be a "licensed acupuncturist" (New York, California, Massachusetts), "certified acupuncturist" (may also be used in California), "registered acupuncturist" (Pennsylvania, Vermont), "doctor of acupuncture" (Rhode Island), "doctor of Oriental medicine" (New Mexico), or "acupuncture physician" (Florida). States that offer the most prestigious-sounding titles, however, do not always require the highest educational standards.

The variation in titles from state to state, along with the varying educational requirements for licensure, can lead to some curious inconsistencies. For example, although most acupuncture and Oriental medicine programs in California grant some kind of master's degree, this degree is not necessary for licensure in California; rather, the state requires that the program attended by the candidate for licensure be approved by a separate state committee on acupuncture. In Rhode Island any individual who obtains a license to practice acupuncture automatically receives the title "doctor of acupuncture," without regard for his or her educational background. In New Jersey, on the other hand, applicants, who are granted only the modest title "licensed acupuncturist," must have a bachelor's degree and be a graduate of an accredited acupuncture program, yet the state requires that anyone seeing an acupuncturist first get a diagnosis from a physician.

Most states permit licensed physicians to perform acupuncture as part of their medical practice, but again the specific provisions vary widely from state to state. In New York physicians and dentists may practice acupuncture in connection with their clinical practice once they have completed 300 hours of training. In California a physician, dentist, or podiatrist may practice acupuncture without any additional training. In Montana medical doctors must pass the NCCAOM examination, while in Hawaii they must be licensed as acupuncturists. Some states have not yet determined whether acupuncture is within a physician's scope of practice. A national organization, the American Association for Medical Acupuncture, provides a 200-hour training program for physicians and is developing a standardized examination.

Several states provide for the practice of acupuncture by chiropractors on the basis of an additional 100 to 200 hours of training. Doctors of naturopathy, podiatrists, physical therapists, physician's assistants, and nurses are permitted to practice in some states, but the training requirements for these different groups are highly variable.

Uses and efficacy

Acupuncture has been applied to myriad ailments over the more than 2,000 years of its practice. In the late 1970s a World Health Organization committee developed a list of diseases that lend themselves to acupuncture treatment (*see* Table, page 167). The list is not based on strict scientific evidence, and the reference to specific diseases is meant to indicate not acupuncture's efficacy in treating them but rather that it has the potential to relieve associated symptoms and in some cases produce a cure. The list is short when compared with the range of conditions discussed in clinical acupuncture manuals and texts, but it is useful in that it provides a sense of the range of conditions that have repeatedly been shown to be amenable to this form of treatment.

Michael S. Yamashita—Corbis

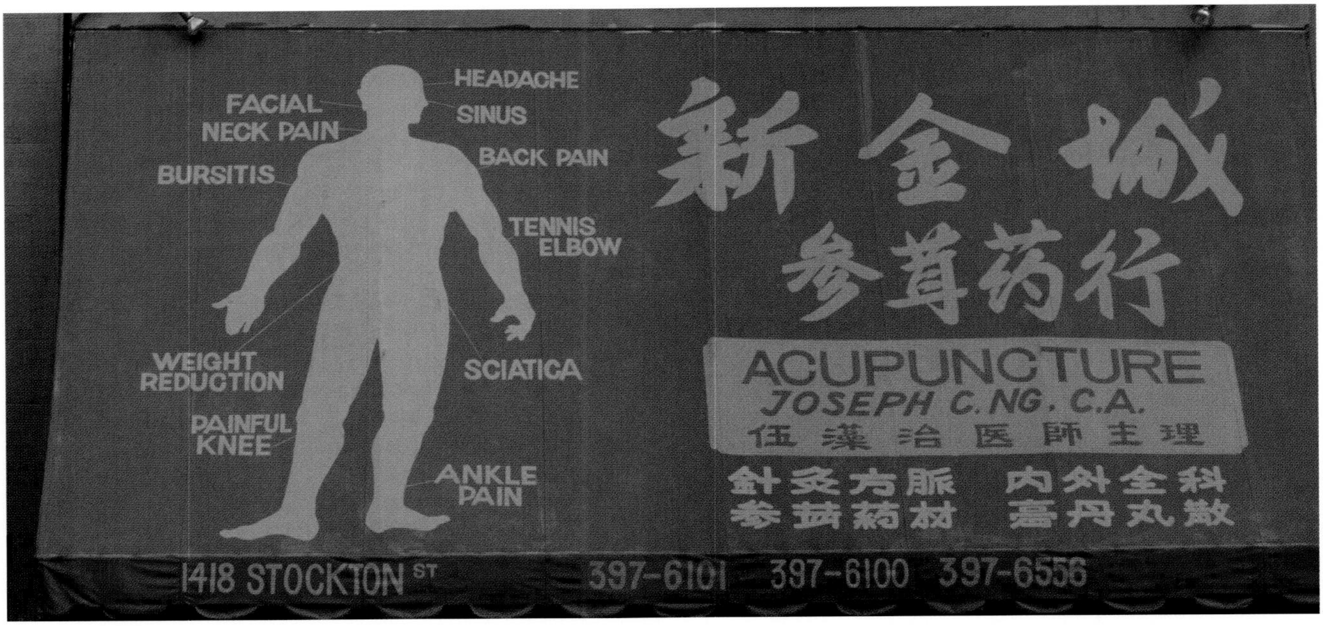

A certified acupuncturist advertises his services in the Chinatown neighborhood of San Francisco. In the U.S. 34 states and the District of Columbia have statutes regulating the practice of acupuncture. Licensing laws vary from state to state, as do the titles license holders are allowed to use.

As mentioned above, acupuncture has been the object of clinical and scientific research in Asian countries, especially China and Japan, since the mid-20th century. Because many of the Chinese studies are what Western scientists term "anecdotal reports" (the observed results of selected cases) rather than controlled clinical trials (in which the intervention under study is compared with either another treatment or a placebo in two or more randomly chosen patient populations), authorities in the West are hesitant to accept the Chinese findings. They have, therefore, begun to subject acupuncture to the kinds of scientific trials typically used in Western countries to evaluate new drugs and medical procedures.

A number of these studies have convincingly demonstrated the efficacy of acupuncture. Many have shown the procedure to be highly effective in the management of a variety of pain conditions, acute and chronic, including headache, migraine, facial pain, menstrual discomfort, osteoarthritic joint pain, and low back pain. Other trials support the usefulness of acupuncture in the management of respiratory diseases such as asthma and chronic obstructive pulmonary disease, treatment of substance abuse, and rehabilitation of stroke patients.

Safety concerns

Although there is clearly the potential for serious harm anytime the human body is penetrated with a sharp instrument, a sterilized acupuncture needle in the hands of a properly trained professional will rarely do substantial damage. Nonetheless, many professional acupuncturists carry professional liability—*i.e.,* malpractice—insurance.

Probably the two most common adverse effects of acupuncture are slight bruising at the site of needle insertion and transient sensations of numbness and tingling. Infection—from inadequately sterilized or improperly handled needles—is a more serious complication. Most acupuncturists use disposable needles that have been presterilized with ethylene oxide gas. Others employ autoclaving or other sterilization methods. Most states that have adopted the NCCAOM examination also require acupuncturists to pass a separate course on the principles of infection control and the proper handling of equipment.

A few isolated instances of transmission of the hepatitis B virus via acupuncture needles have been reported, but overall, infection is quite rare, given the frequency with which acupuncture is used. Apart from one unverified report originating in Europe, there have been no cases of the transmission of HIV infection through acupuncture.

Organ puncture is another potentially serious complication of acupuncture treatment. Pneumothorax (lung collapse), for example, can occur if acupuncture points in the chest and back are penetrated too deeply. (Acupuncture needles range in length from 1.3 cm [0.5 in] to 15.2 cm [6 in].) Like infection, however, organ puncture occurs relatively rarely in acupuncture treatment.

Practice issues

Professional acupuncturists in the U.S. have widely varying scopes of practice. As mentioned above, some states require that patients receive a diagnosis or a referral from a physician before they can be seen by an acupuncturist. Others recognize the acupuncturist as a primary provider of medical care and in some cases describe the professional acupuncturist as a "doctor" or "physician." In certain states certified practitioners of acupuncture may order laboratory tests and diagnostic imaging studies, while in others they are not authorized to do so. There is also considerable variation in the range of modalities that acupuncturists are allowed to employ; techniques that may be legal in one state, such as the application of laser light or magnetic fields, may be forbidden to the professional acupuncturist in another state. Such regulations and the resulting restriction on the scope of practice do not seem to correspond to educational standards for licensure. The ambiguities produced by these different standards present a challenge for both patients and practitioners.

Acupuncture services are now covered by many forms of health insurance. Some states require health plans that cover acupuncture services to pay for these services whenever they are provided by a licensed provider. Other states do not have these regulations, and in these cases some plans distinguish between acupuncture delivered by a physician and that performed by a professional acupuncturist. Some plans treat acupuncturists as specialists who must be seen through referral, and others treat them as fully accessible independent providers of therapy. Recently health maintenance organizations have begun to incorporate acupuncture into the range of services they offer to their members. Oxford Health Plans, a large provider based in the northeastern U.S., has embarked on an ambitious project of credentialing professional acupuncturists and making their services widely available to plan members.

A growing acceptance

In the past 20 years, acupuncture has assumed an important role in U.S. health care. Many uses of acupuncture therapy have been validated by scientific study, and many more await investigation. Despite a variety of challenges facing the practitioners and proponents of acupuncture, the technique will undoubtedly continue to find new applications.

The 16 U.S. states that do not currently provide for the professional practice of acupuncture will probably do so within the next decade. A number of trends contribute to the likelihood of this development, including the continued elevation of educational standards, the Food and Drug Administration's recognition in 1996 of the acupuncture needle as a medical device, and the availability of standardized testing provided by the NCCAOM. Perhaps most important to the future of acupuncture, however, are the widespread popular acceptance of this treatment and the growing willingness of managed-care organizations to provide it.

—Kevin V. Ergil, M.A., M.S., L.Ac.

Disorders for Which Acupuncture Treatment May Be Appropriate

Upper respiratory tract	**Eye**
Acute inflammation of sinuses (sinusitis)	Acute inflammation of mucous membrane (conjunctivitis)
Acute inflammation of lining of nose (rhinitis)	Central inflammation of retina (retinitis)
Common cold	Nearsightedness (in children)
Acute inflammation of tonsils (tonsillitis)	Cataract (without complications)
Respiratory system	**Mouth**
Acute inflammation of airways (bronchitis)	Toothache
Bronchial asthma	Pain following tooth extraction
	Inflammation of gums (gingivitis)
	Acute and chronic sore throat
Neurological and musculoskeletal systems	**Gastrointestinal system**
Headache and migraine	Esophageal spasm
Facial pain due to irritation of trigeminal nerve (trigeminal neuralgia)	Hiccups
Facial palsy (early stage)	Sagging of stomach into abdomen (gastroptosis)
Paralysis following stroke	Acute and chronic inflammation of stomach (gastritis)
Peripheral nerve pain	Excess stomach acid
Early aftereffects of poliomyelitis	Chronic duodenal ulcer (pain relief)
Ménière's disease (inner ear disorder)	Acute duodenal ulcer (without complications)
Bladder dysfunction due to nerve disorder	Acute and chronic inflammation of colon (colitis)
Bedwetting	Dysentery
Chest pain originating in nerves between ribs (intercostal neuralgia)	Constipation
Nerve pain in neck and shoulder (cervicobrachial syndrome)	Diarrhea
"Frozen shoulder," "tennis elbow"	Bowel obstruction due to intestinal muscle paralysis
Pain in sciatic nerve (sciatica)	
Low back pain	
Osteoarthritis	

Source: Adapted from R.H. Bannerman, "The World Health Organization Viewpoint of Acupuncture," *World Health—The Magazine of the World Health Organization*, Dec. 24–29, 1979.

SOURCES OF INFORMATION

Books

- Kaptchuk, Ted J. *The Web That Has No Weaver.* New York: Congdon & Weed, 1983. A comprehensive explanation of the clinical world view of Chinese medicine.
- Micozzi, Marc S., ed. *Fundamentals of Complementary and Alternative Medicine.* New York: Churchill Livingstone, 1996. Contains a chapter on traditional Chinese medicine by Kevin V. Ergil.
- Unschuld, Paul U. *Medicine In China: A History of Ideas.* Berkeley: University of California Press, 1985. An outstanding history of the practice of Chinese medicine.

Organizations

- National Acupuncture and Oriental Medicine Alliance
  14637 Starr Rd SE
  Olalla WA 98359
  253-851-6896
- American Association of Oriental Medicine (AAOM)
  433 Front St
  Catasauqua PA 18032-2526
  610-266-1433
- American Academy of Medical Acupuncture (AAMA)
  5820 Wilshire Blvd Suite 500
  Los Angeles CA 90036
  213-937-5514
- National Academy of Acupuncture and Oriental Medicine (NAAOM)
  Box 62
  Tarrytown NY 10591
  914-332-4576
  E-mail: naaom@acor.org
- Council of Colleges of Acupuncture and Oriental Medicine (CCAOM)
  1010 Wayne Ave
  Suite 1270
  Silver Spring MD 20910
  301-608-9175
- Accreditation Commission for Acupuncture and Oriental Medicine (ACAOM)
  1010 Wayne Ave
  Suite 1270
  Silver Spring MD 20910
  301-608-9680
- National Certification Commission for Acupuncture and Oriental Medicine (NCCAOM)
  Dept 0595
  Washington DC 20036
  202-232-1404

Sickle-Cell Disease Update

Sickle-cell disease (SCD), or sickle-cell anemia, used to be considered a disease of childhood, but thanks to noteworthy advances in patient care, made possible by intensive research, this is no longer the case. The eminent jazz trumpeter Miles Davis had SCD, though this fact was not widely known during his lifetime. Davis died in 1991 at the age of 65, having suffered an instructive list of SCD-related complications: episodic bouts of pain, jaundice, gallstones, hip disease, recurrent pneumonia, and stroke among them. Yet the jazz artist's life illustrated not only the serious medical consequences that patients face but also the stunning degree of accomplishment that is possible for some despite this formidable condition.

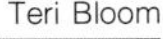

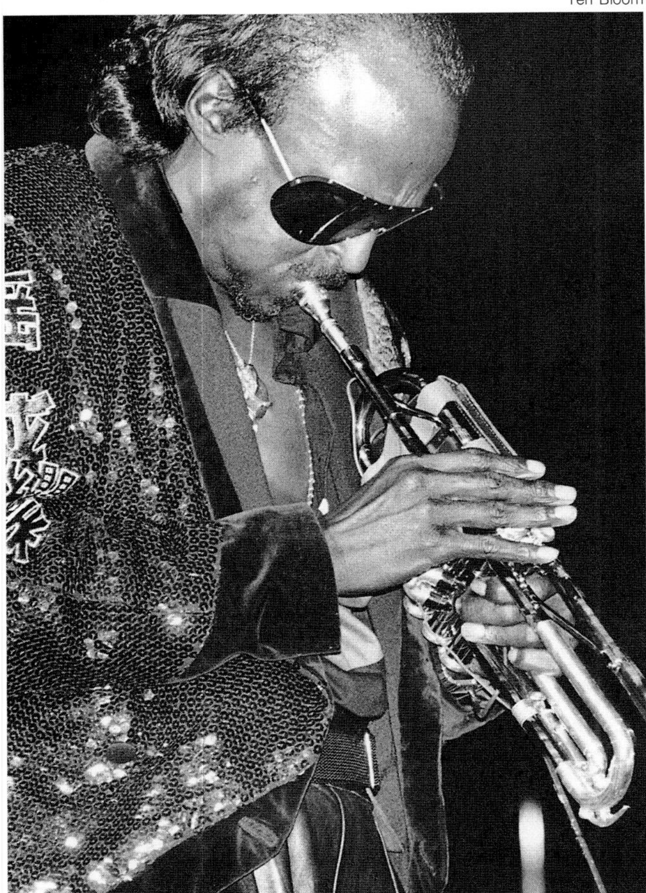

Jazz legend Miles Davis, who began playing trumpet at age 13, was a brilliant innovator, bandleader, composer, and recording artist; few knew he suffered from serious complications of sickle-cell disease.

SCD is a disease of the blood. Since blood flows to all parts of the body, every organ system can be affected. Yet there are remarkable differences in the character and severity of symptoms between individuals. Having no simple cure, it is a chronic illness, whose course is punctuated by relapsing and sometimes catastrophic events.

SCD is among the most common serious genetic diseases in the world, though its first clear description in Western medical literature did not appear until 1910. Its tendency to run in families and cause recurring pain and early death in some victims had long been recognized within African cultures. Persons of African ancestry remain the most commonly affected, though from a global perspective it is a multiethnic condition.

Despite the fact that scientists know a great deal about the genetic and molecular basis of SCD, research into treatments had been quite limited in scope. Recently, however, prospective studies of large numbers of newborns diagnosed with sickle-cell disease at birth have shed considerable light on the basic biology and natural history of the disease and suggested meaningful treatment approaches. Consequently, patient care and survival have been vastly improved by a combination of newborn diagnosis, preventive drugs, prompt and appropriate therapy for acute medical episodes, timely utilization of blood transfusions, and in some cases carefully devised surgical procedures. A few patients have even been cured by bone marrow transplantation.

Basis in the blood

Blood is composed of a liquid, nutrient portion called plasma and a cellular portion that is suspended within the plasma and has three main cell types. *White cells* help to fight infection. *Platelets,* which are smaller and more numerous, help to prevent bleeding. *Red cells,* which give blood its color and are more numerous still, pick up oxygen in the lungs and carry it to the tissues; at the same time, these cells carry the waste product carbon dioxide back to the lungs, where it is expelled in the breath. It is the protein called hemoglobin inside the red cells that is primarily responsible for these special functions.

In order to perform their functions properly, red blood cells must be soft and flexible. In people with SCD, these cells may acquire a bent, crescent (or "sickle") shape, which makes them both rigid and fragile. The sickled red cells may adhere to the walls of blood vessels, interrupting the flow of nutrients and oxygen, causing chronic tissue damage and unpredictable bouts of bone pain. Many parts of the body may be affected by this process, including the lungs, brain, spleen, kidneys, retinas, penis, and liver. Damaged and misshapen by the sickling tendency of their abnormal hemoglobin, the red cells also come apart prematurely in the circulation. This chronic and excessively rapid loss of red cells results in anemia, or low hemoglobin, a characteristic (though not universal) feature of the disease.

In 1949 the U.S. chemist Linus Pauling realized that it is the hemoglobin molecule inside the red cell that is uniquely abnormal in SCD patients. A slight chemical difference in the hemoglobin structure causes an immense change in its behavior. Molecules of sickled hemoglobin stick together (polymerize) inside the red blood cell, forming crystals. It is this polymerization of hemoglobin inside the cell that changes the cell's shape and damages its membrane. Besides blocking blood vessels (vaso-occlusion) and causing pain and tissue damage, these sickled cells have a shortened life span in the circulation. An individual cell affected by sickling may survive only 20 days, compared with the usual 120. With this perpetual loss of red cells, the body strives to produce replacements. The bone marrow, where blood cells are made, is maximally stimulated by chemical signals demanding more hemoglobin to carry oxygen that will nourish the tissues. The newly produced red cells, however, contain only abnormal hemoglobin

(Below) Gopal Murti—Science Source/Photo Researchers; (bottom) Walter Reinhart—CNRI/Phototake

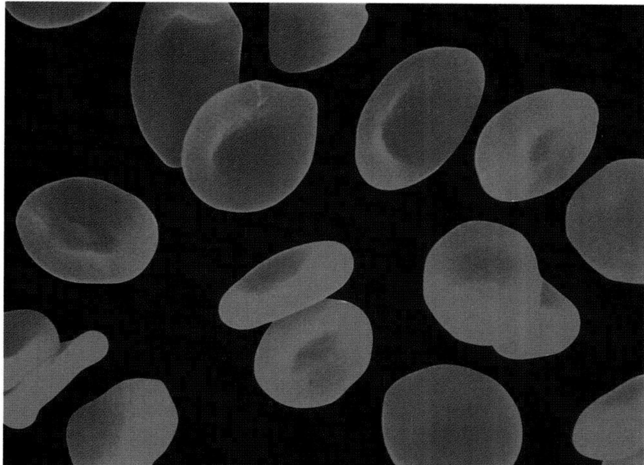

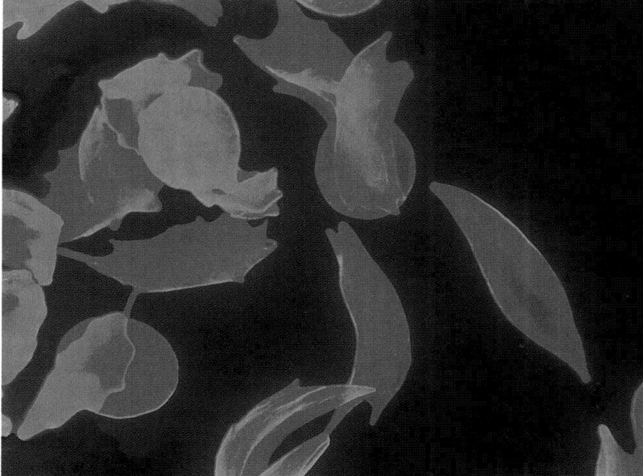

Scanning electron micrographs show normal red blood cells (top), which are round, soft, and flexible, and the typically crescent-shaped cells seen in sickle-cell disease (above). Sickled red blood cells are rigid and fragile; by impeding the vital flow of nutrients and oxygen to the tissues, they can cause chronic tissue damage and unpredictable bouts of bone pain.

and are not able to carry out this function. The increased production of new but defective red cells does not compensate for the ongoing destruction of mature red cells (hemolysis) in the circulation, which produces the low-hemoglobin condition anemia.

Sickle-cell trait

To manufacture hemoglobin—and all other proteins—the body requires specific instructions from specific genes. These genes are inherited from parents in pairs. An individual with SCD has inherited two abnormal hemoglobin genes, one from each parent. Individuals who have only a single abnormal hemoglobin gene have what is known as sickle-cell trait (also called the genetic carrier state). Because their red cells survive and function normally, persons with sickle-cell trait are entirely healthy under ordinary circumstances. Only when their bodies are deprived of oxygen might those with sickle-cell trait develop problems. Drastic exercise undertaken without prior conditioning or proper fluid intake is one such oxygen-depriving condition that may induce red-cell sickling. In a study of military recruits, subjects with sickle-cell trait were found to have a slightly higher death rate during rigorous basic training than controls (healthy recruits without the trait). In a few rare instances, individuals with sickle-cell trait have developed damage to the spleen at high altitudes. But on the whole, studies of large populations of persons with sickle-cell trait—including trained athletes—show no increased risk of illness or death. Sickle-cell carriers can prevent complications by simply avoiding dehydration, altitude extremes, and intense exercise without adequate conditioning.

Both SCD and sickle-cell trait are genetically determined and inherited. Neither is contagious. Neither can be acquired after birth. Moreover, the trait does not develop into the disease, nor does the disease become the trait. If both parents are carriers, each offspring has a one-in-four chance of having SCD, a two-in-four chance of having sickle-cell trait, and a one-in-four chance of having neither (*see* Figure, page 170).

The malaria connection

In the United States there are more than 60,000 individuals with SCD. In the United Kingdom there are between 5,000 and 6,000 patients. Internationally, an estimated 100,000 newborns inherit the disease every year. Those of African descent are by far the most commonly affected. Approximately one in every 400 African-Americans inherits this abnormal hemoglobin gene from both parents (and thus has SCD); one in 12 is born with sickle-cell trait.

There are regions of Africa where the carrier frequency is as high as one in every three to four individuals. This remarkably high prevalence of the sickle-cell trait led scientists to ask why the trait had become so common among Africans and those of African ancestry. The answer probably lies in SCD's relationship to malaria, a sometimes fatal parasitic infection transmitted by mosquitoes.

Genetic diseases are caused by abnormal genetic material (DNA). The mutated gene that causes SCD arose independently in different groups of people living across a broad equatorial belt in Africa and other locations where malaria was prevalent. The mutation traveled with migrating populations and is now widely distributed among groups living in many regions of the world. Persons of Mediterranean, Caribbean, South and Central American, Arabian, and East Indian ancestry are also affected.

The malaria parasite spends part of its life cycle inside the red blood cells. As already noted, when sickle hemoglobin is present, red cells break down much more readily than they should—a process that also results in the destruction of the malaria parasite. Those in whom the parasites are unable to complete their life cycle benefit by having a small degree of protection from malaria. Because sickle-cell trait confers this slender survival advantage by rendering affected individuals slightly more likely to attain reproductive age, which enables them to pass on the trait to offspring, over time the trait became extremely common in malarial regions.

Malaria, however, is not benign in individuals with SCD. Someone with sickle-cell disease who is already anemic and is bitten by a malaria-carrying mosquito is likely to be devastated by accelerated hemolysis and without medical care and transfusion may die from rapidly progressive anemia.

Sickle-Cell Inheritance: both parents carriers

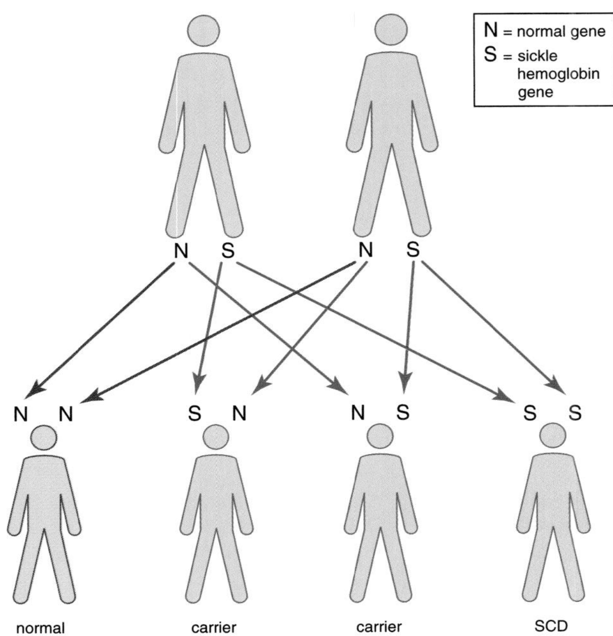

Notable progress

As already stated, SCD is exceptionally variable in both its character and its severity. Nonetheless, there are certain common features. Affected infants are entirely healthy during gestation and at birth because their bone marrow produces only a fetal type of hemoglobin, which is not affected by the genetic abnormality present in SCD. Gradually, however, over the first months of life, the body switches off the manufacture of fetal hemoglobin in favor of adult-type hemoglobin; because children with SCD have an abnormality in their adult hemoglobin gene but not in their fetal hemoglobin, their symptoms then become apparent. The majority of children who have inherited SCD will experience symptoms by age five and usually well before.

Painful episodes. Because of their abnormal shape, relative inflexibility, and sticky consistency, sickled red blood cells can cause chronic and recurring blockages of blood vessels anywhere in the body. Wherever they occur, these blockages (known as vaso-occlusive episodes) deprive tissues of oxygen and nutrients and thereby produce pain along with tissue damage. Skeletal pain due to vaso-occlusion is the most common complaint. Episodes typically last four to six days and may be triggered by infection, dehydration, cold, or emotional distress. Often, however, there is no such identifiable predisposing factor.

About one-third of SCD patients are severely affected by these episodes and require repeated hospitalizations. (A small subset of that group has nearly unremitting complications.) Another one-third are moderately affected, while a final one-third are generally fit and seem well most of the time and seldom need the resources of the hospital. Medical scientists still do not fully understand why there is such conspicuous variability between individuals who have essentially the same genetic disease.

In infancy the small bones of the hands and feet are characteristically affected, which causes a symmetrical, painful swelling known as dactylitis, or hand-and-foot syndrome. The infant may be irritable, difficult to feed, and reluctant to bear weight on limbs. Beyond infancy, youngsters tend to experience painful episodes that involve the longer bones of the arms and legs, as well as the back, chest, or abdomen, but swelling may no longer be observable. In the past such episodes were sometimes mistaken for appendicitis, arthritis, injury, or even malingering (pretended incapacitation). Increasingly, however, health care providers are becoming aware that the absence of external attributes of pain, such as swelling, is common and that patients' complaints of pain should be taken seriously. Heightened awareness is also the result of newborn diagnosis (discussed below).

Compromised immunity. Within the first few months of life, infants with SCD develop subnormal immune function, which predisposes them to serious infections. This occurs because chronic low-grade vaso-occlusion damages the spleen, an organ that is vital to the functioning of the immune system. Its ability to filter bacteria from the blood and manufacture specific antibodies against bacteria is impaired. Overwhelming bacterial infection, therefore, was previously the most common cause of premature death in SCD patients. This, however, is changing, and many serious infections can now be treated early or prevented entirely. SCD patients take daily penicillin in a preventive fashion for at least the first five years of life. All parents of affected children are urged to seek prompt medical attention for their child whenever fever occurs so that antibiotic treatment can be initiated without delay. A study sponsored by the National Institutes of Health demonstrated that this combination of parental attention to initial signs of infection and appropriate treatment can prevent about 85% of serious infections.

As in other areas of medicine, a major cause of concern in the treatment of SCD is that bacteria resistant to common antibiotics are now causing infections with increasing frequency. Patients whose infections do not respond to drug treatment are at increased risk of dying. The key is for the clinician to be vigilant for antibiotic-resistant infections in SCD patients so that appropriate alternative drugs can be administered promptly.

Anemic events. Most patients with SCD have anemia due to a premature demise of red cells in the circulation. In addition to malaria, two other conditions commonly produce a precarious worsening of anemia. Parvovirus B19 can infect red cell precursors in the bone marrow, where blood cells are formed. When this happens, production of new red cells can fall quickly to naught—a life-threatening situation known as an aplastic episode. Blood transfusion is usually necessary to prevent death.

Epidemics of parvovirus often occur within communities during the spring months, causing clusters of illness. Siblings with SCD are at particularly high risk. People who do not have SCD may develop fever, rash, and joint swelling but generally do not develop severe anemia because they are not affected by chronic red-cell breakdown. Although an effective vaccine is routinely given against canine parvovirus (a virulent infection in dogs), none is yet available for the comparatively small group of SCD patients and others with chronic hemolytic anemia at special risk from this viral illness because their bodies constantly break down red cells.

The second cause of severe anemia is known as splenic sequestration, which occurs mainly in children under age three. In this condition blood is blocked from leaving the spleen but not from entering it. Consequently, the spleen, normally the size of a baby's fist, swells dramatically. With a major portion of the child's red blood cells trapped in the spleen, the heart has little to pump. Again, if an episode is severe, blood must be quickly replaced through transfusion to prevent death.

Parents of youngsters with SCD are taught to recognize an enlarged spleen so that early diagnosis and treatment are possible. Since this condition tends to recur, it often becomes necessary to remove the spleen following a major episode of sequestration. Recently surgeons have attempted to prevent sequestration by removing only part of the spleen; though this is a much more difficult operation than splenectomy (excision of the entire spleen), for selected younger patients it may have the advantage of preserving some of the immune function.

Stroke. At least 25% of school-age children and young adults with sickle-cell disease experience a diminished supply of blood to the brain, resulting in stroke. Much less commonly, bleeding into the brain from abnormal vessels causes a drastic stroke. Initial symptoms of stroke can vary greatly—ranging from subtle behavioral changes to seizures, severe neurological impairment, and even death. Unlike most cases of stroke in adults, SCD-related stroke is not associated with atherosclerosis (arteries clogged by deposits of cholesterol and other fatty substances) or high blood pressure. Once a stroke has occurred, there is a high probability of recurrence. Frequent blood transfusions are necessary for prevention and rehabilitation. Although motor skills usually improve with aggressive transfusion and rehabilitative therapy, learning difficulties and neuropsychological deficits (*e.g.,* memory and concentration problems) are often permanent and severe.

Ultrasound evaluation of arteries carrying blood to the brain can detect a developing blockage before stroke occurs. A clinical study of early intensive blood transfusion to prevent stroke in appropriately selected patients was ended in September 1997, 16 months early, when it was shown that such treatment reduced the risk of stroke by 90%.

Respiratory illness. More than half of all patients with SCD suffer from so-called acute chest syndrome (ACS), a complication that can be triggered by a variety of events. In younger children lung infection can severely compromise the ability of these organs to perform their role of oxygenating the blood, which leads to sickling of hemoglobin within the lung. This sickling in turn blocks the blood flow and further impairs oxygenation, perpetuating the destructive cycle. In older children and adults, damage to the marrow tissue (from vaso-occlusion due to sickling) sometimes results in the release of fat into the circulation. This fat travels to the lungs and other organs, where it incites tissue damage. The same cycle of sickling, blockage of blood flow, and decreased oxygenation occurs.

Whatever the trigger, recurrent episodes of ACS can lead to irreversible lung damage. Heart failure may occur as the organ strains to pump blood through stiff, damaged lungs. Again, transfusion of normal red blood cells is often needed. Recently, a newly devised blood test has been able to recognize some patients with impending ACS. A trial of early transfusion therapy in selected ACS-prone patients is under way.

Other organ systems. In patients with sickle-cell disease, the kidney is prone to infection and chronic low-grade sickling. Since the normal job of the kidney is to filter the entire fluid content of the blood every 45 minutes, progressive loss of kidney function

W. Reed and D. Jett

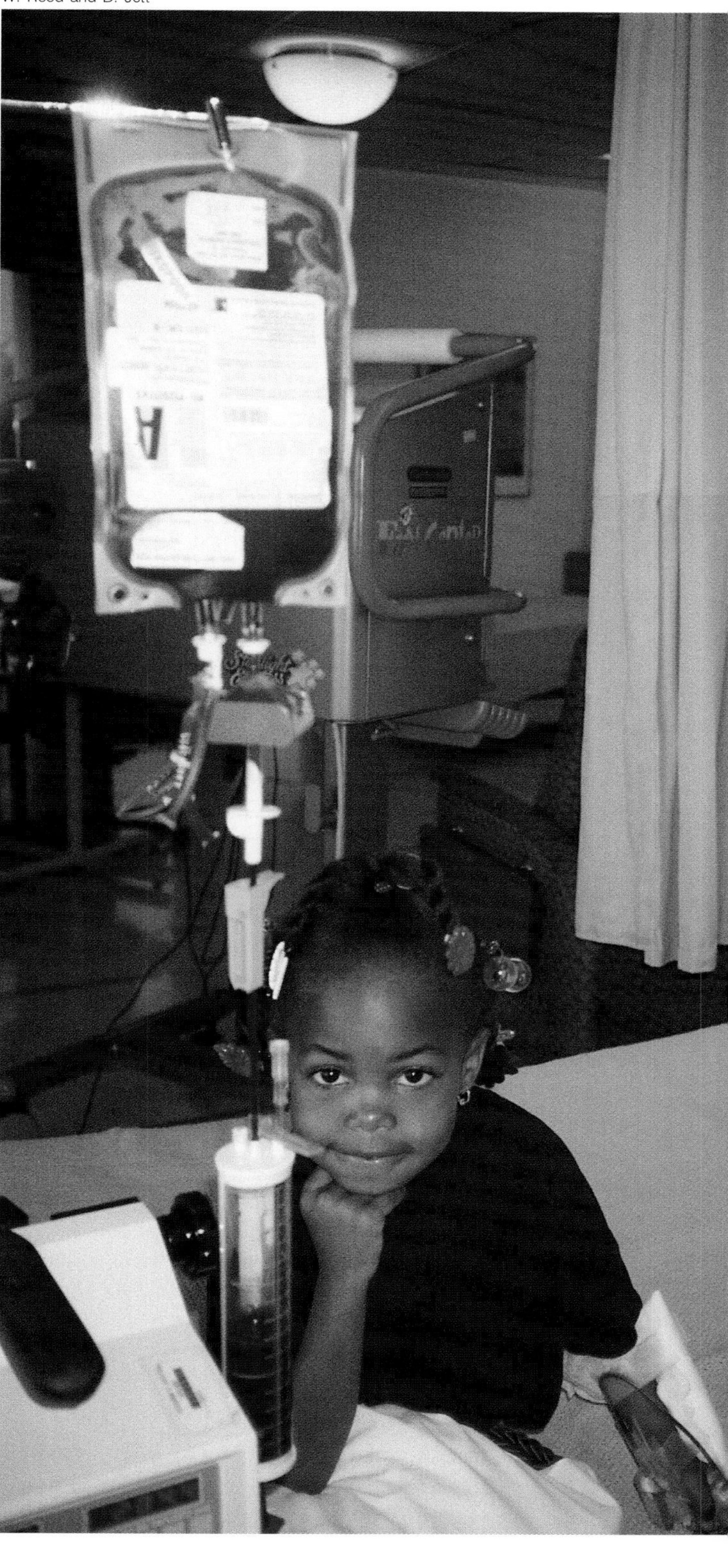

A six-year-old with sickle-cell disease (SCD) received monthly blood transfusions at Children's Hospital in Oakland, Calif., as part of a recently concluded study sponsored by the National Institutes of Health. The trial determined that the proactive use of transfusions reduced the risk of strokes in selected SCD patients by 90%.

due to chronic sickling makes the need for dialysis (artificial cleansing of the blood by a machine) during adulthood commonplace.

The constant breakdown of red cells releases a yellowish pigment, bilirubin, into the blood. This substance may accumulate in the gallbladder (causing gallstones) or in the skin and eyes (causing the yellowish discoloration known as jaundice).

Chronic sickling in the circulation of the eye may damage the retina and impair vision. Such damage usually does not occur before age 10.

In boys and young men, the penis may become engorged with blood whose circulation is sluggish or nil. This results in priapism, a persistent, unwanted painful erection. More often than not, therapy for priapism is unsatisfactory.

Newborn diagnosis and other lifesaving measures

Careful studies of the typical course of SCD in Jamaican and African-American children showed that early deaths (during the first three years of life) were common and usually due to an overwhelming bacterial infection of the bloodstream or severe anemia. Because fatality would often precede a diagnosis of sickle-cell disease, death would be attributed to sudden infant death syndrome (also known as crib death) or to anemia that was not recognized as a complication of underlying SCD. Investigators came to realize that diagnosing SCD in newborns—before symptoms occur—would be critical to improving patient care and preventing such early deaths. In the past decade much progress has been made toward that goal. In the U.S. today 42 of the 50 states screen nearly all newborns for SCD. While most states find an efficient economy of scale in testing all newborns, some programs attempt to test only those infants considered to be at risk because of their ethnic background. These targeted screening programs, often mired in political controversy, fail to diagnose many affected newborns. In parts of the country where newborn diagnosis is routine and where parents are educated to spot early signs of sickle-cell crises and children receive comprehensive medical care, mortality has been reduced from between 15% and 30% of children aged 3 years and younger to well under 5% by age 10.

Presently all laboratory techniques used to detect SCD in newborns also, unavoidably, identify the sickle-cell carrier state. The affected infant derives no known direct benefit from this information, though family members may benefit from the identification of the gene within the family. In fact, identifying newborns with sickle-cell trait can be detrimental because it may lead to stigmatization, delayed adoption, disclosure of nonpaternity, and erroneous attribution of symptoms.

Even with newborn screening for SCD, geographic differences in mortality persist and may correspond to the availability of comprehensive medical care. Successful management of SCD depends on the ability to provide the most comprehensive care possible by health care providers experienced with the disease's protean manifestations. Newborn diagnosis, parent education, daily preventive penicillin for the first five years of life, and transfusions are all components of such care. Presently, it is of considerable concern to clinicians and affected families that with the emergence of managed care in the U.S., sickle-cell patients will be deprived of the full range of services they need. In fact, there have already been documented instances of unnecessary deaths of children due to such lack of access to care.

Blood transfusion

Normal red cells from a healthy volunteer blood donor can correct anemia, increase the oxygen-carrying capacity of the blood, dilute the patient's own sickle hemoglobin, and, by decreasing the activity of the patient's bone marrow, limit the production of abnormal red cells. When malaria, splenic sequestration, or parvovirus causes severe anemia, early transfusion preserves life. Stroke, priapism, growth failure, relentless pain, and ACS all may be improved by transfusion. In some circumstances, most often following stroke, blood transfusions are given regularly at three- to four-week intervals. Such a regimen (known as hypertransfusion) leaves the recipient's bone marrow virtually inactive, so it produces very few new sickled cells. With this continuous substitution of normal red cells for the patient's own blood, SCD usually becomes quiescent. Occasionally, though, severe complications occur despite even the most intensive transfusion.

While indispensable for preventing many complications of SCD, transfusion therapy is limited by certain obstacles. Patients are prone to developing antibodies against transfused red cells. When this happens, delayed but sometimes serious reactions can result, in part because there are predictable differences between the typical pool of donor blood and those needing transfusions. Often the development of such antibodies can be prevented by a special extended-matching process of donor and recipient blood types. In the U.S. certain blood types that are relatively rare in the population at large but are common among SCD patients of African ancestry may be unavailable when they are needed. In that regard, increased voluntary donation of blood by *any* and *all* African-Americans would be of particular value.

Another obstacle that restricts the application of transfusion therapy is the high iron content of blood. Because the body is unable to excrete iron, toxic amounts of the substance accumulate in the heart, liver, and other tissues whenever transfusions are continued over a period of many years. Current methods of removing iron in recipient tissues and/or preventing its accumulation, unfortunately, have some serious limitations.

Every country has its own blood-banking system. Currently, the U.S. blood supply is derived almost exclusively from healthy volunteer donors and is exhaustively tested for infectious agents, which have made it safer than at any time in the past. Still, there is a small residual risk, and presently unforeseen problems may emerge. In parts of the less-developed world, neither recruitment of donors nor testing of blood is as rigorous as it is in many developed countries—a situation that raises very great concerns about blood safety.

Progress and breakthroughs (in perspective)

In Europe and the U.S., a few patients have been cured of sickle-cell disease by bone marrow transplantation. Powerful but toxic drugs are used to eradicate blood-forming cells in the patient's own bone marrow. Healthy stem cells (undifferentiated cells in the bone marrow that give rise to all blood cells and some blood-derived tissue cells), usually from a sibling, are then infused to replace the eradicated cells. At the present time the selection of appropriate patients for transplantation is difficult, in part because the procedure is risky and in part because transplantation is probably safest during infancy, *before* an individual can be recognized as one who is likely to be severely affected and for whom the transplant risk may be appropriate. Also, few patients have the needed matched sibling donor. Placental blood (umbilical cord blood) may soon prove to be an excellent alternative source of stem cells for transplantation. This resource, which has been routinely discarded with the placenta (afterbirth), can be stored frozen, creating banks of stem cells from unrelated donors. Early results from placental blood transplants are promising, which suggests that less-stringent tissue matching and utilization of unrelated donors may be acceptable.

Gene therapy, the introduction of a normal hemoglobin gene into stem cells to replace the abnormal sickle gene, is intriguing for its theoretical simplicity. Stem cells can be readily isolated and removed from the patient's circulating blood. Then, in the laboratory, they can be genetically altered by the introduction of a normal hemoglobin gene. A virus serves as the delivery vehicle, carrying the gene to the cell. Though the process may sound straightforward, there are significant technical hurdles that need to be overcome—particularly difficulties with the stability and control of the inserted genes and the fact that very large amounts of hemoglobin must be made under the genes' direction. As a routine cure, this very promising therapy is still on the distant horizon. As with transplantation, many ethical, as well as scientific, problems remain to be addressed.

Hydroxyurea, an old anticancer drug that interferes with cell division, and a few other drugs, including butyrate (derived from a simple fatty acid) and erythropoietin (a natural hormone that stimulates red-cell production), can help increase fetal hemoglobin production and thereby partially return the red cells to their less-troublesome state. Some form of drug therapy is likely to become common for SCD patients in the near future. Like other new therapies, these drugs require very close monitoring. Moreover, because they are new, their long-term effects are not yet fully appreciated.

The results of a large U.S. study of hydroxyurea therapy in adult patients with SCD were greeted with enthusiasm by patients and the physicians who treat them. The trial, involving nearly 300 patients with severe disease, was ended in 1995 several months earlier than planned. The drug's benefits had become strikingly apparent. The treatment reduced the occurrence of ACS and the need for blood transfusions. There was a 50% decline in the frequency of painful episodes. One of the authors of the study reported that some subjects "were really reborn—just amazing. Some people who were so sick they couldn't do anything went back to work." Hydroxyurea may also render sickle cells less sticky and thus less likely to block blood vessels. Some patients in the trial, however, realized no benefit.

Many attempts to produce a blood substitute are under way, but success has been limited thus far. One class of blood substitute, solutions in which single normal hemoglobin molecules are intentionally chemically modified, or polymerized, holds particular theoretical interest for SCD patients. Having no large blood cells to get stuck in the circulation, these hemoglobin polymers might be able to circumvent obstructions created by sickled cells. This would allow oxygen, carried by the hemoglobin polymer, to reach the deprived tissues and would mitigate vaso-occlusive episodes. Such blood substitutes have both advantages and limitations. On the plus side, they would not require compatibility testing. They also could be stored at room temperature for many months. On the other hand, such polymers are short-lived in the circulation and may be toxic to certain organ systems. In SCD, early trials are under way; these hemoglobin solutions may prove useful during episodes of pain or in transfusion prior to surgery.

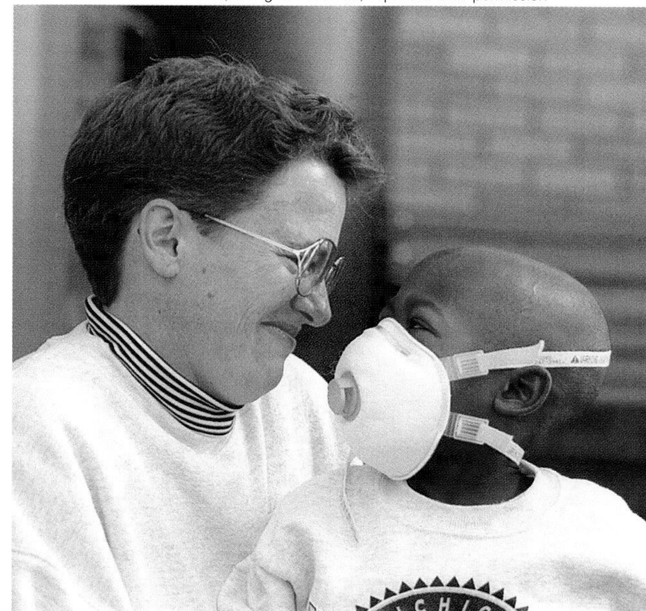

In early 1997 a five-year-old SCD patient in Michigan recovers after a bone marrow transplant. A handful of youngsters in the U.S. and Europe have been cured after undergoing the experimental procedure.

In the past half century, the investment in research on sickle-cell disease has paid off substantially. Currently, scientific investigators are zeroing in on many aspects of SCD. Hip problems, stroke, ACS, and the potential for preventing infections by vaccination are all under intensive study. New preventive and therapeutic approaches to priapism, retinal disease, and chronic organ failure are greatly needed.

A recent study estimated the overwhelming costs of the disease; in the U.S. alone an estimated 75,000 SCD patients are hospitalized annually, and each hospitalization costs an average of $6,300. The costs in suffering are beyond estimation. Perhaps the most important step that has been taken in the right direction in the last few years is that this intriguing systemic disease is being widely acknowledged not only for its striking genetic and molecular characteristics but also for the profound effects it has upon those who continue to live with it.

—William Reed, M.D., and Elliott P. Vichinsky, M.D.

Placental Blood Transplantation

As a primal source of life, the human placenta—the blood-vessel-filled organ that nourishes the developing fetus—has long had mystical connotations. Even today some of the most expensive skin-rejuvenating products on the market claim to derive their efficacy from "placental extracts." While it is doubtful that these ingredients genuinely reverse the ravages of time, there is no question that the placenta does contain substances that have therapeutic value—for example, hormones used in the treatment of infertility.

In recent years blood from the placenta and the umbilical cord (the structure that connects the developing fetus with the placenta) has been found to possess genuine lifesaving properties in the form of "stem" cells—undifferentiated cells capable of developing into mature blood cells. For purposes of transplantation, placental and cord blood stem cells have many advantages over bone marrow collected from family members of the prospective recipient or from unrelated donors; perhaps most important is that they can be stored for extended periods and used without delay in patients who lack a suitable bone marrow donor.

Stem cells: primitive but powerful

Blood cells originate not in the bloodstream but rather in specific blood-forming, or hematopoietic, tissues and organs. In adult humans the bone marrow is by far the most important of these. Human blood cell development begins with a small number of stem cells. These are primitive, self-renewing cells, which, through a series of gradual transformations, give rise to all of the different types of blood cells—red cells, white cells (including the infection-fighting lymphocytes, granulocytes, and monocytes), and platelets. Hence, in principle, a few stem cells can generate sufficient numbers of cells of all types to reconstitute an individual's entire hematopoietic system.

This remarkable property has led to wide use of stem cell transplantation as a treatment for life-threatening blood diseases. Patients with leukemia or lymphoma (cancer of the lymphatic system), for example, are sometimes treated with extremely high doses of chemotherapy that kill not only the cancerous cells but also normal stem cells in the bone marrow. Such therapy would be lethal without subsequent transplantation of healthy stem cells capable of producing new blood cells of all types. Stem cell transplants are also used to correct genetic disorders due to abnormalities in any of the cells that arise from stem cells—inherited immune deficiencies due to defective white blood cells, for example, or diseases of the red cells such as sickle-cell anemia.

Traditionally, stem cells for transplantation have been extracted from either the blood or the bone marrow of a living donor. Removing, or "harvesting," bone marrow is a costly procedure. Donors must be hospitalized and undergo general anesthesia. A hollow needle inserted into the donor's hip bones removes 500–1,000 ml (1–2 pt) of marrow. Usually the procedure is accompanied only by mild soreness for two or three days, but in rare cases more serious complications may occur.

It has always been known that a small number of stem cells circulate in the blood, but recovering a sufficient number for transplantation was a problem. Recently, with the development of

Using a hollow needle, a physician drains blood from an umbilical cord shortly after childbirth. For purposes of transplantation, stem cells from placental and umbilical cord blood have a number of advantages over stem cells derived from other tissues.

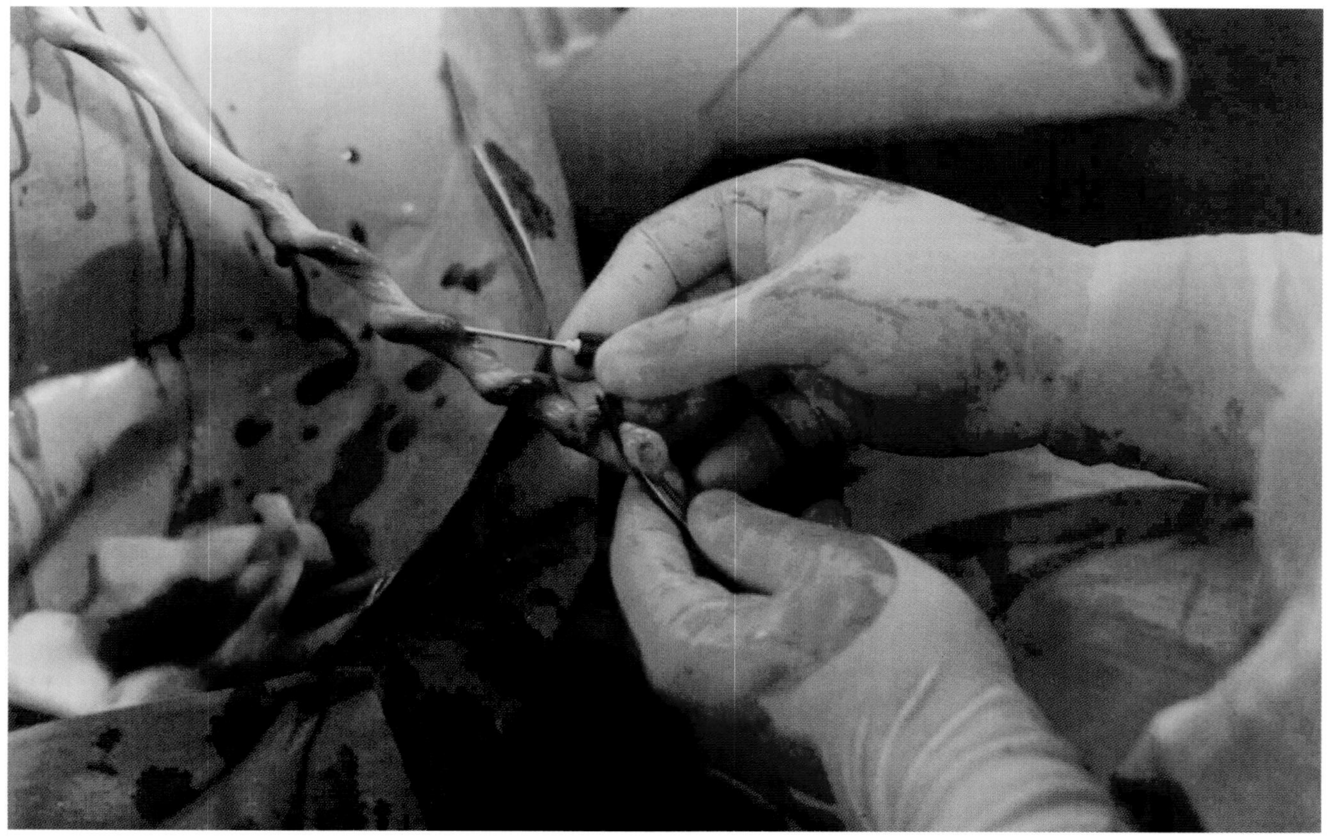

Associated Press

synthetic compounds capable of stimulating stem cell proliferation, it has become possible to increase the number of stem cells in blood by mobilizing them from the marrow. Collecting stem cells from donor blood has the immediate advantage of not requiring hospitalization.

The fetal liver is another potential source of stem cells for transplantation, but, in the U.S. especially, ethical issues surrounding the use of fetal tissues have limited this approach. Blood remaining in the placenta and umbilical cord after childbirth is also a rich source of stem cells and one that, although still experimental, holds great promise.

Making a match

Until recently the majority of successful allogeneic stem cell transplants (those in which the donor and recipient are of the same species but are not genetically identical) involved siblings who had identical human leukocyte antigens (HLA), also known as transplantation antigens. (Antigens are substances capable of triggering an immune response. HLA are a group of antigens involved in the identification and rejection by the body of foreign tissues.) As with blood typing in transfusion, determining the HLA types of prospective donors and recipients is a routine step in all transplantation procedures, whether of whole organs, tissues, or cells. Matching the HLA types of donor and recipient reduces the risk that the transplant, or graft, will be rejected. It also minimizes the chances of the recipient's tissues being attacked by immune system cells in the graft, a potentially lethal condition known as graft-versus-host disease (GVHD).

Recent advances in HLA-typing techniques, better methods of preventing GVHD and other posttransplantation complications, and larger numbers of prospective donors have done much to abolish past discrepancies of transplantation outcome based on the source of stem cells. Currently, the results of allogeneic stem cell transplantation vary only slightly by donor type (sibling or unrelated volunteer). Why, then, has placental blood generated so much interest as a source of stem cells?

Advantages of placental stem cells

One of the major problems in using stem cells from the bone marrow of an adult donor not related to the recipient is the unavoidable delay involved. Although the HLA types of registered donors are stored in computer databases, the subsequent steps—locating the donors, examining their cells by high-resolution typing techniques, counseling them about potential risks, examining them to make certain they are healthy, and harvesting their marrow—can take an average of four months, a delay that can be fatal to a seriously ill patient. Moreover, for many patients, especially members of racial and ethnic minorities, whose HLA types are different from those in the population at large, only a small number of prospective donors may be registered.

For these reasons, fewer than half of those who might benefit from unrelated-donor stem cells actually receive them. Some of these patients could receive transplants from HLA-mismatched family members, but in many cases the immunologic disparity is so great that this course of action would be extremely risky. It is for these individuals that placental blood transplants offer the greatest hope. Rather than storing only the tissue types of potential donors (and, perhaps, small samples of their blood), the placental blood bank stores the graft itself. The volume of the sample is small—only 50–150 ml (2–5 oz)—and the collection process, performed in the delivery room at the time of birth, causes no inconvenience to the donor. In principle, therefore, placental blood cells can be made available for transplantation as soon as HLA typing has been confirmed.

As noted above, in conventional allogeneic stem cell transplants, close matching of HLA types is essential. The use of placental blood stem cells, however, may permit a greater degree of antigenic disparity between donor and recipient. This advantage seems to reflect the immunologic immaturity of placental stem cells. Scientists who study biological development distinguish between animals that are *altricial* at birth, which means that they are born in a primitive, helpless state, and those that are *precocial,* or born in a relatively well-developed state and able to fend for themselves soon after birth. Humans are a curious mixture of these two states; at the time of birth, they are largely altricial, although individual organs differ in their stages of development. If the human immune system were entirely precocial, successful transplantation with placental blood cells would require the same close HLA matching as is now required for stem cells from other sources. Most current evidence indicates, however, that the T lymphocytes (immune system cells that act in concert with the HLA system) of newborns are relatively immature and are more tolerant of mismatches than are T lymphocytes from a mature donor. In addition to reducing the overall incidence of graft rejections and GVHD, the immunologic immaturity of placental stem cells makes them suitable for use in an ethnically diverse population.

Placental blood stem cells also hold promise for use in autologous transplantation (in which donor and recipient are the same). Cells collected at the time of an individual's birth could be frozen and stored in case that person eventually needed to be treated for, say, leukemia or other blood diseases. Infants born with certain genetic disorders might be able to undergo gene therapy using their own placental stem cells. A few youngsters with inherited immunodeficiency syndromes have already received experimental therapies using stem cells that have been modified to carry normal versions of the defective gene. Since placental blood cells are thought by some authorities to be more receptive than other cells to the introduction of new genes, and since, theoretically at least, they would go on to generate a population of new cells containing the normal, functioning gene, they may prove to be the ideal vehicles for gene-replacement therapy.

Early but encouraging results

The results of early trials of sibling umbilical cord blood transplants were so encouraging that within the past year or so, several teams of researchers have applied the process to cases involving unrelated donors. In 1996 investigators at the Duke University Medical Center, Durham, N.C., working in collaboration with the New York Blood Center, reported on 25 such cases. A majority of the patients were children with leukemia and other cancers of the blood. All but one were mismatched with their donors at as many as three HLA sites. Patients with more than one mismatch would be expected to have a high risk of graft rejection or GVHD, but in these cases the grafts were successful in all but two patients, and severe GVHD occurred in only two. Close to half of the patients survived for 7–32 months, a result comparable to that obtained in conventional stem cell transplants from fully matched but unrelated donors. Other transplant centers have reported higher rates of graft failure and GVHD in patients who received placental transplants from unrelated donors, but overall, findings have been promising enough to provide impetus for further study of the procedure in patients with no suitable related donors.

Some caveats

Although placental blood transplantation has been successfully performed in well over 200 children and young adults worldwide, the procedure should not yet be viewed as a substitute for conventional stem cell transplantation. It does have certain drawbacks and disadvantages. One of these is that the infant donors of placental and cord blood necessarily receive less-extensive medical scrutiny than that given to adults who donate blood or bone marrow. As a consequence, the risk of transferring an infectious agent or inherited disorder through a placental blood transplant is higher than that for a transplant from an adult donor. In the U.S., for example, although the collection and testing of placental blood are closely regulated, it is still possible that a placental blood sample that tests negative for HIV has, in fact, come from a virus-positive infant whose infection was not yet in a detectable stage. In many European countries where placental and cord blood are already being collected, new mothers cannot receive full maternity benefits until they take their infants back to the hospital for further blood tests, usually three months after birth. Because such precautions add significantly to the cost of preparing and storing placental blood, the total cost of a placental blood transplant can be expected to equal that of a marrow graft from an unrelated donor, at least for the next few years.

A problem of more immediate concern is the small volume of blood that can be extracted from the placenta and cord. As noted above, the sample size ranges only from 50 to 150 ml. While such small samples are convenient to store, they may not contain sufficient numbers of stem cells for the successful treatment of adults, who require larger volumes of cells than do children. Some preliminary studies indicate that stem cells from placental blood proliferate more readily than marrow-derived cells, which could mean that fewer would be required. At the present time, however, scientists do not have enough experience with the procedure to judge how well it will work in average-size adults. For this reason,

Five-month-old Robbie Turner was born with infantile osteopetrosis, a potentially fatal genetic bone disease. In August 1995, three months before this photo was taken, Robbie became the first patient with this rare disorder to receive a placental blood transplant.

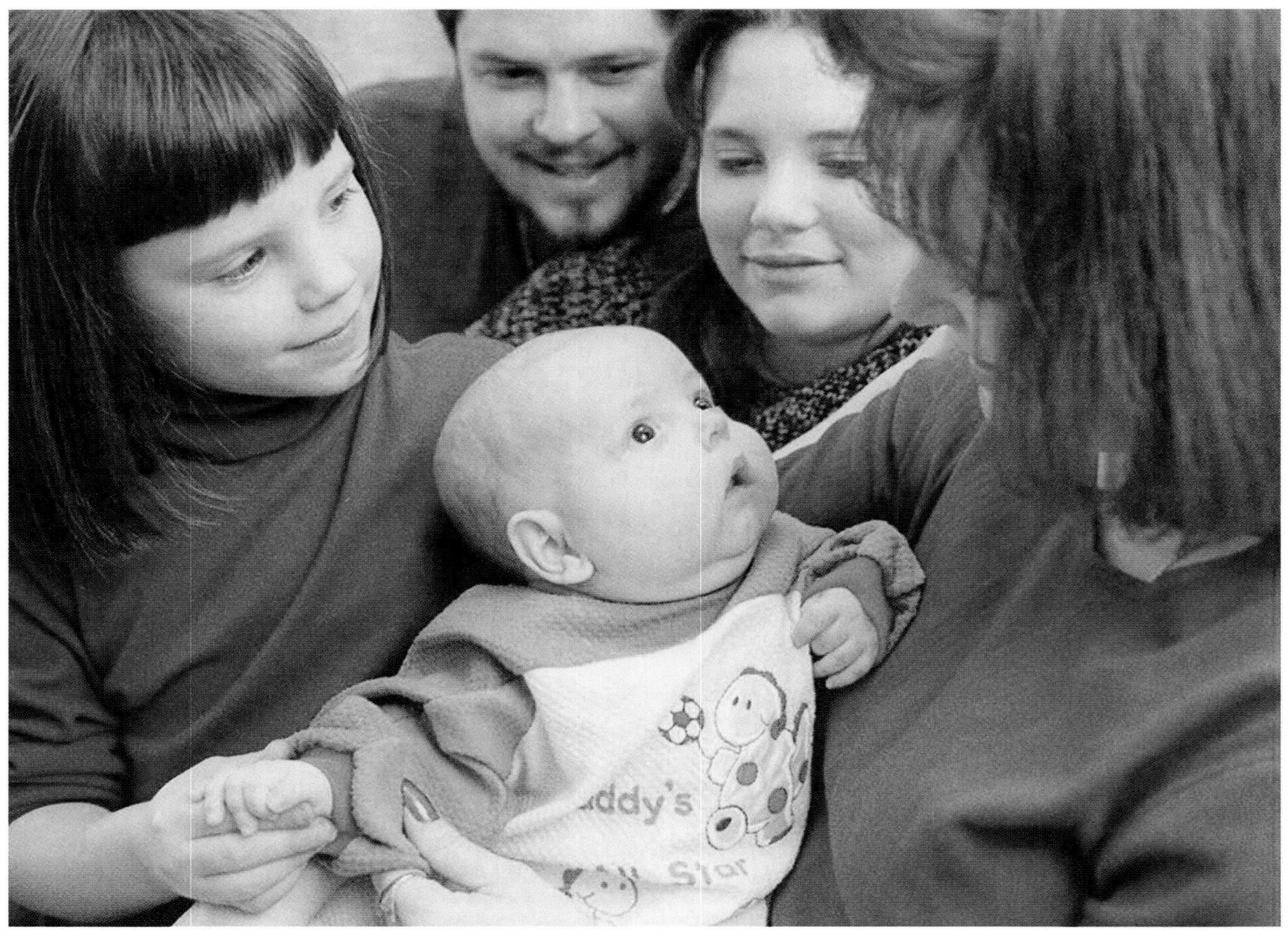

Chris Polydoroff—KRT

Betty Udesen—KRT

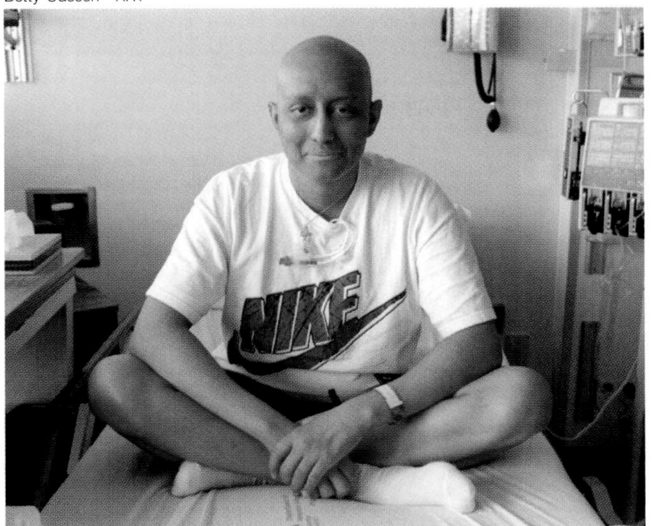

Like many other people with leukemia, Robert Gomez was unable to find an immunologically compatible bone marrow donor. Gomez is unique, however, in that he is one of only a very small number of adult leukemia patients to be treated experimentally with placental blood transplantation.

placental blood transplantation has been limited to use in children and small adults. It may soon be possible to circumvent this obstacle by expanding the placental blood stem cell population in laboratory cultures before transplantation.

As noted above, placental blood transplants have a relatively small capacity to trigger an immune response. This property, which is welcomed when the concern is to avoid rejection of the transplant or occurrence of GVHD, is highly undesirable when the purpose of the transplant is to eradicate malignant cells that have escaped the effects of high-dose chemotherapy. Most transplant specialists now agree that the graft-versus-host effect eliminates a substantial number of leukemic cells from recipients' bodies after conventional allogeneic stem cell transplantation. They have observed, for example, that when the T lymphocytes are removed from grafts, the rate of relapse often increases. On the other hand, when donor T lymphocytes are infused into patients who have relapsed after allogeneic transplantation, a sustained remission from leukemia may occur without further therapy. It is not yet clear how the T lymphocytes target leukemic cells, but whatever the explanation, if the T lymphocytes in placental blood are too immature to reliably identify antigens and destroy the cells displaying them, then patients with leukemia may have an increased risk of relapse after placental blood transplantation. It will therefore be essential for researchers to monitor the recipients of placental blood grafts for extended periods.

Still another drawback is that maternal consent to store placental blood—especially from women in minority groups—has not been as easy to obtain as was predicted several years ago. This means that in at least some cases, it will continue to be difficult to find close HLA matches between placental blood donors and patients needing stem cell transplants.

Ethical dilemmas

Traditionally, researchers who have used bone marrow, blood, or other tissues to obtain stem cells for transplantation have not attempted to patent their tissue source, on the grounds that such an action would be unethical. This position was recently challenged by a U.S. corporation seeking to gain exclusive rights to the "making, keeping, selling, disposing, importing and exporting of stem cells from cord blood, as well as their therapeutic uses." A group of scientists in the European academic community oppose the patent application because, in their view, a placental blood donation represents a noncommercial, nonpatentable gift from a donor to a recipient. Their legal argument centers on the fact that the concept of placental blood transplantation and its application in practice have been in the public domain for almost a decade. The outcome of this case will have important implications for the future practice and study of stem cell transplantation.

In addition to these commercial and intellectual property concerns, placental blood transplantation raises a host of difficult questions for both society as a whole and the individuals directly involved. Should placental blood banking be a public or private function? How will it be monitored and regulated? If testing of placental blood reveals that an infant has a genetic disorder, should the parents be told? How can such information be kept confidential?

Perhaps the most difficult of all questions facing parents is whether to have their infant's placental and cord blood donated to a tissue bank for general use or stored privately in case of need by their own child. With current techniques, frozen blood stem cells are expected to survive less than 10 years. Although there is only a remote possibility that a child will require a stem cell transplant during the first 10 years of life, parents still face a choice between the selfless and the selfish option, which raises a moral issue that would have been unimaginable before the advent of this new technology.

Associated Press

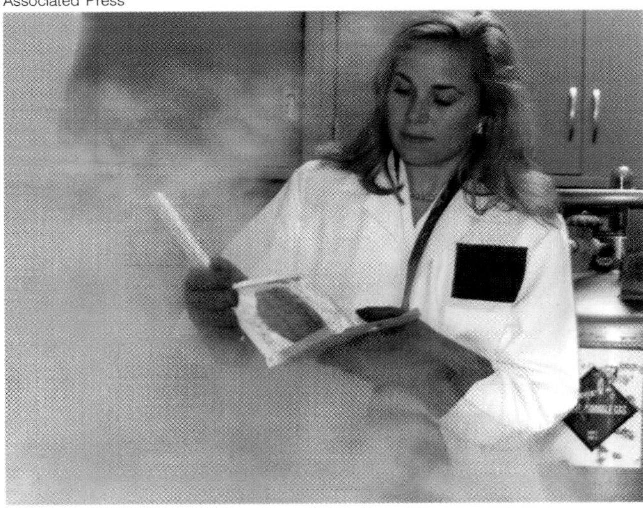

A placental blood sample is prepared for freezing at the Hoxworth Blood Center in Cincinnati, Ohio. Whether the banking of placental and cord blood should be a public or private function and who will oversee and regulate this new technology are issues still to be resolved.

—Malcolm K. Brenner, M.B., Ph.D., and John R. Gilbert, M.A.

P53: Key to Many Cancers

The human body is composed of trillions of cells living in harmony. They are organized in a precise fashion into tissues and organs, and they are strictly regulated as to numbers and location. When cells cease to operate by these biological rules, cancer develops. In cancer, rogue cells reproduce out of control, eventually invading surrounding tissues.

The control of cell reproduction is governed by two classes of genes, the proto-oncogenes and the tumor suppressor genes. Proto-oncogenes normally act to promote cell division and do so in a tightly controlled fashion. Mutations, or alterations, in proto-oncogenes can make them hyperactive, which can result in inappropriate cell proliferation. Once such a mutation has occurred, the proto-oncogene becomes a cancer-promoting gene, or oncogene. Tumor suppressor genes, in contrast, normally act as brakes on the cell-division process, instructing the cell to cease dividing at the appropriate time. Like nearly all other genes in the body, genes of these two classes exist in pairs, one inherited from each parent. The nucleus of virtually every cell in the human body, therefore, contains two of each of the tumor suppressor genes and two of each proto-oncogene. In the case of tumor suppressor genes, both members of a given pair must be inactivated for control of cell division to go awry. With oncogenes, on the other hand, a mutation in one of the pair suffices to promote cell proliferation. Mutations in both of these classes of genes are important in cancer development.

Cancer is generally a multistep process occurring over the course of many years. Specifically, the development of a tumor usually occurs in a series of discrete stages, each one being more aggressive than the last. Transition from one stage to another is thought to be caused by a mutation in one or more genes of the tumor cells, which somehow changes their character, making them progressively more abnormal. This theory of cancer progression is supported by the observation that the risk of developing the disease increases dramatically with age, a finding that has been interpreted to mean that cancer occurs when there is an accumulation of mutations over time. In general, mutations in particular combinations of tumor suppressors and proto-oncogenes result in specific types of cancer.

The most common mutation

Approximately 15 different tumor suppressor genes have been identified to date. One of these, the *p53* gene, has received particular attention because it is the most commonly mutated gene in human cancer; studies have found that more than 50% of all human tumors carry mutations in *p53*. The *p53* gene was first identified in 1979 when scientists found unusual quantities of a 53-kilodalton protein in cultured cells to which a tumorigenic (tumor-causing) virus had been added. (A kilodalton—1,000 daltons—is a measure of molecular weight; some proteins are designated p53, p75, p21, and so forth, according to their molecular weight.) The function of genes generally is to encode—or provide instructions for the synthesis of—proteins. Often, as was the case for p53, the isolation of the protein precedes identification of the gene itself. (By convention certain genes and the proteins they encode are given similar or identical names, but the gene is differentiated by italic type.)

Initial studies of the *p53* gene showed that introducing the gene into cells resulted in the transformation of those cells from normal to malignant, a property typical of oncogenes. Subsequent experiments demonstrated, however, that the *p53* gene used in the early studies was mutated and interfered with the function of the normal p53 protein. Once the normal form of the gene was isolated, it was shown to have the opposite property—the capacity to suppress malignant transformation. Further support for its role in tumor suppression came in 1989 when a team headed by Bert Vogelstein at the Johns Hopkins University Oncology Center, Baltimore, Md., showed that the *p53* gene is inactivated by mutation in approximately 80% of human colon cancers.

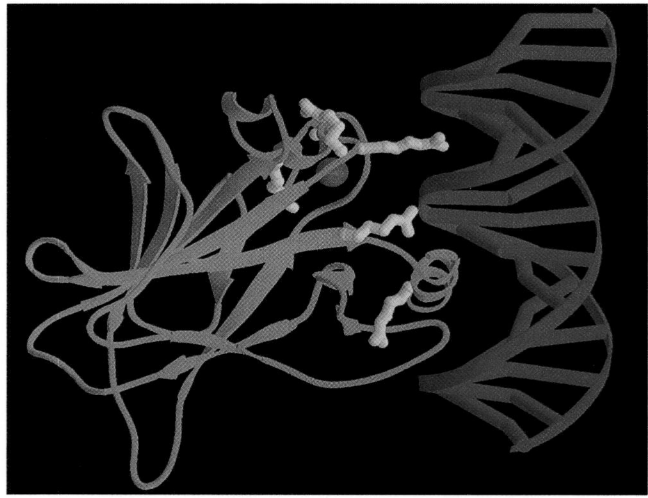

Once they were able to visualize the three-dimensional structure of the p53 protein, scientists discovered that the most frequently mutated amino acids (yellow) lie close to the site where the protein binds to DNA (blue helix, right). This finding confirmed their suspicion that p53's activity as a tumor suppressor is directly related to its ability to bind to DNA.

Subsequent examination of the status of *p53* in tumors showed that the gene is mutated in a wide variety of cancers—in at least 52 kinds, in fact—but particularly in breast, lung, pancreatic, liver, bladder, colon, and brain cancers. These observations strongly suggest that the p53 protein is important for tumor suppression in many cell types. In the majority of the tumors studied, subtle mutations in one member of a pair of *p53* genes were accompanied by the complete loss of the other member, which resulted in an absence of functional p53 protein. Taken together, these findings suggest that loss or inactivity of *p53* is a common prerequisite for tumor development.

After recognizing the importance of *p53* loss in sporadic (*i.e.*, nonhereditary) cases of cancer, researchers began to examine its role in hereditary cancer syndromes. One such disease, called Li-Fraumeni syndrome (named after the physicians Frederick Li and Joseph Fraumeni, who first described it), is characterized by the development of several kinds of tumors similar to those sporadic ones commonly displaying *p53* mutations. Individuals with Li-Fraumeni syndrome have an approximately 50% risk of developing cancer by the age of 30. They have especially high rates of breast cancer, bone and soft-tissue sarcoma (a type of cancer that develops only in certain tissue layers), brain tumors, adrenocortical carcinoma (a malignancy of the adrenal gland), and leukemia. Upon testing the DNA of Li-Fraumeni patients, oncologist Stephen Friend and colleagues at Massachusetts General Hospital Cancer Center, Boston, discovered that the syndrome is caused by the inheritance of only one functional *p53* gene. Individuals who have only a single functional *p53* gene per cell are just one mutational event away from lacking this important tumor-suppressive function, which explains their dramatic predisposition to developing cancer.

Experiments with mice have provided unequivocal support for the role of *p53* in tumor suppression. Using a method known as gene targeting, or knockout technology, several teams of investigators have created strains of mice that carry *p53* mutations. To their surprise, these scientists found that inheritance of two nonfunctional *p53* genes has little effect on growth and development in mice. Nonetheless, as expected, the *p53*-deficient animals have a markedly higher-than-average risk of developing cancer. While normal mice generally live two to three years, the *p53*-deficient mice die from cancer, especially lymphoma (a malignancy of the lymph system), within six months of birth. Animals carrying one defective and one normal *p53* gene, called heterozygous mutants, represent a genetic analogue for Li-Fraumeni patients, and, indeed, they too develop cancer, usually between one and two years of age. Also like Li-Fraumeni patients, *p53* heterozygous mutant mice tend to develop sarcomas, which suggests that these mice may be a good animal model for the human disease and could be useful for designing treatments. It is clear from these studies that inactivation of *p53* greatly facilitates the process of tumor formation, although other mutational events are also important.

A milestone in *p53* research was the elucidation of the protein's biochemical function. In 1990 researchers noted that part of the p53 protein is similar to a class of proteins known as transcriptional activators. These proteins bind to specific sites in the DNA of other genes and stimulate the transcription of these genes, the first step in the creation of proteins. Such stimulation ultimately results in increased production of the proteins encoded by those genes. Subsequently, it was demonstrated that p53 does indeed bind to specific DNA sequences and activate transcription of specific genes.

Cellular damage control

Studies in both cell cultures and mice have suggested two possible mechanisms for the action of p53 protein in tumor suppression, both of which implicate the protein as a sensor of cellular damage. In the first mode of action, the protein induces a temporary halt in the cycle of cell proliferation, allowing for damaged DNA to be repaired. The existence of this function was first suggested when scientists observed that the low level of p53 protein normally present in cells increases rapidly upon exposure to radiation or other DNA-damaging agents. Then in 1991 Michael Kastan and colleagues at Johns Hopkins University showed that in some cell types an increase in p53 levels (and, therefore, p53 activity) causes a pause in the cell cycle just prior to DNA replication. (Replication is the duplication of a cell's DNA.) Replicating damaged DNA would have dire consequences, as mutations in the genetic material of the parent cell would then be passed on to subsequent generations of cells. Hence, p53 has been dubbed the "guardian of the genome."

The second suggested mechanism involves an even more dramatic response to DNA-damaging environmental stresses. In some types of cells, *p53* initiates a programmed process of self-destruction, or cellular "suicide," which scientists call apoptosis. Several different cell types have been shown to undergo *p53*-dependent apoptosis upon treatment with DNA-damaging agents. Scientists speculate that the absence of normal apoptosis following *p53* mutation enables the survival of cells that have sustained DNA damage and thus facilitates tumor formation. For its activity in protecting the body from retaining defective cells, *p53* has been given the nickname "guardian of the tissue."

Using cell cultures and experimental animals, several researchers have shown that emerging tumor cells are highly prone to apoptosis if they contain normal *p53*. If the *p53* gene is mutated, however, the tumor cells fail to self-destruct and can continue to proliferate unchecked. Other studies have shown that the process of *p53*-dependent cell death in tumors can be enhanced by stresses like oxygen deprivation (hypoxia), which occurs when a tumor outgrows its blood supply. On the basis of these experiments as well as some observations from human cancer, it appears certain that escape from apoptosis represents one of the steps in the development of cancer.

The process of cellular suicide normally triggered by *p53* seems to be a mechanism by which many cancer treatments act. In a similar fashion to hypoxia, these agents can stimulate *p53*-dependent apoptosis in tumor cells, which leads, at least temporarily, to tumor regression. For example, in a study conducted by Scott Lowe, Tyler Jacks, and colleagues at the Massachusetts Institute of Technology's Center for Cancer Research, experimentally induced tumors formed by cells containing functional *p53* were shown to be sensitive to treatment by radiation or chemotherapy, both of which are capable of damaging DNA, whereas the tumors formed by cells lacking *p53* failed to respond to treatment. The investigators noted, however, that tumors that regressed in response to therapy sometimes recurred and were no longer responsive to therapy. Some of these refractory tumors were found to have developed *p53* mutations and thus could no longer initiate apoptosis. These findings suggest that loss of *p53*-dependent apoptosis not only promotes tumor development but also interferes with tumor treatment. Indeed, it is commonly observed in clinical cancer treatment that tumors with *p53* mutations are particularly resistant to therapy (*see* below).

Mutation "hotspots"

The ability to pinpoint the location of mutations in the *p53* gene is critical for understanding tumor origins. Once scientists have located the gene and sequenced it—*i.e.,* determined the linear order of the nucleotides, the subunits that constitute genes—they can compare the sequence of the normal gene with that of the gene isolated from tumor cells. In this way, they can determine the location and nature of any mutations in the genes of the tumor cells.

Such studies have revealed that the vast majority of *p53* mutations affect a part of the protein called the central domain, which is known to be involved in DNA binding. In particular, mutations are concentrated in four regions within the central domain; these mutation "hotspots" are very likely sites critical to the normal function of p53 protein.

Epidemiological studies have shown that certain cancers are associated with particular carcinogens—lung cancer with cigarette smoking, for example, and skin cancer with exposure to sunlight. Moreover, many carcinogens are known to be mutagens, substances that induce characteristic changes in DNA. Studies of *p53* carried out by Curtis Harris and colleagues at the National Cancer Institute, Bethesda, Md., among others, have provided significant insight into the effects of mutagens on this particular gene. By determining the exact type of *p53* mutation in a specific tumor associated with particular environmental conditions, researchers can trace the cause of the disease. For example, the majority of skin cancers are known to be associated with ultraviolet (UV) light exposure. UV light is unique in that it damages DNA by causing the fusion of two adjacent nucleotides and thus creating a distinct, identifiable lesion called a pyrimidine dimer. Molecular biologists examining the *p53* gene sequence in skin cancer specimens have indeed found pyrimidine dimers. These results not only implicate ultraviolet light as the cause of *p53* mutation but suggest that *p53* loss is important for the development of skin cancer.

Another example comes from lung cancers, the majority of which occur in cigarette smokers. In *p53* genes isolated from human lung tumors, a particular kind of mutation (in which one nucleotide is substituted for another) is especially prevalent. In October 1996 investigators in Texas and California reported in the journal *Science* that this very same mutation is characteristic of exposure to benzo[*a*]pyrene, a compound in cigarette smoke. This finding provided the first direct evidence—at the cell biology level—of a causal link between cigarette smoking and lung cancer.

In certain areas of the world such as China and Mozambique, there is a high correlation between liver cancer and the consumption of aflatoxin, a harmful natural product of a mold that frequently contaminates improperly stored nuts and grains. Examination of the *p53* gene sequence from liver tumors reveals a striking phenomenon; essentially all cases show a specific nucleotide substitution at a particular site in *p53* that is known to be mutated by exposure to aflatoxin in a laboratory culture.

The p53 protein may be inactivated in ways other than by direct mutation of the gene. In breast cancer, for example, the normal protein is produced, but by some poorly understood mechanism, it is retained in the cytoplasm of the cell (the region outside the nucleus). Since p53 needs to enter the nucleus of the cell to activate gene transcription, exclusion from the nucleus in essence incapacitates the protein. In soft tissue sarcomas, p53 is inactivated by an oncoprotein (the protein product of an oncogene) that

NEWS CAP MHA 98

Cancer Deaths: A Turning Point?

While it is too early to declare victory in the 25-year U.S. "war on cancer," success on some fronts is finally making an impact on the country's cancer death rate. Three recent studies showed that cancer deaths, after having increased for decades, have finally begun to decline—the first sustained turnaround in cancer mortality in the 20th century. Even this heartening finding was controversial, however. The author of one of the studies disputed the contention of other leading researchers that improved treatment was in part responsible for the drop in deaths.

According to statistics released in November 1996 by the National Cancer Institute (NCI), the cancer death rate fell by nearly 3% between 1991 and 1995. This trend was in contrast to an increase of more than 6% between 1971 and 1990. A University of Alabama study published at the same time as the NCI analysis found a similar decline—3.1%—in the first half of the 1990s and projected that the trend would continue, and probably accelerate, for at least 20 years. The Alabama investigators, Philip Cole and his colleagues, published their findings in *Cancer,* a scientific journal of the American Cancer Society (ACS).

Officials of the NCI and ACS hailed the two studies as evidence that the nation's concerted cancer research effort, begun under the administration of Pres. Richard M. Nixon, was finally paying off. They attributed the declining cancer death rate to a variety of factors, including smoking cessation, earlier detection of cancer, and better treatment for those diagnosed with the disease. Cole said the evidence suggests that both prevention and improved medical care have made major contributions. In an editorial in *Cancer,* Curtis J. Mettlin of the Roswell Park Cancer Institute in Buffalo, N.Y., agreed, noting that while the long-sought "magic bullet" had not materialized, there was clear evidence of "meaningful progress" in preventing, detecting, and treating cancer.

This assessment was challenged by a longtime critic of the federal cancer research effort, health policy expert John C. Bailar III of the University of Chicago. In April 1997 Bailar published a study that also showed a trend toward declining cancer mortality beginning in the early 1990s, but the amount of the decrease was much smaller—only about 1%. Bailar disputed the impact of improved treatment on cancer mortality, contending that the results of new therapies have been "largely disappointing." He attributed the decline to early detection and a drop in the number of smokers.

All of the studies found that reductions in deaths from several key cancers—including lung, colon, and prostate cancer in men and breast, colon, and gynecologic cancer in women—were largely responsible for the trend. For reasons that are not well understood, mortality from non-Hodgkin's lymphoma, a cancer of the lymph system, continued to increase among both men and women.

is present in abnormally high levels in these tumors. Finally, 90% of cervical cancers are caused by infection with the human papillomavirus. The virus encodes a protein that promotes tumor formation by inducing the degradation of p53 protein.

These findings suggest that the *p53* gene may be inactivated in more than the 50% of cancer cases in which *p53* mutations have been found. Given that the *p53* gene does not have to be mutated to be inactivated, it may be the case that the protein is nonfunctional in the majority of human tumors.

Application for diagnosis and prognosis

The identification of mutations in *p53* is a sensitive method for detecting tumor cells among a large number of normal cells and therefore could be the basis of lifesaving diagnostic tests. Recent research indicates that if such a method had been available 30 years ago, it might have saved the life of former U.S. vice president Hubert Humphrey, who died from bladder cancer in 1978. Humphrey reported finding blood in his urine as early as 1967, yet studies of bladder cells present in urine specimens failed to detect abnormalities. It was not until 1976 that he underwent surgery and radiation therapy for what was then recognized to be bladder cancer. Unfortunately, the cancer recurred.

In 1994 David Sidransky and his colleagues at the Johns Hopkins Oncology Center, who had already shown that *p53* mutations were common in bladder cancer, obtained permission from Humphrey's widow to test DNA from his tumor and from a 1967 urine sample. Indeed, *p53* mutations were detected in the tumor cells, as well as in a small percentage of bladder cells found in the urine. If this test had been available in 1967 and Humphrey's physicians had determined that the cells were in the process of becoming malignant, they might have been able to intervene early and prevent the disease from taking its course.

Not only is *p53* testing useful in diagnosis, but it can also be a sensitive indicator of prognosis. A variety of studies have shown that mutations in *p53* generally signal increased tumor aggressiveness, increased potential for metastasis (spread to other parts of the body), and a lower patient survival rate. At least part of the poor prognosis is due to poor response to standard radiation and chemotherapies. Owing to their ability to initiate apoptosis, tumors containing *p53* are usually more responsive to therapy than tumors lacking *p53*. Wilms' tumor (a childhood kidney cancer), testicular cancer, acute lymphoblastic leukemia, retinoblastoma (a tumor of the eye), and neuroblastoma (a nerve cell tumor), which rarely display *p53* mutations, are among the most curable cancers. In contrast, leukemia, lymphoma, soft-tissue sarcoma, lung carci-

The magnitude of the decline differed greatly by sex, age, and race; men, adults under 65, and African-Americans benefited most. The NCI reported, for example, that the five-year decrease was 4.3% for U.S. men, compared with only 1.1% for women. The disparity was attributed in large part to gender differences in the prevalence of smoking, the primary cause of lung cancer.

The drop in cancer mortality was generally greater among African-Americans than among whites, with an overall decrease of 5.6% in the former versus 1.7% in the latter. Still, cancer death rates remain about 40% higher in black men than in white men and 20% higher in black women than in white women, according to the NCI.

The update on cancer death rates coincided with the 25th anniversary of the National Cancer Act of 1971, which poured increased federal funding into a national cancer effort inspired by the success of the American initiative to send a man to the Moon. The tactics and results of the "war on cancer" have long been debated. A particular point of contention has been the relative importance of basic research, prevention, early detection, and treatment. Cancer remains the number two killer in the U.S., accounting for nearly one-fourth of all deaths. Despite the recent decline in the mortality rate, the total number of cancer deaths continues to climb as the elderly population increases. The ACS estimates that about 560,000 Americans will die of cancer in 1997 and that 1,382,400 new cases of invasive cancer will be diagnosed.

Writing in *The New England Journal of Medicine* in May 1997, Bailar urged a stronger national commitment to prevention, including stepped-up research on risk factors that contribute to cancer, on behavioral techniques to help people change unhealthy habits such as smoking, and on the understanding of specific diet-cancer links. Bailar's report updated his controversial 1986 analysis, in which he had concluded that the federal focus on cancer treatment was a "qualified failure." In the 1997 report he stated that there was "little reason" to alter his earlier conclusion. Bailar noted that despite the short-term decline, overall cancer mortality was 6% higher in 1994 than in 1970. Nonetheless, he tempered his criticism with recognition of the achievements of the past 25 years: progress in treating children and young adults with cancer, a better understanding of the underlying biology of cancer, and significant improvements in imaging techniques for detecting small, early-stage cancers.

Would more vigorous preventive efforts be likely to have an impact? A study published in late 1996 by scientists at the Harvard School of Public Health suggested that this is so. The Harvard researchers found that about two-thirds of all U.S. cancer deaths are linked to unhealthy personal habits, such as smoking (30%), poor diet (30%), and lack of exercise (5%). They suggested that only about 10% of cancer mortality is due to genetic predisposition and only about 2% to exposure to environmental pollutants.

—*Cristine Russell*

Archive Photos

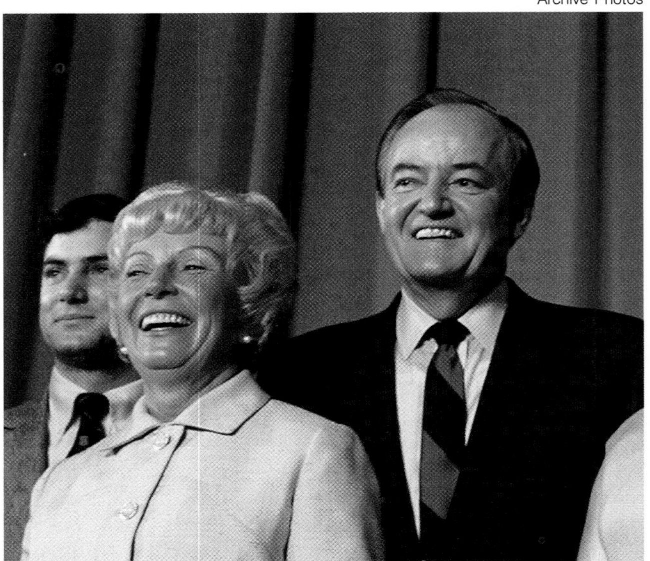

If a test to detect mutations in p53 *had been available in 1967, when the late U.S. vice president Hubert Humphrey (pictured with his wife, Muriel) first experienced symptoms of bladder cancer, his disease might have been diagnosed at an early—and potentially treatable—stage.*

noma, and breast carcinoma (carcinomas are tumors that arise in the tissues that line organs and ducts) often contain *p53* mutations, and patients with these cancers often have a poor prognosis. In some cases tumors that produce normal p53 protein are responsive to therapy, but they may eventually acquire a *p53* mutation, upon which they may become refractory to treatment. The prevalence of *p53* mutations in human cancer raises the question of whether there are cancer therapies that work independently of *p53* and, if not, how such treatments could be developed.

The promise of gene therapy

In addition to searching for *p53*-independent cancer therapies, researchers have focused their efforts on establishing methods for restoring *p53* function in tumors. *P53* gene therapy—the introduction of the normal *p53* into tumor cells—is one means of achieving this goal. Viruses offer an effective way of delivering genes to cells, and certain retroviruses and adenoviruses are being extensively tested for this purpose. First, of course, the viruses must be altered so that they are incapable of causing disease in the recipient. Next, *p53* genes must be inserted into the disabled viruses. These genetically modified viruses are then introduced into tumor cells in a laboratory culture to see if they have the capacity to suppress cell growth. If these experiments are successful, the viruses are tested in experimental animals into which human tumor cells have been transplanted. If infection with *p53*-expressing viruses suppresses tumor-cell growth in these model systems, then—and only then—can the viruses be tested in humans.

In 1996 a team led by Jack Roth and colleagues at the University of Texas M.D. Anderson Cancer Center reported the preliminary results of the first clinical trial of *p53* gene therapy in human lung cancer. The investigators constructed a retrovirus containing the *p53* gene and injected it directly into the lung tumors of nine patients who had previously failed to respond to therapy. The goal was to provide enough p53 protein to induce apoptosis in the tumor cells without killing normal cells. Although all lung cells could potentially be infected by the virus, only tumor cells would be sensitive to apoptosis. In fact, injection of the *p53*-containing viruses did result in increased tumor cell death. Although one patient died and one did not continue treatment, in six others the tumors either ceased to grow or regressed, with no notable side effects. These initial results are quite promising, and future studies will build on this approach by attempting to increase the efficacy of treatment. In particular, scientists will focus on designing combination treatments using both *p53*-expressing viruses and DNA-damaging agents to stimulate a greater degree of *p53*-dependent apoptosis in tumor cells. Viruses that express the *p53* gene are also being explored for the treatment of head and neck cancers, which commonly have *p53* mutations and are quite refractory to standard therapies. Early clinical trials in humans are now under way.

Other therapy strategies rely on the possibility that mutant p53 molecules in tumor cells might be returned to normal by introducing "activating agents," such as antibodies that bind to p53 or small protein fragments known as peptides. Such strategies may hold the key to treating and potentially curing over half of all cancer patients.

Still to come

The role of *p53* in the development of human cancer is now widely recognized. Between 1991 and 1995 alone, more than 4,000 research papers on *p53* were published, and in 1993 it was recognized by *Science* as the "molecule of the year." Despite intense interest and experimentation, however, numerous questions remain. For example, how do p53 protein levels rise in response to cellular damage? How does the protein trigger apoptosis? These and related questions will have to be answered if the basic understanding of *p53* function is to yield more effective means of cancer prevention and treatment. The quest is certain to keep cancer researchers busy for many years to come.

—Tyler Jacks, Ph.D., and Laura D. Attardi, Ph.D.

Cardiovascular Disease Update

> *Diseases of the heart and circulation...kill more people than any others, accounting for over 15 million deaths, or about 30% of the global total....They cause grief in families and...a loss of valuable talent that many countries need for economic development....These diseases are emerging rapidly as a major public health concern in most developing countries, where they now account for about 25% of all deaths.... In developed countries, almost half of all deaths...are attributable to them.*
>
> —*The World Health Report 1997,* issued by the World Health Organization, Geneva, May 1997

The prevention and treatment of cardiovascular diseases remain top research priorities because coronary heart disease, stroke, and other forms of atherosclerotic vascular disease (conditions characterized by fatty deposits in arteries) continue to take such a huge toll. This is true in virtually all industrialized countries and increasingly in less-developed countries.

While new medical and surgical procedures, advances in technology, and new drugs with a truly innovative role capture considerable public attention, these "breakthroughs" actually arrive on the medical scene only infrequently. Most research and most developments in the field of cardiovascular medicine instead have to do with defining the best use of established treatments. If two treatments are known to be effective for a given heart condition, then which one is best? Are there subsets of patients for whom one treatment is preferable? If an effective surgical treatment can be refined to be safer and less expensive, should it then be offered to a wider range of patients? If an adverse effect of an established cardiovascular drug therapy comes to light, must not all of the risks and benefits of that particular treatment then be reexamined carefully? These and many other similar questions are constantly being asked and answered through clinical research studies, and it is the results of these studies that actually shape the practice patterns of physicians who regularly treat cardiovascular disease.

Controversy over calcium channel blockers

Calcium channel blockers are a group of popularly used drugs that work by blocking the passage of calcium into the heart and smooth muscles. (Muscles depend on calcium to contract; by interfering with contraction, the drugs encourage the muscles within blood vessel walls to dilate, or relax, which in turn lowers blood pressure.) Calcium channel blockers can control angina pectoris (a type of chest pain related to poor oxygen supply to heart muscle) and certain kinds of cardiac arrhythmias (abnormal heart rhythms) and have even been used to treat migraine headaches. The most common use of calcium channel blockers, however, is in the treatment of high blood pressure (hypertension). In fact, for multiple reasons, they have become a virtual mainstay of antihypertensive therapy. They are highly effective in lowering the blood pressure; many of the available formulations can be taken conveniently as a single daily dose; and they have a low incidence of side effects.

With such positive characteristics, it is not surprising that the drugs are so widely prescribed. But should their use be favored over that of other antihypertensive agents? Questions about the safety of the calcium channel blockers first arose a few years ago when they were tested on patients with acute myocardial infarction (heart attack). The drugs did not increase survival in these patients and in some instances were associated with a slight increase in mortality.

Then, in 1995, researchers reported that hypertensive patients treated with short-acting preparations of the calcium channel blockers nifedipine, diltiazem, or verapamil were 1.6 times more likely to have a myocardial infarction than patients using other medications to treat high blood pressure. This was a case-control (or retrospective) study; *i.e.,* it looked back at clinical outcomes in a large number of patients who had been treated with various medications. Although a prospective, randomized study (in which patients and controls are randomly assigned a particular medication or a placebo at the *beginning* of the investigation, and their course is then followed) would have provided the most accurate comparison of treatments, the 1995 report raised considerable concern and sparked professional debate. Then, in the same year, a meta-analysis (a comprehensive evaluation of the results of several studies that pooled all the patient data) also implicated one type of calcium channel blocker; patients who had confirmed coronary artery disease (determined by the presence of angina or a history of myocardial infarction) and were using short-acting nifedipine had 1.16 times the death rate of similar patients who were not using this drug.

The validity of those studies was questioned by experts, and some subsequent studies did not find adverse effects associated with calcium channel blockers. The controversy, however, was stirred further in 1996 when a high-quality randomized study of hypertensive patients showed that those treated with the immediate-release short-acting calcium channel blocker isradipine experienced more frequent major vascular events (*e.g.,* heart attack, stroke, or sudden death) than patients receiving another type of antihypertensive drug, the diuretic hydrochlorothiazide. Moreover, additional studies have raised concerns about calcium channel blockers' potential to cause excess postsurgical bleeding, increased gastrointestinal bleeding, and even an increased incidence of cancer in elderly patients.

It has been theorized that short-acting calcium channel blockers provoke cardiovascular events by abruptly lowering blood pressure, reducing coronary artery blood flow, and activating the sympathetic nervous system, which in turn increases the heart rate and levels of circulating adrenaline (a hormone that stresses the heart). Calcium channel blockers that have a more gradual and prolonged effect (the long-acting variety) and those formulated for delayed release theoretically should not provoke these adverse reactions.

Several randomized, controlled trials addressing the safety of various long-acting and controlled-release calcium channel blockers are now under way, with results due in a few years. In the meantime, the consensus of experts is that the short-acting calcium channel blockers should be avoided altogether. Patients with well-controlled blood pressure who are taking the longer-acting drugs need not change their therapy. In most cases the use of beta-adrenergic blocking drugs (commonly called beta-blockers) and angiotensin converting enzyme (ACE) inhibitors should be favored over calcium channel blockers in the initial treatment of hypertension, as the drugs in both these classes have been shown to prevent heart attack and other adverse cardiac events.

A corollary of the calcium channel blocker debate is a recurring series of warnings against the oral administration of rapid-acting nifedipine to treat hypertensive emergencies. To induce rapid lowering of high blood pressure, physicians have made it a very common practice to prescribe nifedipine, administered sublingually (under the tongue) or in a capsule that is swallowed. Patients have been treated by this method in emergency rooms (whether or not their hypertension is truly an emergency), in postsurgical settings, and even in doctors' offices. The drug, however, was never approved for this use by the Food and Drug Administration (FDA). Furthermore, there have been reports of serious reactions, including precipitous drops in blood pressure, stroke, acute heart attack, and death, from such "emergency" use of the drug. In light of these observations and in the absence of systematic proof that the treatment is clinically beneficial, there is broad agreement among physicians that this particular use of short-acting nifedipine should cease.

Matthew McVay—AllStock/PNI

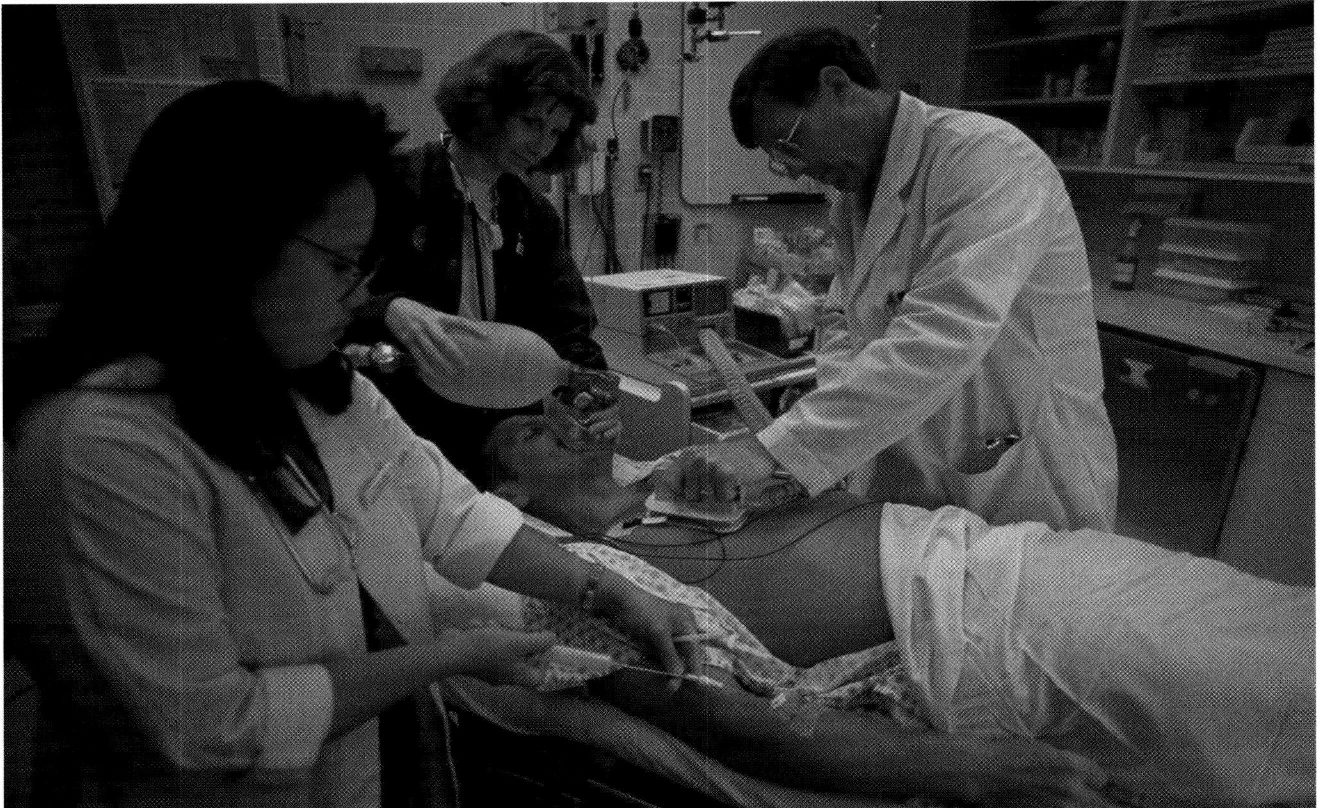

New guidelines specify prompt and aggressive treatment of all suspected heart attacks. A crucial first step is the reestablishment of blood flow through blocked coronary arteries, generally accomplished by injecting a clot-dissolving drug (foreground) within 10–30 minutes of arrival at the hospital.

Time is muscle: lifesaving guidelines

A trend in medicine for the last several years has been for specialty organizations to issue "practice guidelines" for the treatment of major conditions. The American College of Cardiology (ACC) and the American Heart Association (AHA) issued their first joint guidelines for the management of acute myocardial infarction in 1990; in 1996 those guidelines were substantially revised. A joint task force of 13 cardiovascular disease experts reviewed some 5,000 published studies and then made recommendations intended for doctors, nurses, and other medical personnel who care for patients with a suspected or established heart attack. The new ACC/AHA guidelines, which have been officially endorsed by other specialty groups, including the American Society of Echocardiography, the American College of Emergency Physicians, and the American Association of Critical-Care Nurses, were notable in that they brought the existing recommendations into line with the current protocol of treating heart attacks *promptly* and *aggressively*. Considering that about 900,000 people in the U.S. alone experience acute myocardial infarction each year, these guidelines should have a major impact.

The need for guidance on appropriate therapy was underscored by a recent study of physicians' patterns of prescribing for elderly patients after a heart attack. Death rates among those who received beta-blockers (drugs that block the activity of beta-receptors and thereby decrease blood pressure and heart rate) were 43% lower than among those who did not receive beta-blockers. Treated patients also had 22% fewer rehospitalizations. Unfortunately, however, only 21% of patients who might have benefited from taking beta-blockers ever were given such a prescription.

Several features of the new guidelines deserve highlighting. Roughly 225,000 of the 900,000 heart attack sufferers each year die, and of those about 125,000 die before they have received any medical care. Heart attacks result when one or more of the coronary arteries are blocked and the supply of blood to a portion of the heart muscle is interrupted. A major treatment objective is early reperfusion (reestablishment of blood flow through the blocked artery). Thus, public education is vital to ensure prompt recognition of heart attack symptoms and the most-rapid-possible transport of the patient to a hospital.

Reperfusion is most often accomplished by giving clot-dissolving (thrombolytic) drugs (*e.g.,* tissue plasminogen activator, streptokinase, urokinase, anistreplase). An alternative to thrombolytic therapy is immediate balloon angioplasty, a procedure used to enlarge the inner hollow portion of a partially obstructed artery by passing a thin tube (catheter) with an attached balloonlike device through the narrowed artery portion, then inflating the balloon. Direct angioplasty is appropriate when it can be accomplished in an expedient manner by experienced personnel in a suitably equipped hospital. Because these lifesaving methods are now known to be so successful, it is more important than ever before that pretreatment delays be minimized. Once the patient has arrived at the hospital emergency department, there is a 10–30-minute window during which reperfusion therapy ideally should be initiated. When compared with standard medical therapy (*e.g.*, nitroglycerin, analgesics, aspirin, oxygen), immediate thrombolytic therapy reduces the 35-day mortality rate in heart attack patients by 21%. With earlier reperfusion, less heart muscle is damaged. In other words, time is muscle.

The new ACC/AHA guidelines also specify that aspirin, beta-blockers, and ACE inhibitors are recommended to prevent additional cardiovascular events in the acute heart attack patient. The pharmaceuticals in these classes have all been shown to enhance survival following heart attack and have a long-term therapeutic role as well. Calcium channel blockers are not recommended as standard therapy.

Another part of the ongoing management of heart attack survivors is the modification of well-established risk factors. Smoking should cease immediately, and moderate exercise is advised. The new guidelines establish the goal of achieving a low-density lipoprotein (LDL) cholesterol level of less than 130 mg/dl (milligrams per deciliter) by altering food choices. If such dietary efforts are not successful, drug therapy is recommended to bring the LDL (or so-called bad cholesterol) level to less than 100 mg/dl. This aggressive cholesterol-lowering recommendation is based on a series of recent studies that found clear benefits of such an approach in previous heart attack sufferers.

Sensitive test for cardiac damage

Heart attacks are usually diagnosed by measurement of the heart's electrical activity with an electrocardiogram (EKG). When this test is done in the emergency room on a patient who is having symptoms suggestive of myocardial infarction and the EKG recording shows sharp irregularities, there is little doubt that a heart attack is occurring, and prompt treatment should be initiated. With many heart attacks, however, particularly the smaller, milder ones, the EKG recording shows only minor changes or is essentially normal; therefore, an accurate blood test is needed to make an early diagnosis.

A blood test commonly used to detect heart damage measures the enzyme creatine kinase MB, which is released into the bloodstream by damaged cardiac muscle. This test is not always reliable, however, because creatine kinase MB can be released by damaged skeletal as well as heart muscle. Fortunately, a simple new blood test can diagnose mild heart attacks that traditional tests have failed to detect.

Substances in the heart muscle known as troponins control the interaction of the proteins actin and myosin, which affect the contractility of heart muscle. Two forms of cardiac troponin, troponin T and troponin I, are released by dying heart muscle cells and are easily detected in the bloodstream. Since troponin T and troponin I originate *only* in cardiac muscle, their detection in the blood is a clear indication of heart muscle damage. Moreover, the cardiac troponins provide increased accuracy by showing elevated blood levels soon after the onset of chest pain, whereas creatine kinase MB levels can take hours to rise.

The new troponin tests are so sensitive that slight amounts of heart muscle injury are being confirmed in patients who would formerly have been regarded as having an accelerated pattern of angina. Troponin elevations in these patients suggest a poor prognosis; thus, the cardiologist is alerted that an aggressive treatment approach is warranted.

Pulmonary artery catheters: right or wrong?

A recent study of the effectiveness and safety of pulmonary artery catheters, also known as Swan-Ganz, or right-heart, catheters, has questioned the appropriateness of their widespread use in intensive care units. Popular in critical care units for over 25 years, these catheters are positioned through the right heart chambers and into a pulmonary artery for the purpose of measuring the heart's output and monitoring the pressures within the heart's chambers as they fill with blood. Adjustments of cardiac medication and of intravenous fluids are based on readings from the catheter.

At least one million of these catheters are sold by manufacturers to hospitals in the United States annually, but no large clinical study ever demonstrated that their use improves patient outcomes. In the recent study, carried out in five teaching hospitals across the country, 2,184 patients who underwent pulmonary artery catheterization were compared with other critical care unit patients with similar degrees of illness. Patients in the former group had a higher mortality rate, and they spent more days in the intensive care unit at a higher cost.

The main weakness of the study (published in the *Journal of the American Medical Association* [*JAMA*] in September 1996) lies in the obvious possibility that patients receiving pulmonary artery catheters were actually sicker than those managed without the catheters, despite the investigators' rigorous efforts to study patients whose conditions were comparable. The authors of the report themselves recognized this limitation. They and others are calling for a randomized controlled trial to answer with certainty the concerns that have been raised about this popular medical device.

Coronary stents: getting better all the time

Coronary stents are small, tubelike, expandable metal cylinders with a meshlike structure that are implanted in coronary arteries to keep them wide open. They are inserted after a balloon angioplasty or a rotational atherectomy ("roto-rooter") procedure (in which a rotating knife tunnels through fatty deposits in a

The ability of stents to keep coronary arteries wide open over a long period is impressive. The tiny, expandable cylinders are placed in an artery after plaque blocking the blood flow to the heart muscle is removed.

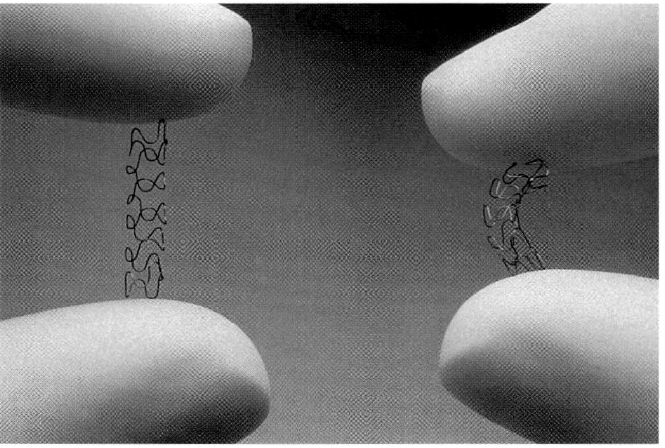

Courtesy of Medtronic, Inc., Minneapolis, Minn.

Photographs courtesy of Medtronic, Inc., Minneapolis, Minn.

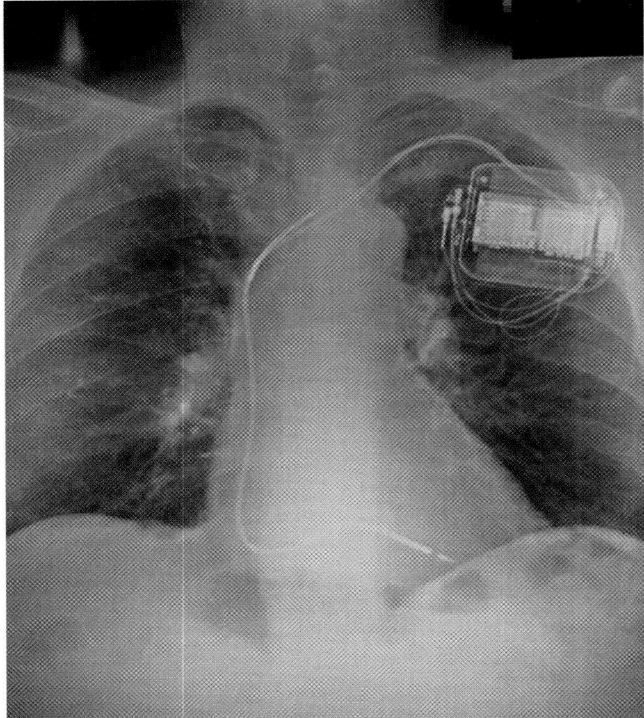

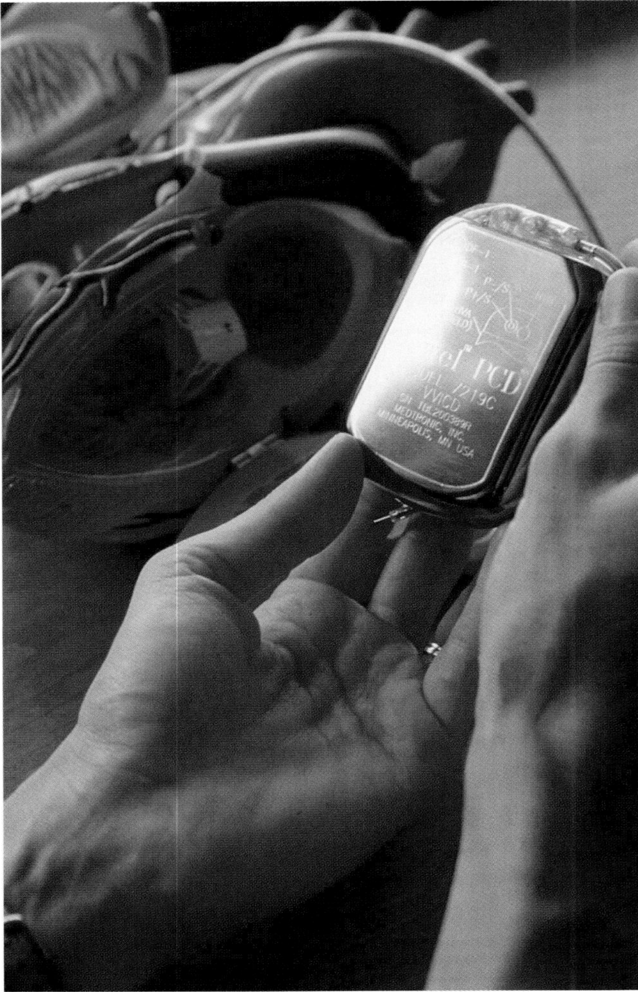

The automatic cardioverter-defibrillator (left) is remarkably effective at preventing sudden cardiac death in patients with life-threatening arrhythmias. (Left top) An X-ray shows the defibrillator's battery-powered generator in place just under the skin of the chest. Increasingly, the devices are being implanted prophylactically in symptomless patients.

clogged artery). Stents were quickly shown to prevent acute closure of treated vessels and thus reduce myocardial infarctions and the need for emergency coronary bypass surgery after angioplasty. More and more studies have decisively shown the advantages of stents for keeping coronary arteries open over the long term. A recent study compared coronary artery stenting with conventional angioplasty in patients with stenosis (narrowing) of the left anterior descending artery, a particularly important coronary artery. This vessel supplies blood to a large area of muscle at the front of the heart and is associated with some of the most serious heart attacks. Patients in the study had a narrowing at the beginning portion of the artery, which further increases the seriousness of the condition. One year after the procedure, 13% of patients in the stenting group had experienced a cardiac event (angina, myocardial infarction, or death), compared with 30% of regular angioplasty patients. The rates of restenosis (renarrowing) demonstrated by angiography (X-ray motion pictures of the heart) were 19% after the implant of a stent and 40% after angioplasty alone.

The advantages of stenting are quite significant, and implant rates have been steadily increasing. Further, the stenting process has become considerably safer and more effective in the past few years with the replacement of the potent anticoagulant (blood-thinning agent) warfarin, which can cause serious bleeding complications, by the antiplatelet agents ticlopidine and aspirin. This change in therapy has also permitted shorter hospital stays for patients receiving stents.

Various new types of stents, including plastic ones, that have a wider range of diameters and lengths are coming onto the market. The increased flexibility of the new stents will permit the cardiologist to implant these devices within particularly tortuous arteries that previous devices could not reach.

A radical new approach to stenting has stirred the interest of cardiologists. In a pilot study of 55 patients undergoing balloon angioplasty and stent implantation, 26 patients also received radiation therapy. A ribbon containing radioactive seeds of iridium-192 was positioned into the implanted stents for 20 to 25 minutes. The intention is to inhibit the proliferation of scarlike cells in the artery wall that contribute to restenosis. Initial results are encouraging, and a larger, long-term study is anticipated.

Implantable defibrillators: new use, new questions

Two types of life-threatening arrhythmias are associated with sudden cardiac death. *Ventricular tachycardia* causes the heart to beat extremely rapidly. In *ventricular fibrillation,* impulse conduction in the heart's ventricles is chaotic and ineffective. The latter may be preceded by the former, or it may occur alone, suddenly and without warning. Since the early 1980s automatic implantable cardioverter-defibrillators have been used to prevent sudden cardiac death. These surgically implanted devices monitor the heart rhythm and interrupt a life-threatening arrhythmia by either rapidly pacing the heart or delivering a lifesaving shock.

The current devices consist of an electrical wire lead placed through veins into the heart chambers and a battery-powered generator that is placed under the skin of the chest wall or abdomen.

Even though implantable defibrillators have been in use for over 17 years and the implantation rate in the U.S. alone has soared to over 25,000 per year, the first prospective randomized study of the effectiveness of implantable defibrillators was published only in December 1996. This study, called the Multicenter Automatic Defibrillator Implantation Trial (MADIT), compared defibrillator implantation with conventional medical therapy in patients who were determined to be at high risk of sudden death. Specifically, these patients had a history of myocardial infarction, weakened heart muscle function, and nonsustained, symptomless ventricular tachycardia (documented on an EKG recording). None had ever experienced a spontaneous episode of *sustained* ventricular tachycardia or cardiac arrest, but during electrophysiological testing using electrode catheters, life-threatening ventricular arrhythmias could be triggered in these patients.

After an average follow-up of 27 months, the frequency of death in patients with an implanted defibrillator was less than half of that observed in patients without the implant. Not surprisingly, this announcement suggested great promise for the high-tech and expensive devices, but at the same time, cogent criticisms of the study were voiced. The "conventional" medical therapy used in MADIT was not truly conventional by today's standards. Most of the medically treated patients were given antiarrhythmic drug therapy early in the observation period, yet such medications have never been shown to prolong survival following myocardial infarction. Of these patients, 10% were given a particular type of antiarrhythmic agent (class I drugs), which are now known to increase the risk of death following a heart attack. Beta-blockers, which are clearly effective in preventing death after heart attacks, were given to only a few of the study patients. Perhaps the advantages of a defibrillator implant would not be so clear if the medical treatment group had been given medical therapy of proven value—namely, aspirin, beta-blockers, ACE inhibitors, and cholesterol-lowering drugs.

Implantable defibrillators were originally approved for survivors of sustained ventricular tachycardia or ventricular fibrillation—patients who had been successfully resuscitated from these life-threatening emergencies. The FDA has now liberalized the indications for defibrillator implantation to include symptomless patients similar to those in MADIT. Since these patients have never had life-threatening episodes of ventricular tachycardia or actual cardiac arrest, their implants are truly prophylactic. It is not absolutely clear what the best therapy is for the patients in this category; this, however, should be well clarified by three research trials that are currently in progress in North America and Europe.

Cardiovascular health: measuring progress

> ***The coronary heart disease epidemic began in North America, Europe and Australasia in the early decades of this century. In many industrialized countries, death rates peaked in the 1960s and early 1970s and have since declined dramatically—by over 50% in some countries....Decades of research have shown conclusively that a number of determinants—most of them associated with lifestyle—operating from childhood onwards, are responsible for coronary heart disease.***
>
> —*The World Health Report 1997*

The financial cost of coronary heart disease in the United States alone approximates $80 billion a year and accounts for 15% of health care expenditures. In the face of such a burdensome national health problem, it is somewhat encouraging that coronary disease incidence in the U.S. has declined about 1% annually over the last three decades, while coronary mortality has declined between 2% and 4% a year.

(continued on page 189)

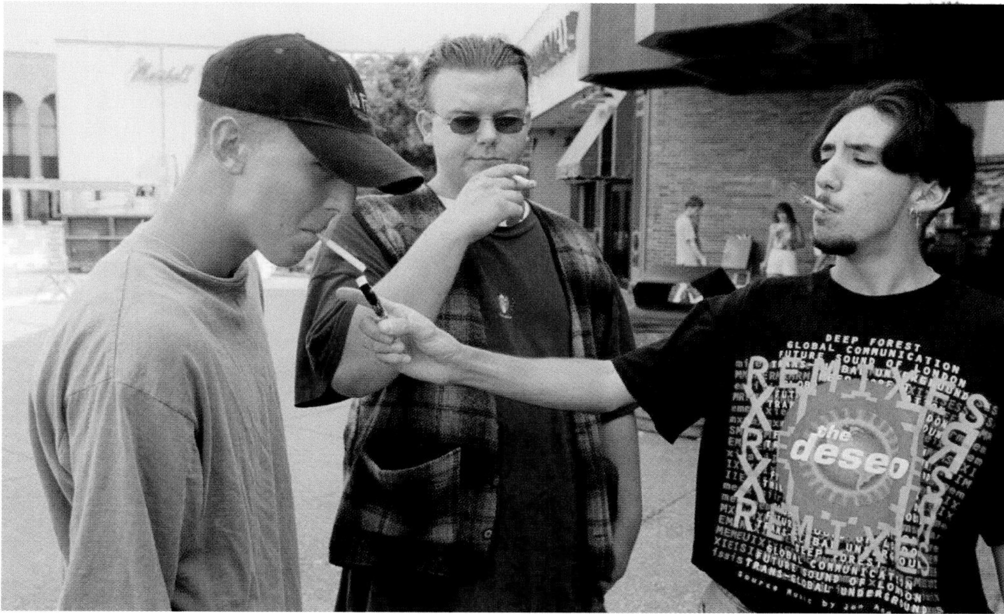

Young people who smoke cigarettes predispose themselves to coronary heart disease (CHD). To the chagrin of the public health community, declining CHD mortality has more to do with treatment advances than with the success of primary prevention efforts.

Chuck Berman—KRT

NEWS CAP MHA 98

Hitting Stroke Below the Belt

Called "apoplexy" by the ancients, stroke—damage to the brain due to either blockage or rupture of a blood vessel—has been known for centuries but has long lacked effective treatment. Within the past year or so, however, this situation has changed.

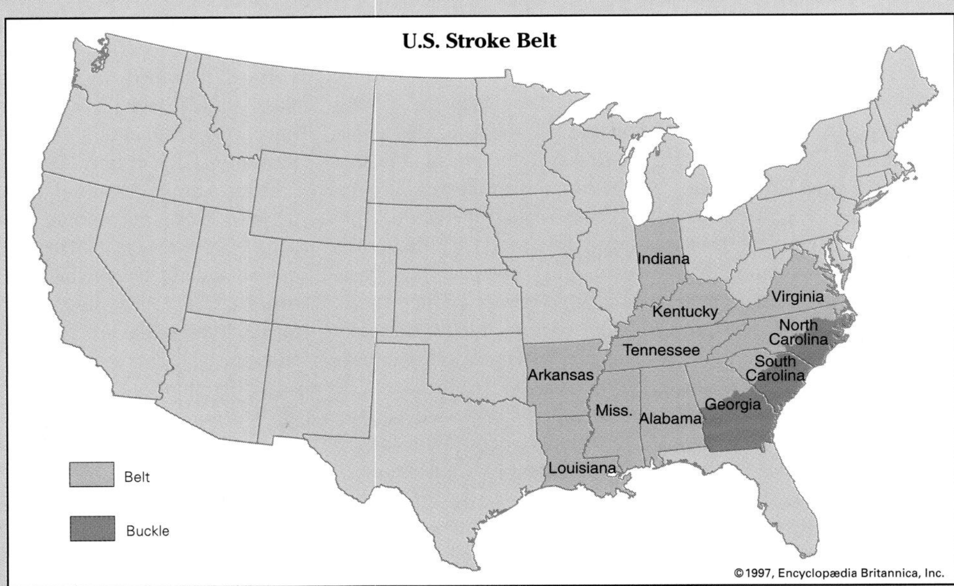

In 1996 the first drug for the treatment of ischemic stroke (*i.e.,* a stroke in which part of the brain is deprived of blood flow by a vessel-blocking clot) was approved by the U.S. Food and Drug Administration. The agent, tissue plasminogen activator (t-PA), is a clot-dissolving (thrombolytic) substance already being used successfully as an emergency treatment for acute heart attack. Although t-PA carries risks—particularly of cerebral hemorrhage—clinical trials have shown that it substantially lowers the severity of disabilities in stroke survivors. (Interestingly, however, in early trials of t-PA therapy, the death rates of treated and untreated stroke patients were the same.)

According to guidelines issued by the American Heart Association in October 1996, t-PA can be administered for stroke only if certain conditions are met; it must be given within three hours of the onset of symptoms, and because of the increased risk of bleeding, it can be used only after a computed tomography scan of the patient's brain has ruled out hemorrhagic stroke (*i.e.,* a stroke caused by rupture of a blood vessel). Further, some patients—for example, those who are being treated with anticoagulant drugs—are not approprate candidates for t-PA therapy.

The three-hour period is a very brief window of opportunity, and as more hospitals become equipped to provide t-PA therapy, individuals at risk of stroke must be prepared to act quickly if symptoms occur. The most common indications of stroke include weakness and/or numbness (usually unilateral—*i.e.,* affecting one side of the body), abnormalities in speech and vision, dizziness, confusion, and difficulties in walking. According to a February 1997 report, however, most people—and especially those at greatest risk, such as the elderly and persons with high blood pressure—are not familiar with these signs.

The investigators, from the University of Cincinnati (Ohio) Medical Center, surveyed patients admitted to emergency facilities for evaluation of potential stroke. They found that 39% did not know a single stroke symptom. An even larger proportion could not name one risk factor—*e.g.,* hypertension, stress, high cholesterol levels, diabetes, smoking, use of alcohol. The researchers concluded that further public education is indeed needed.

This lifesaving knowledge may be especially important for Americans who live in the so-called stroke belt, a group of states (*see* map) in which the rate of death from stroke is significantly higher than elsewhere in the country. While this epidemiological phenomenon has been recognized since the 1960s, scientists at Wake Forest University's Bowman Gray School of Medicine, Winston-Salem, N.C., announced in 1997 that they had found the "buckle" of the stroke belt—a group of 153 counties in Georgia and the Carolinas where the death rate from stroke among the middle-aged population (those between the ages of 35 and 54) is twice as high as in the rest of the country. While low socioeconomic status has long been presumed to be the major risk factor operating in the stroke belt, the new report suggested that poverty is not the sole explanation for the region's high stroke mortality rate. The researchers speculated that other influences—including environmental exposures, genetic predisposition, and lifestyle factors (notably, smoking and lack of exercise)—probably play a part.

—*Robert Rauch*

(continued from page 187)

What accounts for this progress? Public health professionals might hope that basic prevention efforts are the chief reason. Basic (or primary) prevention involves such measures as lowering cholesterol and other blood lipids, controlling blood pressure, and ceasing tobacco use *before* coronary disease has manifested itself. Researchers who analyzed the U.S. decline in mortality from coronary heart disease between 1980 and 1990 published their findings in *JAMA* in February 1997. Using a unique computer model to perform their statistical study, the researchers found that only 25% of the decline in mortality was due to primary prevention and that 71% was due to improved treatment of coronary patients. Secondary prevention (modifying risk factors in patients with an *established* diagnosis of coronary disease in order to prevent further problems) accounted for 29% of the mortality decline. Other improvements in treatment, including the use of clot-dissolving drugs, other cardiovascular medicines, angioplasty, and bypass surgery, were responsible for 43% of the decline. (For methodological reasons, the total decline reflected by these statistics is not 100%.)

These findings speak well for the effectiveness of contemporary medical management of patients who have already developed symptoms of coronary disease. It is unfortunate that a similar mortality reduction has not yet been achieved through primary prevention. Moreover, with treatment saving more and more lives, there are growing numbers of coronary disease survivors, most of whom will continue to require costly medical care.

There is still considerable room for further improvement in cardiovascular disease prevention. Cigarette addiction by early adulthood continues as a major public health problem. Elevated blood cholesterol levels are still inadequately treated in all age groups, even though cholesterol-lowering drug treatments that are well tolerated and have a proven ability to prevent coronary events are widely available. Beta-blocker drugs are still underprescribed for hypertension and after myocardial infarction.

Progress in cardiovascular disease management is often measured by the introduction of sophisticated technologies and heroic therapies. *Real* progress, however, could be fairly easily achieved—simply by making better use of well-established forms of prevention and readily available treatments.

—*Marc K. Effron, M.D.*

Cholesterol Counts—More than Ever

The past year has seen several important developments pertaining to cholesterol and its control. Exciting new evidence emerged regarding the effectiveness of cholesterol lowering in reducing the risk of coronary heart disease (CHD); the latest U.S. survey results showed a continuing decline in cholesterol levels; and, paradoxically, a flurry of controversy arose over who should have their cholesterol levels measured. In the end, however, the case for cholesterol consciousness was substantially strengthened.

Clinical trial results

Recent results of two clinical trials—the Cholesterol and Recurrent Events (CARE) trial and the Post Coronary Artery Bypass Graft (Post-CABG) trial—extended the line of evidence showing that lowering cholesterol is beneficial in patients with and without CHD. All of these studies used a new class of drugs, the "statins," to lower cholesterol to a greater degree than had been possible with older drugs. These drugs, which inhibit the enzyme HMG-CoA reductase, essential to the synthesis of cholesterol in the liver, include lovastatin, pravastatin, simvastatin, fluvastatin, and the most recent of these medications, atorvastatin, approved by the U.S. Food and Drug Administration in early 1997.

In 1994 the Scandinavian Simvastatin Survival Study had shown that in men and women who had elevated cholesterol levels and already had CHD, lowering total cholesterol by 25% and low-density lipoprotein (LDL, or "bad") cholesterol by 35% reduced heart attacks by 34%, deaths from CHD by 42%, and the overall death rate from all causes by 30%. The Scandinavian study was actually the first trial to prove that lowering cholesterol levels prolongs life. In 1995 the West of Scotland Coronary Prevention Study found that lowering cholesterol in patients without CHD reduced the risk of first heart attacks and deaths from CHD by 31% and overall deaths by 22%.

Building on these results, the CARE trial showed for the first time that even in CHD patients with relatively average cholesterol levels, lowering cholesterol resulted in a 24% drop in heart attacks and CHD deaths. The Post-CABG trial found that aggressive lowering of LDL-cholesterol to below 100 mg/dl (milligrams per deciliter) in patients who had undergone coronary artery bypass surgery—an open-heart procedure involving blood vessel grafts from other parts of the body to bypass coronary arteries that have become obstructed by cholesterol deposits (plaque) and thereby restore the blood supply to the heart—slowed the growth of plaque in the grafts significantly better than did a more moderate degree of LDL-cholesterol lowering.

Taken together, these trials have proved that lowering cholesterol in patients with or without known CHD will greatly reduce the risk of suffering a heart attack or dying from heart disease and will actually prolong life for many people. These studies also provide strong support for the recommendation that people with CHD lower their LDL-cholesterol levels to 100 mg/dl or less—a target level that is lower than that for people without CHD. That widely accepted recommendation was issued by the National Cholesterol Education Program (NCEP) of the National Heart, Lung, and Blood Institute in 1993. The table below shows the initiation and target LDL levels for diet and drug treatment in patients with or without CHD. In people without CHD, a trial of therapy that involves diet, physical activity, and weight control should be carried out (usually for about six months) before drug treatment is added. In patients with CHD, diet and drug treatment may have to be started together, depending on how high above the target level of 100 mg/dl the person's initial LDL level is.

Cholesterol Lowering: When, How, and for Whom?

Health status	(LDL-cholesterol levels in mg/dl) Initiate diet[1]	Initiate drug	Goal
Coronary heart disease (CHD)	over 100	130 or higher	100 or less
No CHD, two or more risk factors	130 or higher	160 or higher	under 130
No CHD, one or no risk factors	160 or higher	190 or higher	under 160

[1]Regimen should include exercise and weight control.
Source: National Cholesterol Education Program of the National Heart, Lung, and Blood Institute.

National Heart, Lung, and Blood Institute/National Institutes of Health

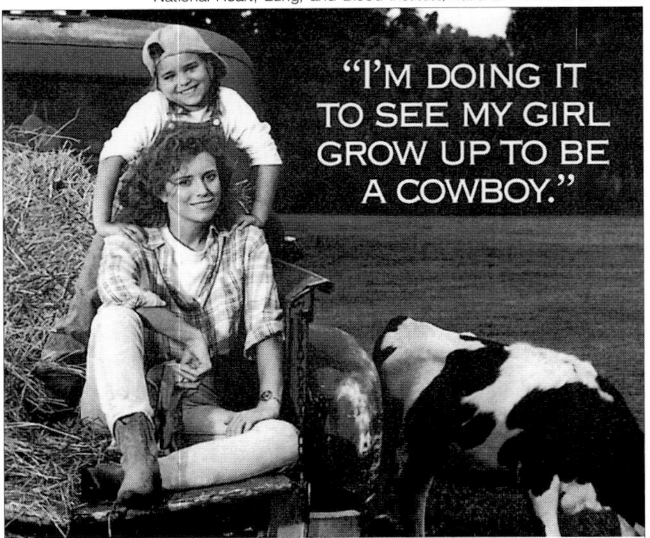

"I'M DOING IT TO SEE MY GIRL GROW UP TO BE A COWBOY."
You've got big reasons to lower your cholesterol. So eat foods low in saturated fat and cholesterol, be physically active, watch your weight, and know your cholesterol numbers. 'Cause you've got a lot to stick around for. Call 1-800-575-WELL for more information.
EVERY HEART COUNTS. CARE ABOUT CHOLESTEROL.
NATIONAL CHOLESTEROL EDUCATION PROGRAM • NATIONAL HEART, LUNG, AND BLOOD INSTITUTE

For nearly 15 years, the National Cholesterol Education Program has been raising the public's awareness of high blood cholesterol as a major risk factor for coronary heart disease.

Safety of cholesterol lowering

The cholesterol reductions produced by the statin drugs in the Scandinavian, West of Scotland, and CARE trials were larger than had been seen in earlier trials. As a result, the benefits in terms of reduced rates of heart attacks, CHD deaths, and total deaths were more clear-cut than in previous studies. These large cholesterol reductions were not associated with an increase in deaths from noncardiovascular causes, such as cancer, suicide, or fatal accidents. This result strongly indicates that lowering cholesterol itself is safe, and it goes a long way toward offering the reassurance that the statin drugs (the first of which, lovastatin, became available in the late 1980s) are safe. Of course, one cannot be absolutely certain that taking a cholesterol-lowering medication for 30 or 40 years might not produce some adverse effect. Nevertheless, the track record of the statins to date is quite good. For an individual who is at high risk of having a heart attack and whose cholesterol remains unacceptably high despite therapy with a combination of diet, physical activity, and weight control, the proven benefits of taking a cholesterol-lowering drug clearly outweigh any theoretical risks.

Preventing heart attacks: new insights

The dramatic benefits seen in the Scandinavian and CARE trials raised an important question: How does lowering cholesterol prevent heart attacks? Previous studies using angiograms (X-rays of the coronary arteries, which supply blood to the heart) had shown that lowering cholesterol slows the progression of plaque buildup and even leads to shrinkage of existing deposits in some cases. As a result of these findings, it was thought that the reduced size of the cholesterol plaques in the arteries lessened the chances that an artery would become completely blocked and thus lowered the rate of heart attacks. The 30–40% reduction in the heart attack rate observed in these same studies, however, was too great a change to be caused by the mere increase in the size of the arterial blood channel (usually in the range of one millimeter [0.04 in]) that was achieved.

Recent studies have shown that the large plaques visible on angiograms (some of which grow more slowly and others of which actually shrink in size as a result of cholesterol lowering) are *not* the main cause of heart attacks. The chief culprits, in fact, appear to be smaller cholesterol-rich plaques that are unstable and have a tendency to rupture. When the thin cap overlying such a plaque ruptures, the plaque contents burst into the bloodstream and trigger blood clotting. The resulting blood clot blocks the artery completely, depriving the heart muscle of oxygen; a heart attack then ensues. When the level of LDL-cholesterol is lowered, however, the cholesterol content of plaque is reduced; the plaque is then less likely to rupture. Thus, the main mechanism by which lowering cholesterol is now thought to reduce the likelihood of heart attacks in people with extensive cholesterol deposits is through plaque stabilization. Lowering the level of LDL-cholesterol in such people is a very effective way to reduce the risk for a heart attack.

Measuring cholesterol: relevant to *all* adults

Ironically, just as the clinical trials were yielding incontrovertible evidence that lowering cholesterol will reduce heart attacks and CHD deaths and even prolong life, a flurry of controversy arose over who should have their cholesterol levels measured. In March 1996 the *Annals of Internal Medicine* published a recommendation that cholesterol be measured only in middle-aged people (35–65-year-old men and 45–65-year-old women) and not in young adults, premenopausal women, or the elderly. The authors supported their view by saying that young adults do not suffer heart attacks, that there is time to find and treat high cholesterol at a later age, that measuring cholesterol in young adults will inevitably lead to the overuse of cholesterol-lowering drugs, and that the benefits of lowering cholesterol are uncertain in women and the elderly.

This view represented a sharp dissent from the prevailing guideline that all adults 20 years of age and older should have their total and high-density lipoprotein (HDL, or "good") cholesterol levels measured at least once every five years. This guideline has been endorsed by representatives of more than 40 medical and health organizations participating in the NCEP, including the American Heart Association, the American College of Cardiology, and the American College of Preventive Medicine. The reason this position is widely shared is that it is based on a large and diverse body of scientific evidence.

The case for young adults. The scientific evidence shows that although heart attacks do not usually occur until middle age, the atherosclerotic process—*i.e.,* the accumulation of cholesterol and other deposits that thickens the walls of the coronary arteries and eventually blocks the flow of blood to the heart—actually begins in late adolescence or early adulthood. The Pathobiological

Determinants of Atherosclerosis in Youth study, which reported its final results in early 1997, confirmed that atherosclerotic plaque is already present in the arteries of young adults, and the amount of plaque is related to the levels of "bad" and "good" cholesterol in the blood.

Measuring the cholesterol level of a young adult predicts that individual's risk for CHD over the following 30–40 years. A study conducted by researchers at Johns Hopkins University, Baltimore, Md., showed that 22-year-olds with cholesterol levels in the top 25th percentile had nine times as many heart attacks in the subsequent 40 years as their counterparts with cholesterol levels in the lowest 25th percentile. The Framingham Heart Study, which has been among the most instructive of all large epidemiological studies to date on the risk factors for CHD, found that young men and women with high cholesterol levels had an increased risk of dying of cardiovascular disease and an increased overall death rate in the ensuing 30 years. In the short term, a young adult's CHD risk is usually quite low; however, because a young person is likely to live many years, what really matters is having an accurate picture of his or her *long-term* risk for CHD. It is thus essential to measure cholesterol in young people.

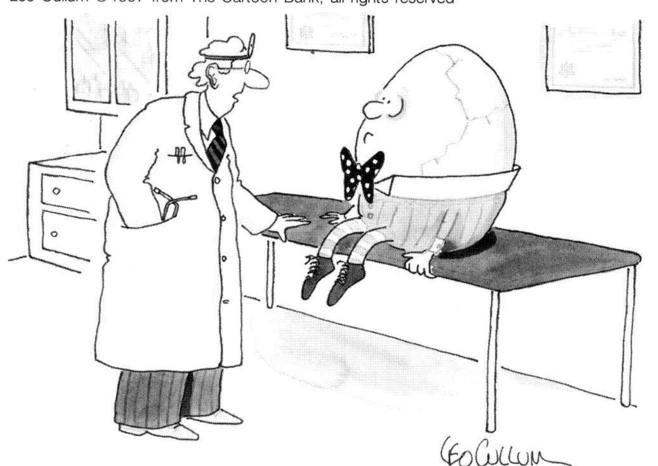

"The cracks can be fixed—it's your cholesterol level that worries me."

Not measuring cholesterol in young adults denies them meaningful information that could help motivate them to alter their lifestyles in ways that reduce CHD risk. There is strong evidence that diet can have a significant effect on cholesterol levels and CHD risk. Studies show that for the average person a switch from the typical American diet to the diet recommended by the NCEP, which is lower in saturated fat and cholesterol, will produce about a 10% reduction in LDL-cholesterol levels. Individuals who start with higher intakes of saturated fat and cholesterol or higher blood cholesterol levels will probably experience greater reductions, and more intensive dietary therapy will also produce a bigger drop in cholesterol levels.

The best proof that diet works comes from the experience of the overall U.S. population. Surveys show that over the past two decades, the American public has reduced its intake of saturated fat, total fat, and cholesterol. At the same time, the average levels of total cholesterol and LDL-cholesterol in the blood have declined markedly. The latest survey data, released in December 1996 by the National Center for Health Statistics, show that the average total cholesterol level declined from 213 mg/dl in 1978 to 203 mg/dl in the period 1988–94, and that level is continuing to drop.

The decline in average cholesterol levels has occurred at the same time that there has been a marked increase in the proportion of people who have had their cholesterol checked and have been told what their levels are. Those who know their own cholesterol levels are more likely to modify their dietary behavior, which in turn affects the amount of cholesterol lowering they achieve. It is very likely that the documented increase in cholesterol measurement has played a major role in raising the public's cholesterol awareness and has contributed to the decline in average cholesterol levels.

Waiting until midlife to measure cholesterol exacts a price in several ways. First, the older the age at which lowering cholesterol is begun, the less benefit it produces. It has been estimated that a 10% reduction in cholesterol levels will reduce CHD risk by over 50% if the reduction is accomplished before age 40; if such a reduction is not accomplished until age 50, CHD risk is reduced by only 39%, and at age 60 a 10% cholesterol reduction lowers CHD risk by just 27%.

Moreover, if the basic message to the public is that cholesterol measurement can wait until middle age, many people will have some manifestation of CHD before they ever get their cholesterol measured. About 25% of first CHD events are fatal, so for these people it will be too late to do anything about their cholesterol levels. As the Scandinavian and CARE trials demonstrated, for those who survive the first CHD event, lowering cholesterol will dramatically reduce their chance of having a subsequent heart attack. Nonetheless, people with a diagnosis of CHD already have so much accumulated plaque in their coronary arteries that even after a large reduction, their risk of a heart attack and death from CHD is still unacceptably high compared with that of someone without CHD. It is thus vitally important to keep cholesterol levels low from an early age to keep the risk of CHD low.

Many people with elevated cholesterol levels will be missed if cholesterol measurement is delayed until midlife. One category of such individuals who will be overlooked is the approximately 79,000 young adults in the U.S. with familial hypercholesterolemia, an inherited condition that produces extremely high cholesterol levels, who will not be detected by family history. Because many of these individuals will develop premature CHD, they should all begin lowering cholesterol at as early an age as possible. In addition, about 35% of young adult men and about 28% of premenopausal women have elevated cholesterol levels that increase their risk of developing premature CHD. If these millions of people are found and informed of their risk, they will have the opportunity to make the kind of lifestyle changes that will ultimately increase their quality and length of life.

The concern that cholesterol measurement will necessarily lead to overuse of cholesterol-lowering drugs runs against the known evidence. Only 0.2% of U.S. adults aged 25–34 years currently take cholesterol-lowering medications, despite the fact that 61% have had their cholesterol measured. Among 35–44-year-olds, only 1% are on cholesterol-lowering drugs, although 76% have had their levels checked. These data support the view that there

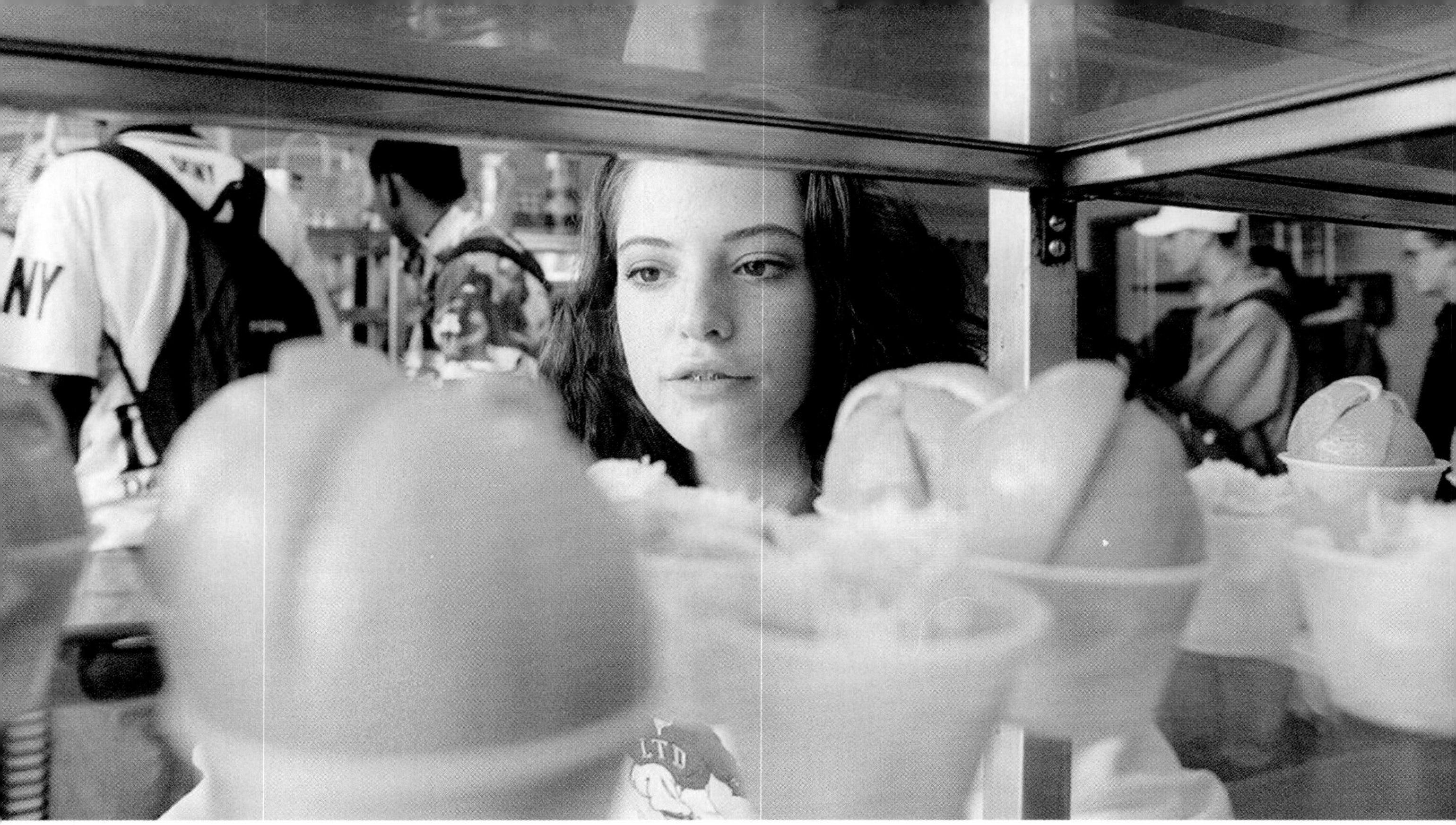
Surveys indicate that over the past two decades, the American public has reduced its intake of saturated fat, total fat, and cholesterol; at the same time, average levels of total cholesterol and low-density lipoprotein cholesterol in the population at large have declined.

David Carson—KRT

is no reason to fear the consequences of measuring cholesterol in young people. On the contrary, members of this group will benefit if they know what their long-term CHD risk is and are given individualized advice that will help them make diet and other lifestyle changes to reduce that risk.

The case for women and older people. The evidence favoring cholesterol measurement in older persons and women is also persuasive. An analysis that pooled the results of 22 studies, including Framingham, showed that an elevated total cholesterol level powerfully raises the risk of dying from CHD in men and women under the age of 65. After the age of 65, elevated cholesterol multiplies CHD risk to a lesser extent. But CHD is much more common after age 65 than before, and many of those in the older group who do not have obvious CHD are on the threshold of it. Consequently, elevated cholesterol is actually responsible for more cases of CHD in older people than in younger groups. Furthermore, there is good evidence that a low HDL-cholesterol level continues to be a powerful predictor of CHD risk at least until the age of 80, especially in women.

Direct evidence from recent clinical trials—the Scandinavian, West of Scotland, and CARE trials—shows that lowering cholesterol significantly reduces CHD risk in older persons. Older individuals with elevated cholesterol who are otherwise in relatively good health and have a reasonable life expectancy are good candidates for cholesterol lowering. Reducing the amounts of saturated fat and cholesterol in the diet, becoming more physically active, and controlling weight are the main steps necessary for most seniors to lower their cholesterol; only a minority will need medication.

In women the basic process of atherosclerosis does not differ from that in men, and total and HDL-cholesterol are important predictors of CHD risk. The women who participated in the Scandinavian study had significant reductions in their risk of a heart attack. In CARE the women actually derived a greater benefit than the men. All in all, there is no justification for denying people the benefits of cholesterol lowering on the basis of their age or sex alone.

On the horizon

Looking ahead, there are important developments under way that are likely to have a major impact on the approach to cholesterol lowering in the 21st century.

- **New drugs.** New, more powerful drugs are in the pipeline, and they promise to lower LDL-cholesterol more effectively than has ever been possible before. It will be important to see whether the reductions in heart attacks and deaths produced by such large degrees of cholesterol lowering will be correspondingly large.
- **Raising HDL.** To date, the clinical trial results have primarily shown the benefits of lowering LDL-cholesterol. If the evidence from trials now in progress confirms that raising HDL-cholesterol actually reduces CHD risk, as is thought to be the case, that information will have a powerful effect on the way doctors approach cholesterol problems.
- **Women and the elderly.** The existing scientific evidence, as already noted, supports cholesterol lowering in women and the elderly. There remains, however, a need to determine the extent to which CHD will be reduced as a result of lowering cholesterol in these groups, especially in people free of CHD. A trial that is designed to demonstrate the size of the benefit that lowering cholesterol produces in women and older individuals is currently under way and should yield specific results in five to six years.

- **Subclinical disease.** New noninvasive techniques for detecting plaque at a stage that is fairly advanced but has not yet reached the point of causing the symptoms of CHD (called "subclinical disease") are being developed and studied. These approaches may enable doctors to identify individuals who are on the threshold of CHD and who would be especially likely to benefit from cholesterol lowering.
- **New risk factors.** Several new risk factors for CHD have been identified. They include fibrinogen, a blood-clotting factor; lipoprotein(a), a combination of cholesterol and other fatlike substances with protein, which may promote blood clotting as well as plaque formation; and homocysteine, a substance produced in the metabolism of amino acids (the basic building blocks of proteins). Although the presence of elevated blood levels of these factors is associated with an increased risk for CHD, not enough is yet known about their precise roles in CHD or the benefits of reducing their levels to warrant their incorporation into the standard assessment and treatment protocols aimed at lowering CHD risk. New scientific findings about any of these, however, could change the situation in the near future.

Aiming low

The exciting scientific developments of the past several years underscore the necessity of applying what has been learned. People with CHD should aggressively lower their LDL-cholesterol levels. As worthwhile as this will be, however, it will still leave an unacceptable burden of illness and death from CHD. Reducing that burden will require measuring and lowering cholesterol levels in people free of CHD to prevent its development in the first place. The combination of cholesterol reduction in people with and without existing CHD promises to have the greatest impact on reducing the toll from heart disease and thereby improving the health and prolonging the lives of millions of people.

—*James I. Cleeman, M.D.*

Getting to the Heart of Homocysteine

Charles Gupton—Stock, Boston

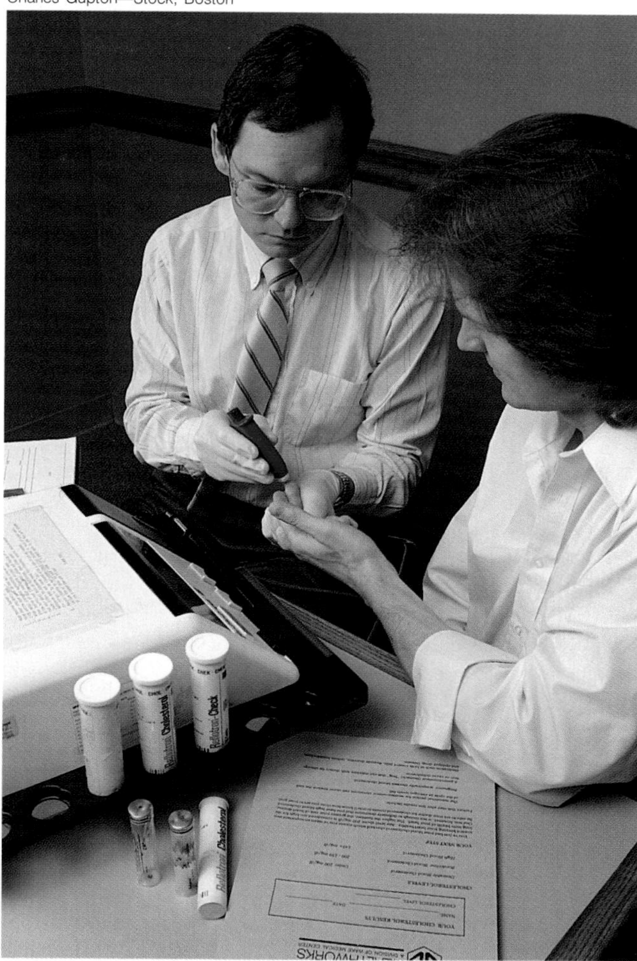

Will measurement of blood homocysteine eventually become as common as cholesterol testing? Many authorities who have studied the evidence linking elevated homocysteine levels and cardiovascular disease believe the answer is "yes."

Disorders of the heart and blood vessels—collectively termed cardiovascular disease—are a major cause of illness and death around the world, and many countries have launched ambitious public health campaigns to prevent these ailments. Such efforts typically focus on strategies to reduce known risk factors—for example, persuading people to quit smoking or reduce their consumption of unhealthy foods. Until quite recently, the dietary risk factors receiving the most attention were fat and cholesterol. A growing body of evidence suggests, however, that another naturally occurring substance—homocysteine—may be an underappreciated but significant diet-related risk factor for cardiovascular disease. These data show that high blood levels of homocysteine are associated with increased rates of coronary heart disease, stroke, and blood vessel disorders.

In many ways the understanding of homocysteine is at much the same stage as that of cholesterol 20 years ago. Epidemiological studies have implicated homocysteine as a factor in cardiovascular disease, but the underlying mechanisms are still being elucidated. Scientists know that supplementing the diet with certain B vitamins, particularly folic acid, can reduce blood homocysteine levels. What they do not yet know, however, is whether efforts to lower homocysteine levels will result—as cholesterol-lowering treatments so clearly have—in lower rates of cardiovascular disease.

Homocysteine and the body

Homocysteine is produced when the amino acid methionine is metabolized, or broken down. Amino acids are the building blocks of protein. Some amino acids can be synthesized within human cells from simpler compounds, while others, including methionine, must be ingested in foods. (The amino acids that must be obtained from the diet are called *essential* amino acids.) The amount of homocysteine within the cells is tightly regulated; when intracellular homocysteine rises above a certain level, homocysteine is released into the blood. Extremely high blood levels of homocysteine result in excretion of large amounts of homocysteine in the urine.

Methionine is ingested in protein-containing foods. Once in the body, methionine, which contains sulfur, is incorporated into proteins within cells or is converted to *S*-adenosylmethionine (SAM), a substance that eventually is converted into homocysteine. Homocysteine is metabolized by two pathways; it is broken down into cysteine via the vitamin B_6-dependent enzyme cystathionine β-synthase (CBS) or regenerated to its precursor, methionine, via another enzyme, methionine synthase, which cannot be produced without folic acid and vitamin B_{12}. The active form of folic acid required for this process can be derived from dietary sources or regenerated from inactive forms of folic acid via yet another enzyme, methylene tetra-hydrofolate reductase (MTHFR). Thus, intracellular—and, in turn, blood—levels of homocysteine can be affected by both vitamin deficiencies and genetic defects in the ability to synthesize certain enzymes.

Homocysteine exists in the blood in free and protein-bound forms. Most studies have measured total homocysteine, which includes both. Homocysteine levels can be measured after fasting or after the ingestion of a measured amount of methionine, a process known as methionine loading.

Following the research trail

The first suggestion of a role for homocysteine in cardiovascular disease came from investigations into a rare inherited metabolic disorder known as homocystinuria. Children born with homocystinuria are mentally retarded and have certain characteristic physical abnormalities. In 1964 researchers demonstrated that the disorder could be due to a nearly complete lack of activity of the enzyme CBS. A short time later scientists recognized that affected children also had a high incidence of occlusive vascular disease (narrowing and/or obstruction of blood vessels).

In 1969 Kilmer S. McCully, then a pathologist at Harvard Medical School, reported on an unusual case. The patient was an infant with a rare inborn error of vitamin B_{12} metabolism. McCully observed that the baby also had homocystinuria and widespread severe atherosclerosis (narrowing of the arteries due to fatty deposits in the arterial walls) similar to that caused by CBS deficiency. Both the homocystinuria and the atherosclerosis could be attributed to lack of vitamin B_{12}, which is required along with folic acid for converting homocysteine back to methionine. Observing that an elevated blood homocysteine concentration was the single metabolic abnormality common to homocystinuria and the vitamin B_{12} metabolic defect, McCully proposed the "homocysteine theory" of atherosclerosis. The high rate of venous thromboses (blood clots in veins) in children with these inherited metabolic disorders would later be recognized as a clue that elevated homocysteine exerts its effects on vascular disease not only by promoting atherosclerosis but also by encouraging the formation of blood clots.

Until the early 1970s only extremely high blood levels of homocysteine, sufficient to cause high levels in the urine, had been linked to vascular disease. In 1976, however, investigators in Sydney, Australia, found that middle-aged individuals with coronary artery disease had modestly elevated homocysteine levels after methionine loading. It was believed at the time that this condition indicated a defect in one of the two copies of the CBS gene. (Humans have two copies of each gene, one inherited from the mother and one from the father.)

It has since been recognized that moderate elevations of homocysteine may also be due to nutritional deficiencies. Nevertheless, the report from Australia was the first to document an association between moderate elevations of blood homocysteine and premature vascular disease among adults. In the meantime, numerous other case-control studies (investigations that compare people who have a given disease, called *cases,* with unaffected individuals, or *controls*) have confirmed this association, initially among young adults but subsequently among older people as well.

In case-control studies homocysteine is measured after the onset of disease among the cases. Such investigations are, by definition, retrospective. (In contrast, prospective studies follow a population of initially healthy people, noting which ones go on to develop the illness in question.) The problem with a retrospective study of the association between high homocysteine levels and vascular disease is that it cannot show whether elevations in homocysteine are a precursor of the disease or a consequence of it.

The first prospective study showing a link between increased homocysteine levels and subsequent heart attacks was published in 1992. The subjects were nearly 15,000 male physicians, aged 40–84, who were followed medically for five years. The data showed that individuals with baseline homocysteine levels (*i.e.,* measured *before* disease onset) above 15.8 micromoles/liter had a threefold greater risk of heart attack than those with lower levels. Subsequent prospective studies of heart disease in Norway and of stroke in England have shown that baseline homocysteine levels not only are predictive of vascular disease but also show a graded, or dose-response, relationship—that is, the risk of disease increases progressively as homocysteine levels rise.

Finally, the results of a multicenter European case-control study that examined the strength of the homocysteine–vascular-disease relationship were published in June 1997. The investigators found that the graded relationship between homocysteine and the risk of vascular disease was present both for fasting homocysteine levels and for levels after methionine loading.

Defining "elevated"

Hyperhomocysteinemia—the condition of having an elevated homocysteine level—bears several resemblances to other cardiovascular risk factors, including hypertension (high blood pressure) and hypercholesterolemia (high cholesterol). First, in all of these conditions, the concept of normal versus abnormal is, in itself, an oversimplification. As noted above, the association between homocysteine level and risk of vascular disease is graded, and there is no threshold (*i.e.,* the dose-response relationship extends throughout the entire range of homocysteine values). Second, moderate hyperhomocysteinemia, like moderate elevations in blood pressure and cholesterol levels, is extremely common in elderly people, particularly those with atherosclerosis.

In one large Norwegian study of middle-aged and older men and women with no history of hypertension, diabetes, coronary heart disease, or stroke, the mean total homocysteine among those 40–42 years of age was 11.3 micromoles/liter in men and 9.6 in women; among those aged 65–67, the corresponding values were 12.9 in men and 11.6 in women. In other words, in this apparently healthy population, homocysteine levels were higher in men than in women and increased slightly with age.

In a study of elderly residents of Framingham, Mass., aged 67–96, researchers defined high plasma homocysteine as greater than

14 micromoles/liter. With this criterion, some 29% of the subjects had elevated levels. In general, about 50% of people who are diagnosed with vascular disease will have elevated levels by this definition.

Diet, genes, or both?

As described above, there are two primary determinants of homocysteine level, genetic variation in the activity of the various enzymes needed for homocysteine metabolism and dietary intake of B vitamins. Homocystinuria is usually due to defects in both copies of the gene for CBS. It is much more common, however, for a person to have one defective gene and one normal gene. In fact, between one in 70 and one in 200 individuals is born with this combination of normal and defective CBS genes, which is associated with moderate elevations in homocysteine level.

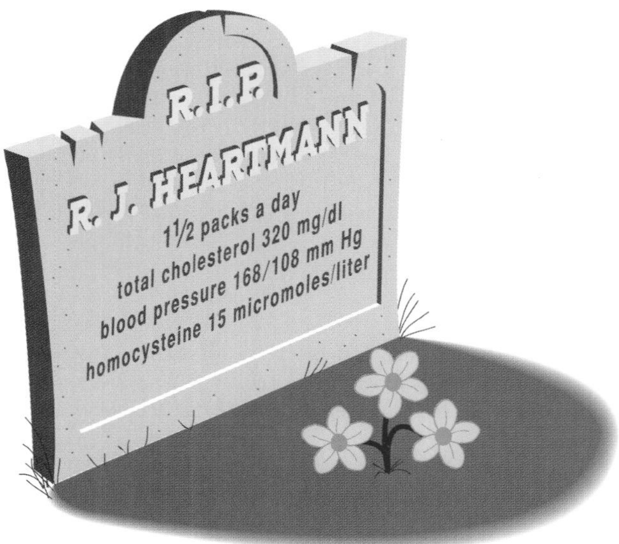

Of probably greater importance as a cause of hyperhomocysteinemia are variant forms of the gene for the enzyme MTHFR. About 10–15% of U.S. Caucasians and a smaller percentage of African-Americans have a common variant that is associated with much lower than normal enzyme activity and a tendency to develop both moderate hyperhomocysteinemia and coronary artery disease. Elevated homocysteine levels develop in these individuals, however, only when two copies of the defective gene are present *and* there is a low intake of folic acid. This finding suggests that some people may have a higher folate requirement than others. (Folate is the natural substance in foods. Folic acid is the synthetic form of folate used in vitamin supplements.) Further, it emphasizes the potential importance of interactions between genetic and dietary factors in determining homocysteine levels and, perhaps, the risk of vascular disease.

The other important factor in hyperhomocysteinemia is low vitamin B status—meaning inadequate dietary intake of B vitamins or low levels circulating in the blood. In the elderly Framingham residents, researchers found that individuals with low blood levels of folate, vitamin B_{12}, and vitamin B_6 had high blood homocysteine levels, while those with moderate or high vitamin levels had markedly lower homocysteine concentrations. Inadequate levels of folic acid, vitamin B_6, or vitamin B_{12} appeared to contribute to 67% of the cases of elevated homocysteine. More than 50% of persons with low levels of at least one of the three vitamins had homocysteine levels higher than 14 micromoles/liter.

Elevated homocysteine levels have also been shown to be correlated with other risk factors for vascular disease. The Norwegian study, for example, showed that plasma homocysteine level was positively associated with male gender, older age, cigarette smoking, total cholesterol, blood pressure, and heart rate and inversely associated with physical activity. These results were not substantially changed by adjustment for intake of fruits, vegetables, and vitamin supplements. As noted above, individuals with a history of high blood pressure, diabetes, coronary heart disease, or stroke were excluded from the study to avoid potential effects on homocysteine, either direct or indirect, of medical treatment or changes in lifestyle.

This study raises fundamental questions about the association of elevated homocysteine with vascular disease. Is homocysteine merely a marker for increased risk of blood vessel disease due to other factors? Does homocysteine mediate the effect of other factors such as cigarette smoking or physical inactivity? A detailed understanding of how homocysteine affects the cardiovascular system would go a long way toward answering these perplexing questions.

Underlying mechanisms

While the mechanism by which homocysteine induces vascular disease is still unknown, several clues to the process have come from animal and human experiments and in vitro studies (those conducted outside the living body). Scientists now believe that moderate elevations in homocysteine may promote both atherogenesis (thickening of the arterial wall due to fatty deposits) and thrombosis (the formation of blood clots, which, in turn, may block narrowed arteries).

In vitro studies have suggested that homocysteine promotes atherogenesis in one of two ways. The first is by direct toxic effects on the endothelium, or lining, of blood vessels. The second is by encouraging the proliferation of smooth muscle in the walls of vessels, which causes thickening of the walls. In experiments with baboons, animals that were given homocysteine showed changes in the aortic endothelium (the lining of the major vessel carrying blood from the heart to the arteries), increased turnover of the blood cells called platelets (indicating an increased tendency for clotting), and early signs of atherogenesis. In another, more recent experiment, specially bred miniature pigs were fed a methionine-rich diet to induce high homocysteine levels. After four months of moderate hyperhomocysteinemia, the animals had clear damage to the walls of their arteries.

Epidemiological studies in humans have also shed light on the means by which homocysteine may damage blood vessels and promote clots. In one large study of adults who were free of cardiovascular disease, even a mildly elevated homocysteine level of 10.5 micromoles/liter was independently linked to thickening of the walls of the carotid arteries (the paired vessels in the neck that supply blood to the brain), a condition that is a precursor of carotid atherosclerosis and, potentially, stroke. In the elderly Framingham subjects, plasma homocysteine levels of 14.4 micromoles/liter or more were strongly associated with narrowing (stenosis) of the carotid arteries in elderly subjects. The Framingham researchers also found that blood levels of folate and vitamin B_6 were inversely related to the presence of carotid stenosis, which illustrates the clinical relevance of vitamin deficiency to the development of hyperhomocysteinemia and atherosclerosis in the elderly.

As noted earlier, the first clue that elevated homocysteine levels might predispose people to thrombosis came from the observation that children with homocystinuria frequently developed blood clots in their veins. Thrombosis occurs when there is an imbalance between factors that promote clot formation, factors that inhibit clot formation, and factors that promote fibrinolysis (clot dissolution). Studies indicate that elevated homocysteine may affect all three.

Homocysteine has also been shown to induce changes in the lining of the blood vessels that have the effect of promoting thrombosis. In the laboratory the addition of homocysteine to vessel-lining cells depletes endothelium-derived relaxing factor (EDRF), a substance that causes vessels to dilate (widen) and prevents platelets from aggregating, or clumping. Platelet aggregation is an important step in the formation of blood clots, and constriction of vessels contributes to narrowing and blockage. A deficiency of EDRF could, therefore, impair the capacity of vessels to dilate in response to a need for increased blood supply—during exercise, for example, or when blood flow is blocked by a clot. Lack of EDRF also may contribute to abnormal platelet aggregation and, hence, clot formation.

Cause or marker?

The evidence gathered to date shows that elevations in homocysteine precede the occurrence of vascular disease. The strength of association of high homocysteine levels and disease is similar to that of other established vascular risk factors. Many studies have documented a progressive, dose-response relationship between homocysteine level and vascular disease. Furthermore, the relationship has been relatively consistent in studies involving different populations, in a variety of study designs (both retrospective and prospective), and in studies with different end points (*e.g.*, occurrence of stroke or heart attack, diagnosis of blood vessel disease). Still, there is always the possibility that elevations in homocysteine are simply a marker, or sign, of preclinical disease or of other, already established risk factors.

While observational investigations of large populations can never conclusively demonstrate a causal relationship, three additional lines of evidence further support a causal link between homocysteine and vascular disease. First, the "natural experiment" of severe inherited homocystinuria, in which very young individuals develop arterial or venous thrombosis, is unlikely to be explained by confounding factors or by the presence of preclinical disease. Second, as summarized briefly above, a substantial body of evidence has identified several plausible mechanisms by which elevated blood levels of homocysteine can lead to both atherosclerosis and thrombosis. Third, in experiments with the minipig—the best animal model yet developed for this condition—a high methionine diet has been shown to lead to both modest elevations in homocysteine and early signs of atherosclerosis.

B vitamins: how much is enough?

Of the three vitamins principally involved in homocysteine metabolism—folate, vitamin B_6, and vitamin B_{12}—folate appears to be the one most strongly and consistently correlated with homocysteine. Indeed, virtually every observational study that has examined the impact of nutrition on homocysteine levels has demonstrated that low dietary intake or low blood levels of folate are associated with high levels of fasting homocysteine.

Other than fortified cereals, the most common sources of folate in the American diet are leafy vegetables, orange juice, and certain fruits. The recommended dietary allowances (RDAs) for folate in adult men and women are 0.2 mg and 0.18 mg per day, respectively; the average dietary intakes are 0.32 mg and 0.24 mg per day, respectively. Some nutrition authorities believe that the RDAs for folate are too low (they were revised downward in 1989) and that an intake of nearly 0.4 mg/day is desirable, at least to reduce homocysteine. On the basis of investigations demonstrating the role of folate in preventing certain birth defects, the U.S. Public Health Service recommends a daily intake of 0.4 mg (often expressed as 400 micrograms) for all women of childbearing age.

Several studies have examined the impact of folic acid supplements on homocysteine levels. The results indicate that doses of one milligram per day or more can reduce fasting homocysteine levels by 20% to 50% from baseline levels, particularly in persons with elevated homocysteine. Even doses of only 0.4 mg, an amount commonly found in multivitamins, have been shown in preliminary trials to have an impact on homocysteine. In response to the persuasive evidence that folate can help to prevent birth defects, the Food and Drug Administration passed a regulation requiring that as of Jan. 1, 1998, manufacturers of enriched grain products (*e.g.*, bread, flour, cornmeal, rice, pasta) add folic acid to their products. The level of folic acid fortification will range from 0.43 to 1.4 mg per 454 g (one pound) of cereal-grain product, an amount that will not raise average daily intake beyond the recommended upper limit of one milligram per day. The effect of fortification on homocysteine levels is uncertain.

Folate is generally considered safe, even in high doses, but there are a few caveats. First, there is concern that in people with vitamin B_{12} deficiency, high doses of supplemental folic acid may mask this condition and allow irreversible neurological disease to progress. For this reason, vitamin pills with more than 0.4 mg of

Vitamins That Influence Homocysteine Levels

	Folate	Vitamin B_6	Vitamin B_{12}
Food sources	leafy vegetables, orange juice, fortified cereals, legumes, whole grains	meat, poultry, fish, fruits, brown rice	foods of animal origin
Average dietary intake (mg/day)	0.32 (men) 0.24 (women)	2.1 (men) 1.5 (women)	0.006 (men) 0.004 (women)
Recommended dietary allowance for adults (mg/day)	0.20 (men) 0.18 (women)	2.0 (men) 1.6 (women)	0.002
Adverse effects of supplementation	progression of neuropathy in vitamin B_{12} deficiency; seizures after rapid injection of high dose in epileptics	reversible neuropathy at very high doses	none

(Opposite page) Steve Hansen—Stock, Boston

folic acid per pill are not available without prescription. A second concern pertains to the impact of supplemental folic acid on seizure control in persons taking anticonvulsant drugs. Intravenous infusions of large doses of folic acid (typically seven or more milligrams) have precipitated seizures in persons with epilepsy who take certain of these medications. (The relatively small amounts in fortified foods and pill supplements pose no danger to this group.)

Vitamin B_6 also influences homocysteine metabolism. It attenuates the rise in homocysteine after methionine loading but has little impact on fasting levels of homocysteine. Foods that are good sources of vitamin B_6 include bananas, brown rice, and chicken. The adult RDA for vitamin B_6 is 2 mg per day for men and 1.6 mg per day for women. The average intakes are 2.1 and 1.5 mg, respectively. Supplemental vitamin B_6 at doses up to 250 mg per day is generally considered safe, even if taken for an extended period of time. Higher doses can cause neurological problems, however, but these are reversible upon discontinuation of the vitamin.

Vitamin B_{12} is yet another micronutrient that may have an impact on fasting levels of homocysteine. In studies of patients with vitamin B_{12} deficiency, blood levels of vitamin B_{12} have been inversely associated with homocysteine levels. The principal dietary sources of vitamin B_{12} are foods of animal origin (meat, including liver and other organ meats, eggs, and dairy products). The RDA is 0.002 mg per day in both men and women; average daily intakes are 0.006 and 0.004 mg per day, respectively. While even high-dose supplements (0.4 mg of vitamin B_{12} per day) have not had an impact on fasting homocysteine levels in healthy populations, vitamin B_{12} supplementation may be effective in lowering homocysteine in persons with vitamin B_{12} deficiency. High doses of vitamin B_{12} have no known adverse effects.

Waiting for answers

In 1996 the National Institute of Neurological Disorders and Stroke launched a multicenter clinical trial, the Vitamin Intervention for Stroke Prevention (VISP) Trial, to test whether a B-vitamin supplement can reduce the risk of stroke recurrence, heart attack, or death in individuals who have already had a stroke. Participants will receive a regimen of 2.5 mg of folic acid, 25 mg of vitamin B_6, and 400 micrograms of vitamin B_{12}. (Multivitamins typically contain 0.4 mg of folic acid, 2 mg of B_6, and 6 micrograms of B_{12}, doses that may be sufficient to reduce blood levels of homocysteine.)

Could lowering homocysteine levels in the general population prevent many cases of heart disease and stroke from occurring in the first place? The answer to this question will come only from trials of vitamin supplements in people who are initially free of cardiovascular disease. Until the results of such studies are in,

Eat a healthy diet or take a pill? While scientists debate the merits of vitamin supplements for lowering homocysteine levels, consumers can buy low-cost "health insurance" in the produce departments of their local supermarkets.

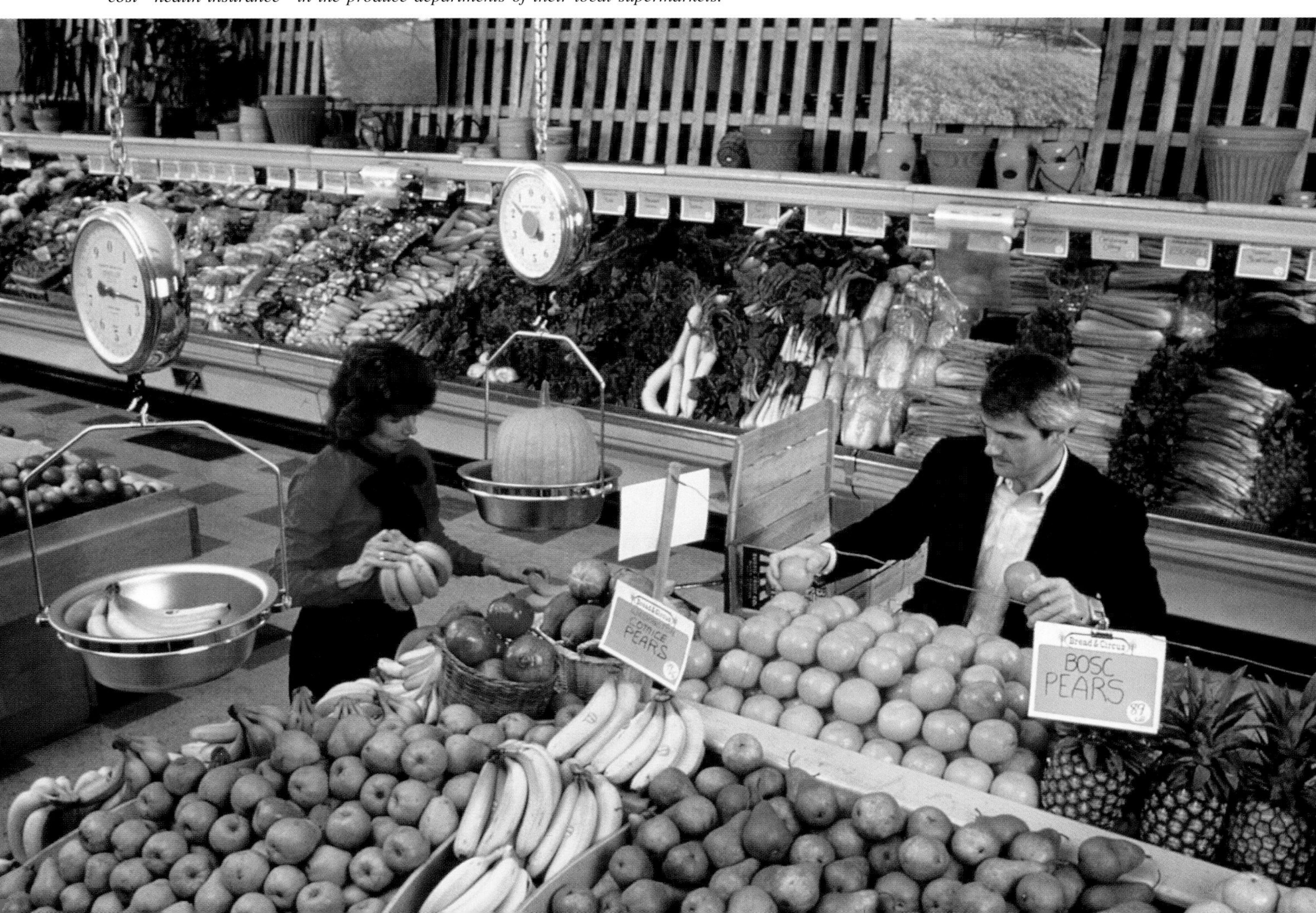

there will be no public policy recommendations on the use of homocysteine-reducing vitamins. In the meantime, people with cardiovascular disease and those at risk for it must act on available knowledge. Diets rich in fruits and vegetables provide natural sources of folate and are accepted to have myriad other health benefits, with more being discovered all the time. Most Americans are already aware that they should be increasing their consumption of these healthful foods. Whether the "homocysteine hypothesis" is ultimately confirmed or not, eating more fruits and vegetables is a wise course of action for people with cardiovascular disease and those trying to avoid it.

—Steven J. Kittner, M.D., M.P.H., and Lawrence J. Appel, M.D., M.P.H.

Sex and the Heart

Is sexual activity strenuous enough to cause a heart attack? That question is commonly asked, especially by middle-aged and older people who have reason to be concerned about their cardiovascular health. A study published in 1996 should reassure those who have such fears. Researchers from Harvard Medical School and the Harvard School of Public Health sought to find out what events had triggered the myocardial infarctions (heart attacks) of 1,774 patients in 45 U.S. hospitals. Among all the patients interviewed, 858 reported that they had been sexually active in the previous year; of those, 79 (9%) had had sexual activity in the 24 hours preceding their attack, and 27 (3%) reported having had sexual intercourse in the two hours prior to the onset of myocardial infarction symptoms. After a careful statistical analysis of the data, the investigators concluded that sexual activity was a probable contributor to heart attacks in fewer than 1% of the total patients. Their results were published in the *Journal of the American Medical Association* (May 8, 1996).

The authors also determined that in the two hours after sexual activity, the relative risk of a heart attack was doubled. That finding, however, needs to be put in perspective. (The risk of having a heart attack after sexual activity is referred to as "relative risk"—*i.e.,* it is relative to the likelihood of having a heart attack during periods of lighter activity or no exertion, known as the "absolute risk.") One of the longest-running and most comprehensive epidemiological studies, the Framingham Heart Study, has shown that the absolute risk of a 50-year-old, nonsmoking, nondiabetic man's having a heart attack during *any one-hour period* is one in a million; thus, the chances of having a heart attack in the two hours after sexual activity would be two in a million—still extremely low.

A subject in the ongoing Framingham Study has an electrocardiogram as part of his biannual checkup. Framingham has shown that a 50-year-old man's risk of having a heart attack is about one in a million during any one-hour period—if he does not smoke and is not diabetic or obese.

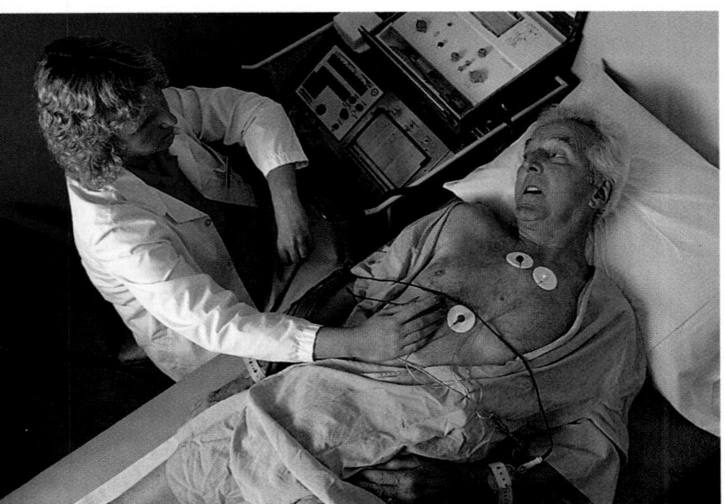

Nathan Benn—Stock, Boston

Sex as exercise

Another interesting finding from the Harvard study was that the risk of a heart attack after sexual activity was lower in patients who regularly engaged in heavy physical exertion. The authors defined "heavy physical exertion" as exercise that required six or more metabolic equivalents (METs). One MET is the rate of energy expended when a person is at rest (*see* Table). The relative risk of having a heart attack after sexual activity was 3.0 in those who exercised once a week or not at all, 1.9 in those who exercised two times a week, and 1.2 in those who exercised three or more times a week. In other words, regular physical activity reduced the risk of a heart attack's being precipitated by sex.

Those results confirmed previous studies done by exercise physiologists and cardiac rehabilitation experts. One study showed that even when people exercised up to their peak capacity for 10–15 minutes during an exercise stress test, the risk of cardiac death was one in 10,000. Another study found a rate half as great—0.5 deaths per 10,000 exercise stress tests performed. Exercise stress testing generally requires an exertion level of more than six METs. The average young to middle-aged adult can achieve 10 to 12 METs at peak, or maximal, exercise.

Just how strenuous then is sexual activity? For most people it involves sustained physical exertion at only one-third or less of their physical capacity for a relatively short time. One of the earliest studies of heart disease and sexual activity found that the mean maximal heart rate during sexual intercourse was 117 beats per minute and systolic blood pressure increased by 30–40 mm Hg (millimeters of mercury). Achieving a similar heart rate and rise in blood pressure during an exercise stress test would require 3.5 to 4.5 METs—the exercise equivalent of walking one kilometer in about 10 1/2 minutes without discomfort.

In fact, the heart rate may rise to fairly high levels during sex, but this does not necessarily correspond to the exertion level. Factors such as emotional stress, excitement, and anxiety about performance can increase sympathetic nervous system activity and thereby quicken the pace of the heart. The *actual* energy expenditure during intercourse may be as low as two to three METs.

Exercise as medicine

Although sexual activity does not require a lot of energy, it may exceed the exertional tolerance of some inactive people who have had a heart attack or who have been diagnosed with coronary heart disease (CHD). In addition to prescribing medications for patients after a heart attack or a diagnosis of CHD, physicians may recommend an endurance-training program. Among the important effects of endurance training (*e.g.,* walking, jogging,

Energy Expenditure in Pleasurable Activities

METs[1]		
Men	**Women**	**Activities**
1.6–3.9	1.2–2.7	walking, reading a book, driving a car, shopping, bowling, fishing, golfing, pleasure sailing, ♥
4–5.9	2.8–4.3	pleasure cycling, dancing, playing volleyball or badminton, doing calisthenics, ♥
6–7.9	4.4–5.9	ice skating, water skiing, playing competitive tennis, novice mountain climbing, jogging
8–9.9	6–7.5	fencing, playing touch football or basketball, swimming (most strokes), scuba diving
10 and over	7.6 and over	playing handball, squash, or paddleball, cross-country skiing, running (fast pace)

[1]METs=multiples of amount of oxygen required for various levels of physical activity (1 MET=sitting at rest) for untrained men and women.

♥ Estimated energy expenditure for sexual activity.

Source: Frank I. Katch and William D. McArdle, *Nutrition, Weight Control, and Exercise*, Lea & Febiger, 1983.

swimming, cross-country skiing, and bicycling) are that it increases the amount of oxygen available during exercise (referred to as "maximal oxygen consumption," which is an important measure of cardiorespiratory fitness) and lowers the heart rate, blood pressure, and perceived exertion required for doing the same amount of exercise. These physiological responses have been studied to determine how the effects of regular exercise translate to sexual activity.

For example, one researcher had 16 cardiac patients exercise on stationary bicycles for 16 weeks. Once before the exercise program and twice afterward, they wore Holter monitors (ambulatory electrocardiographic devices) during sexual activity to record their heart rate. Another six men (the control group) did not exercise. The men in the control group did not experience any changes in maximal oxygen consumption and heart rate during sex, but the men who had exercised did; from the preprogram recording to the postprogram recordings, they had an average increase in maximal oxygen consumption of 11.5% and a 5.5% decrease in heart rate. This suggests that sexual activity required the use of a smaller percentage of their total exercise capacity and left them with greater cardiovascular reserve.

In another study of heart attack survivors, patients who participated in an exercise program reported that their frequency and quality of sexual activity stayed the same as before their heart attack or improved. Although the physiological effects of exercise training are important, the *psychological* benefits should not be underestimated. The ability to exercise strenuously on a regular basis proves to the cardiac patient that he or she is not a "cardiac cripple"; patients gain confidence in their physical recovery process and are less likely to be fearful about what they can and cannot do. Sex is more enjoyable when the patient knows he or she can engage in it without ill effects.

Concerns beyond the cardiac

The actual cardiac stress induced by sex is not the only factor a person who has had a heart attack must consider. Most people who have had a heart attack experience some depression, at least during the first few months of recovery, and depression inevitably affects sexual desire. Despite research showing the relative safety of sexual intercourse in cardiac patients, one study showed that the frequency of sexual intercourse decreased by 24% to 75% in middle-aged men who had had a heart attack. Among the reasons given were fatigue, angina (chest pain), psychological fears, and medication-related sexual dysfunction.

Needless to say, a heart attack is a scary event, and it changes a person's life in many ways. Some people make drastic changes—they stop smoking, start exercising, alter their diets, lose weight, learn stress-reduction techniques, reduce the number of hours a day they work, and so forth. Others who suffer a heart attack may be so traumatized by the event that they fear almost any activity. They may give up regular sports activities, socialize less, or quit their job. Some may be afraid to travel. Many people stop having sex. When a man or a woman who has had a heart attack avoids sex, it can cause stress, hurt, and resentment in the spouse or partner, which may establish a pattern of fear, sexual abstinence, guilt, and anger that inevitably takes a toll on the relationship. Very commonly, neither partner is willing to talk about the problem or seek help. (This should not be surprising; people tend to be reluctant to seek counseling for sexual problems of *any* nature.)

The concerns about sex after a heart attack or a CHD diagnosis may be complicated by the fact that many other factors affect sexuality. Typically, as people get older, they do not have sexual intercourse as often as they once did. Men may need more stimulation to maintain an erection, and women may have problems associated with diminished vaginal lubrication. In addition, chronic illnesses, such as diabetes and arthritis, can affect sexual activity.

Medications also affect sexual performance. After a heart attack or heart disease diagnosis, a person may take medications to lower the heart rate, reduce the blood pressure, prevent anginal pain, or control arrhythmias (irregular heartbeats). Psychoactive drugs may be prescribed to relieve depression. Many of these medications have unwanted side effects—most notably, impotence in men and diminished sex drive in both women and men. A less-well-appreciated fact is that medications prescribed for post-heart-attack patients may also *enhance* sexual activity. For example, the drugs that relieve angina during exertion—beta-blockers or nitroglycerin—also reduce chest discomfort that might occur during sexual intercourse; thus, patients may be advised to take them beforehand. Drugs that control irregular heartbeats may relieve the anxiety of people who otherwise have palpitations during sexual activity. Antihypertensive medications can improve the quality of sex by reducing blood pressure, which in some patients may decrease the workload on the heart and the likelihood of exertional angina. Antidepressants often relieve anxiety and improve mood, which makes it easier to approach and enjoy sexual activity.

Smart sex

After a heart attack, resuming sexual activity without information and advice is like starting on a heart-healthy diet without knowing which foods are high in fat. However, with knowledge of the physiological requirements of sexual intercourse, a lot of patience, and a little common sense, most patients will be able to resume sexual activity safely and pleasurably. Fear and myths should not stop the cardiac patient from having a full and rewarding sex life.

Nathan Benn—Stock, Boston

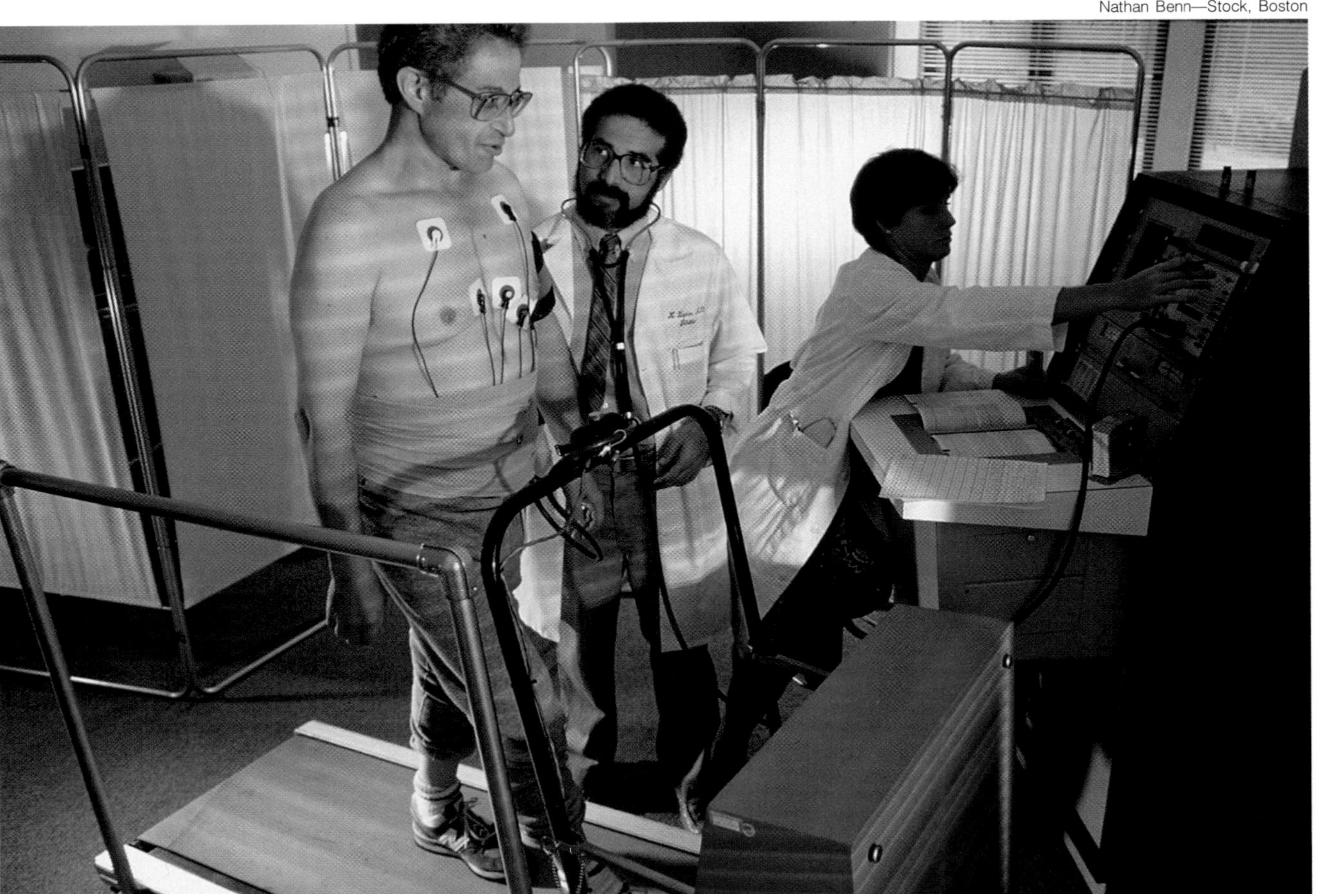

A supervised workout on a treadmill helps a post-heart-attack patient regain his strength and vigor. Most cardiac rehabilitation programs provide excellent guidance on all aspects of recovery, including diet, exercise, stress management, and the safe resumption of sexual activity.

The following tips for heart attack survivors also apply to individuals with a CHD diagnosis.

- In general, a person can resume sex within a few weeks of a heart attack or coronary artery bypass operation and within a few days of a balloon angioplasty procedure. As already noted, having sex is comparable to walking a kilometer in about $10^1/_2$ minutes, so anyone who can do the latter can probably engage quite safely in the former.
- People who have had heart attacks should be patient about resuming sexual activity. A relaxed setting with one's regular partner is best. People should avoid eating heavy meals or consuming a lot of alcohol before sexual intercourse. (One study showed that 80% of deaths precipitated by sexual intercourse occurred during extramarital affairs, and most of the victims had been eating and drinking heavily.)
- Cardiac patients—like all adults—should maintain a healthy lifestyle. This includes regular exercise, a low-fat diet, not smoking, and moderate (if any) alcohol consumption. Most cardiac rehabilitation programs provide guidance about diet, exercise, stress management, *and* sexual activity. Unfortunately, a majority of patients do not engage in formal rehabilitation after a heart attack. They would be wise to ask their physicians for help in making suitable lifestyle adjustments. To find out about specific cardiac rehabilitation programs, people can contact their local chapter of the American Heart Association, the American College of Cardiology, or the American Association of Cardiovascular and Pulmonary Rehabilitation.
- Many patients assume that the bottom position during sexual intercourse is easier for a cardiac patient, male or female. Studies have shown, however, that the cardiac response is similar in the bottom or top position. Couples should experiment to find out which position is most comfortable.
- As mentioned above, medications can be helpful for relieving symptoms and helping decrease anxiety. Men whose medications cause problems such as impotence should not discontinue taking the drugs but should discuss the problem with their physician. Often a change in medication can solve the problem, or various available impotence treatments can help.
- Although sexual activity after a heart attack or CHD diagnosis is generally safe, problems may arise. Cardiac patients should be aware of potentially serious symptoms and know what to do about them. Warning symptoms include: (1) chest pain or pressure, (2) a rapid or irregular heartbeat, (3) extreme shortness of breath, and (4) dizziness. People who experience any of these should discontinue the activity and not resume it until they have consulted a physician.

—Barry A. Franklin, Ph.D., and Frances Munnings

Pediatric Perspective on a Lousy Problem

The pattern is familiar and tends to present itself in one of two ways: an elementary-school nurse discovers lice eggs in a student's hair and calls the youngster's home to report the news, or a mother or father, while combing a child's (usually a daughter's) hair, notices a live creature scurrying across the scalp. In either case, the parents are usually distraught. Epidemics of head lice (pediculosis) are being reported across the United States and the world. These creatures know neither geographic nor socioeconomic bounds. Homes are infested; schools are infested—and posh private schools are no exception. As a practicing pediatrician in a large metropolitan area, this author is indeed very familiar with the problem.

What are these creatures that have made so many youngsters miserable and parents frantic? Are all lice the same? How are they transmitted? Are they a danger or simply a social nuisance? Are they eradicable? Are all treatments the same? Are there things that families, schools, and day-care centers *should* be doing but are not?

Since biblical times

> ***Ye ugle, creepin, blastit wonner,***
> ***Detested, shunned by saint an sinner,***
> ***How daur ye set your fit upon her,***
> ***Sae fine a lady***
> ***Gae somewhere else and seek your dinner***
> ***on some poor body***
>
> —Robert Burns (1759–96), written after watching a louse move across a lady's bonnet during a kirk (Scottish church) service

Lice have been with the human race since at least biblical times. Egyptian priests are said to have shaved their heads and bodies to prevent infestations. By Roman times, "nit combs" were in use. In the late 1980s a parasitologist and a curator of antiquities in Israel described wooden combs dating to the 2nd century that were found at Qumran, near the site of the discovery of the Dead Sea Scrolls. The combs were obviously intended for louse removal (having a coarse-toothed edge that served to straighten hair and a fine-toothed edge to delouse the hair). Lice in broken-up pieces were noted in every stage of development on the combs.

Morphologically, lice then and now are the same, but much of what scientists know about the parasites was learned only in the early part of the present century. All plans for the eradication of lice have failed; not only are they still a problem, but since the 1960s there have been sharp increases in head lice reported worldwide and in pubic lice reported in the United States and Western Europe. The National Pediculosis Association (NPA) estimates that in the U.S. alone 12 million children are infested with head lice annually.

Basic biology and epidemiology

Human lice are parasitic insects of the order Phthiraptera and suborder Anoplura; the latter contains about 560 bloodsucking species that live only on mammals. Each species is very host-specific. Humans are the only natural host for the head louse (*Pediculus humanus capitis*), the body louse (*Pediculus humanus corporis*), and the pubic louse (*Phthirus pubis*). Lice are so-called ectoparasites: they live on, not in, the human host. Thus, humans are "infested," not "infected." All three forms of lice survive by piercing the skin and taking a blood meal from their host.

The head louse is about two to four millimeters long (the size of a sesame seed), wingless, and colorless when hatched but reddish brown after feeding and has six legs ending in claws that readily grasp hair. Adult females live up to two or three months, and they lay about six eggs (nits) per day. Although there can be hundreds of lice on a head, the average population is only 10. The head louse lays her eggs at the base of the hairs, about one millimeter from the skin; the whitish, oval-shaped nits become "glued" to the hair. The egg hatches into a nymph 7–10 days later. After hatching, the louse passes through three nymphal stages, molting its skin at each stage. Finally, approximately three weeks after the start of the cycle, the now-mature lice mate, the females lay eggs, and the cycle repeats.

How long head lice can live without a human host is a matter of debate. A report from the 1980s suggested that lice could survive for 10 days off the body, while nits, in ideal conditions, could survive for three weeks. The NPA estimates that a head louse will not survive more than a day without a human host.

P.h. corporis is a larger version of *P.h. capitis* and appears to have evolved from the latter as humans began to wear clothes.

*(Below) A false-colored scanning electron micrograph shows a head louse (*Pediculus humanus capitis*), magnified about 88 times, clinging with its six clawlike legs to a human hair. The adult female louse lays about six eggs (known as nits) a day. (Top) Each nit becomes glued to an individual shaft of hair very close to the scalp.*

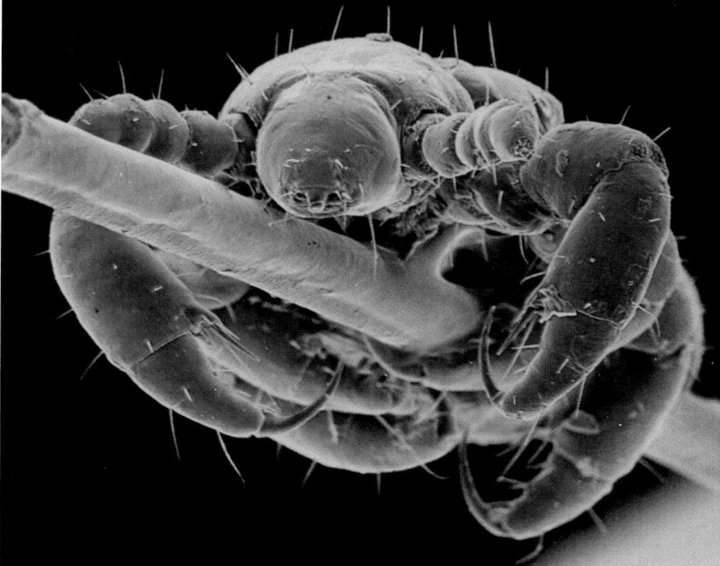

(Top) Christian Gautier—Science Source/Photo Researchers; (above) CNRI/Science Source/Photo Researchers

The body louse lays its eggs on the seams of clothing. In addition to being heftier, the body louse is also more independent than the head louse in that it can live off the body for somewhat longer. Body lice are rare in the United States and other industrialized, wealthier nations. They are associated most frequently with overcrowding, lack of sanitation, and poverty.

Body lice are the only lice known to transmit disease under natural conditions. Historically, most widespread infestations of body lice have occurred during times of war or famine. The diseases most recently known to be transmitted by body lice include trench fever (seen during World Wars I and II), classic typhus, and relapsing fever.

The pubic, or "crab," louse looks quite different from the other two forms. It is crablike and almost square. Its front two legs are delicate and end in tiny hooks. The posterior four legs are heavier and end in powerful claws. The adult female life span is about one month, and she is much more reliant on the host for food and body heat than either the head or body louse. At room temperature

Oliver Meckes—Science Source/Photo Researchers

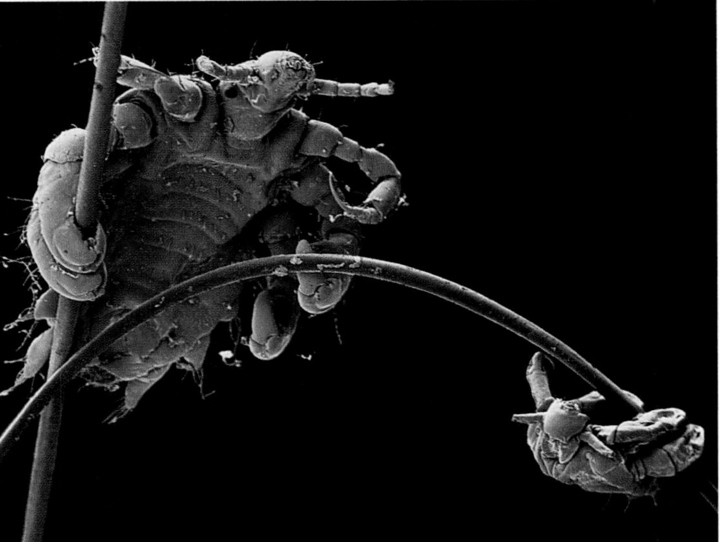

An adult pubic louse (Phthirus pubis) *and one that is newly hatched (right) grasp onto individual pubic hairs.* P. pubis *have squarish bodies that closely resemble those of crabs, hence the common designation "crabs." Pubic lice are usually sexually transmitted.*

she can survive for only 12 hours off the host. The adult female lays three eggs per day and cements these to the base of the pubic hair shaft. After seven days the eggs hatch, and the adults emerge after two more weeks.

P. pubis is seen most commonly in people aged 15–40 years. These lice are typically transmitted during sexual activity, and they often coexist with other venereal (sexually transmitted) diseases. One sexual exposure is all that is necessary. Bedding and clothing can also be a source of transmission.

Pubic lice prefer the pubic region but can wander to other body parts. In people with a great deal of body hair, the crab louse can infest the beard, mustache, and hair on the legs or under the arms. In children, lice that appear on the eyebrows or eyelashes are usually pubic lice and may come from an infested adult in the household.

Head lice epidemic

Head lice affect all groups of people but appear to have their preferences. According to the *Canadian Journal of Public Health, P.h. capitis* tend to like: "children more than adults, females more than males (especially after childhood)... whites more than blacks, clean heads more than dirty or dandruffed heads, [and] large families more than small families." Some experts consider long hair an attraction for lice, but the parasites are well known to infest short-haired hosts as well.

Schoolchildren are often the first persons in a household to be identified as having head lice; family members of an infested schoolchild typically also have lice. Infestation with head lice may therefore be seen as a community problem.

Transmission of head lice is usually by direct, personal (hair-to-hair) contact. A single louse might spend one day on several heads within a classroom or crowded household, getting as many meals as it can. Another reason a louse will leave one host for another is if the former dies or has a high fever. Inanimate objects such as brushes, combs, hats, towels, sheets, and pillowcases have been implicated as agents of transmission, but not all studies looking into this mode of spread agree. Head lice do *not* infest pets, nor do they hop, jump, or fly.

Symptoms. Itchy scalp is the hallmark of pediculosis, although in its early stages infestation with head lice is frequently "silent." Head lice usually stay on the scalp, and in children they especially like the postauricular (behind the ears) and occipital (nape of the neck) regions. Excessive scratching can lead to secondary infection of the skin.

Diagnosis. Diagnosis is usually based on the observance of nits or the live adult lice on the scalp. Nits can be distinguished from dandruff by their gluelike attachment to the hair shaft. Dandruff (unlike nits) slips along the hair with little resistance. Also, nits attach to the hair shaft on one side only, whereas dandruff surrounds the hair. A specific diagnosis of pediculosis can also be made by taking the suspected louse or hair on which it appears, placing it on a glass slide with a drop of oil, and examining it under the microscope. Whether they are viewed under a microscope or live on the scalp, the characteristic nits and lice are not hard to detect.

Public health. Unlike body lice, head lice and pubic lice have not been associated with transmission of disease. In the U.S., school nurses have routinely inspected youngsters' heads for lice since 1890. Before insecticides were available for treatment, control of lice was mechanical. In the 1920s a family of barbers promoted a fine-toothed comb that removed both eggs and egg casings. So-called environmental control was advocated in 1941, when it was demonstrated that treating children but not their home contacts did not effectively eliminate the parasite problem. Many health officials, however, ignored this important method of management until the 1980s.

Insecticidal treatments. DDT, the first modern insecticide, was used in Italy during the 1940s to halt a lice-spread typhus epidemic. All chemical treatments kill lice by damaging their nervous system on contact. Newly laid louse eggs have no nervous system. Therefore, an insecticide must have residual activity—that is, it must continue working so that nymphs are killed once eggs have hatched.

Present-day treatments are mainly chemical formulations that are used topically. Medications in common use for lice include pyrethrins (sold without prescription under the trade name Rid), permethrin (Nix and Elimite), malathion (Prioderm), lindane (Kwell), and ivermectin (Mectizan, Stromectol).

- Pyrethrins, a natural extract of chrysanthemums, are easy to apply and may work, but treatment failures are relatively common. The medications are poor at killing nits and have no residual activity to kill newly hatched nymphs.
- Permethrin is a synthetic compound of insecticidal components of pyrethrins. It has residual activity (for two weeks or more), is

NEWS CAP MHA 98

Puberty in U.S. Girls: New Norms

Puberty is the time of life when a child is transformed into an adult capable of procreation. In girls the beginning of breast development is usually the first sign of puberty. A period of relatively rapid growth and the appearance of pubic and axillary (underarm) hair follow. The ovaries begin producing estrogen, which leads to an increase in fat on the hips and thighs, while the adrenal glands manufacture hormones that contribute to the hair and physical growth. The first menstrual period is generally the final event and usually occurs two or more years after puberty's onset.

It had been widely assumed, on the basis of past evidence, that this stage in a girl's development occurred normally between the ages of 11 and 16. A recent study, however, indicates that girls in the United States are beginning puberty at younger ages, with nearly half of African-American girls and almost 15% of white girls beginning to develop sexually by age eight.

The study, published in the April 1997 issue of *Pediatrics,* was conducted by 225 clinicians belonging to the Pediatric Research in Office Settings (PROS) network of the American Academy of Pediatrics (AAP). Hitherto, no large-scale studies on sexual maturation had focused specifically on racially diverse groups of girls under the age of 12. The study described the occurrence of menses and the development of secondary sexual characteristics—breasts, pubic hair, and axillary hair—in 17,077 U.S. girls between the ages of 3 and 12, of whom 90.4% were white and 9.6% were African-American. Hispanic girls were assigned to either the white or the African-American group, while girls of other races were excluded from the study because they provided too small a sample. The subjects were examined in 65 pediatric practices around the country during routine "well-child" visits or when receiving care that required a complete physical examination. Although the researchers recognized that girls who visited pediatricians would not necessarily reflect the U.S. preadolescent female population as a whole, they believed their findings would help to provide more accurate sexual-maturation norms.

The study revealed that girls as young as three can begin developing secondary sexual characteristics. At age three, 1% of white girls and 3% of African-American girls exhibited breast and/or pubic hair development. By the time the girls had reached the age of eight, those figures had risen to 14.7% and 48.3%, respectively. On average, the African-American girls began puberty between the ages of 8 and 9 and the white girls by age 10.

By age 12, 62.1% of African-American girls and 35.2% of white girls had reached menarche (the onset of menstruation). In addition, all of the African-American girls and 96.6% of the white girls had some breast and/or pubic hair development. At the same age, however, only 68.3% of the white girls, as compared with 93.4% of the African-American girls, exhibited a prevalence of axillary hair.

The onset of menses per se in white girls appears to have remained stable at 12.88 years over the past 45 years, but African-American girls' age of onset had decreased slightly, from 12.52 to 12.16 years over the past 30 years.

Why are girls growing up in the United States reaching puberty at younger ages than before? Previous international studies had shown that pubertal development is influenced by nutrition, general health status, environmental conditions, geographic location, and race and ethnicity. Authors of the AAP–PROS study speculate that a newer factor may be the environmental prevalence of certain chemicals (*e.g.,* industrial compounds and the breakdown products of pesticides) that are believed to mimic the effects of estrogen on the body (so-called environmental estrogens). Another factor may be African-American girls' use of certain hair products that contain estrogen and placenta.

The findings of the AAP–PROS study have important medical, educational, and social ramifications. For one, racial differences in the pubertal process have now been clearly established. Practitioners may need to revise their criteria for the referral of girls with precocious puberty to gynecologists, with attention to racial differences. The newly established norms may also lead to a better understanding of subsequent female health problems—including the prevalence of breast cancer. Owing to the occurrence of puberty at young ages, sex education may need to begin sooner than it has, and its content may need to be revised.

—*Jackie Orihill*

Corbis/Bettmann

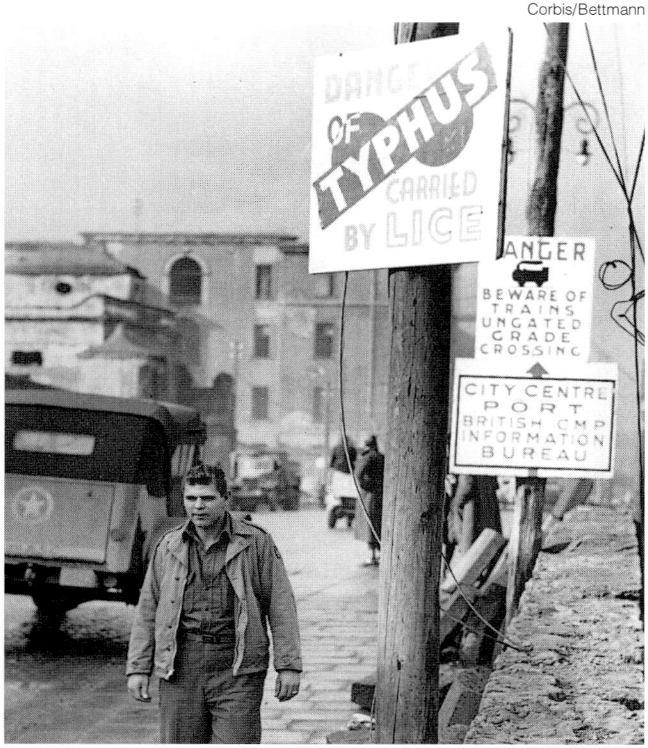

An American soldier stationed in Naples during World War II passes under a newly posted sign warning of a new enemy—a lice-spread typhus epidemic. Historically, widespread infestations of body lice, capable of transmitting infectious diseases, have been associated with war or famine.

more effective than the parent compound, and is as safe. Recent reports of resistance to the over-the-counter 1% compound (Nix) have emerged. According to consultants to *The Medical Letter* (Jan. 17, 1997), 5% permethrin (Elimite), which is sold by prescription only, can be applied to clean, dry hair, covered by a shower cap, and left on overnight (8–14 hours). (The Food and Drug Administration [FDA] has not approved Elimite for this use, and the NPA does not support this approach.)

- Malathion is a very effective insecticide but was removed from the U.S. market by its manufacturer because of its flammability and objectionable odor, among other reasons. It is still used outside the U.S.
- Lindane 1% shampoo is sold by prescription and is effective in most cases, but high doses have been associated with central nervous system toxicity, including seizures. If it is used as directed, however, it is generally considered safe.
- Ivermectin, available by prescription only, is an antiparasitic drug now available for use in the United States. It is the only available drug that is taken orally (200 micrograms per kilogram of body weight). Reports claim it is "highly effective for treatment of head lice with virtually no adverse effects." It is not presently approved by the FDA for head lice, however. A topical solution of ivermectin has worked well in a trial, but at the current time no such formulation is commercially available for human use.

There are reports in the current literature about increasing resistance of lice to the available chemicals. The aforementioned issue of *The Medical Letter* stated: "Available data are insufficient to judge whether head lice have truly become resistant to [conventionally] recommended drugs." If 1% permethrin fails, it suggests that 5% permethrin, used as indicated above, may be effective. It also states that a single dose of ivermectin, followed by one repeat dose after 10 days, "may be worth trying" if other modes of therapy do not work.

Practically speaking, what is a parent to do? Most physicians (this author included) still recommend over-the-counter permethrin (Nix) as a first-line treatment for head lice. Every family member should be treated, not just the infested person. Like all medications, permethrin should be used according to its label's directions; the treatment should be repeated in 7–10 days. It is also recommended that all nits be removed diligently from the infested person's head after each treatment.

The use of this medication should be coupled with good environmental management. Environmental controls include washing all bed linens, towels, clothes, and head gear in hot water, followed by drying in a hot dryer. The reason for the high heat is that exposure of nits or adult lice to temperatures of 50° C (125° F) for more than five minutes is lethal to the parasites. It is also recommended that nonwashable items such as coats, hats, stuffed animals, etc., be sealed and stored in plastic bags; one source suggests storage for a month, but most experts agree that two weeks is enough. Combs and brushes should be soaked in

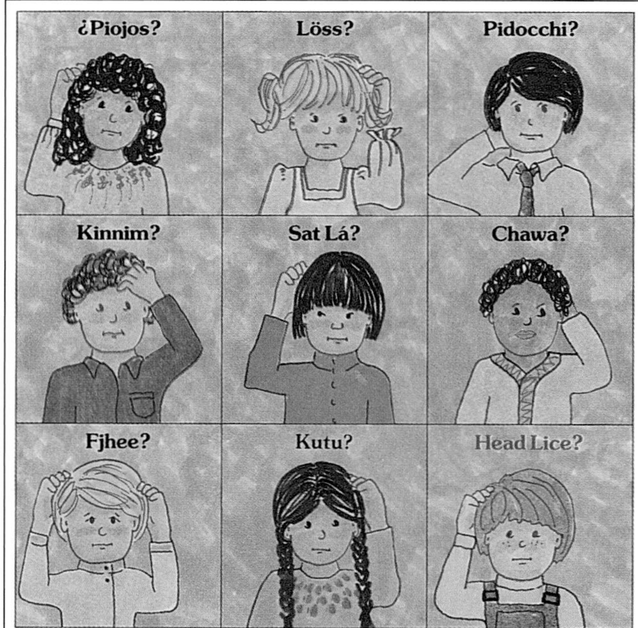

Courtesy of the National Pediculosis Association, Inc.

Through education and early-detection efforts, the National Pediculosis Association seeks to dispel myths about head lice among schoolchildren, which know neither geographic nor socioeconomic bounds.

permethrin or boiled for 20 minutes. Careful vacuuming is appropriate for carpets, rugs, couches, car seats, and the like.

What should *not* be done? Pesticide sprays should not be used on people, clothing, furniture, or objects. The *Archives of Diseases of Children* states: "Under no circumstances should a home or school be fumigated with general pesticides by the pest control industry. The effort is wasted, and possibly harmful."

A nonmedicinal solution? Some parents become quite frustrated about the amount of time and money spent on applying Nix or any of the other recommended medications, especially when treatments must be repeated many times as a result of recurrent infestations. Their frustration led physicians in England to come up with an alternative approach that relies on nonmedicinal measures. While their approach has not yet been endorsed by the American Academy of Pediatrics or other U.S. doctors' groups, it deserves scrutiny.

This management approach is based on the understanding of the louse's life cycle and an awareness that combing dripping wet hair with a fine-tooth plastic comb after ordinary shampooing is a simple and effective way to lift out lice. The protocol requires a nontoxic regular shampoo, a regular conditioner, a wide-tooth comb, and a fine-tooth comb. The shampooing slows the activity of the lice. This is followed by application of the conditioner, which makes the hair slippery to the lice. Liberal amounts of conditioner are recommended. After rinsing out the conditioner, the wide-tooth comb should be used to straighten out the hair. Finally, the fine-tooth comb is used to thoroughly and carefully remove the lice.

Because hatched lice need at least six days to spread and seven days to reproduce, the nonmedicinal protocol should be repeated twice a week for two weeks. The first treatment and combing should remove lice at every stage. The second, third, and fourth treatments should remove all subsequently hatched nymphs. It should be noted that along with this nonmedicinal approach, as with the more established application of insecticidal medications, it is still extremely important to take the environmental steps described above and to remove nits.

Wearing rubber gloves and using Popsicle sticks, Stephanie Troyan, a parent-volunteer lice inspector, routinely checks the scalps of Palo Alto, Calif., schoolchildren. She coordinates a team of very willing nitpickers, who are helping to prevent a P. humanus capitis *epidemic.*

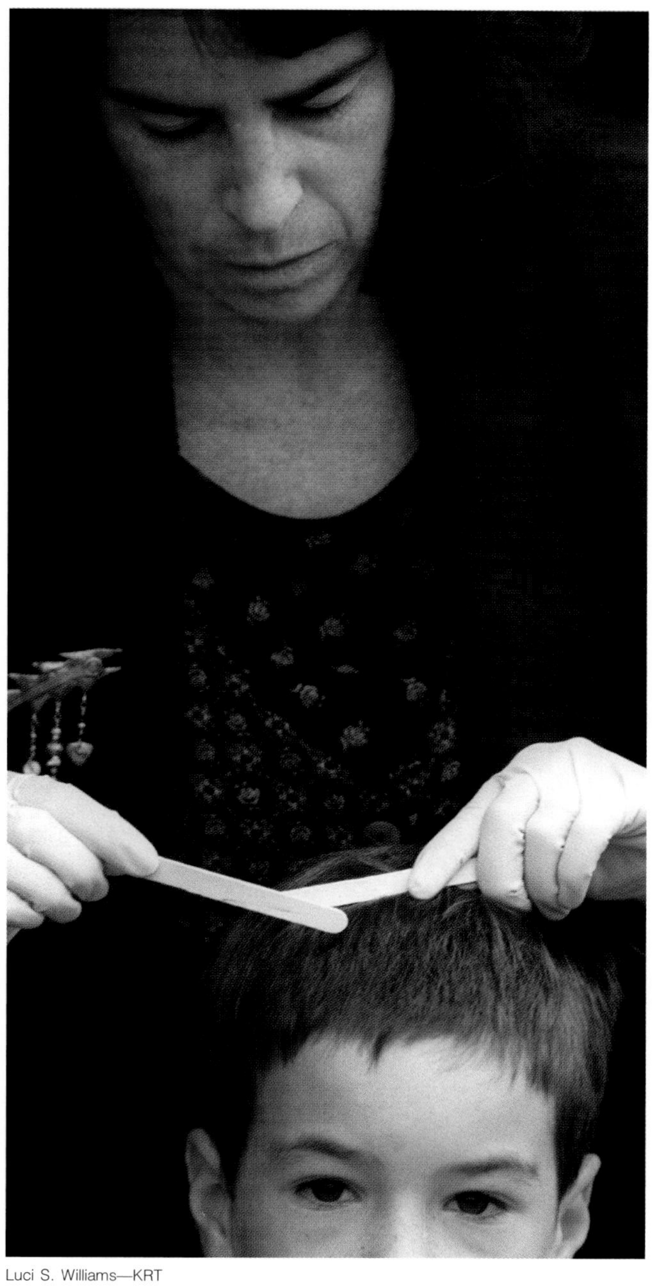

Luci S. Williams—KRT

Plenty to nitpick about!

With the spectacular rise of lice infestations worldwide, a new effort is needed to educate the public and prevent the problem. Unfortunately, there remains much confusion about lice both in the public mind and in the medical literature, and treatment recommendations often conflict. Clearly needed is a proactive approach that involves child-care centers, drugstore chains, individual pharmacies, health departments, camps, professional organizations, hair salons, health maintenance organizations, school nurses, physicians, and especially schools and parents.

Schools can formally screen children at least three times a year—for instance, at the beginning of each new school year and before winter and spring breaks. Just as important, grammar schools must set and strictly enforce a "no nit" policy; that is, no child found to have pediculosis should be allowed to attend school and mingle with other children until he or she has been adequately treated.

Ideally, coats and clothing should be hung widely spaced in cloakrooms or separately in lockers. If a school is in the middle of an epidemic of head lice, children's coats and gym clothes should be stored in plastic bags.

Though schools must take an active part in pediculosis prevention and control, parents have an even bigger role to play. They can detect head lice at home, stresses the NPA, "before infestations reach outrageous proportions. This should help minimize the need for crisis intervention and the disruption that can occur with outbreaks."

—Judith Anne Turow, M.D.

NEWS CAP MHA 98

A Tangled Web: Medical Advice in Cyberspace

Health experts worldwide are growing increasingly concerned over the reliability of medical information available to the general public on the Internet. A revolutionary communications tool that provides computer users with a wealth of data at their fingertips, the Internet is a decentralized and largely unregulated medium, and the credibility of many on-line sources is often difficult to gauge. "At first glance," declared an editorial in the April 16, 1997, issue of the *Journal of the American Medical Association (JAMA),* "science and snake oil may not always look all that different on the Net."

The need to check the spread of incorrect or misleading health care information on the Internet was underscored by a recent study conducted by the Laboratory for Mother and Child Health, Istituto di Ricerche Farmacologiche "Mario Negri" in Milan and published in the *British Medical Journal* (June 28, 1997). Taking to their computers, researchers scrutinized on-line medical advice regarding a common ailment, childhood fever. Boolean searches for "fever management" *and* "child" *and* "parent information," using two popular search engines, Yahoo! and Excite, yielded a total of 41 relevant Web sites. Although searches were also performed in French, Spanish, Italian, and German to reduce the potential for a language bias, most of the sites originated in the U.S. While a few of them were sponsored by individual practitioners, clinics, universities, or educational organizations, 32 of the sites were maintained by commercial ventures.

Treatment recommendations offered by the Web sites were compared with those given by an authoritative medical text, A. Sahib El-Radhi and James Carroll's *Fever in Paediatric Practice* (1994). Aspects of fever management on which the study focused included drug treatment, temperature measurement, sponging procedures, nondrug remedies, and the appropriate time to call a doctor. Since professional opinions differ on certain aspects of treatment, the researchers expected some inconsistencies, but they were surprised to find that only 4 of the 41 Web sites closely followed the published guidelines! The four sites were: American Housecall Network, Kids Health, Microsoft Pregnancy and Child Care Preview, and Sistema de Emergencia Medico Movil (Web site addresses are available at http://www.bmj.com).

More alarming, however, was the fact that some sites suggested potentially dangerous treatments. One was cold sponging. Although sponging a child to reduce body temperature is sometimes recommended when a fever is excessively high, most authorities advise using tepid water. Two of the sites recommended using cold water, which may cause shivering and can actually raise body temperature, or using alcohol, which can induce hypoglycemia (low blood sugar) and even coma in children who inhale the alcohol. One site also suggested dipyrone as an antipyretic (fever-reducing) drug for children, even though dipyrone has been taken off the market in the U.S., Great Britain, and other countries because of its potential to cause agranulocytosis, a condition characterized by severe sore throat, chills, and exhaustion. Two sites advised parents to use aspirin, which may put children at risk of Reye's syndrome, an often fatal neurological disease that can develop following a minor viral infection. Moreover, though most of the sites mentioned paracetamol (acetaminophen), which is a widely recommended drug for treating childhood fever, only a quarter of the sites that recommended the drug gave specific dose and frequency instructions.

While it is not known whether or how information gleaned from the Web sites has affected the decisions of parents, the study's findings make it clear that medical advice on the Internet should be looked at with a critical eye. In order to help Net users evaluate sources of information they may run across, the writers of the aforementioned *JAMA* editorial proposed four "core standards" that all Web sites should meet:

- **Authorship:** Authors of on-line articles, along with their credentials and affiliations, should always be cited.
- **Attribution:** Authors should list their references and sources. Copyright information should also be noted.
- **Disclosure:** Ownership or sponsorship of the Web site should be disclosed prominently and fully. If links to other sites are posted as the result of financial arrangements, this should also be indicated.
- **Currency:** Viewers should know how often the content on a particular site is updated. Sites should note the date that the information it provides was posted.

Other groups and government agencies also began to address the need for improving the quality of medical information on the Internet. The Geneva-based Health on the Net Foundation, a nonprofit organization dedicated to promoting the effective use of the Internet by patients and physicians alike, established a six-point code of conduct for health-related Web sites (available at http://www.hon.ch).

—*Afrodite Mantzavrakos*

UNICEF: 50 Remarkable Years

The United Nations Children's Fund—better known as UNICEF, the acronym for its original name (United Nations International Children's Emergency Fund)—celebrated its 50th anniversary on Dec. 11, 1996. In all, it has been a remarkable 50 years for the organization. It has been uniquely successful in drawing together countries and groups that have often been at loggerheads in other forums: the superpowers of the East and the West as well as the nations of the industrialized North and the less-developed South. UNICEF has been remarkably adept in raising the consciousness of the world to the problems of children, as well as in raising funds to support its work. Its stability of leadership, soundness of governance, and heartening ability to function on a small budget have been unusual for an international organization. Most important, of course, UNICEF has been singularly successful in accomplishing its mission, which is improving the health and well-being of the world's most cherished resource, its children.

Postwar relief and mass immunization

Originally established after World War II, UNICEF was scheduled to shut down operations in the 1950s, having provided

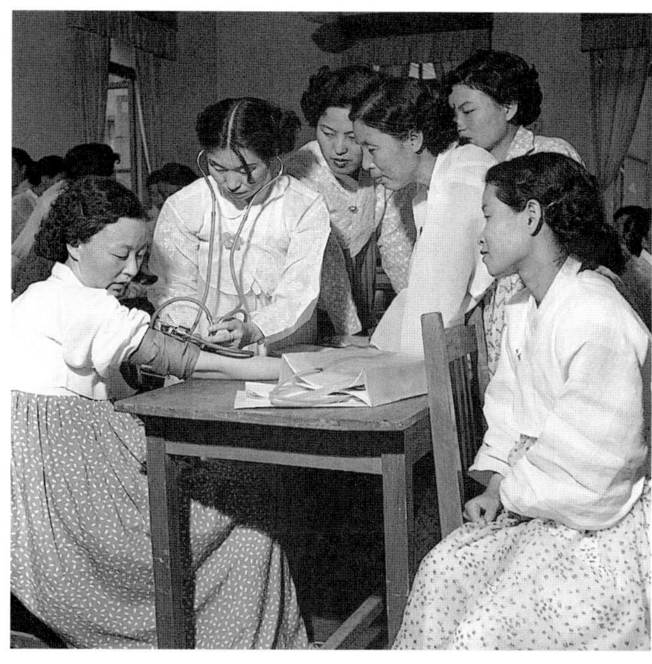

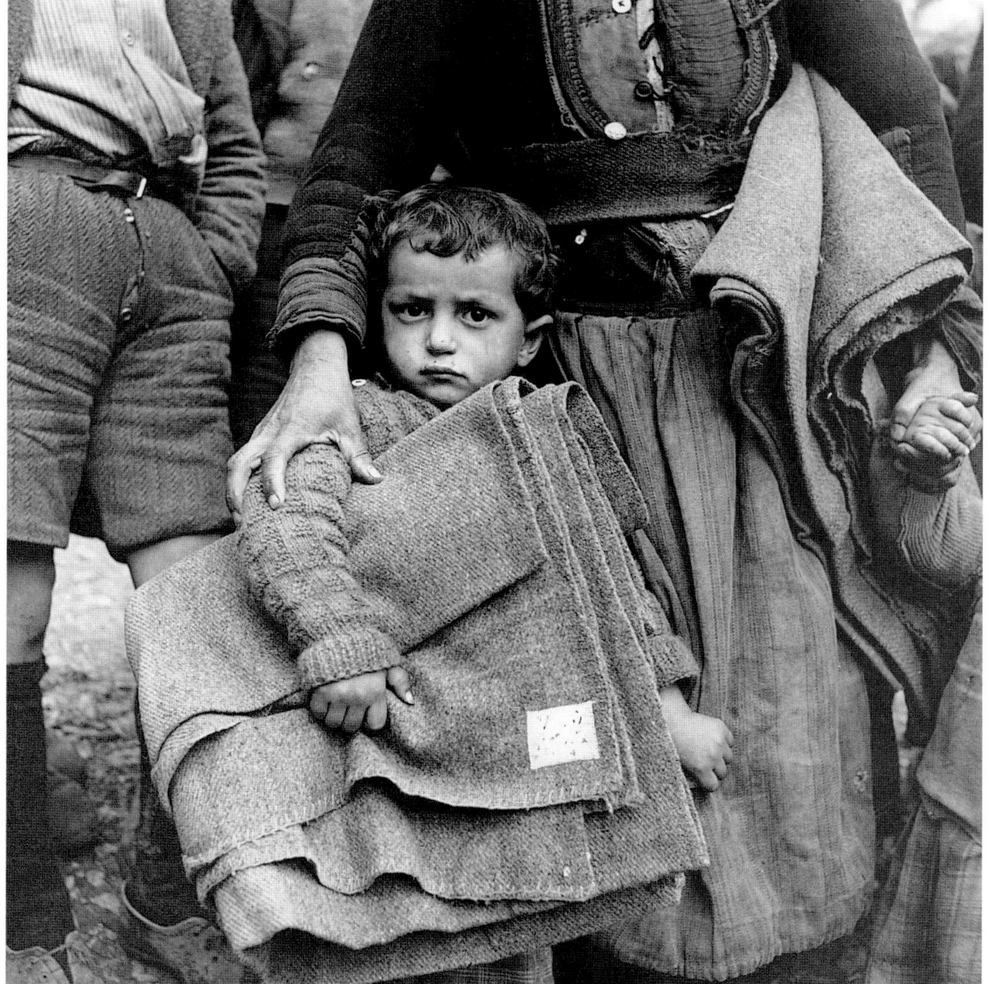

(Above) A refresher course for village midwives in Seoul, South Korea, c. *1955, was part of an ongoing international UNICEF campaign to improve maternal and child health services. (Left) A child, displaced from his Greek mountain village during World War II, holds a blanket furnished by UNICEF along with other relief supplies, including soap, daily food and milk rations, and medicine.*

Photographs, UNICEF; (top) ICEF-2090/Breitenbach; (above) ICEF-0318 adequate relief, largely in the form of powdered milk from the U.S., to the children of war-devastated Europe and China. The UN General Assembly quickly realized, however, that the need for international assistance would persist as long as children around the world continued to suffer from poverty, hunger, and sickness. In 1953 UNICEF was confirmed as a permanent part of the UN family of organizations.

During the 1950s UNICEF's key activities focused on massive vaccination campaigns to control epidemics of infectious diseases such as yaws and tuberculosis (TB). Health care workers in Indonesia were treating 100,000 yaws cases a month with penicillin, while 3.5 million children worldwide were being tested for TB and over one million vaccinated for that disease. UNICEF continues to support immunization programs that, ultimately, prevent the deaths of millions of children each year.

Toward a monumental convention

The 1960s—the UN's first "Decade of Development" and a time when many poor nations were becoming independent states—saw

Health workers in Indonesia examine a child for signs of yaws, a highly contagious and disfiguring tropical disease that primarily affects youngsters. UNICEF helped lead the fight against yaws, contributing both medical assistance and large supplies of penicillin, which easily cures the infection.

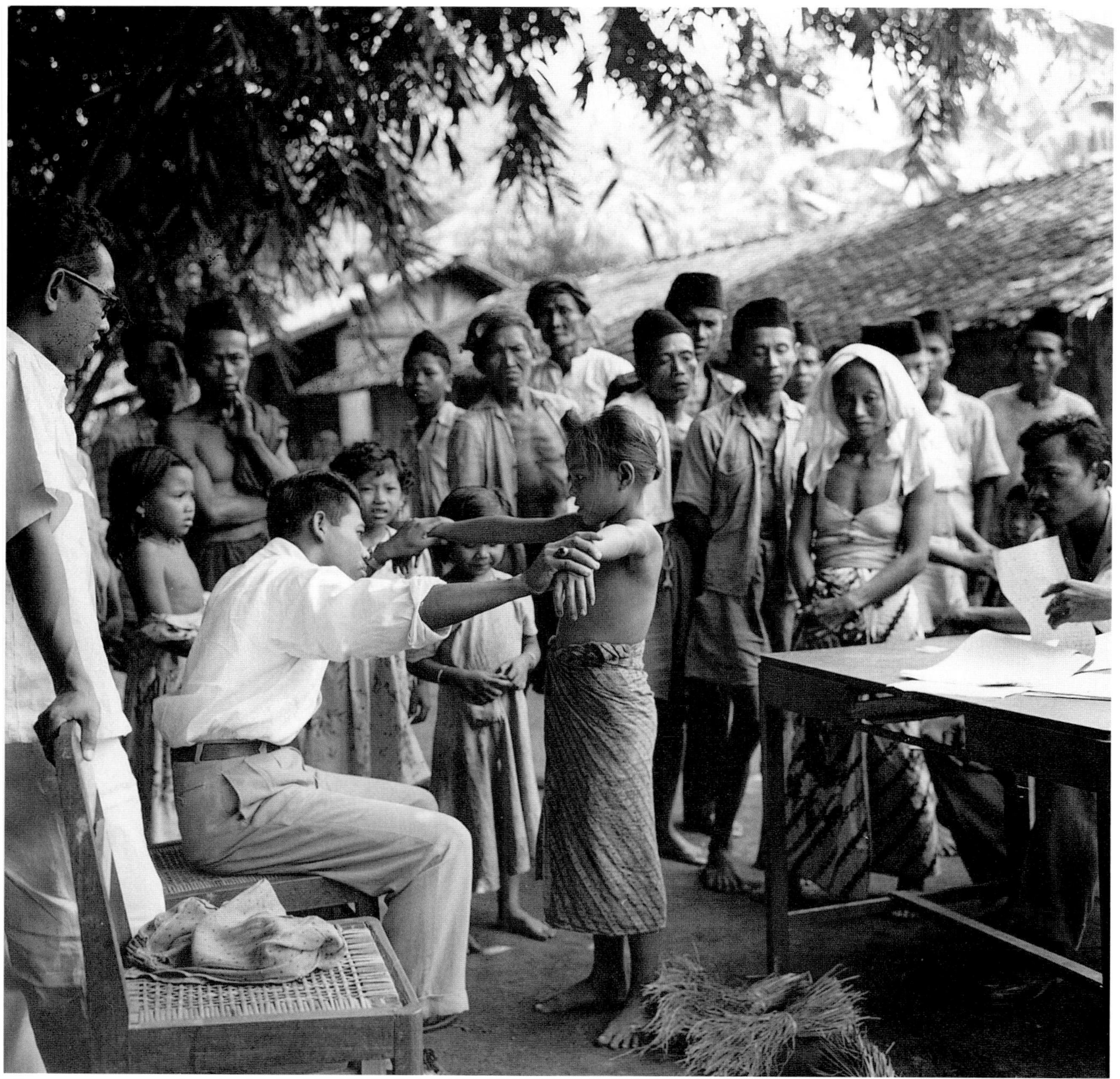

UNICEF/ICEF-3895/Jack Ling

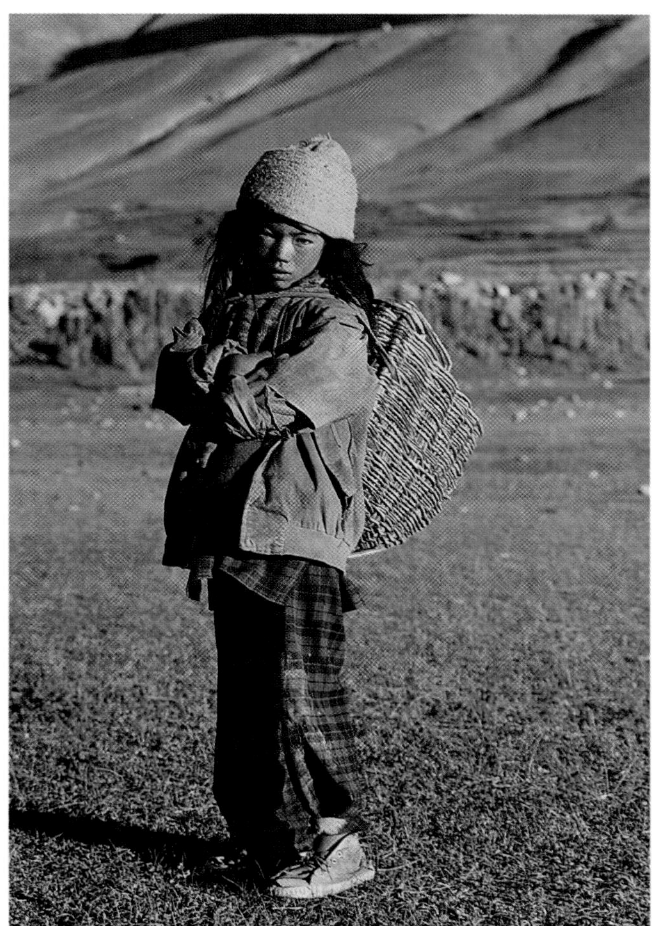

UNICEF take on a broader role. In its wider focus the organization continued to combat childhood diseases but also concerned itself with the "whole" child, sponsoring diverse public health and educational programs. In the 1970s rich-versus-poor and developmental issues were still at the forefront, during which time UNICEF adopted a basic-services approach to help poor communities. The 1980s saw a return to primary concern for children's health issues through the application of appropriate—and inexpensive—technology. Some 12 million children, who might otherwise have perished, lived to see the end of the decade. By the end of the '80s, children's rights issues were being added to UNICEF's already full plate, and the landmark 1989 Convention on the Rights of the Child provided an international framework for concerted action that would continue through the 1990s. To date, the convention on children's rights has been ratified by all but two UN member states: Somalia and the United States.

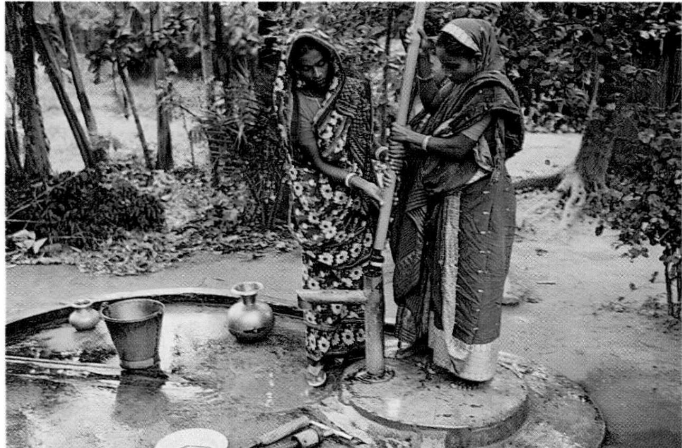

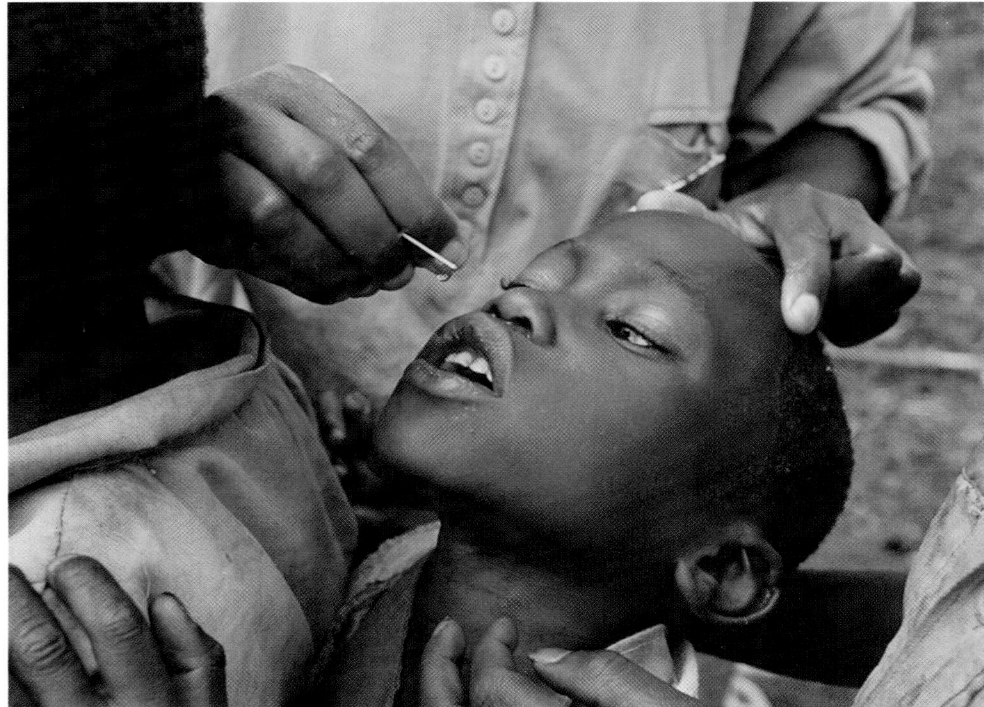

UNICEF upholds the most fundamental rights of children: to receive an education and not be forced into labor, to have access to clean water and proper sanitation, and to be protected against major preventable childhood diseases. (Clockwise from above) A child laborer in a remote mountain hamlet of India gathers fuel rather than attending school; Bangladeshi women install a freshwater pump in a village near Mirzapur; a Rwandan child in the Ndosho refugee camp in Zaire receives vitamin A drops to protect against blindness.

Photographs, UNICEF; (top) C114-17/Franck Charton; (center) 90-227/Jorgen Schytte; (above) DOI94-0243/Betty Press

Above politics

From its inception, UNICEF was declared to be above politics, and its founders insisted that material aid go wherever it was needed, to the children of the victorious as well as the vanquished. Accordingly, in the early years its work advanced in Eastern and Western Europe and on both sides of the civil wars in China and Greece. Even in the tense Cold War years of the 1960s and '70s, UNICEF resisted pressures from the contending sides. Acknowledgment for its wartime work came in 1965 when UNICEF was awarded the Nobel Prize for Peace.

The organization has always had remarkable success in attracting public attention and enrolling broad segments of the public to raise funds for its work. "Trick or Treat for UNICEF" has been a mainstay of Halloweens in the United States since 1950. UNICEF greeting cards are lovingly sent and received around the world. Who could have been more representative of the world's children than actor and comedian Danny Kaye, appointed UNICEF's first goodwill ambassador in 1954? Over the years the likes of Sir Peter Ustinov, Liv Ullmann, Harry Belafonte, Audrey Hepburn, Tetsuko Kuroyanagi, and others also served in this capacity, while Sir Edmund Hillary, Youssou N'Dour, Julio Iglesias, Johann Olav Koss, and Judy Collins, among others, have served as UNICEF special representatives. In 1997 the popular American actor Laurence Fishburne went to Liberia on an ambassadorial mission to visit children who had suffered grievously during years of factional conflict in that West African country.

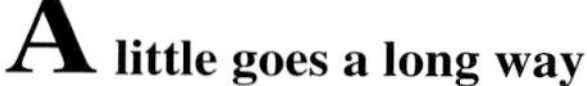

A little goes a long way

UNICEF has always excelled at making a little aid go a long way. The organization helped provide nutrition, medicines, clean water,

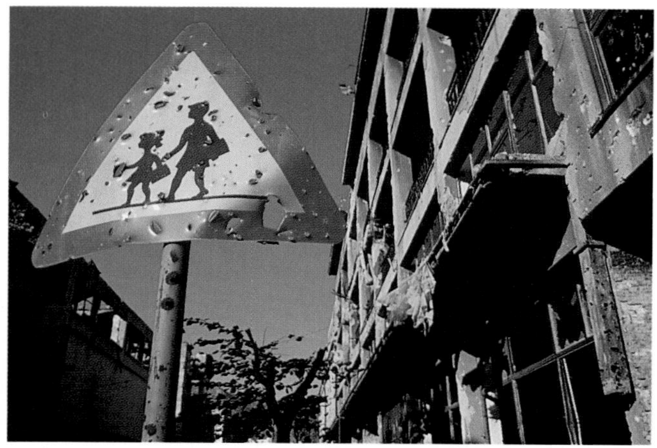

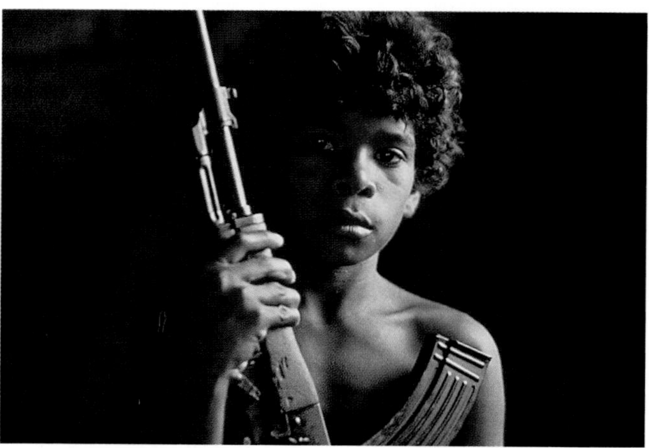

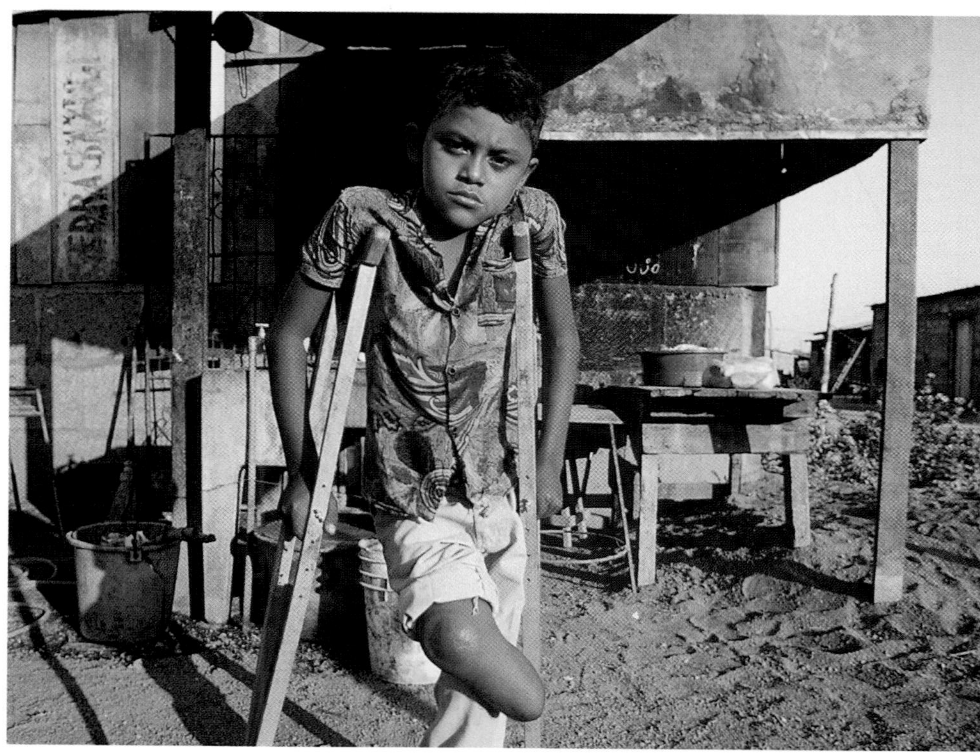

(Top) Amid rows of destroyed buildings in the war-torn city of Mostar, Bosnia and Herzegovina, a street sign advising drivers to proceed with caution and watch for crossing schoolchildren is riddled with bullet holes. (Center) A rifle-bearing Nicaraguan boy-soldier and (right) a 10-year-old whose foot was blown off in a land-mine explosion in Nicaragua's capital, Managua. UNICEF believes that no child under age 15 should take direct part in armed conflict and that children should not be the hapless victims of warring parties.

Photographs, UNICEF; (top) HQ94-091/Roger Lemoyne; (center) 88-091/Aslak Aarbus; (above) C112-4/Jeremy Horner

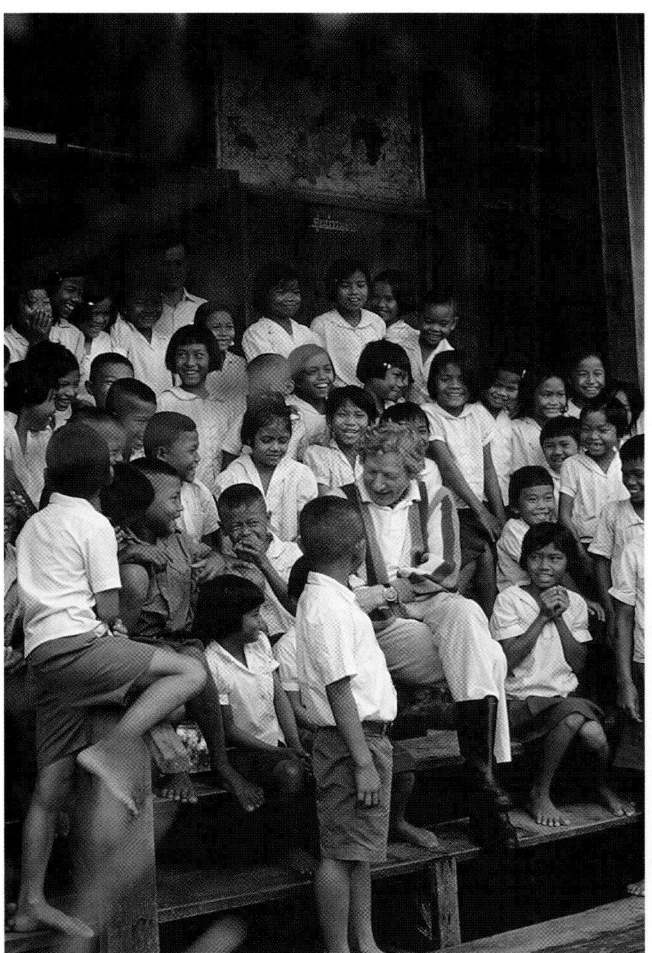

and education to children in 161 countries in 1996 at the cost of almost $1 billion, about one-third of what the Chicago school system spends.

As one example, in 1982 James P. Grant, UNICEF's energetic executive director from 1980 until his death in 1995, launched the "Child Survival and Development Revolution" to demonstrate that high child-mortality rates can be significantly decreased by simple and effective low-cost methods. The four remedies of this program, best remembered by the acronym GOBI—growth monitoring, oral rehydration therapy, breast-feeding, and immunization—are responsible for preventing more than six million deaths annually. One premeasured package of oral rehydration salts, used to treat diarrheal dehydration—among the most common killers of children in the less-developed world—is simple to administer, prevents fatal outcomes under even the most adverse circumstances, and costs only eight cents.

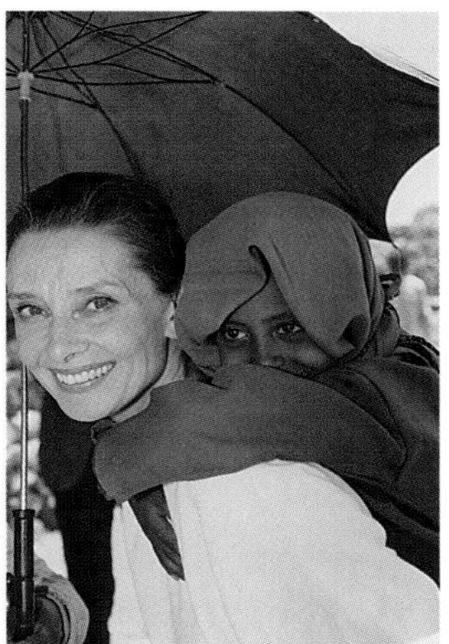

(Far left) Danny Kaye, UNICEF's first goodwill ambassador (1954), brings smiles to the faces of children in Thailand. (Left) Audrey Hepburn, a UNICEF ambassador from 1988 until her death in 1993 and a tireless advocate for Third World children, carries a child in Ethiopia. (Bottom) In August 1994 singer Harry Belafonte paid a six-day goodwill visit to Rwanda, where he visited children in refugee camps and met with Pres. Pasteur Bizimungu. Here he holds nine-month-old Serge, whose mother was injured in the war between the rival Hutu and Tutsi and thus was forced to leave her infant son to be cared for at a UNICEF-assisted center for unaccompanied children.

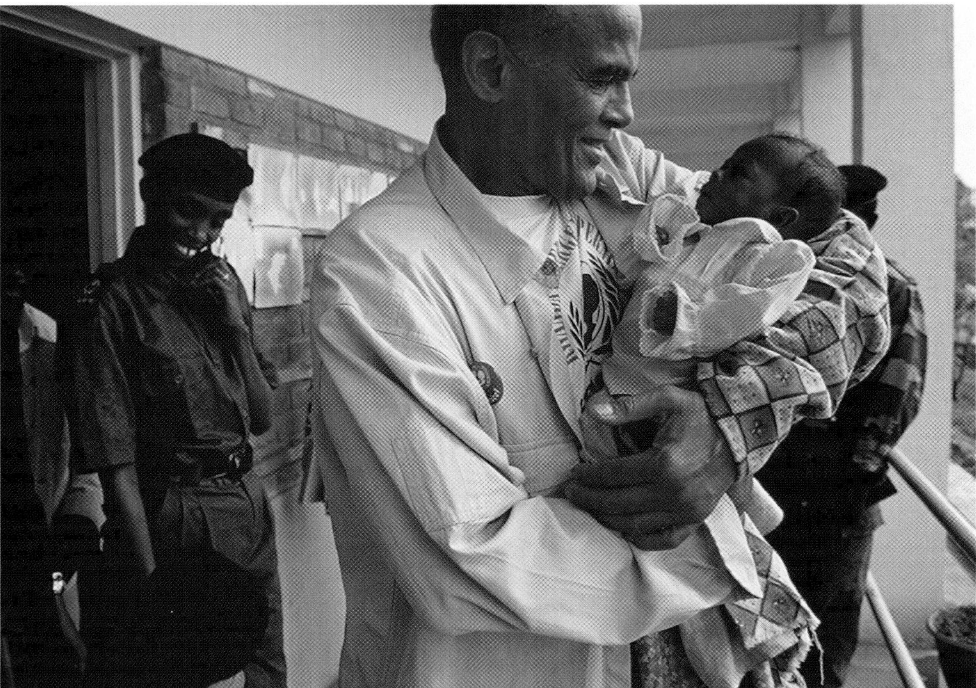

Photographs, UNICEF; (top left) 71-054/Kaufman; (top right) C29-1/John Isaac; (above) 94-0294/Betty Press

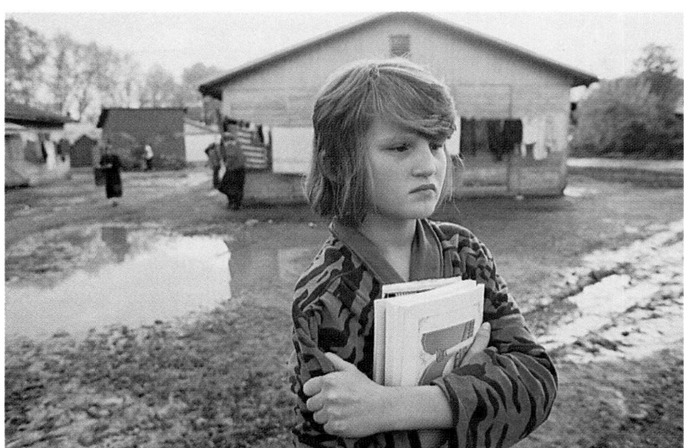

New challenges

Like many other international agencies, UNICEF has recently come under the scrutiny of some who are concerned by swelling bureaucracies and rising administrative costs within the UN system. The organization's executive director, Carol Bellamy, acknowledged those concerns in her address to the executive board in January 1997: "To do our work effectively, UNICEF must be an efficient and well-managed agency, and we continue to work towards that end."

UNICEF *is* set to continue its child-centered work into the next century. Meantime, millions upon millions of children and under-50 adults around the world have good reason to celebrate. They owe their lives to the work of this singular organization.

—Afrodite Mantzavrakos

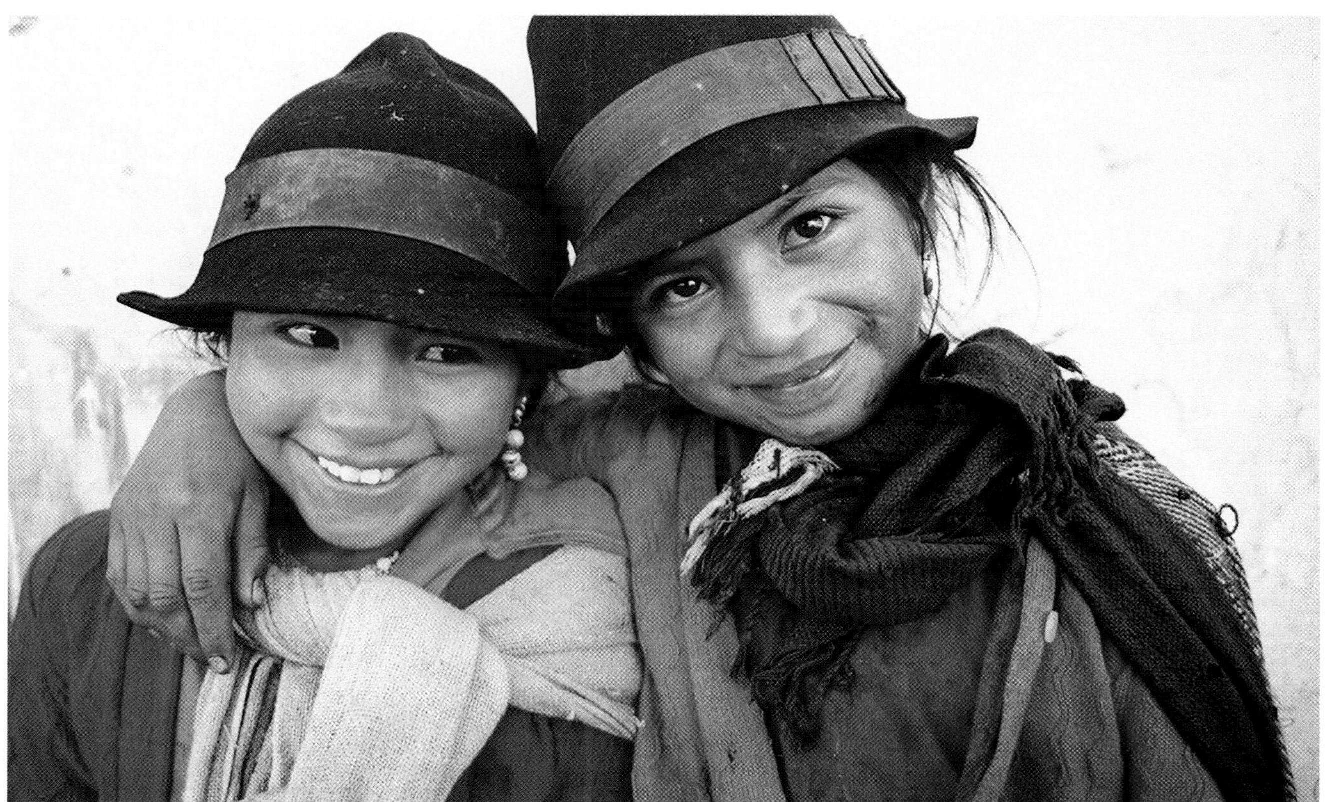

Thanks in large measure to the leading role played by UNICEF, "a century that began with children having virtually no rights is ending with children having the most powerful legal instrument [the landmark Convention on the Rights of the Child] that not only recognizes but protects their human rights." So said Executive Director Carol Bellamy on the occasion of the organization's 50th anniversary. Enjoying their freedoms: (top) an 11-year-old Muslim child in Bosnia and Herzegovina returning home from a religion class; (above) basking in friendship, girls of the Quechua indigenous group in Ecuador; and (right) Moorish girls attending a primary school in Nouakchott, Mauritania.

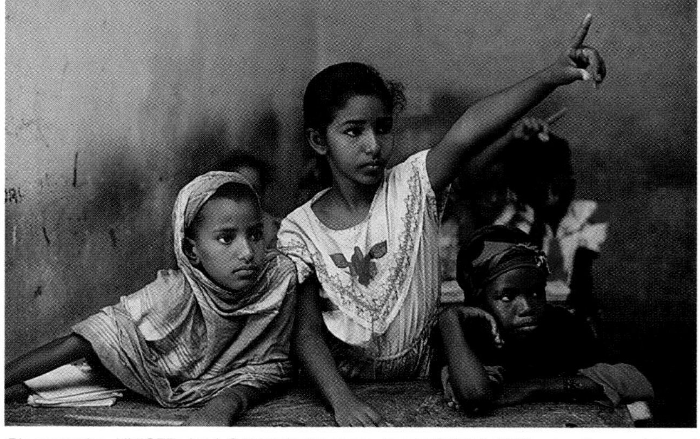

Photographs, UNICEF; (top) C100-6/John Isaac; (center) C104-19/Jeremy Horner; (above) C88-17/Lauren Goodsmith

Itching

Itch is one of the most important, annoying, and mysterious skin sensations. It is related to other common touch sensations—including tickle and pain—but it is different. Itch undoubtedly serves some useful purpose, but aside from triggering scratching, which can dislodge bugs or other irritants from the skin, it is not clear why, for example, a mosquito bite should continue to itch long after the insect has gone. Itch is a common feature of many skin disorders, ranging from poison ivy to eczema to psoriasis (*see* Table, page 215). It also occurs as a consequence of certain diseases of internal organs such as the liver or kidney. Occasionally, generalized itching may occur as the earliest sign of a serious condition such as hyperthyroidism or Hodgkin's disease (a cancer of the lymphatic system). Itching as a sign of serious internal illness is extremely uncommon, however, and can present difficult diagnostic challenges to the physician.

Any person who has had an unexplained itch or an itchy rash for more than a few weeks should consult a physician. At some point a specialist—a dermatologist—may need to be consulted as well. Dermatologists are medical doctors with special training and expertise in diseases of the skin, hair, nails, and mucous membranes. Some skin diseases can be diagnosed simply by their clinical appearance; some require a biopsy (removal of a small piece of skin for examination under the microscope); and others may require a variety of other laboratory tests. In some cases skin scrapings can be examined microscopically to diagnose fungal infections such as ringworm or infestations with mites or other parasites.

The itch sensation

In medical jargon itching—the symptom—is called *pruritus.* Itch is defined as an unpleasant sensation that provokes the desire to scratch. One of the curious mysteries of itching, though, is that it is not always entirely unpleasant. How else to explain the adage "One scratch is too many; a thousand are not enough"?

The skin is the body's major interface with and barrier to the external environment. Nerves in the skin detect heat and cold, touch, pressure, vibration, and pain. For many years scientists thought that itching was merely a variety of pain. It now appears that although it is related to pain, itch is a separate sensation. For one thing, scientists have found that some drugs that relieve pain (morphine, for example) can actually cause itching. For another, experiments have shown that very severe itching does not turn into pain. Furthermore, while the normal reaction to a sudden pain is a quick, reflexive withdrawal, the normal reaction to itching is simply to scratch. These are just some of the facts that support the conclusion that itch is not just a "little pain."

Cutaneous sensations are carried from the skin to the central nervous system by a number of different kinds of nerves. The nerves for some sensations, such as pressure and vibration, have special structures at their endings in the skin. Under the microscope some of these look like tiny onions. The nerves for both itch and pain, however, end simply by branching into progressively smaller fibers. These so-called free nerve endings can be activated by a variety of chemicals and physical stimuli. Once triggered, the nerve endings for itch send a signal along nerves that travel to the spinal cord. Nerves in the spinal cord then transmit the itch sensation to the brain. Once the signal has reached the spinal cord or brain, scratching may occur as either a conscious or an unconscious (reflex) response.

Partly because of the mistaken notion that itch is just a minor form of pain, and partly because research dollars are directed toward more pressing problems such as cancer and heart disease, itch research has been something of a neglected field. Other reasons for the slow progress in itch research include the difficulties inherent in studying a subjective sensation and the fact that there is no particularly good animal model for itching. Over the past 10 years, however, advances in biochemistry, pharmacology, neurophysiology, and clinical medicine have resulted in new understanding of the underlying causes of itching—and, most important, improved treatments for those troubled by itch. Indeed, the study of itch is a very good example of a field in which close clinical observation has yielded as many useful insights as laboratory research.

One of the most exciting recent advances has been the discovery that a group of molecules called opioid peptides seem to play an important role in several types of itching, such as the severe itching that accompanies primary biliary cirrhosis (an autoimmune disease of the liver). Even more exciting is the recent observation

Sensations are carried from the skin to the brain by many different kinds of nerves. A cross-sectional diagram of the skin shows the branching structure of the free nerve endings that transmit the itch and pain sensations.

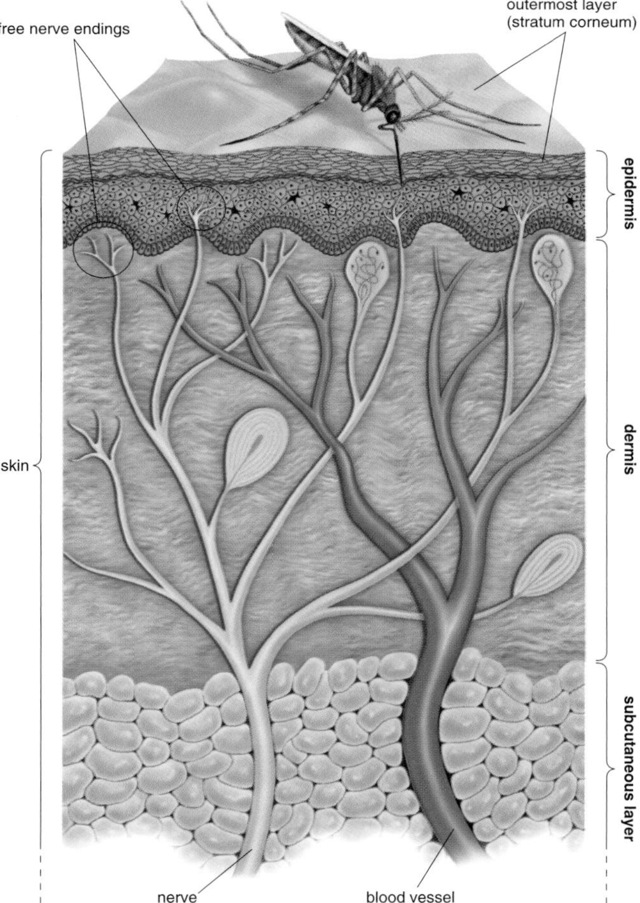

Sheila Terry—Science Source/Photo Researchers

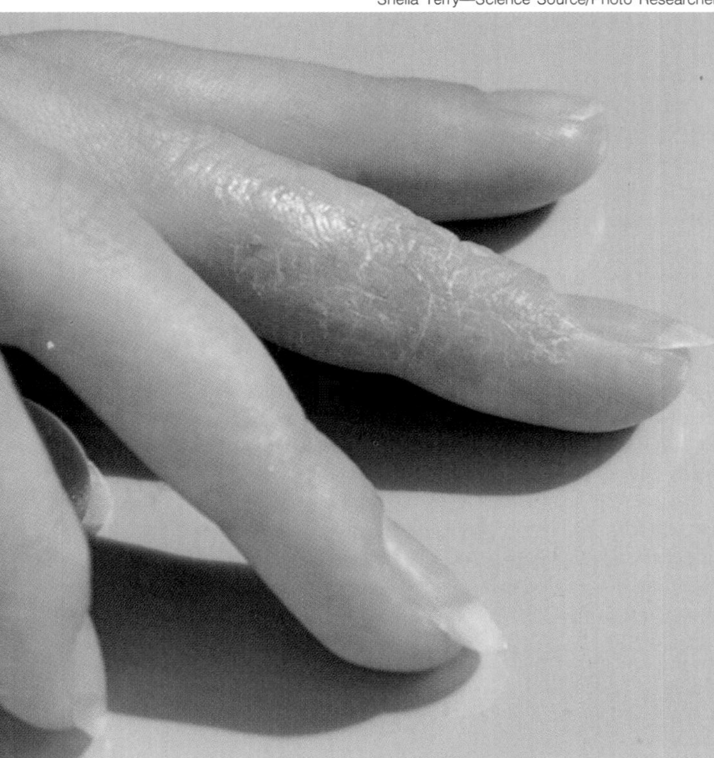

The skin on the third finger of this woman's hand has the scaly redness that is characteristic of atopic dermatitis, or eczema, one of the most common dermatologic conditions associated with the symptom of pruritus—or, more simply, itching.

that substances that interfere with the action of opioid peptides, the so-called opiate antagonists (*e.g.,* naloxone, naltrexone), can block itching in certain experimental settings. Before these exciting findings can be translated into relief for patients, however, much clinical research remains to be done.

Other naturally existing chemicals involved in the itch sensation include histamine, the prostaglandins, certain enzymes, and, almost certainly, a number of other substances that play a part in inflammation. The number and diversity of chemical substances involved help explain why antihistamines alone are almost never enough to control itching and why the inflammation present in many skin diseases probably causes itching in a variety of different ways. There is, however, one condition, hives (urticaria), in which antihistamines alone often are quite an effective treatment; this is because histamine is the single most important chemical mediator of the localized red, raised wheals seen in this skin reaction.

Why scratching works

> *Scratching is one of the sweetest gratifications of nature, and as ready at hand as any.*
>
> —Michel de Montaigne in "Of Experience"

According to one theory, scratching stimulates a set of nerves that seem to block or short-circuit the nerves carrying the itch signal. Another theory is that scratching simply produces a different, stronger sensation that replaces or overshadows the itch. The latter hypothesis might explain why some people will scratch a mosquito bite to the point of pain rather than put up with the unbearably annoying itch. It might also explain why a variety of remedies—for example, rubbing the area around an itch or applying cool compresses—seem to offer at least temporary relief to some people.

In many skin diseases, however, scratching only increases inflammation and the risk of secondary infection and thus makes things worse. The urge to scratch can, of course, be irresistible; rather than chastising the individual who cannot help scratching, doctors and family members can help most by suggesting ways to reduce the itch.

Cutaneous causes

Perhaps the most common cause of generalized itching is the parching effect of dry, heated indoor air in winter, especially when excessive bathing or the use of harsh soaps adds insult to injury. This condition is often called "winter itch." The physical appearance of extremely dry, itchy skin may be quite normal, giving no clue as to the cause of the discomfort. For this reason it is usually worthwhile for the affected individual to adopt a regimen of less-frequent bathing and liberal application of skin moisturizers before consulting a physician and undergoing expensive diagnostic tests. If skin dryness has led to obvious redness and inflammation as well as itching, a mild topical corticosteroid lotion or cream can be helpful in relieving discomfort. Over-the-counter products may suffice, but prescription-strength corticosteroids, such as triamcinolone or fluocinolone, may sometimes be required.

People who are prone to skin dryness can develop "winter itch" during the summer when they are chronically exposed to the drying effects of air-conditioned and dehumidified air. Other summertime itches include prickly heat (miliaria), which occurs when sweat glands malfunction during exposure to excessive heat, and chafing (irritation due to a combination of sweating and friction). Another fairly common cause of summer itch is "sun poisoning," or polymorphic light eruption, a condition in which itchy red bumps develop on sun-exposed skin several hours after exposure.

Skin diseases, including reactions to external substances such as fiberglass or chemicals, are frequently the cause of itching. Infestation with the scabies mite deserves mention, as it is widespread and often difficult to diagnose. Scabies occurs in people of all socioeconomic groups and can cause itching out of all proportion to the rash that eventually occurs in most people. The scabies mite is transmitted by close, usually intimate, skin-to-skin contact.

Other common skin diseases in which itching plays a significant role include psoriasis, atopic dermatitis (eczema), urticaria, and allergic contact dermatitis. In the latter condition an individual develops an allergic reaction to something he or she has touched or handled—for example, cosmetics, soaps, jewelry, poison ivy, or chemicals encountered on the job. The rash is usually red and scaly, but, when acute, it may include small to large blisters, as are seen in poison ivy. The main clues to the diagnosis of allergic contact dermatitis, aside from the history of exposure, are the tell-tale shape of the rash and its localization to areas where the offending agent is known to have come into contact with the skin.

Such reactions have become increasingly less common as the cosmetics and toiletries industries have developed better skin-care products. Most such products now undergo extensive testing, and known chemical culprits are avoided. However, new chemicals and preservatives are constantly being introduced, and a product a person has trusted for years may be reformulated without warning. Ironically, a number of over-the-counter skin-care products, even including some products specifically intended to relieve itching, contain ingredients to which some people become allergic. Certain preservatives, antibiotics such as neomycin, and topical anesthetic agents are examples of such ingredients. Nickel in earrings and other jewelry can cause an allergic reaction in some people.

Itching induced by elastic waistbands, bra straps, and the like can have a variety of causes. Some people are allergic to certain ingredients of clothing, elastic, or rubberized fabrics; in these cases the rash of allergic dermatitis will almost always be apparent. In a rare condition called delayed pressure urticaria, patients develop hivelike swelling and itching at pressure sites, often several hours after the pressure has been released. It is not unusual, however, for people who do not have this condition to experience itching at pressure points as soon as a tight or binding garment has been removed. Such itching is probably related to a rebound firing of cutaneous nerves that were previously suppressed by pressure, although no one knows for sure if this is the explanation.

Some of the less-common dermatologic diseases that are associated with itching include lichen planus (an inflammatory condition characterized by the development of tiny papules, which may coalesce to form larger scaly patches), mastocytosis (a disorder of the histamine-releasing mast cells), and the immunologic diseases dermatitis herpetiformis and bullous pemphigoid. Of course, hundreds of other skin diseases, too numerous to list here, can also cause itch.

Other causes

As noted above, in rare instances itching may be a sign of internal, sometimes serious, illness. In some such cases a rash may be present as a result of continued rubbing and scratching. In others there is no rash at all, even though the itching is severe. The absence of any recognizable specific skin disease may be an important clue that some other cause is to blame. Since the visible signs of winter itch, external irritants, and subtle skin diseases may be quite similar, it is important that individuals with unexplained itching not panic or jump to conclusions about the cause of the problem.

Drug reactions are an important cause of unexplained itching. Almost any drug, even aspirin, can cause itching, with or without a rash. Drug reaction should be suspected any time a person notices that itching started within a few weeks of starting a new medication. Some of the agents most commonly linked to itching (without a rash) are opiate analgesics such as morphine, hormones such as estrogen, antimalarials such as chloroquine, and antibiotics such as sulfonamides.

Kidney failure is another very important cause of itching, although itching is almost never the first symptom. Certain liver diseases, especially those associated with cholestasis (obstruction of bile flow), also may have among their symptoms generalized itching. The blood disorder polycythemia vera (a disease of the bone marrow that affects primarily middle-aged and older men) causes a very curious itch that characteristically occurs after bathing. But most people who itch after a shower or bath do not have a blood disorder; they have a "pruritic curiosity" called aquagenic pruritus (*i.e.,* itching caused by water). As noted at the outset, hyperthyroidism, Hodgkin's disease, and parasitic infestations are among the other systemic causes of itching, but again, these are quite uncommon.

Pruritic curiosities

It is often said that everyone has his or her "own little itch." For some people it may be a spot on one foot that itches as soon as they take off their shoes or lie down to go to sleep. For others it may be an itch that begins only when it is time to practice the piano or violin. (Many children experience this phenomenon.) Or it may be an itch that cannot be scratched because the person's hands are full or he or she is giving a lecture or is in the middle of performing brain surgery. This desire to scratch at times when it is not possible to do so has been called "pruritus prohibitus." Another curious itch is the *mitempfindungen,* or "referred itch," that occurs in a certain spot every time another specific spot is scratched. Referred itch is probably related to neural pathways in the central nervous system that are triggered unintentionally when a particular itch is scratched.

Some itches seem to be related to the unique pathways of nerves that supply certain areas of the skin. One such sensation, called "notalgia paresthetica," occurs around the upper middle of the back. U.S. cartoonist and writer Shel Silverstein wrote a poem, "Unscratchable Itch," about it. Although these itches are annoy-

Itching: Some Dermatologic Causes

Infestations
- Scabies (mites)
- Lace

Inflammatory disorders
- Dermatitis herpetiformis (chronic eruption marked by papules and small blisters; may be autoimmune)
- Bullous pemphigoid (chronic eruption marked by blisterlike lesions; autoimmune)
- Atopic dermatitis (eczema)
- Allergic contact dermatitis
- Psoriasis
- Lichen planus (eruption characterized by papules that may combine into larger scaly patches)
- Urticaria (hives)
- Drug reactions

Infections
- Chicken pox
- Fungal infection
- Folliculitis (inflammation of follicles)

External causes
- Fiberglass
- Irritants (detergents, cosmetics, wool, urine)
- Insect bites

Miscellaneous
- Dry skin
- Miliaria (prickly heat)
- Anogenital itch (many causes)
- Sunburn
- Mastocytosis (proliferation of mast cells)

Adapted from Jeffrey D. Bernhard, M.D. *Itch: Mechanisms and Management of Pruritus.* New York: McGraw-Hill, 1994.

ing, they are not serious, and some helpful topical treatments are available.

Roles of stress and aging

Stress-related itching is extremely rare. Although it is entirely fair to say that stress can exacerbate itching, it is more often a triggering factor than an underlying cause. Certain psychiatric illnesses and psychiatric medications are known to cause itching. In delusional parasitosis patients develop a delusional belief that they have a parasitic infestation. This condition can be difficult to diagnose and treat. In some cases itching may be a consequence of another mysterious problem called tactile hallucinosis, in which the presence of an underlying itchy, crawly, or tingly sensation convinces patients they must have an infestation. A number of medications (*e.g.,* pimozide) seem to be effective in treating either the underlying tactile hallucinosis, the delusion, or both, which is why psychiatric consultation can be critical in such cases.

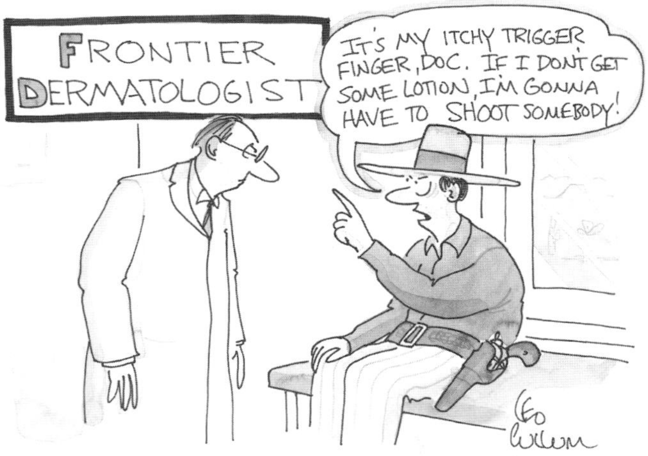

Most dermatology textbooks mention a type of itching in the elderly called senile pruritus. The term is applied when all other known, and more common, causes of itching have been excluded. In practice, most cases of itching in elderly individuals are related to either dry skin (winter itch), drug reactions, skin diseases, or underlying systemic illnesses such as cerebrovascular disease or renal failure. In some cases, however, no such cause can be determined. One theory is that such itching is a result of changes in the nervous system associated with the aging process, which lead to a malfunction of certain cutaneous sensations.

Evaluation and treatment

Itching lasting more than a few weeks with no apparent cause should be brought to the attention of an internist, pediatrician, or family physician or a dermatologist. It is entirely reasonable for either a primary care provider or a specialist to begin an evaluation. The first order of business is careful examination of the skin for primary skin diseases or evidence of an infestation such as scabies. If the skin exam is inconclusive, a complete medical history and physical examination are warranted. Blood tests and X-rays certainly are not indicated in every case but may be considered when the history or physical examination suggests that they may be worthwhile. People whose itching goes on for more than a few months should be periodically reevaluated.

Because itch is a symptom for which there is no specific "cure," correct diagnosis is the cornerstone of treatment. In fact, no symptomatic treatment exists for itching that is as effective as aspirin is for pain. Specific skin diseases respond to specific treatments—for example, topical permethrin for scabies, topical corticosteroids for eczema, phototherapy for certain kinds of psoriasis, and treatment with systemic drugs (oral corticosteroids) for bullous pemphigoid. Because of this specificity and because itching can be a sign of internal disease, self-treatment for more than a few weeks is not a good idea. By providing temporary relief while the underlying cause is ignored, prolonged self-treatment may allow a potentially serious condition to progress unchecked.

Whatever the underlying cause of itching, it is almost always worthwhile to eliminate or at least reduce triggering factors such as skin dryness, exposure to fabrics that may irritate the skin (*e.g.,* wool), stress, and overheating (as from sleeping under too many blankets). Topical agents that may dry out the skin (for example, rubbing alcohol) or products that have the potential to cause allergic contact dermatitis should also be avoided.

Some symptomatic relief can be obtained from moisturizing lotions, and those that contain menthol provide the additional benefit of a cooling sensation. Other helpful ingredients include urea, lactic acid, and glycolic and other alpha-hydroxy acids. Aloe is very popular but can cause allergic reactions in some people. One old favorite, and still one of the most effective remedies for dry, itchy skin, is petroleum jelly, which works by holding moisture in the skin, especially if applied right after bathing. A number of excellent products are available, and many of them are not expensive. Personal preference and trial and error are usually the best guides.

Bathing in tepid water can increase the moisture content of the skin, and adding old-fashioned ingredients like oatmeal, oilated oatmeal, or moisturizing oils to the bath can help by holding moisture in the skin. Anti-itch powders also may provide relief by permitting air to circulate near the skin and by reducing friction. Some powders have soothing qualities in themselves; others contain antifungal agents, which are helpful when itching is due to fungal infection, or hydrocortisone, which has a mild anti-inflammatory effect.

In some cases medical treatment is necessary to relieve itching. Ultraviolet phototherapy, for example, can be very helpful in a variety of itches, especially the kind associated with kidney failure. Conventional antihistamines are sometimes helpful because the drowsiness they cause takes the "edge" off the itch. Certain topical anesthetics and antihistamines help some people, at least temporarily. Capsaicin, the active ingredient of hot peppers, can sometimes provide relief for certain very localized itches such as notalgia paresthetica, but it is not practical for application to large areas. Patients with certain types of liver disease may benefit from a variety of special oral prescription medications, but here again, correct diagnosis and careful ongoing supervision by a physician are essential.

—*Jeffrey D. Bernhard, M.D.*

Carotenoids: Can Carrots Prevent Cancer, Cataracts, and Coronaries?

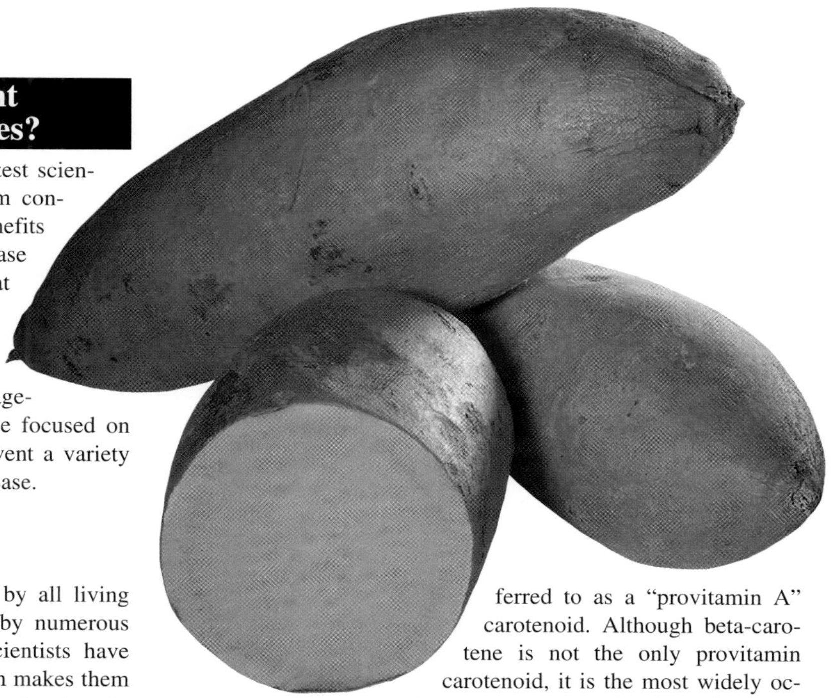

It is ironic that sophisticated inquiries using the latest scientific methodology sometimes serve only to confirm conventional wisdom. Knowledge about the health benefits of the natural substances called carotenoids is a case in point. Generations of children have been told that eating carrots will help them to have good eyesight, but it was only recently that scientists found that carotenoids—chemical compounds present in certain fruits and vegetables—may help prevent age-related vision loss. Other recent investigations have focused on the potential of carotenoid-containing foods to prevent a variety of chronic diseases, including cancer and heart disease.

"Nature's paint"

Carotenoids are natural pigments. They are made by all living organisms that carry out photosynthesis and also by numerous nonphotosynthetic bacteria and fungi. To date, scientists have identified more than 600 different carotenoids, which makes them among the most abundant natural pigments on Earth. Genetic mutations affecting early steps in carotenoid biosynthesis are fatal to plants—evidence that they require these compounds for survival.

As "nature's paint," the carotenoids come in a variety of hues (mainly yellows, oranges, and reds) and can be seen in a variety of species. The most widely known is the orange carotenoid beta-carotene. The characteristic bright orange color of the root of the carrot plant (the portion that is eaten) is a result of the accumulation of beta-carotene and other carotenoids. Other foods that derive color from carotenoids include corn, tomatoes, red peppers, oranges, apricots, cantaloupe, and watermelon. Daffodils owe their colorful yellow flowers to carotenoids. The presence of carotenoids in the leaves of deciduous trees is usually masked by the green pigment chlorophyll but becomes evident in autumn when the chlorophyll begins to break down. Carotenoids are also largely responsible for the vibrant pink and red of salmon, lobsters, crabs, flamingos, and numerous insects. Fish, birds, mammals, and insects do not make their own carotenoids but instead acquire them by eating carotenoid-rich plants and microorganisms.

Provitamins and antioxidants

Research into the relationship of carotenoids to human health began in 1929 when it was discovered that beta-carotene was a precursor to the essential nutrient vitamin A. (A precursor is a substance from which another substance is formed.) For this reason beta-carotene is often referred to as a "provitamin A" carotenoid. Although beta-carotene is not the only provitamin carotenoid, it is the most widely occurring and is considered to have the greatest potential for conversion to vitamin A. The vitamin A value of a carotenoid depends on its chemical structure. In addition to beta-carotene, the other major provitamin A carotenoids are alpha- and gamma-carotene and cryptoxanthin. Alpha- and gamma-carotene often accompany beta-carotene in foods; cryptoxanthin can be found in a variety of foods, including corn, pumpkin, peppers, and squash.

As much as two-thirds of the world's population relies on the provitamin A carotenoids to meet most of their requirement for vitamin A. In the United States, where meats and dairy products are an integral part of the diet, vitamin A deficiency is uncommon. This is not the case in many less-developed nations. The World Health Organization estimates that 230 million children currently suffer from vitamin A deficiency; every year as many as 350,000 children become partially or totally blind as a direct result of this deficiency, and around one million die from deficiency-related conditions.

In addition to serving as a source of vitamin A, carotenoids also contribute to health through their function as antioxidants. Human cells are continuously being challenged by free radicals, unstable molecules (especially oxygen molecules) that seek to achieve stability by giving up electrons; ultimately this process can damage the DNA—the genetic material of the cells—and this damage is believed to play a part in many chronic diseases. Air pollution, radiation, ultraviolet light, and cigarette smoke are among the many substances in the environment that induce the body to form free radicals. Even normal

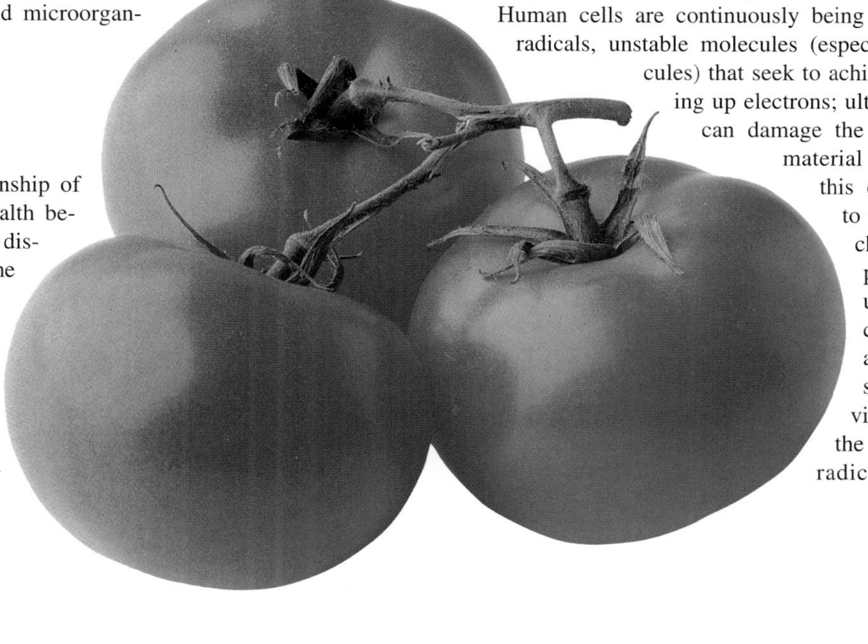

Photographs, Joel DeGrand

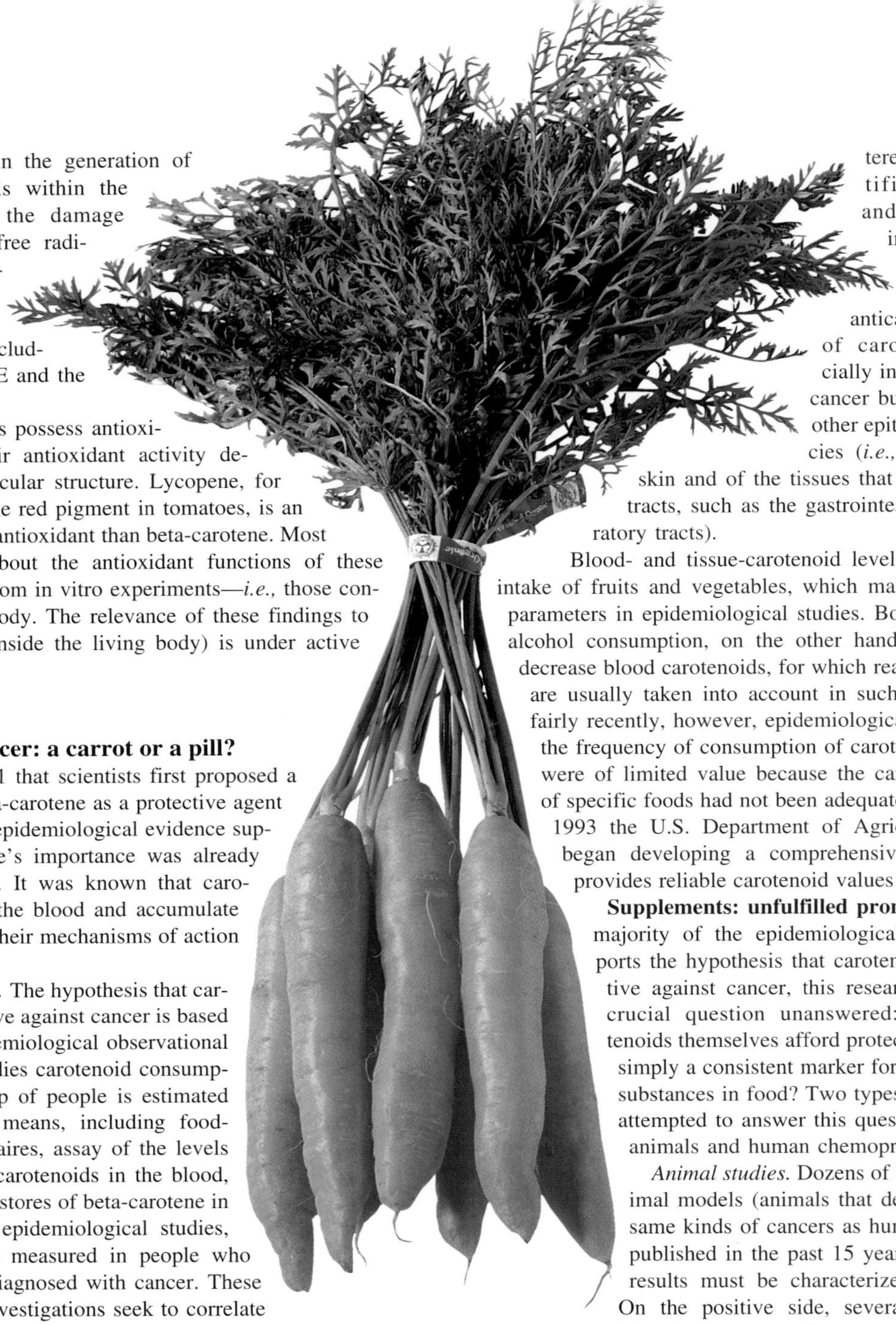

metabolism results in the generation of oxygen free radicals within the cells. To mitigate the damage caused by oxygen free radicals—so-called oxidative damage—the body relies, in part, upon antioxidants, including vitamins C and E and the carotenoids.

Not all carotenoids possess antioxidant properties; their antioxidant activity depends on their molecular structure. Lycopene, for example, which is the red pigment in tomatoes, is an even more effective antioxidant than beta-carotene. Most of what is know about the antioxidant functions of these compounds comes from in vitro experiments—*i.e.,* those conducted outside the body. The relevance of these findings to processes in vivo (inside the living body) is under active investigation.

Combating cancer: a carrot or a pill?

It was not until 1981 that scientists first proposed a possible role for beta-carotene as a protective agent against cancer. The epidemiological evidence supporting beta-carotene's importance was already beginning to mount. It was known that carotenoids circulate in the blood and accumulate in body tissues, but their mechanisms of action were still unclear.

The data on diet. The hypothesis that carotenoids are protective against cancer is based on a variety of epidemiological observational studies. In these studies carotenoid consumption in a large group of people is estimated by any of several means, including food-frequency questionnaires, assay of the levels of beta-carotene or carotenoids in the blood, and measurement of stores of beta-carotene in body fat. In many epidemiological studies, carotenoid intake is measured in people who have already been diagnosed with cancer. These retrospective-type investigations seek to correlate carotenoid consumption with disease incidence. The carotenoid intake of the population with the disease is then compared with that of a similar group who are disease-free. In other, so-called prospective studies, intake of specific food items is evaluated periodically in a group of initially healthy individuals, and occurrence of disease is monitored over time—usually for many years. Prospective studies are often considered less-biased or more reliable than retrospective studies, as dietary intake is determined long before the disease status of participants is known.

In 1992 a group of scientists analyzed the existing epidemiological data on diet and lung cancer. They found that of 25 studies, 24 showed that populations with diets rich in fruits and vegetables had a reduced risk of the disease. According to this research, both smokers and nonsmokers benefited from eating beta-carotene-rich foods. This dramatic finding captured the interest of the scientific community and provided the impetus for further investigation of the anticancer properties of carotenoids, especially in relation to lung cancer but also for many other epithelial malignancies (*i.e.,* cancers of the skin and of the tissues that line organs and tracts, such as the gastrointestinal and respiratory tracts).

Blood- and tissue-carotenoid levels reflect dietary intake of fruits and vegetables, which makes them useful parameters in epidemiological studies. Both smoking and alcohol consumption, on the other hand, are known to decrease blood carotenoids, for which reason these habits are usually taken into account in such research. Until fairly recently, however, epidemiological data based on the frequency of consumption of carotenoid-rich foods were of limited value because the carotenoid content of specific foods had not been adequately measured. In 1993 the U.S. Department of Agriculture (USDA) began developing a comprehensive database that provides reliable carotenoid values for many foods.

Supplements: unfulfilled promise. While a majority of the epidemiological evidence supports the hypothesis that carotenoids are protective against cancer, this research has left one crucial question unanswered: Do the carotenoids themselves afford protection, or are they simply a consistent marker for other protective substances in food? Two types of studies have attempted to answer this question: research in animals and human chemoprevention trials.

Animal studies. Dozens of studies using animal models (animals that develop much the same kinds of cancers as humans) have been published in the past 15 years. Overall, their results must be characterized as equivocal. On the positive side, several investigations have demonstrated that beta-carotene is protective against skin tumors in rats and mice. The carotenoid canthaxanthin has been shown to protect against mammary tumors in rats exposed to an environmental carcinogen. Alpha-carotene inhibits certain liver tumors in rats as well as several skin cancers in mice, and lutein and lycopene have been found to protect against some animal tumors. On the negative side, several studies of colon cancer in rats have found no protective effect for beta-carotene (although they did confirm the preventive role of other carotenoids such as lycopene and alpha-carotene). Adding to the confusion, experiments repeated in different strains of laboratory animals have had contradictory results.

Rats and mice have been extensively studied in cancer research, and many strains have been bred exclusively for this purpose. More is known about the disease in these animals than in any other species. An inherent problem in using rodents as models, however, is that they metabolize beta-carotene differently from humans. Humans can absorb beta-carotene intact and can readily accumulate substantial amounts in their blood and tissues. Rats and mice, in contrast, do not readily absorb beta-carotene. Instead, they convert it to vitamin A in the small intestine with tremendous efficiency. In order for beta-carotene to be detectable in the blood or tissues of these animals, they must be fed very large doses—doses greatly exceeding what humans would consume in foods or take as supplements. The development of an experimental animal model that metabolizes beta-carotene similarly to humans and that could be adapted to the study of cancer would be of enormous value in this field.

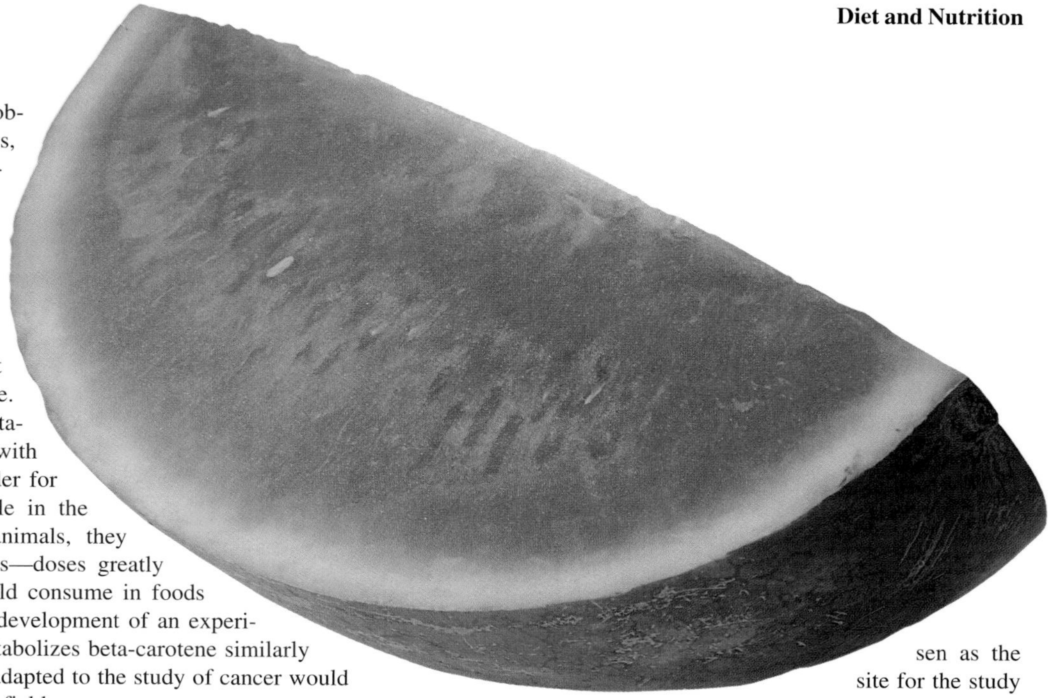

Human trials. Interest in human cancer chemoprevention—the use of synthetic compounds to ward off the disease—grew in the mid- to late 1980s, and by 1990 several chemoprevention trials had been launched. Encouraged by the possibility that a pill could prevent cancer, consumers began taking beta-carotene supplements with increasing frequency. As the results of the scientific trials started to appear, however, it quickly became clear that the enthusiasm for supplements was premature.

The findings of the first and perhaps most publicized controlled human cancer chemoprevention trial, widely known as the Finnish smokers study, were published in 1994. Finland was chosen as the site for the study because of the unusually high rate of lung cancer in men in that country. In the trial some 29,000 Finnish men, aged 50–69 years at the outset and all of them longtime smokers, were given a supplement containing beta-carotene alone or in combination with vitamin E (alpha-tocopherol) or a placebo. The groups receiving beta-carotene took 20 mg per day (about four times the recommended intake from fruits and vegetables) for an average of 6.1 years. Upon conclusion of the study, it was revealed that the men who took the beta-carotene supplement had 18% more lung cancers and an 8% higher death rate than those in the other groups. This result most certainly was not what the researchers had expected, and their findings served as a wake-up call for all those who were hoping that dietary supplements would prove to be the proverbial "magic bullet" for cancer.

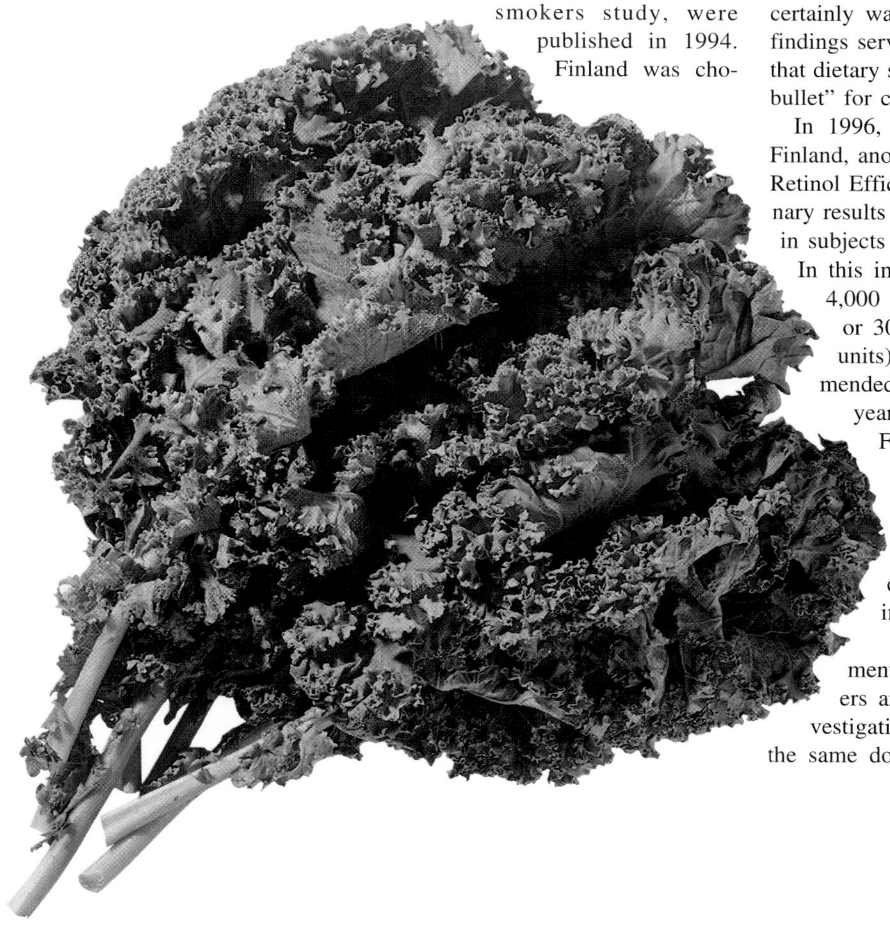

In 1996, a short time after publication of the report from Finland, another human intervention trial, the Beta-Carotene and Retinol Efficacy Trial (CARET), was halted early when preliminary results revealed a 28% higher rate of lung cancer incidence in subjects receiving beta-carotene and vitamin A supplements. In this investigation 14,000 current and former smokers and 4,000 asbestos-exposed workers received either a placebo or 30 mg of beta-carotene plus 25,000 IU (international units) of vitamin A (the latter is five times the recommended dietary allowance). The trial was ended after four years. A common denominator in both CARET and the Finnish smokers study was that the supplementation was begun only after years of exposure to a proven cause of lung cancer (cigarette smoke or asbestos fibers). Most authorities now believe that if beta-carotene supplementation is to be effective in reducing this cancer, it will have to be started earlier in life and prior to harmful exposures.

While the above-cited research showed that supplementation may actually increase lung cancer risk in smokers and asbestos-exposed workers, another long-term investigation, the Physicians' Health Study, demonstrated that the same does not hold true for nonsmokers. The male health professionals in this study who took 50 mg of beta-carotene with or without aspirin every other day for 12 years showed no negative effects. Only 11% of the 22,000 participants were current smokers, however. Taken together, the results of these three studies clearly suggest that beta-carotene supplementation offers little benefit to nonsmokers and could be harmful to people who are heavy smokers.

New directions. Given the disappointing results of the supplementation trials, scientists have had to reevaluate their thinking about cancer chemoprevention. Some authorities point out that the initial trials used extremely high doses of carotenoids, in some cases providing as much as 10 times the recommended daily intake of beta-carotene. The five daily servings of fruits and vegetables all Americans are advised to eat contain only about five milligrams of beta-carotene. (Half a cup of broccoli provides about one milligram of beta-carotene and a medium raw carrot the full five milligrams. In the U.S. most people get an average of only 1.5 mg per day from food.) Future studies will likely focus on smaller doses of beta-carotene—closer to the recommended level—along with increased intake of other carotenoids and antioxidants. For example, in one trial currently under way in France, participants are receiving six milligrams of beta-carotene per day in combination with vitamin C, vitamin E, selenium, and zinc.

Several of the non-provitamin A carotenoids are also being studied for their anticancer potential. At least 14 carotenoids can be found in the blood, the predominant ones being, in addition to beta-carotene, lycopene and lutein. In 1995 researchers analyzing data from the Physicians' Health Study reported that participants whose diets included relatively large amounts of tomatoes and tomato products had lower-than-average rates of prostate cancer. As a result of this report, lycopene is now being tested as a protective agent against this form of cancer.

The impact of cooking and food processing on the chemical structures of carotenoids is also under investigation. Heating causes physical and chemical changes in carotenoids, and scientists suspect that such changes have an impact on both absorption and physiological effects.

Counting Carotenoids*

Food source	Alpha-carotene	Beta-carotene	Crypto-xanthin	Lutein/zea-xanthin	Lycopene
Apricot halves, 6 dried	0	3.7	0	0	0.2
Broccoli, ½ cup cooked	0	1.0	0	1.4	0
Cantaloupe, 1 cup chunks	0.1	4.8	0	0	0
Carrot, 1 medium raw	2.6	5.7	0	0.2	0
Collard greens, ½ cup cooked	0	3.5	0	10.4	0
Grapefruit, pink, ½ medium	0	1.6	0	0	4.1
Kale, ½ cup cooked	0	3.1	0	14.2	0
Mango, 1 medium	0	2.7	0.1	0	0
Mustard greens, ½ cup cooked	0	2.0	0	7.4	0
Orange, 1 medium	0	0.1	0.2	0	0
Papaya, ½ medium	0	0.2	1.1	0	0
Pepper, red, ½ raw	0	0.8	0	2.5	0
Pumpkin, ½ cup cooked or canned	4.7	3.8	0	1.8	0
Romaine lettuce, 1 cup	0	1.1	0	3.2	0
Spinach, ½ cup cooked	0	5.0	0	11.3	0
Spinach, ½ cup raw	0	2.3	0	5.7	0
Sweet potato, ½ cup mashed	0	14.4	0	0	0
Tangerine, 1 medium	0	0	0.9	0	0
Tomato, 1 medium	†	0.6	0	0.1	3.8
Tomato sauce, ½ cup	†	1.2	0	0.2	7.7
Watermelon, 1 cup cubed	0	0.4	0	0	6.6

*All quantities in milligrams.
†Not available.
Source: U.S. Dept. of Agriculture/National Cancer Institute carotenoid database.

Preventing heart attacks

Cardiovascular disease is the leading cause of death among adults in the U.S. and most other industrial countries. Oxidation of the fatty substances in the blood known as low-density lipoproteins (LDL) is believed to be an important factor in the development of atherosclerosis (the buildup of fatty deposits in the arteries interfering with blood flow). Epidemiological studies show that populations whose diets are rich in fruits and vegetables not only have lower rates of cancer than those who consume little of these foods but also have a reduced risk of cardiovascular disease. This observation has led to the hypothesis that the antioxidant properties of carotenoids may play a part in preventing heart attack, stroke, and blood vessel disorders. The exact mechanism is unknown, but some scientists hypothesize that beta-carotene works synergistically with vitamin E, which also has strong antioxidant activity. Beta-carotene is believed to scavenge oxygen free radicals in the interior of lipoprotein molecules; vitamin E is known to reduce oxidation in the outer portion of the LDL molecule.

In the Physicians' Health Study, beta-carotene supplementation had no effect on the rates of death from cardiovascular disease, heart attack, or stroke. Only in one group of participants—those with a history of a particular type of angina (chest pain) or previous coronary bypass surgery—did supplementation produce a significant benefit. Likewise, the Finnish smokers study showed no general improvement in cardiovascular risk among subjects taking beta-carotene supplements; in fact, compared with those taking a placebo, this group had an 11% higher death rate from cardiovascular disease.

The conclusion to be drawn is that consumption of fruits and vegetables—but *not* beta-carotene supplements—is consistently associated with decreased risk of cardiovascular disease. These foods are rich sources of a variety of antioxidants, including both vitamin E and carotenoids, as well as dietary fiber, all of which are associated with decreased cardiovascular risk. As is true for cancer, beta-carotene alone does not appear to be the magic bullet for heart disease and blood vessel conditions.

Spinach and other sight-savers

In the U.S. age-related macular degeneration (AMD), a progressive deterioration of the retina, is currently the leading cause of legal blindness in adults over the age of 65. The origin of the disorder is poorly understood, and no treatment exists for most who are affected, which makes prevention all the more urgent.

The idea that carotenoids may somehow be involved in AMD comes from the discovery that the macula of the retina contains a rich concentration of two carotenoids, lutein and zeaxanthin. The macula is an area in the middle retina that includes the fovea, a tiny depression at the spot where visual acuity is at its greatest. In patients with AMD, the levels of lutein and zeaxanthin in the macula are significantly lower than normal.

A study conducted at five ophthalmology centers in the U.S. evaluated the association between carotenoid consumption and the incidence of AMD. The findings, published in 1994, showed that people with the highest dietary carotenoid intake had a 43% lower risk for AMD than those with the lowest intake. People whose diets included the largest amounts of dark green, leafy vegetables such as spinach and collard greens (the primary dietary sources of lutein and zeaxanthin) were the least likely to develop AMD. This promising finding provided an impetus for the recommendation that all Americans increase their consumption of leafy green vegetables.

Hypercarotenemia: too much of a good thing

Three carotenoids are approved by the U.S. Food and Drug Administration (FDA) for use as food colorants: beta-carotene, beta-apo-8-carotenal, and canthaxanthin. For use in the food industry, these substances are synthesized rather than being extracted from vegetable sources. Most beta-carotene supplements sold over the counter are also products of laboratory synthesis. The only consistently observable adverse effect reported from taking beta-carotene supplements is hypercarotenemia, the presence of higher-than-normal concentrations of beta-carotene in the blood and tissues. Hypercarotenemia is characterized by a yellowing of the skin, often most marked in the palms of the hands. It has also been reported in people, especially children, who drink carrot juice or eat an excessive amount of carrots or squash over a period of several weeks or longer. No adverse health consequences have been reported in people diagnosed with hypercarotenemia, and the condition is completely reversible. Beta-carotene supplements in doses of up to 180 mg per day or more are a safe and often effective treatment for certain photosensitivity disorders (excessive sensitivity of the skin to the effects of sunlight). People with these disorders have taken such supplements for years. While they do develop hypercarotenemia, which helps to protect their skin from sunburn, they experience no other ill effects.

Supplementation with canthaxanthin, by contrast, has been reported to have negative effects. In addition to its FDA-approved use as a food colorant, canthaxanthin also has an unapproved use as the active ingredient in "tanning pills." These pills contain at least 100 times more canthaxanthin than is found in foods colored with canthaxanthin. Megadoses of canthaxanthin result not only in a tanned appearance but sometimes in a form of retinopathy (damage to the retina) due to the formation on the retina of crystalline deposits of carotenoid. Studies indicate that the retinopathy is reversible upon discontinuation of the pills, but in some individuals the eye condition may persist for years afterward.

Mother was right after all

So far, the majority of the evidence for the health benefits of carotenoids comes from observational studies of people who eat diets rich in fruits and vegetables. Taking supplements has not been shown to be beneficial and, for some people, may even be harmful. If all Americans followed the dietary guidelines of the National Cancer Institute and the USDA, they would consume five milligrams or more of beta-carotene daily. They would also eat at least five servings a day of fruits and vegetables. As government nutrition surveys show, however, a large gap exists between recommendation and practice.

It is always possible, of course, that high levels of carotenoids in the blood are simply a marker for a healthful diet and, perhaps, other health-promoting habits (like exercising regularly and not smoking). As scientists learn more about phytochemicals—chemical compounds found in

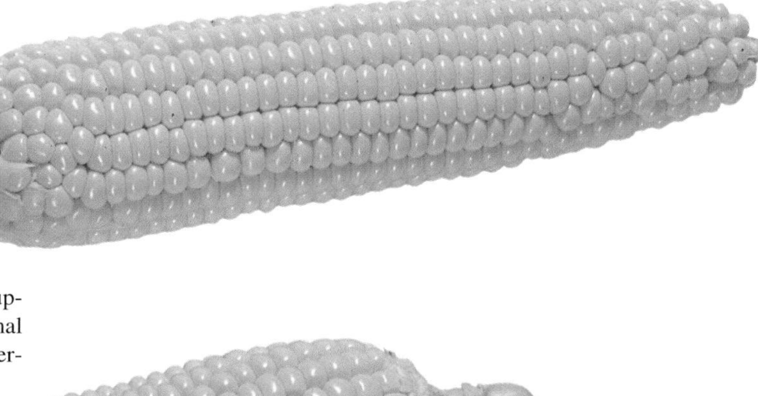

plants—they are also finding hitherto-unknown food components with important disease-fighting capacities. Perhaps carotene-rich diets derive their protective effects from a combination of nutritional factors working together and present only in whole foods. Clearly, a great deal more research will be necessary to test these theories. For now, the best advice for those who want to reduce their risk of chronic diseases is pretty much what nutrition experts—and mothers—have been saying for many years: eat more fruits and vegetables.

—John W. Erdman, Jr., Ph.D., and Amy C. Moore, B.S.

Is Everything Coming Up Roses for Garlic?

> *Since Biblical times in all parts of the earth*
> *It has cured countless sufferings and ills.*
> *If we understood what the garlic is worth*
> *We would throw out our poisonous pills....*
>
> —from Ruthie Gordon's "Garlic Song" in the motion picture *Garlic Is as Good as Ten Mothers* (1980)

Because of its reputation as an herb with numerous medicinal properties, garlic, nicknamed the "stinking rose," is a top-selling food supplement, with worldwide annual sales in excess of $200 million and the number of garlic and garlic-derived products on the market ever growing. Does the herb itself or any of the commercial garlic products truly offer any health benefits? If so, how have these been documented? When a product is labeled "aspirin," its main ingredient is acetylsalicylic acid, but when the term *garlic* appears on a label, what does this tell the consumer about the contents of the product? To appreciate the answers to these questions, one needs to know something about the chemical compounds that are present in the intact plant and the various processed garlic products.

Garlic and its relatives: basic botany

Botanically, garlic (*Allium sativum*) is classified as a member the genus *Allium,* which consists of more than 600 widely distributed species. Plants of the genus *Allium* are typically herbaceous perennials that form bulbs and are now classified in the family Alliaceae (order Asparagales), rather than in the Liliaceae, as they long had been. While some members of the genus are little more than botanical curiosities or nuisances for farmers (*e.g., A. vineale* [crow garlic], which, when eaten by cows, gives milk a garlicky taste), others are attractive ornamental and garden plants of diverse sizes and hues (*e.g., A. moly, A. carinatum, A. stellatum,* and *A. textile*). Still others are economically important spices and vegetables (*e.g.,* onion [*A. cepa*], leek [*A. porrum*], shallot [*A.*

(continued on page 224)

Selected members of the genus Allium, *all popular spices and vegetables: onions (*A. cepa*), leeks (*A. porrum*), shallots (*A. ascalonicum*), chives (*A. schoenoprasum*), scallions (*A. fistulosum*), and, probably the most ennobled member, garlic (*A. sativum*)—sometimes called the "stinking rose."*

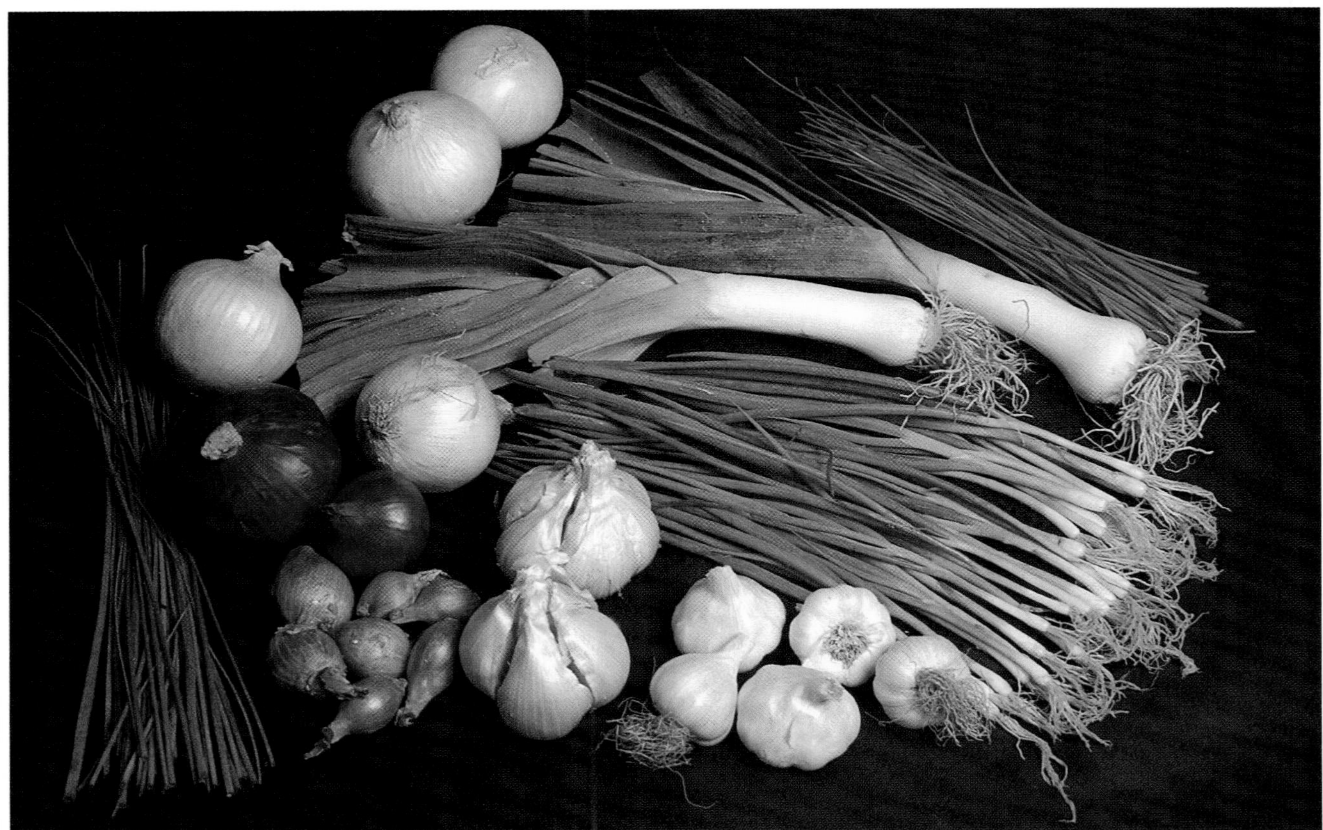

Mark Schmidt

NEWS CAP MHA 98

Selenium: A Supplement to Watch

A long-term study designed to test the effect of selenium supplementation on skin cancer rates came up with unexpected results in 1996. Selenium is a trace element found in varying amounts in soil and, consequently, in the food supply. The Nutritional Prevention of Cancer Study, a clinical trial lasting more than a decade, found that a selenium supplement may significantly reduce the chances of developing common cancers, such as prostate, colon, and lung cancer, in people with a history of skin cancer. To the researchers' surprise, however, increased selenium intake did not protect against the development of basal or squamous cell skin cancers, which was the original premise of the study.

The trial involved 1,312 skin cancer patients at seven dermatology clinics in Connecticut and several southeastern states. Half were randomly assigned to take a daily tablet containing 200 micrograms of selenium in the form of brewer's yeast, while the other half took a placebo. At the study's conclusion, the investigators found that the total number of cases of cancer was nearly 40% lower in the group that took selenium as compared with the placebo group. Those taking selenium had a 63% lower rate of prostate cancer, a 58% lower colon cancer rate, and a 46% lower rate of lung cancer. No differences were observed in the rates of skin cancer or cancers of the bladder, head and neck, or breast. (The number of deaths from other cancers was too small for adequate analysis.) Overall cancer mortality in the treatment group was also lower, by nearly 50%.

The study was largely conducted in areas of the U.S. where the natural levels of selenium in soil and crops are relatively low. Before treatment, the study participants, who ranged in age from 18 to 80, had lower-than-average blood-selenium levels. The supplements consumed in the study raised their selenium levels by two-thirds, and their average daily selenium consumption doubled.

The results, reported in the *Journal of the American Medical Association* (Dec. 25, 1996), led independent scientists and government cancer officials to express optimism about selenium's potential to prevent cancer. But both groups cautioned that the findings were preliminary. Further research is needed before recommendations can be made for the general public, stressed Larry C. Clark, associate professor at the Arizona Cancer Center at the University of Arizona, who headed the Nutritional Prevention of Cancer Study. Peter Greenwald, director of the Division of Cancer Prevention and Control of the National Cancer Institute (NCI), said that the study needed to be repeated in a larger group and in subjects living in a more representative area of the country. An editorial in the same issue of the journal noted that the findings may have limited applicability to women, since three-fourths of the participants were men.

The primary sources of selenium in the American diet include grains, meat, fish, and dairy products. Most people consume enough of these foods to meet the recommended dietary allowance for selenium of 70 micrograms per day for men and 55 micrograms per day for women.

The Environmental Protection Agency has set a level of 350 micrograms per day as the maximum safe intake, but the NCI said that safe limits for humans have not been fully established. According to the Arizona Cancer Center, doses of selenium higher than 1,000 micrograms daily may have adverse, even deadly, effects. Early signs of selenium toxicity include hair and nail loss, gastrointestinal problems, and garlicky-smelling breath.

Several previous studies had produced conflicting evidence about the relationship between selenium and cancer. Some had shown an inverse relationship between cancer deaths and selenium levels in the soil or in the body, finding, for instance, that overall cancer mortality and death rates for certain cancers were lower in areas with high soil-selenium levels. Other research showed no association whatsoever, and a few studies even found that cancer risk increased with high selenium levels. Animal and laboratory tissue studies had suggested that selenium has antitumor activity, but according to the NCI, the levels involved were far higher than the amounts needed—or normally consumed in dietary sources—by humans.

Earlier international trials of selenium also had mixed results. The Finnish government began supplementing fertilizer with selenium in 1984 in order to increase the amount in crops, but no significant impact on cancer rates has been reported thus far. A trial of dietary selenium supplementation conducted in Linxian, China, had no impact on the high incidence of esophageal cancer seen in that region or on overall cancer incidence or mortality; a second, larger Chinese investigation found a significant drop in stomach cancer cases and deaths in people who received daily pills that included a high selenium content. The recent U.S. trial provides the strongest evidence to date of the anticancer effects of selenium.

—Cristine Russell

(continued from page 222)
ascalonicum], chive [*A. schoenoprasum*], and scallion [*A. fistulosum*]).

Garlic, now known solely in the cultivated form and grown in most parts of the world, probably originated in central Asia. About 90% of garlic in the U.S. comes from Gilroy, Calif. Argentina and Mexico are other major garlic producers in the Americas.

Garlic bulbs come in many sizes, shapes, and colors, ranging from white to pink to light purple, and consist of a tightly packed assemblage of 4–20 individual cloves, enclosed in a papery membrane. Out of the cloves develops a quill-like stalk (or scape) 30–90 cm (12–35 in) high with 5–9 leaves. The scape is topped by a cluster of 5–7 whitish-red or greenish-white blossoms that develop into 20–30 egg-shaped bulblets. The two main subspecies of garlic are softneck and hardneck. The latter variety, sometimes called serpent garlic, is distinguished by an oddly curled flower stalk. Softneck garlic normally does not produce a stalk of bulblets. The plant known as elephant garlic is actually not garlic but a variety of leek that has fewer but larger and milder cloves than garlic.

Cultivated in most parts of the world, garlic has long been reputed to have medicinal properties. A 6th-century Greek medical treatise prescribed a regimen for gout sufferers that included "pure wine every morning" in January, "sweets" in March, and "garlic" in October.

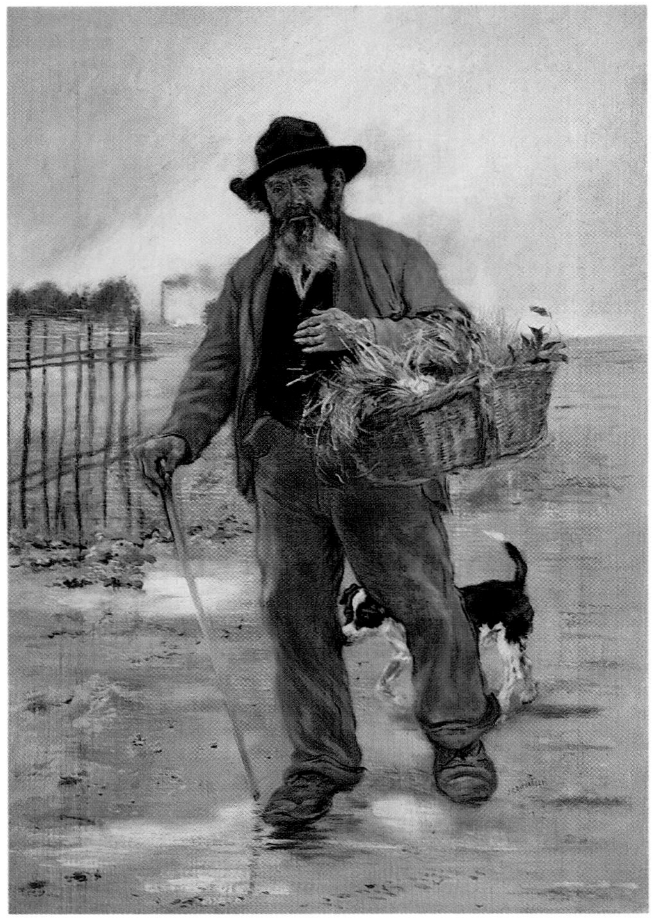

"The Garlic Seller," oil on paper mounted and extended on canvas by Jean François Raffaelli (1850–1924), 71.8 x 49 cm; The Henry C. and Martha B. Angell Collection (19.103); courtesy, Museum of Fine Arts, Boston

On the menu

Garlic is, of course, a classic ingredient in the cuisines of many countries. A garlic and oil sauce, *allioli* (Spanish) or *aïoli* (French), common throughout the western Mediterranean, is made by combining a cup of olive oil with six or more cloves of garlic (crushed), salt, egg yolks, bread or nuts, and lemon juice or vinegar. *Pesto* (Italy) is made by blending garlic with fresh basil, parsley, pine nuts, olive oil, salt, pepper, and grated Parmesan; garlic vinegar is simply crushed garlic and white wine vinegar. Garlic is also featured in *sopa de ajo* (garlic soup; Spain) and is an important ingredient in *gazpacho* (cold vegetable soup; Spain); *escargots* (snails; France); leg of lamb Arlesienne (France); stuffed eggplant, or aubergine (Turkey); *hummus* (a blend of chickpeas, sesame-seed paste, and seasonings; Middle East); *tzatziki* (cucumber-yogurt dip; Greece); and *kimch'i* (cabbage, white radish, chili pepper; Korea). Among the most popular garlic dishes in the U.S. are shrimp scampi and 40-clove chicken, not to mention garlic bread and garlic bagels.

Garlic's chemistry

Garlic should always be stored in a cool, dry place with good air circulation (*e.g.,* in a perforated crockery pot). The natural flavor of garlic is not present as such in the intact plant but is produced when the plant is crushed or cut. This method of flavor formation may actually help garlic survive, since the strong-smelling sulfur-containing aroma compounds work as natural chemical defense agents that keep predators and microorganisms away from the bulbs. When garlic cells rupture, rapid chemical reactions occur as the separate flavor precursors and enzymes commingle. In intact garlic cloves, a compound called alliin and related aroma and flavor precursors are located in the abundant storage compartments (mesophyll cells), while the enzyme alliinase is concentrated in vascular bundles (sheath cells), which are fewer in number. In a mature plant alliinase activity is 10 times higher in the bulb than in the leaves and stems.

The principal flavor precursor in garlic, alliin (compound **3** in the figure on page 226), is derived from the essential, sulfur-containing amino acid cysteine (**2**), which in turn is manufactured within the cells of the garlic bulb from sulfate ions (**1**) found in soil. Disruption of the bulb cells—by cutting or crushing—results in release of alliinase and subsequent breakdown of alliin, creating a volatile and odorous compound called allicin (**5**). Allicin, a member of a class of sulfur compounds termed thiosulfinates, possesses the characteristic aroma and taste of fresh garlic. The flavorant allicin was discovered in 1944 by Chester J. Cavallito at the Sterling-Winthrop Chemical Co. in Rensselaer, N.Y., in connection with research on antibiotics derived from plants. Allicin is formed by the rapid splitting of alliin by the enzyme alliinase into a very reactive chemical intermediate, 2-propenesulfenic acid (**4**). Two molecules of this intermediate rapidly combine to form one molecule of allicin plus water. In addition to alliin, garlic also contains several dozen more cysteine-containing peptides (**6**), as well as several other related flavor precursors (**7**). Like alliin, these flavor precursors are cleaved (chemically split) by alliinase; this process yields thiosulfinate flavorants (**8**). Cysteine-containing peptides function as storage compounds of the elements nitrogen and sulfur and can be enzymatically transformed into flavor precursors under conducive conditions as the plants approach maturity. With a total sulfur content of 0.35%, garlic is considerably higher in sulfur than most other common vegetables. The level of the essential micronutrient element selenium in garlic is also relatively high.

During cooking with garlic, additional flavors are formed by thermal breakdown of initial enzymatically produced flavorants, in either an aqueous (water-based) or a nonaqueous medium (*e.g.,* cooking oil). Some compounds may be lost through evaporation. Heating in an aqueous medium can lead to hydrolysis (chemical breakdown). If the breakdown products themselves are unstable, further compounds can be formed that may also make important contributions to aroma and taste, particularly if these substances have low taste thresholds (*i.e.,* microscopic quantities can be tasted). Allicin itself is quite reactive and unstable, undergoing hydrolysis in water, producing diallyl polysulfides (compound **9** in the figure, page 226). If a large quantity of garlic is subjected to steam distillation (boiling with water and condensing the steam in a separate container), a small amount of "distilled oil of garlic" is collected. This oil, first isolated in 1844 by the German chemist Theodor Wertheim, consists primarily of diallyl polysulfides and has a pungent odor that differs from the fresh aroma characteristic of allicin. Distilled oil of garlic is sometimes used as a substitute for fresh garlic.

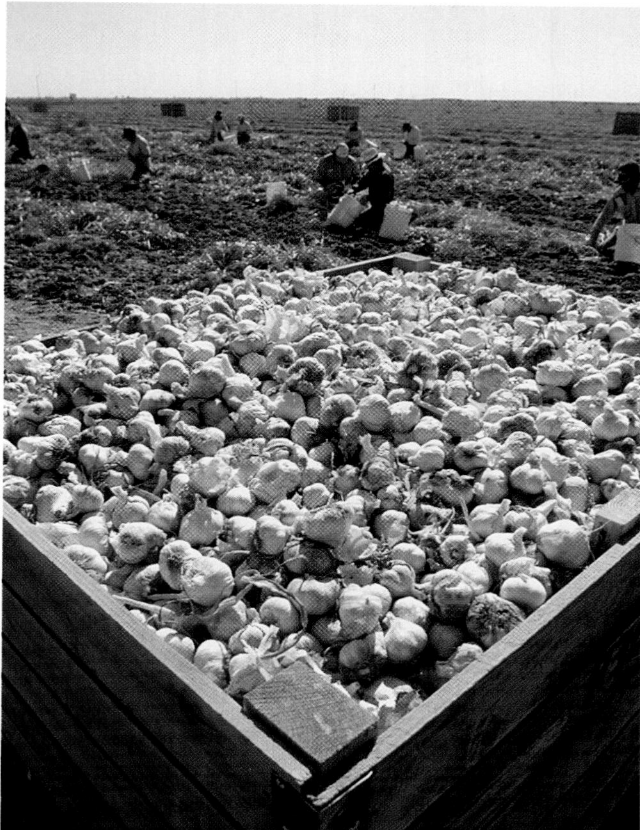

About 90% of garlic used in the United States is grown in California, near the town of Gilroy, about an hour's drive south of San Francisco. Here the fragrant herb is harvested on the 1,400-ha (3,500-ac) Christopher Ranch, founded by Don Christopher, a former prune rancher.

On gentle heating, especially in the presence of cooking oils, allicin is transformed into ajoene and the dithiins (**10** and **11,** respectively, in the figure). These substances were discovered in 1983 by a team of investigators that included Mahendra K. Jain and Roger W. Crecely at the University of Delaware, Rafael Apitz-Castro and María R. Cruz at the Venezuelan Institute of Scientific Investigations, Caracas, and this author along with Saleem Ahmad at the State University of New York at Albany during a search for the compounds in garlic responsible for the inhibition of blood clots. Owing to the instability of *Allium*-derived compounds, it is difficult to distinguish the genuine flavorants from artifacts (compounds not actually present to begin with but formed by the analytic techniques and sampling methods). This difficulty and the fact that such a wide variety of sulfur and selenium compounds are present in cut and uncut garlic make it particularly challenging to investigate *Allium*'s chemistry.

Because garlic is eaten cooked more often than raw, the effects of cooking on flavorants merit discussion. All varieties of garlic have a strong aroma and taste when crushed. Boiling unpeeled whole cloves for 15 minutes or cooking them in a microwave oven at 650 w for 15–30 seconds deactivates alliinase. Before this happens, a small amount of allicin is formed, probably as a result of physical contact between the individual cloves or between the cloves and their container. Upon exposure to boiling water, allicin is converted to diallyl polysulfides. If garlic is chopped or crushed and then heated in a closed container at 100° C (212° F) for 20 minutes, the initially produced allicin and other thiosulfinates are converted into diallyl polysulfides. Frying garlic (which involves temperatures above 100° C) converts alliin to the amino acid cysteine and allyl alcohol. When chopped garlic is stir-fried in hot oil for one minute, some polysulfides, but no allicin, remain. When a mixture of garlic, water, and soybean oil is boiled, considerable allicin survives. Without the soybean oil, the major sulfur-containing products of boiled garlic are polysulfides. This suggests that allicin remains stable when garlic is cooked in oil at moderate temperatures.

Salivating patrons flock to San Francisco's Stinking Rose restaurant, among the most sizzling attractions of the North Beach neighborhood, to sample such gustatory delights as 40-clove chicken and, yes, even rich, creamy, and garlicky ice cream.

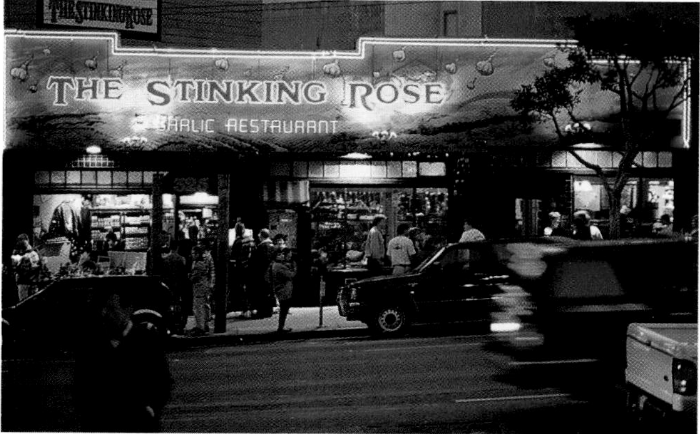

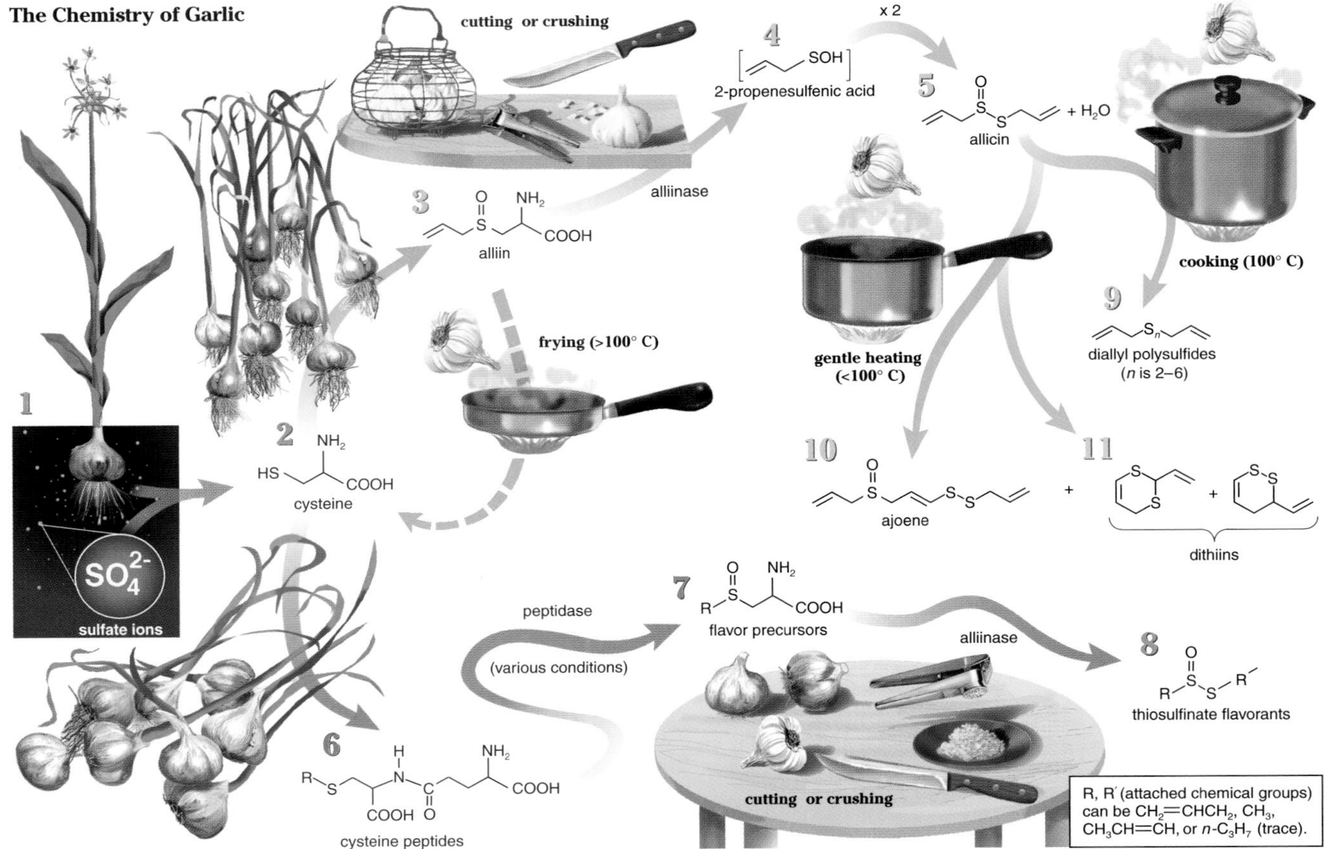

Garlic metabolism

> *Garlic then have power to save from death*
> *Bear with it though it maketh unsavory breath,*
> *And scorn not garlic like some that think*
> *It only maketh men wink and drink and stink.*
>
> —from "The Englishman's Doctor" by Sir John Harington, 1609

The substance 2-propenethiol, detected in the breath within one hour of eating garlic, is probably a primary metabolite of most garlic-derived compounds. Diallyl polysulfides and the selenium-containing dimethyl selenide are other metabolites that can be measured on the breath. In the body, garlic-derived compounds such as allicin and diallyl polysulfide are likely to react rapidly with cysteine, producing *S*-allyl mercaptocysteine. Because of this reaction, allicin itself has never been found in blood after ingestion of garlic. Nor are garlic cysteine peptides or their metabolites found in blood; they, too, undergo conversion in the body (to the compound *N*-acetyl-*S*-allyl-cysteine, which is excreted in urine).

It remains to be established which of these transformation products has the greatest physiological activity and which might therefore explain the biological activity of garlic. About 10% of the sulfur-containing compounds from garlic are excreted through the lungs, while smaller amounts are excreted through the skin. Garlic components such as allicin apparently possess the ability to penetrate skin. This would explain why rubbing garlic on the soles of the feet (or putting a garlic clove in one's sock) produces "garlic breath."

Commercial garlic formulations

In addition to the numerous dried or pickled varieties of garlic sold in food stores, garlic health supplements, sold in pharmacies and health-food outlets, are available in at least four different forms:

1. powder tablets or capsules containing dehydrated garlic powder that consists of alliin and related flavor precursors, alliinase, and cysteine-containing peptides; on exposure to water these products yield up to five milligrams of allicin per gram (the yield is known as the "allicin potential")
2. steam-distilled oil of garlic, consisting of allyl polysulfides
3. garlic vegetable oil macerate extract (garlic crushed in oil), containing ajoene, dithiins, and allyl polysulfides
4. garlic extract aged in dilute alcohol, consisting primarily of *S*-allylcysteine and cysteine-containing peptides; no allicin is formed on exposure to water

Compared with the cost of fresh garlic, which affords the same compounds under different conditions of food preparation and consumption, these products are not inexpensive. There is considerable variation in the amounts of the various garlic components in different commercial products. At the present time there are no requirements for standardization or for the listing of components or their quantities on product labels. Since crushing and processing garlic generate various pharmacologically active compounds (*see* below), the manufacturing process used to make a particular product is a major consideration. It should be noted that the optimum pH (acidity level) for garlic alliinase is 6.5 (lower pH values represent higher acidity); the stomach pH is 1.5 when empty, 3 after a light meal, and 4.5 after a high-protein meal. Alliinase is deactivated at a pH lower than 4.5; thus, dehydrated garlic powder introduced into an empty stomach or into the stomach following a light meal produces no allicin. This is the reason that some garlic tablets are "enterically coated," which enables them to pass through the stomach into the less-acidic small intestine before dissolving.

Ancient remedy, enduring promise

There is an extensive body of scientific literature on the biological activity of garlic and garlic products. Garlic is one of the oldest of all cultivated plants and has been a part of folk medicine for thousands of years. The use of garlic as a remedy for ailments, including bites, worms, tumors, headaches, and heart problems, was described in the Ebers papyrus, an Egyptian compilation of medical writings dating to about 1550 BC. Aristotle, Hippocrates, Aristophanes, Dioscorides, Pliny the Elder, and other prominent writers of ancient Greece and Rome also referred to garlic's medicinal use. The historian Herodutus recorded that garlic and onions were staples in the diet of the builders of the Great Pyramid at Giza and that they went on strike when deprived of their garlic rations. Garlic has been fed to racehorses to improve their stamina.

In modern times the sales of garlic and garlic supplements have benefited immensely from the favorable publicity they have received in the tabloids: "Nature's miraculous healing medicine lowers blood pressure, relieves arthritis pains, guards against major ills...." "Garlic cures man's cancer...it really works, says doctor." "Miracle medicine garlic can make you healthy, happy, and help you to live to be 100."

Several types of research have provided information about garlic's presumed health effects. *Epidemiological studies* have looked at amounts of garlic consumed by people in different countries and cultures to see how consumption correlates with the occurrence of certain types of cancers and cardiovascular disease. In *clinical studies* individuals are given specific doses of commercial garlic products, laboratory-prepared garlic extracts, or the fresh herb. The subjects' blood or urine can then be analyzed; study populations can also be monitored for the occurrence of certain diseases or disease indicators. Both types of studies require control populations—*e.g.,* persons who are in a comparable state of health as the garlic consumers but are not given, or normally do not consume, any of the forms of garlic during the course of the study. *Laboratory studies* also provide information about health effects by looking at the effect of garlic extracts or components of extracts on disease-causing agents (bacteria, viruses, fungi); on specific enzymes, such as those controlling the manufacture of cholesterol in cells; or on blood or other body fluids.

Over the past several decades, the results of numerous studies of the above types have been reported at scientific meetings and published in scientific journals. The fact that so many medical studies on garlic have appeared in print does not by itself validate the claims of health benefits; rather, each study must be judged

NEWS CAP MHA 98

Zinc: Latest Weapon in the "Cold War"?

"A cold will last a week if you treat it and seven days if you don't," says an old adage. All of the known cold therapies—from time-honored folk remedies like whiskey or chicken soup to the hundreds of over-the-counter medications available to the modern cold sufferer—have one thing in common: they treat cold symptoms but do not affect the course of the infection. In July 1996, however, a report in the *Annals of Internal Medicine* suggested that zinc—taken in lozenge form—may actually shorten the duration of a cold.

The report summarized the findings of a study conducted by researchers at the Cleveland (Ohio) Clinic Foundation. The subjects were 100 employees of the foundation. Within 24 hours of developing cold symptoms, half of the subjects were given zinc gluconate lozenges (each containing 13.3 mg of zinc), while the other half received a placebo lozenge with a medicinal taste. All participants were instructed to take the lozenges every two hours while awake. The zinc group recovered from their colds in 4.4 days, compared with 7.6 days for the placebo group. Those taking the zinc lozenges reported one to three fewer days of coughing, sore throat, hoarseness, nasal congestion, and headache, although they experienced no relief from fever, muscle ache, scratchy throat, or sneezing. The zinc group also had some adverse reactions; 20% complained of nausea and 80% of an unpleasant aftertaste. The mechanisms by which zinc may hasten the resolution of the common cold are not known, but it is believed that the metallic element may inhibit replication of rhinoviruses, one of the major families of cold-causing viruses.

Is the efficacy of zinc lozenges now "clinically proven," as the label on at least one of these products claims? Not exactly. Seven earlier clinical studies had tested the usefulness of zinc as a cold treatment. While three demonstrated a beneficial effect, four did not. (Not all of the studies used the same formulation and dosage of zinc, which may account for at least some of the difference.) Moreover, not long after the Cleveland investigators published their findings, reports surfaced of a possible conflict of interest; before the data were released, the physician who headed the trial invested in the company that manufactured the zinc lozenges. Disappointing as it may be to those seeking relief from the misery of a cold, the only conclusion that can be drawn at this point is that more studies are needed.

—Afrodite Mantzavrakos

Courtesy of Nature's Way Products, Inc./Murdock Madaus Schwabe, Springfield, Utah

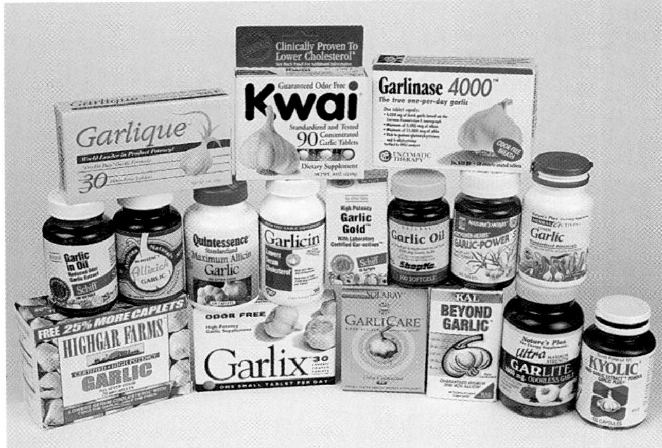

Virtually all health-food stores—and many pharmacies—have shelves brimming with commercial garlic supplements. The products come in tablet, capsule, and liquid extract forms, and their labels claim they do everything from lowering cholesterol to killing bacteria and fungi.

for its scientific design and rigor and for the strength of the evidence presented. Critics in the medical community have found many of the recent garlic studies wanting. Gastroenterologist Graham Woolf at the University of California, Los Angeles, is one such doubter. "There's no evidence that garlic does anything but make your breath smell," he is quoted as saying in *Time* magazine (May 12, 1997). Physician Robert Beaglehole of the Faculty of Medicine and Health Science at the University of Auckland, N.Z., wrote a sharp commentary, published in *The Lancet* (Nov. 2, 1996), in which he said, "At this stage, the evidence does not support use of garlic powder for cardioprotection. Further well-designed controlled studies are required.... In the meantime, garlic should be enjoyed for its culinary, not its cardioprotective, properties." In this author's opinion, a substantial number of the published studies on garlic suffer from "bad science" and unfortunate self-promotion on the part of garlic product manufacturers. Findings of some of the better garlic studies to date are summed up here.

Antibiotic activity

For centuries, garlic preparations have been employed as antibiotics: in India for cleansing wounds and ulcers, in China for treating infection-related fevers and cholera, in Africa (by Albert Schweitzer) for treating amebic dysentery, during both world wars as antiseptics to prevent gangrene, and during epidemics of typhus, diphtheria, and tuberculosis.

- Laboratory investigations reveal that fresh garlic extracts have antifungal activity. Aqueous and organic-solvent garlic extracts and allicin show effectiveness against the fungi *Candida albicans, Aspergillus fumigatus, Cryptococcus neoformans,* and *Histoplasma capsulatum,* among others. In many of these cases, the antifungal activity of garlic is superior to that of the commonly used drugs nystatin, griseofulvin, and amphotericin. In China garlic extracts, including diallyl trisulfide, have been given intravenously to treat fungal (cryptoccocal) meningitis. Ajoene, too, has been shown to inhibit the growth of some pathogenic fungi.
- Lab studies show effectiveness of fresh garlic extracts against a wide variety of bacteria. The growth of streptococci, staphylococci, and the organisms responsible for cholera and typhoid fever—including some antibiotic-resistant strains—is inhibited by allicin, even at very weak concentrations. Ajoene also inhibits the growth of some disease-causing bacteria.
- Limited evidence (largely from China) exists for the antiviral activity of garlic.
- Both allicin and ajoene have very short lifetimes in blood and other body fluids. Thus, the antibiotic activity of garlic is largely limited to topical usage or to activity in the stomach and esophagus, where freshly formed allicin or ajoene comes into direct contact with the treatment site.

Cardiovascular activity

Dioscorides, chief physician to the Roman army in the 1st century AD, wrote, "Garlic doth cleaneth the arteries." Of more than 50 clinical studies, most suggest that consumption of moderate amounts of fresh garlic and certain commercial garlic products has a favorable effect on blood lipids (including low-density ["bad"] cholesterol, high-density ["good"] cholesterol, and the triglycerides). Garlic also promotes fibrinolysis (dissolution of blood clots) and improves blood circulation. In some cases garlic has been found to inhibit the tendency of platelets, tiny disklike bodies in the blood, to aggregate (a process that contributes to the formation of clots) while also increasing blood flow in the capillaries (tiny blood vessels that link arteries and veins).

Studies further show that populations with high levels of garlic consumption are protected from coronary heart disease and that there is an inverse correlation between average garlic intake and incidence of coronary heart disease. The German Federal Bureau of Health is so convinced by the evidence of garlic's cardiovascular benefits that it recommends a daily intake of 4 g fresh garlic (about one clove; equivalent to 1.4 g dehydrated garlic) or its processed equivalent (usually one or two tablets) for prevention of blood clots and atherosclerosis (the buildup of fatty deposits in the arteries).

Prior to 1989 extremely high intakes of garlic (seven cloves, or 28 g, per day) were used in several clinical studies. Recently, more realistic amounts of garlic (3–10 g) have been used, with results showing that treatment for 12 weeks with a commercial dried-garlic tablet (900 mg per day) produced a significantly greater reduction in blood cholesterol than did a placebo. Consumption of one-half to one clove of garlic per day appears to reduce cholesterol levels by approximately 9%. If commercial products are used to lower blood lipid levels, the allicin potential of these products should be high (*i.e.,* about 0.07 mg/kg body weight per day).

- In 1979 an epidemiological study in India compared three populations consuming different amounts of garlic and onions. The subjects were all vegetarians who ate garlic and onions either in liberal amounts (at least 50 g of garlic per week), in relatively smaller amounts (no more than 10 g of garlic per week), or never in their lives. The garlic and onion abstainers had the shortest blood-coagulation time and showed the highest blood level of the clot-promoting protein fibrinogen—both of which are conducive to heart disease (*see* below). The mean fasting cholesterol values for the three groups, respectively, were 159, 172, and 208 mg/dl (milligrams per deciliter), which showed that blood lipid levels are lowest (most favorable) in the garlic-consuming group and highest (least favorable) in abstainers. ("Desirable" cholesterol levels are below 200 mg/dl; borderline-high levels are 200–239 mg/dl; and high levels are 240 mg/dl or above.)

- In clinical studies (also in India) 432 patients who had experienced prior heart attacks were given either 0.1 mg of an ether extract of fresh garlic (mainly dithiins and ajoene) per kilogram of body weight per day or a placebo; there was a 35% lower rate of new heart attacks and a 45% lower rate of total deaths in the garlic group than in the placebo group; the garlic consumers also had lower blood-lipid levels.
- Allicin, ajoene, diallyl disulfide, and 2-propenethiol (a garlic metabolite) can all inhibit cholesterol synthesis; alliin cannot. Over time, water-soluble garlic extracts decreased serum lipid levels in rats and rabbits. In humans long-term intake of garlic-powder tablets led to a reduction in blood cholesterol. Blood samples taken two hours after oral administration of a 300-mg tablet showed decreased cholesterol accumulation in smooth muscle cells cultured from atherosclerotic arteries.
- By contrast, two recent well-designed controlled trials of commercial garlic powders in the treatment of hyperlipidemia (elevated blood lipids), conducted in the U.K. and Australia, failed to show significant differences in lipid levels between treatment and placebo groups after six months. With garlic as well as with many other agents that are clinically tested, there is an evident publication bias, with positive studies more likely to be published than negative studies.
- In five out of six clinical trials involving either fresh garlic or freshly made extracts, fibrinolysis was increased and platelet aggregation inhibited. In healthy individuals the factors that cause the blood to coagulate (and thereby prevent interminable bleeding in the event of injury) are balanced by the factors that promote fibrinolysis (thus, blood clots are prevented from blocking normal circulation). Impairment of fibrinolytic activity enhances blood clotting and consequently increases the risk of heart attack and stroke. Both clinical and epidemiological studies have shown that garlic juice or oil enhances fibrinolysis and that garlic inhibits platelet aggregation in animals and humans. Various substances from garlic are credited with inhibiting platelet aggregation, including allicin, ajoene, and the dithiins; *S*-allylcysteine, however, has no platelet-inhibiting activity.

Anticancer activity

Epidemiological studies associate garlic consumption with diminished risk of gastrointestinal cancers. Garlic may also help prevent several other types of cancers, and active research into the herb's tumor-prevention potential continues.

- A study of 564 patients with stomach cancer and 1,131 controls in Shandong province in China found that high intakes of garlic, scallions, and Chinese chives were associated with a significantly lower stomach cancer risk.
- A related study compared the death rate from stomach cancer in two Shandong province counties with different garlic-consumption patterns. Those living in Cangshan county, where average raw garlic intake was 20 g a day, had a much lower death rate (3 per 100,000) than those living in Qixia county, where the rate was 40 per 100,000 and residents rarely ate garlic.
- An epidemiological study of the incidence of colon cancer over a period of five years among 41,837 women in Iowa aged 55–69 revealed a 35% lower risk for those who frequently consumed garlic.
- Oil-soluble allyl polysulfides have been shown to inhibit the growth of mammary cancer in dogs and cultured human colon cancer cells, but the water-soluble compound *S*-allylcysteine had little effect on these cells. Oil-soluble allyl polysulfides have also been shown to inhibit the carcinogenesis phase (stage at which normal cells are altered by exposure to a potent cancer-causing agent) in skin cancers.
- Because allyl selenium compounds appear to have even greater antitumor activity than other garlic compounds, cancer researchers are currently studying selenium-enriched garlic.

A clove a day?

There is no evidence that the consumption of liberal quantities of fresh garlic or the use of commercial garlic supplements in reasonable dosages is bad for most people. There is very good evidence, on the other hand, that regular inclusion of fresh garlic in the diet can reduce the risk of cancer and cardiovascular disease. Ingestion of excessive amounts of raw garlic on an empty stomach, however, can cause severe irritation; thus, particularly sensitive individuals should limit their intake of garlic or may have to avoid it altogether.

The case for commercial garlic supplements is less clear. Whole and cut garlic contain diverse pharmacologically active components. These are available commercially in various distinct, separate, and in some cases ill-defined formulations. To confuse the situation further, manufacturers of garlic supplements are waging a war of words in advertisements—and now, even on the Internet—challenging the health value of their competitors' products and, in the process, sometimes distorting facts to suit their needs.

—Eric Block, Ph.D.

Salt: Shake the Habit?

With the publication of recent studies reinforcing the link between salt intake and high blood pressure (hypertension), salt is once again in the news. Moreover, blood pressure is no longer the sole issue. A considerable amount of research indicates that salt has many other adverse health effects independent of its influence on blood pressure.

As a result of these findings, many authorities now favor a universal recommendation to limit salt intake. For most people, these experts say, restricting salt intake would require only simple dietary modifications; moreover, most people would quickly become accustomed to—and indeed grow to prefer—the taste of less highly salted foods. And yet this proposal, which hardly seems controversial, has some extremely vociferous opponents. A few are scientists who find the existing studies of salt's cardiovascular effects unconvincing and feel that it would be more worthwhile to draw public attention to other measures—for example, weight loss and reduction of alcohol intake. But by far the most vocal critics are segments of the food industry and trade group representatives who seek to convince the public that the evidence against salt is not compelling enough to warrant a dietary change.

The crucial issue in this dispute is not whether certain people—those who take medication for high blood pressure, for example—should limit their salt intake, a point on which virtually all authorities agree. Rather, the current argument centers on the benefits of salt restriction for people with blood pressures in the normal range—in other words, the vast majority of the population. The following summarizes the studies of salt's adverse effects and the rationale for stricter limitations on salt intake.

The modern "addiction" to salt

The preservative properties of salt were discovered only about 5,000 years ago, which is a relatively recent time in the history of the human race. Because of the difficulty in finding and obtaining it, salt became a precious commodity, often worth more than gold and in some countries (*e.g.,* China and France) a main source of tax revenues. Nonetheless, humans, like most other mammals, have no physiological need to consume more than very small amounts of salt. Indeed, the Yanomami Indians, who live in the Amazon rain forest, eat a diet very similar to that eaten by most human ancestors during millions of years of evolution, are extremely fit, and consume less than a tenth of a gram of salt a day. People in the U.S., the U.K., and many other developed countries eat a hundred times this much. (The average salt intake in these countries is 10 g per day, which translates into about 3,900 mg of sodium, the constituent of salt that is responsible for its physiological effects. By way of comparison, nutrition authorities in the U.S. currently recommend an upper limit of 2,400 mg per day—or about 6 g/day.)

Claus Meyer—Black Star/PNI

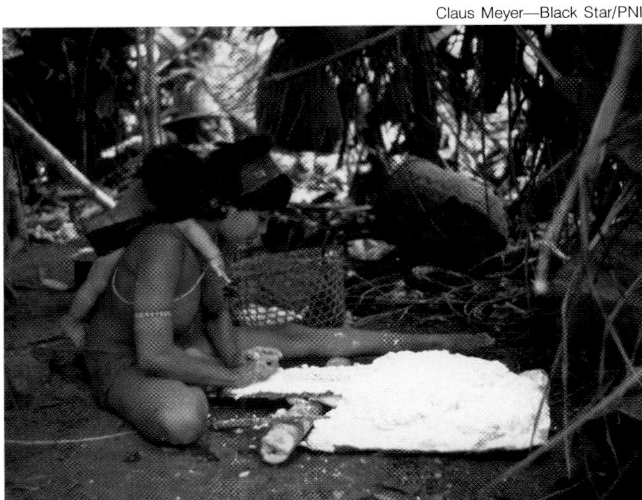

Does the human body have any real physiological need for salt? Apparently not. The Yanomami people of South America eat only about one-tenth of a gram of salt per day—compared with an average of 10 g in many Western countries—and yet are perfectly fit.

With the invention of the refrigerator and deep freeze, the preservative role of salt became redundant, but the use of salt in processed foods persisted. Today about 60–80% of dietary salt comes from these products.

Salt and blood pressure: not just a theory

The higher a person's blood pressure, the greater his or her risk of stroke or heart attack. This observation holds true throughout the entire range of blood pressures. In other words, individuals with pressures in the normal range are at greater risk than those in the low-normal range, and those in the high-normal range are at greater risk than their normal-range counterparts. Although persons with high-normal levels are at lower risk for stroke and heart attack than those with very high blood pressures, there are more of the former; their risk may be less, but the total number of those exposed to the risk is much greater.

In order to reduce the overall rate of stroke and heart attack, it is essential not only to treat each person who is diagnosed with high blood pressure but also to reduce blood pressure levels in the general population. From a public health perspective, then, the factors that determine blood pressure levels in the population as a whole are equally as important as the factors that affect individuals. Evidence that the current high salt intake plays an important role in population—as well as individual—blood pressure levels comes from six different lines of investigation.

Population studies. Studies evaluating salt intake and blood pressure in large groups of people clearly show that populations that do not have access to salt or eat only very small amounts have much lower average blood pressures than those in which salt is widely available. In the former communities, high blood pressure is virtually unknown. Perhaps even more telling, the rise in blood pressure with age—an invariable feature of populations that eat large amounts of salt—is absent.

One of the largest of such investigations ever conducted was Intersalt, an international study whose findings were first published in 1988. The Intersalt researchers compared salt intake and blood pressure in more than 10,000 people in 52 communities in 32 different countries; they concluded that salt is one of the main determinants of blood pressure levels both between and within communities. The data also indicated that high salt intake is the likely cause of the rise in blood pressure with age. Other factors found to be related to elevated blood pressure levels were insufficient potassium intake, excess body weight, and alcohol consumption. Because the Salt Institute (a U.S. trade association) questioned the conclusions of the original Intersalt data, in May 1996 the investigators published an update of their findings, based on more sophisticated methods of analysis than were used in the 1980s. Their conclusions were the same.

Intervention studies. In the intervention studies of salt's relationship to blood pressure, large groups of people are given guidelines for reducing their salt intake and, after some time has elapsed, are compared with a group who have made no changes in their diet. One such study, conducted in The Netherlands in 1980, focused on infants. In this trial about 475 newborns were randomly assigned to two groups, one with a modestly restricted salt intake, the other with normal salt intake. During the course of the study, the two groups showed an increasing difference in systolic pressure (the first, or upper, number in the blood pressure reading). The systolic pressure of six-month-old infants in the reduced-salt group was lower by two millimeters of mercury. The study was discontinued after six months, but 15 years later a subgroup of these children was reevaluated to see whether the early temporary reduction in salt intake had produced a lasting effect. It was found that those in the reduced-salt group still had significantly lower blood pressures. This study clearly illustrates the vital role of salt intake in the first few months of life in determining blood pressure later on.

In Portugal, a country with one of the highest levels of salt consumption in the world as well as one of the highest stroke rates, a similar investigation was conducted, using two villages as the study groups. All of the adults in one village were given advice about reducing salt intake (*e.g.,* not adding salt to food, reducing the amount of salt added during cooking, eating reduced-salt bread); in the other village the adults did not receive dietary counseling. At the end of two years, blood pressure levels had declined significantly in the village that reduced its salt intake.

Migrant studies. The movement of people from one locale or country to another is often accompanied by marked changes in diet, lifestyle, and disease patterns. Such populations make excellent subjects for epidemiological studies and provide data supporting the link between salt and blood pressure. In one such investigation, for example, farmers in rural Kenya who consumed a low-salt diet were studied after they migrated to an urban environment where salt intake was comparable to levels seen in Western countries. When their blood pressure levels and salt and potassium intakes were compared with those of a group that remained in the countryside, it was apparent that the rise in blood pressure seen upon migration to the city was due at least in part to increased salt consumption.

Treatment trials. Studies in which salt reduction is adopted as a treatment are usually shorter-term than intervention or migrant studies and are targeted at specific groups (*e.g.,* normotensive subjects or people with very high blood pressure who are—or are not—taking antihypertensive medications). When the data from all such studies are combined, they show that a reduction in salt intake from 10 g per day to 5 g per day produces a drop in blood pressure in persons with high and normal blood pressures. The extent of the decline seems to depend on the degree of salt reduction, initial blood pressure level, and age of the individual. The greater the reduction in salt intake, the higher the initial blood pressure reading, and the older the person, the more pronounced the response. These studies also provide some evidence that black patients tend to benefit more than whites from salt restriction.

A recent study of people over 60 years of age showed that regardless of their initial blood pressure levels, all of the subjects experienced comparable decreases in blood pressure due to salt restriction. Moreover, reductions in salt intake produced decreases in blood pressure levels equivalent to those seen in studies of blood-pressure-lowering drugs. If this same strategy was applied to the whole of the elderly population and resulted in the same decrease in blood pressure, large numbers of strokes could be prevented in those whose blood pressures are in the upper range of normal and who therefore would not ordinarily be given antihypertensive drugs.

Animal studies. Research in mammals other than humans has produced an enormous amount of evidence of salt's critical role in regulating blood pressure. In all mammals studied, an increase in pressure is either caused or aggravated by a high salt intake.

The results of one of the most elegant of such investigations, a long-term study in chimpanzees, were published in 1995. The researchers showed that when salt was added to the chimpanzee's usual low-salt fruit and vegetable diet, the animals experienced a marked increase in blood pressure even though no other changes were made to their diets or habitat. Likewise, when the chimps' salt intake was later reduced, their blood pressures declined. There seems to be no good reason why humans should differ from their closest animal relative in their response to salt. As a result of this study, the salt content of the diet of chimpanzees in captivity has been reduced.

Genetic research. The majority of people with high blood pressure have what is called "essential hypertension"—that is, high blood pressure with no discernible cause. It is clear, however, that there is a strong familial factor in high blood pressure—*i.e.,* the condition occurs much more frequently in some families than others—and increasing evidence suggests that there are underlying genetic factors that predispose individuals to the development of high blood pressure. Although much current research is focused on the elucidation of these genetic factors, the factors affecting the majority of the hypertensive population remain unclear. A few rare single-gene defects responsible for high blood pressure have been identified. All of those described so far involve either a direct or an imposed defect in the kidney's ability to excrete salt, which leads to retention of salt and water and hence a rise in blood pressure. The increase in blood pressure is in turn aggravated by a high salt intake. The rare genetic causes of low blood pressure also involve the kidney, but the mechanism is exactly the opposite—the kidney cannot retain salt, and the resulting condition can be ameliorated by increasing salt intake.

To act on the evidence or wait for proof?

If so many studies so varied in design have come to roughly the same conclusions, why, one might ask, is salt's relationship to blood pressure still a matter of debate? One answer is that the "definitive" study has not been done and probably never will be. The reason is simply that such a study would be impractical. Ideally, it would require that a group of pregnant women be assigned at the time of conception either to adopt a moderately reduced salt intake or to continue consuming salt at current levels. Each woman's child would then follow the same salt regimen as the mother throughout his or her lifetime, and the blood pressures of both groups of offspring would be measured periodically—for the rest of their lives.

In the absence of definitive proof, measures to improve the public's health have always been—and will undoubtedly continue to be—based on the balance of the evidence. As an example one need only consider the sanitation measures that put an end to the urban cholera and typhoid epidemics of the 19th century. When these measures were first adopted, the exact cause of these diseases was still uncertain and their transmission by contaminated water only a matter of speculation. Nonetheless, the epidemiological evidence in cities like London led health authorities to suspect that water and sewage were involved, and action was taken in advance of firm proof. Lives were saved as a result.

Many expert medical and nutrition committees throughout the world have recommended that as a commonsense public health measure, people reduce their salt intake. Rather than setting an impractical target, these authorities have recommended a reduction from the current average of 10 g per day to 6 g per day. The food industry and its public relations spokespeople have consistently resisted such recommendations, however. Initially, they denounced the studies cited above as flawed. Then they claimed that the existing evidence simply was not sufficient to prompt action. They even went so far as to suggest that for some people reducing salt intake might be harmful. When it was pointed out that the recommended reduction in salt consumption was small and that large numbers of the population had already reduced their salt intake to this level, the industry representatives claimed that (1) reducing salt intake is difficult, and (2) other factors—body weight, alcohol consumption—have a greater impact on blood pressure than salt does, and these factors should be the target of health recommendations.

Other adverse effects

As noted at the outset, the health impact of excessive salt is not limited to blood pressure. Salt intake affects the balance of body fluids, kidney function, and many other physiological functions. There is even preliminary evidence that people who undergo surgery for cataracts are more likely than those without cataracts to have consumed high levels of salt. Some of the research on salt's other harmful effects is summarized below.

Fluid balance and water retention. All of the salt that a person ingests is absorbed into the body and excreted by the kidneys via the urine. Studies show that when salt intake is increased from a low to a high level, some of the additional salt is retained in the body until the kidneys, by a variety of different mechanisms, increase the amount of salt being excreted; thus, within a few days of the dietary change, the output of salt in the urine exactly matches the increase in salt intake, but at the expense of the retention of salt and water in the body and a consequent gain of 1 to 2 liters (about 1 to 2 qt) in body fluid and 1 to 2 kg (2.2–4.4 lb) in weight. Many medical conditions, including congestive heart failure and some forms of kidney disease, are characterized by abnormal retention of salt in the body; all of these problems are aggravated by high salt intake and relieved by a reduction in salt intake.

For unknown reasons women, more than men, tend to develop cyclical swelling due to fluid retention (edema). Many women find that if they reduce their salt intake, their tendency for swelling, particularly the tendency to develop swollen ankles from prolonged standing, is much alleviated.

Kidney disease. In animal models of kidney disease, kidney function is directly influenced by salt intake—increased salt intake speeds deterioration in function, and reduced salt intake slows it. In humans a high salt intake, even in individuals with normal blood pressure, is associated with an increased rate of filtration in the kidneys. A high rate of filtration, which is in itself

NEWS CAP MHA 98

Selling Kids on Poor Eating Habits

While nutrition authorities and government health agencies around the world exhort the public to adopt a healthy diet, television advertisements are bombarding the youngest members of the public with messages promoting foods that are anything but healthful. Such was the conclusion reached by the authors of *A Spoonful of Sugar,* a 1996 report on a comparative survey of advertisements aired during children's TV programs in 13 countries. The study was conducted by Consumers International, a London-based federation of 215 consumer organizations in more than 90 countries.

In most of the developed world high-fat, low-fiber diets and high rates of diet-related chronic illnesses—heart disease, stroke, high blood pressure, certain forms of cancer, etc.—are a major public health concern. Although there is disagreement over the true impact of advertisements on children's dietary habits, most health professionals believe that daily exposure to ads for foods high in fat, sugar, and/or salt may increase young viewers' risks for a number of childhood health problems (including obesity, anemia, and tooth decay), as well as setting a pattern for poor eating habits that may well persist into adulthood.

In almost all of the countries surveyed, food products were the leading category of advertised items during children's programs. The number of food advertisements per hour varied widely, however. Australia, the U.S., and the U.K. topped the list with 10 or more food ads per hour. In contrast, the TV channels monitored in Austria, Belgium, Norway, and Sweden broadcast between 0 and 2 food ads per hour. This wide range is explained largely by national differences in broadcast advertising regulations, which in turn reflect varying cultural attitudes regarding the ethics of advertising to children. Australia, the U.S., and the U.K., for example, do not have very restrictive advertising codes. In Norway and Sweden, on the other hand, TV ads may not be directed at children under 12 years old, nor are they allowed to air at all during children's shows. Other European countries restrict the length of ads run during children's programs.

The three categories of products that appeared most frequently in ads targeted to kids were confections, breakfast cereals (mostly brands with large amounts of added sugar), and restaurants (mostly fast-food chains). The most widely advertised brand names were McDonald's, Nestlé, Kellogg's, Mars, and Cadbury. An analysis of ad content in the U.K. revealed that 62% of ads were for products high in fat, 50% for products high in sugar, and 61% for products high in sodium. Advertisements for fruits, vegetables, and other foods integral to a healthy diet were absent or rare. This lack of balance led the authors of the report to comment that "advertising is a predisposing factor for deterioration in kidney function, is completely reversed by reducing salt intake. Finally, when kidney disease patients restrict their salt intake, the amount of protein in their urine declines. Excessive protein excretion seems to be a marker for the severity of the kidney disease, so a reduction in urinary protein levels would seem to indicate an improvement in disease status.

Most kidney stones either are composed entirely of calcium or have calcium as a major constituent. It would therefore be predicted that a high salt intake, which increases calcium excretion, would exacerbate the tendency for kidney stones to form, and this is exactly what has been found. Indeed, for many years reduction of salt intake has been advocated as a preventive measure for people at risk of developing kidney stones.

Calcium metabolism and bone health. Calcium in the diet is only partially absorbed during digestion, and some of the calcium that is absorbed is excreted in the urine. Salt is the major determinant of the amount of calcium excreted. The increase in salt intake from one-tenth of a gram a day (the amount ingested by early humans) to the current average of 10 g per day causes large increases in calcium excretion, but most authorities have always assumed that this increase was balanced by increased calcium absorption from the gastrointestinal tract, which thus prevented the body's stores of calcium—primarily in bone—from being depleted. Studies show that when urinary calcium excretion rises as a result of increased salt intake, the amount of calcium in body fluids decreases slightly. This reduction in fluid-calcium concentration is the stimulus for compensatory mechanisms that cause increased absorption of calcium from the gastrointestinal tract. Recently, however, scientists have discovered that these compensatory mechanisms include an increased mobilization of calcium from bone. It is possible, therefore, that in the long term a high salt intake will gradually deplete the bones of calcium.

The strength of the human skeleton is greatest around the age of 25–30 years and declines with age as the bones become less dense. Now that people are living longer, osteoporosis (thinning of the bones) is becoming a very widespread problem. Thinning of the bones causes collapse of the vertebral bodies in the spine and compression of the nerve roots, which results in severe pain. Bone thinning also increases the risk of fractures. Several risk factors for osteoporosis have been identified. It is much more common in women than in men and more likely to occur in postmenopausal women, the sedentary, and smokers.

A recent study monitored changes in hip bone density over two years in a group of postmenopausal women. The most important predictor of bone loss was the amount of salt in the urine, which, as noted above, is a consistent reflection of salt intake. Women with the highest salt intake had the greatest reduction in hip bone

often credited with promoting the bastion of consumer freedom—choice. But the choice that food advertising presents children is largely one between one candy bar and another."

The degree to which advertising influences food choices and general health is a matter of heated debate. Not surprisingly, the advertising industry and consumer organizations make opposing claims. A spokesperson for Britain's Advertising Association dismisses the assertion that ads directed at children could have lifelong effects on health, claiming instead that the factors that influence an individual's dietary choices (*e.g.,* culture, family, peer pressure, self-image) are numerous and complex.

The survey report, however, cites sound academic studies that establish a definite link between advertising and children's food choices. It is known that children are brand conscious and often ask their parents to buy specific advertised products. Moreover, studies of children's dietary habits consistently reveal a direct correlation between the amount of time youngsters spend viewing television and their requests for and consumption of advertised foods. Certainly the clients who are willing to pay high prices for TV ad spots believe that advertising is effective.

The authors urge governments and international bodies to develop safeguards for protecting youngsters from the influence of advertisers. Their recommendations call for establishing international standards, obligating broadcasters to comply with the regulations of the receiving country in cross-border TV advertising, mandating that ads be easily distinguishable from programs (*i.e.,* breaks between ads and children's shows should be clear, and cartoon characters or other personalities should not be permitted to appear in ads), and utilizing public-service announcements to relay sound nutritional information to children. In an era of increasing worldwide awareness of the need to protect children and promote their rights, these recommendations are sure to find a receptive audience.

—Afrodite Mantzavrakos

Advertising on Children's TV Programs

Country	Foods, all kinds (average number of ads per hour)	Sweets (number of ads per 20 hours)	Cereals (number of ads per 20 hours)
Australia	12	15	46
United States	11	31	71
United Kingdom	10	54	32
France	8	40	31
Greece	7	64	26
Finland	6	8	...
Germany	6	15	32
Denmark	5	21	11
The Netherlands	4	36	...
Belgium	2	17	3
Austria	1	15	6
Norway	1	5	1
Sweden	<1	2	2

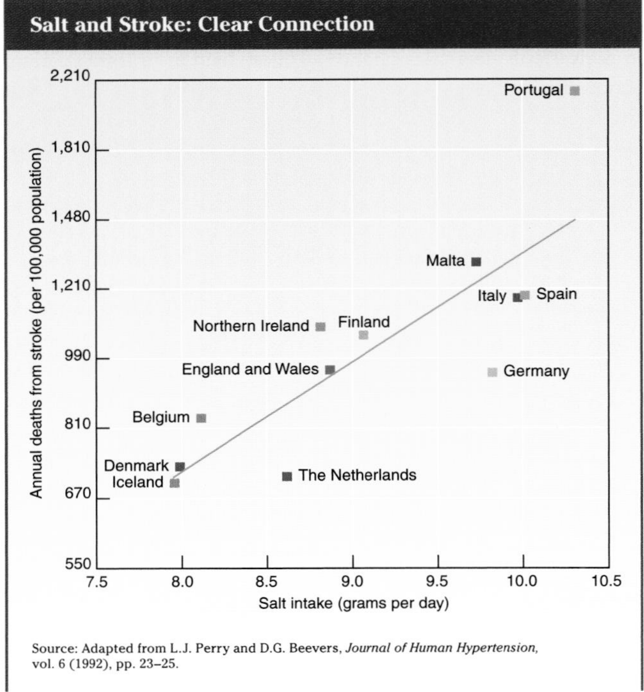

Source: Adapted from L.J. Perry and D.G. Beevers, *Journal of Human Hypertension*, vol. 6 (1992), pp. 23–25.

density. In those women who were eating less than five grams of salt a day, there appeared to be no bone loss from the hip. On the basis of these data, the investigators calculated that a reduction in salt intake from 10 to 5 g per day would have the same beneficial effect on bone density as an increase of approximately one gram per day in calcium. While the reduction in salt intake can easily be achieved with minor dietary modifications, an increase of one gram per day in calcium intake would mean having to take a calcium supplement. Reducing salt intake therefore seems a more practical as well as less-costly means of preventing bone loss. Of particular current concern is that young adolescent girls commonly consume too little calcium and too much salt. Typically, then, this group has relatively high levels of urinary calcium loss. Since women achieve peak bone mass at around age 25—and since failure to reach peak bone mass is a predisposing factor in the development of osteoporosis—inadequate calcium intake in adolescence can increase a woman's risk for osteoporosis. With teenagers eating increasing amounts of high-salt, low-calcium snack foods, it is likely that osteoporosis will be a major problem for this generation as they age.

The effect of salt on calcium excretion is magnified in patients with high blood pressure, who are therefore at increased risk of developing kidney stones. Although this is a rare occurrence, the incidence of kidney stones is higher in hypertensive than in normotensive individuals. Moreover, it stands to reason that they are also at increased risk for osteoporosis. Direct evidence of this effect in humans is lacking, but in animal models of essential hypertension, severe osteoporosis is common. Diuretics, drugs that help rid the body of excess salt and water, not only lower elevated blood pressure but also reduce the amount of calcium excreted in the urine. In both patients with high blood pressure and those with normal pressure, diuretics have been shown to reduce the incidence of fractures due to osteoporosis. Since salt restriction has exactly the same physiological effect as diuretics, it is likely, although not proven, that restriction of salt intake also will reduce the risk of bone thinning and fracture.

Enlargement of the heart. In people with high blood pressure, the heart must pump harder than normal to overcome the resistance of the vessels to the flow of blood. As a result, over time the heart will become enlarged, which further reduces its pumping ability and increases the risk of complications from the high blood pressure. Scientists have studied this vicious circle intensively, and recent investigations have revealed that in addition to blood pressure, salt intake is also an influential—and independent—factor. Indeed, in some studies salt intake was an even more important influence.

Stroke: an independent effect. High blood pressure is very closely associated with strokes. Recently, however, some animal experiments compared stroke rates in two groups of animals with the same blood pressure levels but different levels of salt consumption. The high-salt-intake group had far more strokes, which certainly suggests that a high salt intake may have a direct effect on strokes independent of blood pressure. Again, no comparable direct evidence exists for humans, but population studies of salt intake and stroke mortality show a similar pattern. (*See* graph.)

Cancer of the stomach. Epidemiologists have known for many years that countries with high rates of death due to stomach cancer also have high stroke rates. Recently, scientists seeking a better understanding of the risk factors for stomach cancer reviewed the population studies. Their analysis clearly demonstrated that the strongest relationship was to salt intake. Over the past

A comparison of two typical meals that might be eaten today in any Western country demonstrates how much excess salt—and fat—can be packed onto a plate. The meal that includes sausage, bacon, egg, and fries (below) weighs in at 7.5 g of salt and 130 g of fat, while the turkey dinner (opposite page) has only 0.5 g of salt and 6 g of fat. The total salt and fat in each meal are graphically shown.

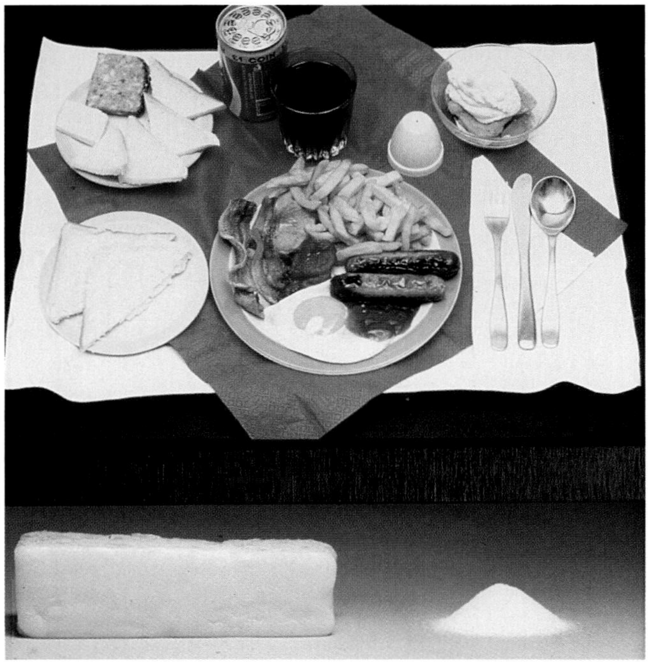

Photographs courtesy of Graham A. MacGregor

100 years, death rates from stomach cancer and stroke have steadily decreased in the U.S. and Western Europe. Many authorities speculate that this trend can be attributed to the reduction in salt intake that accompanied the wider availability of refrigeration. In recent years, however, the decline in stroke rates has begun to outpace the drop in stomach cancer deaths, perhaps because of the success of blood-pressure-lowering treatments in preventing stroke. It would be interesting to see if reductions in salt intake would have a similar impact on stomach cancer mortality.

Asthma. Asthma is usually caused by an allergic response to foreign proteins. The immune reaction triggers constriction of the bronchioles (the small airways in the lungs), which thereby causes the difficulty in breathing. A high salt intake increases the reactivity of the smooth muscle cells lining the bronchioles. In one carefully conducted double-blind study, male asthma patients who reduced their salt by half (from 10 to 5 g per day) had a marked improvement in symptoms, were able to reduce their use of asthma drugs, and had improved scores on objective tests of lung function. Curiously, though, the small number of women in the study did not benefit to the same extent as the men.

Ann McQueen—Stock, Boston/PNI

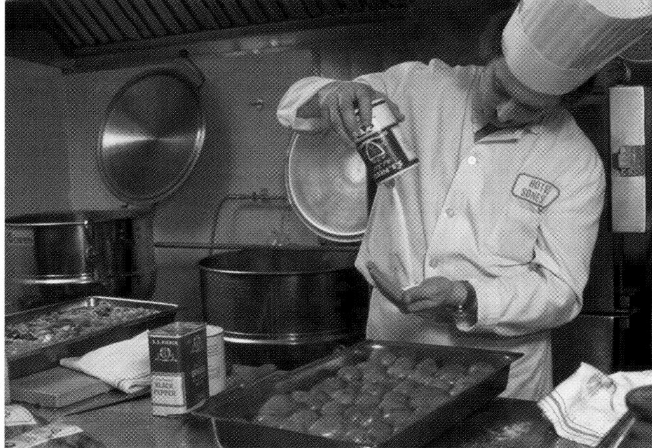

The more salt people eat, the less sensitive they become to its taste. Studies show that individuals who reduce the amount of salt in their diet quickly become accustomed to—and, indeed, grow to prefer—the taste of food without added salt.

Sorting out the issues

Specific taste receptors in the mouth are responsible for the perception of the salt taste. Increasing the saltiness of food blunts the sensitivity of these receptors. Likewise, decreasing the saltiness enhances the receptors' sensitivity. Because of their heightened taste sensitivity, people who have reduced their salt intake typically report that salty foods they formerly would have enjoyed now taste unpleasant. The food industry, however, persists in its claim that the salt added to processed foods is necessary to improve taste and, in fact, that it "makes unpalatable food edible." This may be true of some of the cheapest foods, which consist mainly of animal fat (*e.g.,* sausages) and clearly require some flavoring to make them palatable. Still, it seems unnecessary even for foods like sausages to have a salt concentration of 2.5%—which translates into 1,000 mg of sodium per serving.

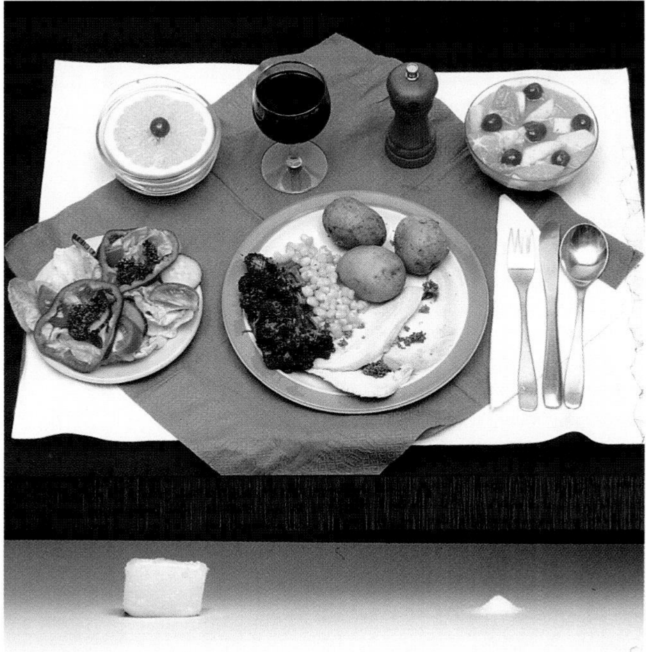

Skeptics say that the main reason so much salt is added to food is not to enhance taste but to allow more water to be added, which increases the weight of the product at very little cost. Critics of the food industry also point out that salty foods make people thirsty, and some of the largest soft-drink manufacturers also own large snack-food companies. It seems, then, that the food industry has a vested interest in opposing recommendations to reduce salt intake. This is the motivation for the industry's campaign to convince doctors, nutritionists, politicians, and the public that the evidence linking salt to blood pressure is flawed. The food industry, the largest single industry in most developed countries, also donates money to political parties, which may explain why governments in many countries have been reluctant to take action to reduce salt intake—in spite of the recommendation of their own health agencies and experts.

The current challenge for nutrition authorities and health professionals is to draw attention to the industry's tactics. One institution that has taken up the gauntlet is the *British Medical Journal* (*BMJ*), which in May 1996 reprinted an article by the president of the Salt Institute criticizing the Intersalt study's methodology and conclusions. An accompanying note from the editor of the *BMJ* read, "We publish this analysis not because we believe it but so as to present readers with an example of how the salt industry works." Another organization that seems determined to expose the salt industry is the Washington, D.C.-based nonprofit Center for Science in the Public Interest.

The food industry too faces a challenge: to continue to do battle with nutritionists and health professionals or to produce processed foods that contain far less salt but that taste (as they are likely to) much better than the highly salted products now being sold. As for the public, their challenge is perhaps the most difficult of all: to evaluate the various different arguments and make the healthiest choices.

—Graham A. MacGregor, M.A., and Francesco P. Cappuccio, M.D., M.Sc.

Medicine in the Middle of Nowhere

Increasing numbers of travelers are leaving modern conveniences behind to explore remote and wild places. From weekend backpackers to high-altitude mountaineers, people with all levels of experience are going to great lengths to surround themselves with natural beauty and discover the rewards of the physical challenges and solitude that come with wilderness exploration.

Far from the reach of physicians

Just as the wilderness offers people opportunities to step out of the familiar routines of daily life, it also leads them out of the reach of physicians—and even of emergency medical personnel, who, of course, can drive their ambulances only as far into the backcountry as there are roads. Still, medical emergencies are inevitable, especially when a person is engaged in wilderness activities that continually challenge the body's levels of endurance, agility, and strength.

By courtesy of SOLO

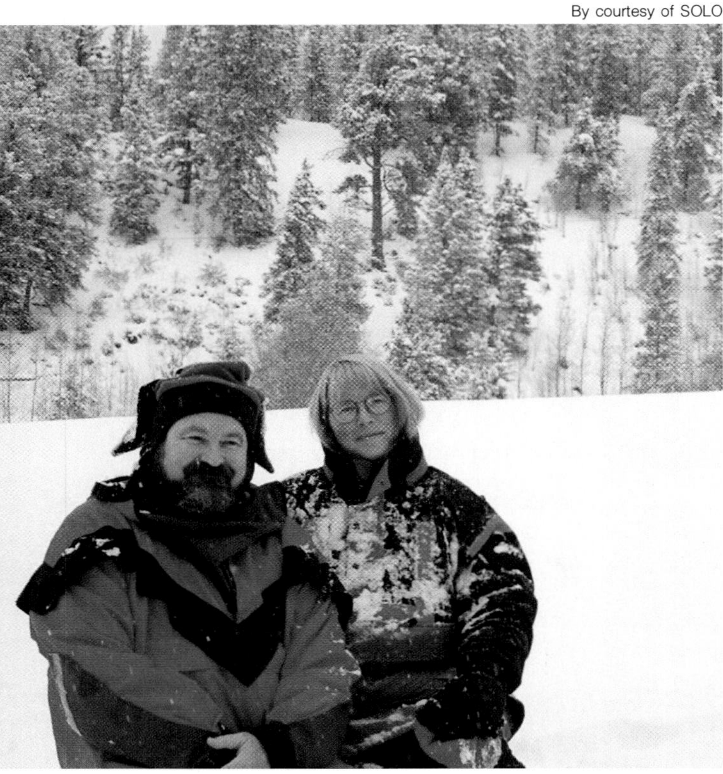

Frank Hubbell (left) and Lee Frizzell are directors of Stonehearth Open Learning Opportunities (SOLO), headquartered in New Hampshire's White Mountains. Since 1976 over 30,000 wilderness emergency medicine providers have been trained in SOLO's state-of-the-art programs.

When a medical emergency occurs hours or days from the nearest hospital, it becomes necessary for someone to assume responsibility for managing the scene, making a diagnosis, providing treatment, coordinating an evacuation, and documenting the case in a way that will be useful to physicians once the patient has been transported back to civilization. These responsibilities, when applied to patient care in remote settings, have helped to define a branch of medicine that is now known as wilderness medicine. Previous to the mid-1970s, a group of people traveling in the backcountry either was fortunate enough to have a physician or nurse among its members or had to rely on the insufficient knowledge of someone in the group who had, at best, taken a course in cardiopulmonary resuscitation (CPR) or basic first aid. At the time, even U.S. Forest Service rangers and other managers of wilderness areas had only the most elementary medical skills.

The boy with the broken arm

In 1975 a paramedic named Frank Hubbell of rural New Hampshire became dismayed by what he was seeing in his daily work. Emergency medical personnel like himself did not have sufficient skills to deal with critical illness or injury in the wilderness, even though they were the ones most likely to provide prehospital care in just such emergencies.

That year, during the rescue of a young boy who had suffered a severe angulated fracture of his arm on a backcountry trail in New Hampshire's White Mountains, Hubbell and his rescue team followed standard protocol and splinted the boy's arm in the position of injury. Tractioning the fracture and straightening the bones would have involved procedures that were reserved for emergency room physicians. These skills were not taught to prehospital emergency care providers, even though, if severe enough, angulated fractures can cut off circulation in adjacent blood vessels. Typically, however, a patient would be in a doctor's care before permanent damage occurred.

The boy's case was not typical. Hubbell and his crew transported him to the nearest hospital as quickly as possible, but the entire evacuation took a total of nine hours. By the time the boy was admitted to the emergency room, his hand was past the point of saving.

After an emergency room physician indicated that the boy's hand could have been saved if the fracture had been straightened in the field by someone who was familiar with the correct procedure, Hubbell felt called to action. A few months after that experience, he helped found Stonehearth Open Learning Opportunities (better known as SOLO), the first school specifically designed for the teaching of wilderness medicine.

The "golden hour"

The term *wilderness emergency medicine* can be somewhat misleading. An ill or injured person does not need to be on the summit of Mt. Everest to be far enough from doctors and hospitals to fall within the purview of wilderness medical care providers. Nor does the patient need to have sustained a traumatic injury for the situation to be considered an emergency, as relatively simple conditions that occur on backcountry outings can lead to quite significant complications (such as infection or dehydration).

The chief determinant of the domain of wilderness medicine is the amount of time it would take in an emergency situation to transport a patient to a medical facility. In areas of the United States that are extremely remote, particularly those bordering wilderness recreational areas—where backcountry travel is common—the emergency medical system (EMS) is stretched beyond its capacity. The EMS in most U.S. communities consists of ambulance crews and other personnel who respond to 911 emer-

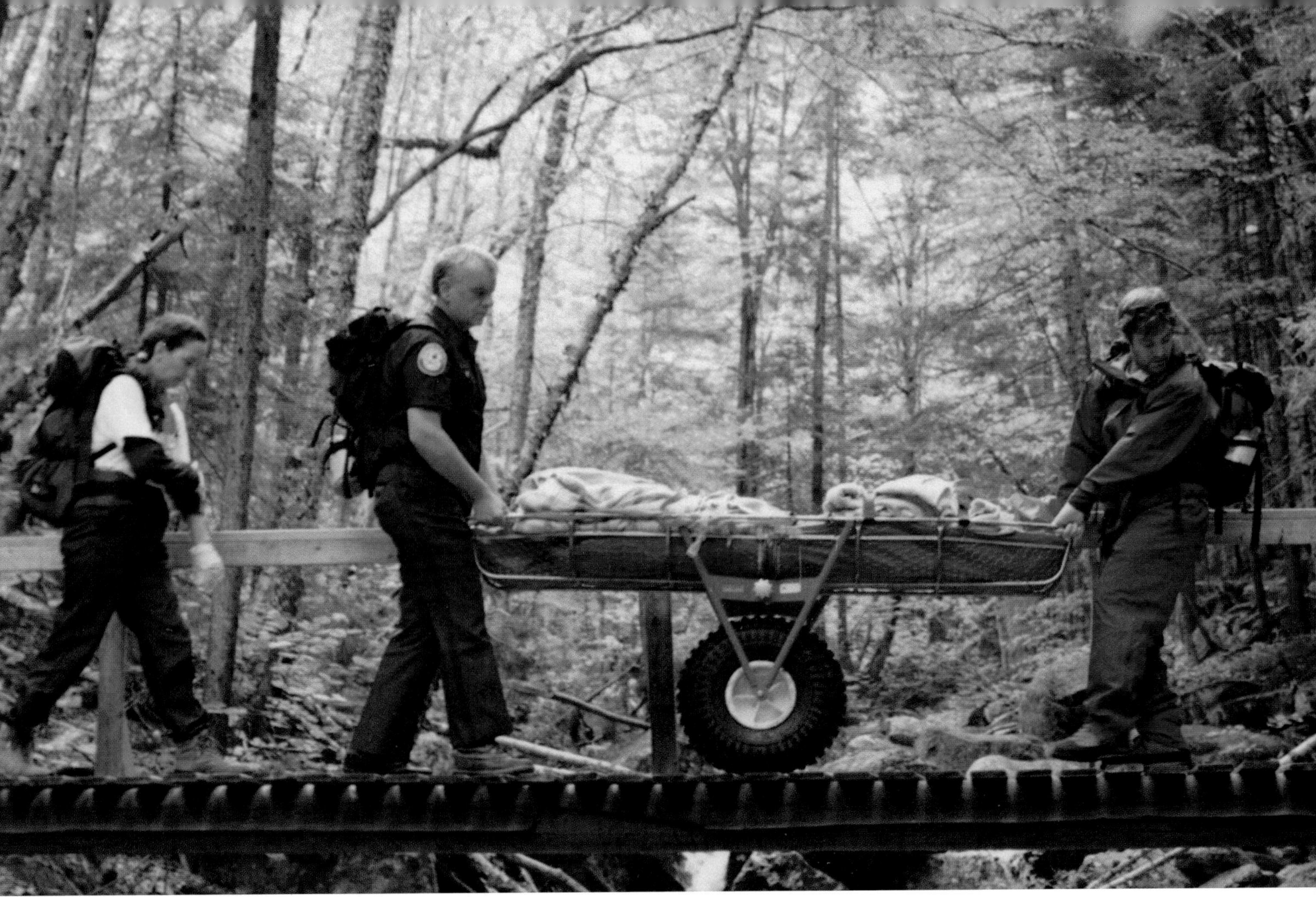

Arethusa Falls is New Hampshire's highest straight-drop waterfall and the site of fairly frequent medical emergencies. SOLO students had a taste of the challenges of carrying out a rescue in a rugged backcountry setting when they helped evacuate a hiker who had fallen 60 m (200 ft) to his death.

gency phone calls. The system was designed around the principle of a short transfer time between the site of a medical emergency and a hospital or clinic where comprehensive care is available. This period of time during which EMS personnel have the medical training, equipment, and support resources to keep most patients alive is referred to by professionals as the "golden hour." Emergency medical technicians (E.M.T.s) and paramedics count on the fact that in almost every case they can transport a patient to a medical facility in less—usually far less—than an hour's time.

Any amount of time that a patient spends in the care of the EMS beyond this one-hour period is, in essence, beyond the bounds of what emergency personnel are able to do as standard protocol. Their medical education has focused on what they can accomplish in 60 minutes with the equipment and resources available to them in an ambulance. This kind of medicine, what paramedics and E.M.T.s can feasibly do in an urban or suburban setting, is often referred to as "street medicine."

The challenges of wilderness medicine

In the U.S. the term *wilderness,* as it applies to emergency medicine, is defined as areas that are more than an hour's travel time from a road. In a wilderness setting, the concept of the golden hour no longer applies, as there can be no expedient transfer of a patient to an emergency ward. As long as the patient is in the wilderness, no matter what the nature of his or her illness or injury, medical care must be as comprehensive as possible with a minimum of resources. In developing curricula for the teaching of wilderness emergency medicine, Hubbell and other innovators in the field had to consider exactly what types of pressures and constraints wilderness medical providers typically face in the course of their work.

Treating patients with a minimum of supplies. A first consideration was that wilderness medical care providers would have to care for their patients without the benefit of extensive medical equipment or supplies. These resources would have to be limited to what members of a group could feasibly transport in the backcountry, often on their backs. Any equipment that required electricity or cumbersome batteries would be out of the question for mobile groups, as would supplies and equipment designed for highly specialized methods of treatment. A realistic wilderness medical kit can contain only a small number of lightweight, durable, and highly versatile items. A wilderness medical care provider thus would have to accomplish a lot with very little.

Providing a diagnosis and treatment with a lack of support. It is typically impossible for a wilderness medical care provider to consult with or receive guidance from medical professionals in the outside world. Citizens band radios are typically too weighty

(continued on page 239)

By courtesy of SOLO

NEWS CAP MHA 98

In-Line in the ER

In-line skating, or Rollerblading, a hybrid of roller-skating and ice skating that requires a pair of ski-boot-structured footgear underlaid with a series of small wheels aligned in the shape of a blade, is the fastest-growing recreational sport in the U.S. By the beginning of 1996, there were an estimated 22.5 million such skaters—a 263% increase over 1991. According to participants, in-line skating is exhilarating. It also provides excellent aerobic exercise (building major muscle groups and conditioning the cardiovascular system). Probably for those reasons, the sport's popularity does not appear to be waning.

Nor, unfortunately, does the number of injured in-line skaters who are landing in hospital emergency rooms (ERs) in need of treatment. ER visits brought on by in-line skating mishaps total about 100,000 a year and consume at least $495 million in medical expenses. Probably more than twice as many injured in-liners a year seek treatment in doctors' offices. As of 1996, at least 25 deaths had been attributed to the sport.

This obviously growing public health problem prompted a team of injury-prevention specialists from the Centers for Disease Control and Prevention in Atlanta, Ga., and the Consumer Product Safety Commission in Washington, D.C., to study in-line skating injuries. Their findings, published in *The New England Journal of Medicine* (Nov. 28, 1996), were illuminating. Injuries tended to be severe, and about half were full-fledged fractures. The most commonly injured body part was the wrist. Other injuries were lacerations (most often of the face and chin), sprained wrists and ankles, and broken elbows and lower legs. Other notable findings were that:

- The skates used by 85% of subjects were in "good" condition.
- Most subjects (75%) had taken up skating "to get exercise"; 31% participated in the sport "to perform tricks" (of whom 40% had sustained injuries while doing tricks).
- In 81% of injuries "spontaneous loss of balance" or "striking a stationary hazard" was the "proximate cause" (*i.e.,* the event immediately preceding the injury).
- Only 7% of subjects wore full safety gear; no such gear was worn by 46% of those sustaining injuries, and the remaining subjects wore only partial gear.

An editorial accompanying the *New England Journal* report speculated that if every in-line skater donned a pair of wrist guards and elbow pads, ER visits would be reduced by 36,000 a year and 80,000 fewer skaters would need treatment in doctors' offices. The cost of a full set of safety gear (about $100 for wrist guards, elbow pads, knee pads, and a helmet) is 10 times less than the average cost of an ER visit. Anyone willing to pay $100–$400 for a zippy pair of skates ought also to get the insurance afforded by good protective apparel.

(Below) Courtesy of Rollerblade, Inc.; (bottom) Wilfredo Lee—Associated Press

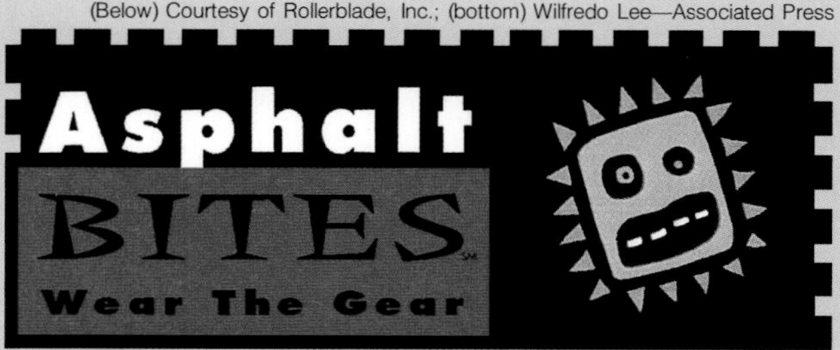

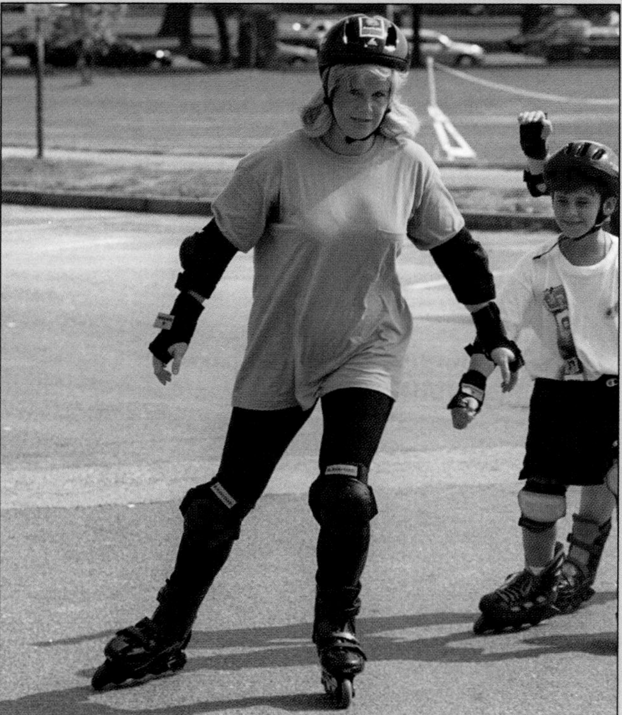

Tipper Gore (above), wife of U.S. Vice Pres. Al Gore, is an avid in-line skater and a leading proponent of safety in the sport. (Top) Rollerblade, Inc., is the sponsor of a major campaign—appropriately named "Asphalt Bites"—promoting the wearing of safety gear.

A major safety crusader is the International Inline Skating Association (IISA) with its "Gear Up! Take a Lesson" campaign. For further information about in-line skating safety, one can visit the IISA's Internet site at http://www.iisa.org or contact the association at 3720 Farragut Ave, Suite 400, Kensington MD 20895 (phone: 301-942-9770).

—Jackie Orihill

(continued from page 237)
to take along, and cellular phones often do not have a wide-enough communication range to function reliably in backcountry situations. Even if a means of communicating with physicians at an urban medical center were available, concerns about the legal ramifications of practicing "telephone medicine" would likely limit them as a resource. An abbreviated medical reference book could easily be taken along, as well as personal notes and reference materials, but beyond these resources, the wilderness medical provider would be working in isolation.

Providing care in a potentially hostile environment. The wilderness is, by nature, an unpredictable place. Throughout the duration of patient care, it could be raining, hailing, or snowing. Proper treatment or evacuation efforts could be hindered or halted by such conditions. There could be lightning, heavy winds, or dense fog, increasing the potential for further injury. The temperature could be dangerously hot or dangerously cold, making it difficult to stabilize a patient's core body temperature. Aggressive wildlife could also be present, posing additional hazards. It could be difficult or impossible to isolate a patient from dangerous allergens in the environment. As well, resources such as fresh water and fuel for heat could become scarce or nonexistent.

Having limited access to the patient. Providing medical care in the wilderness can be as much an issue of accessing the patient as diagnosing and treating the problem. If the patient has fallen from a height, for example, or been carried downriver or become stranded in an area prone to avalanches, it could be difficult or dangerous for a wilderness care provider to address the patient's immediate medical needs quickly without risking additional injury. Wilderness medical care providers, then, would need highly developed backcountry skills to successfully manage emergencies in unstable environments.

Providing extended patient care. A final and critical consideration was the matter of evacuation. In street medicine a patient is typically treated and transported simultaneously in an ambulance. This is virtually impossible during a backcountry evacuation. It is unlikely that even a large group of physically strong people, working in reasonable shifts, could carry a patient in a litter across backcountry terrain faster than a half a kilometer per hour. Time would be needed periodically to halt the evacuation to maintain patient care, take vital signs, administer medications, change dressings, and rest. The wilderness medical care provider would have to be able to make sound judgments about long-term patient care, as well as have the necessary skills to keep a patient stabilized for days at a time.

Furthermore, wilderness medical care providers must be prepared to handle the heightened emotional stress that accompanies working under adverse conditions many kilometers from the nearest road or phone. The stress, for example, of treating a penetration injury to the eye in a tent during a thunderstorm with only a flashlight for illumination can seem overwhelming, yet this is exactly the sort of scenario wilderness emergency medical care providers are trained to handle. In addition, the limited treatment possibilities and delays in transport to a hospital increase the patient's chances of dying or sustaining permanent physical damage. Wilderness medical care providers routinely run the risk of experiencing profound feelings of guilt, anger, failure, and loss, as they must often assume sole responsibility for the outcome of a wilderness medical crisis.

Jean-Marc Giboux—Gamma Liaison

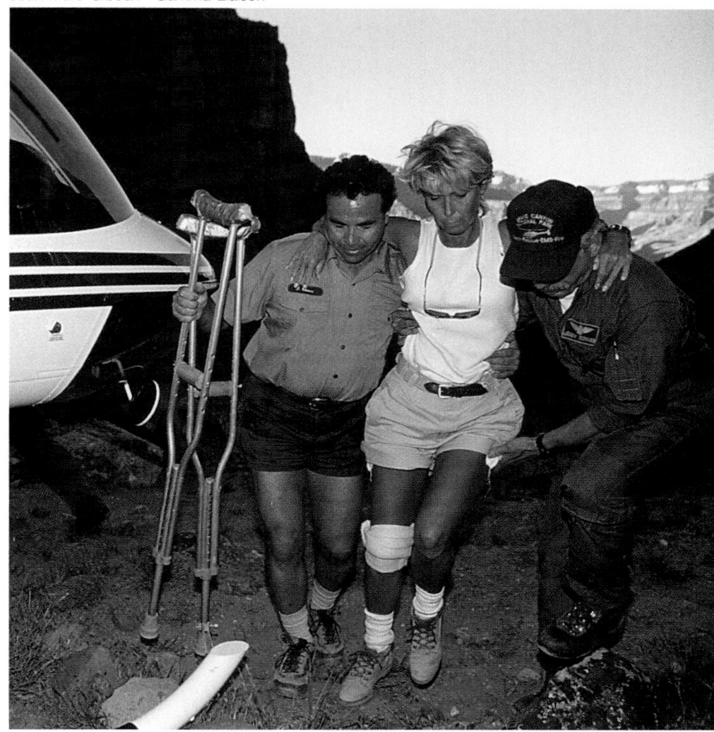

Helicopter rescue of an injured hiker from the Grand Canyon. Backcountry settings challenge the endurance, agility, and strength of adventure-seeking vacationers. Medical mishaps are inevitable.

A unique medical education

It would be unrealistic to expect that every time a person traveled in the backcountry, he or she would be in the company of a physician, with a physician's extensive training and experience. Nor is it necessarily the case that a physician would be the best person to make decisions about managing a medical emergency in a wilderness setting, as a physician is accustomed to working with technology available at a medical facility. E.M.T.s and paramedics may also fall into the same category of having a great deal of knowledge about procedures that are of little or no use in a backcountry environment. Wilderness medicine requires a different sort of medical training as well as a different type of practitioner.

Absent from the education of wilderness medical care providers are the long hours spent examining slides under a microscope, negotiating stacks of pharmacological flash cards, and gaining the technical experience with such tools as electrocardiograms, X-rays, or intravenous appliances. Instead, wilderness medical courses aim to instill in students fundamental sets of skills to help empower them in the backcountry. Therefore, every wilderness medical provider should have excellent training in systems-oriented thinking, in creative problem solving, and in prevention consciousness.

Synergy and the human body. The human body is a highly dynamic collection of systems working in cooperation to achieve optimum health. Wilderness medical care providers need to have an understanding of the ways in which illness and injury can

(continued on page 241)

NEWS CAP MHA 98

Cardiac Emergencies: Nothing to Be Up in the Air About

Airlines in the United States have come under increasing pressure to upgrade the medical kits included on commercial flights and particularly to include new lightweight, portable automatic external defibrillators that have recently come onto the market. Insufficient onboard medical supplies, experts claim, have hindered in-flight emergency care and endangered ill passengers, particularly cardiac arrest victims, for whom speedy care is essential. Cardiac arrest is a condition in which the heart ceases to beat. An attack begins with the heart beating chaotically (ventricular fibrillation) or much too fast (ventricular tachycardia); because the blood stops circulating, the body's organs and tissues are soon deprived of life-sustaining oxygen and the brain is depleted of vital glucose. If resuscitation is not successfully performed within 10 minutes of the attack, death inevitably follows. More than 300,000 Americans die from cardiac arrest every year.

In-flight emergencies, where the victim cannot be quickly transported to a hospital, pose special problems. The policy of U.S. airlines prescribes emergency landing and securing of prompt medical care for the cardiac arrest victim—specifically, automatic defibrillation (the administration of electrical shocks to the heart via electrodes). Many physicians and physicians organizations, however, including the American Medical Association, have long believed that such a policy provides too little too late—approximately 10 minutes too late at best. An emergency landing of a domestic flight takes a minimum of 20 minutes. Airplanes flying over remote parts of a continent or an ocean may not be able to land for hours.

Controversy over medical readiness in the air was stirred in November 1996 when the U.S. Food and Drug Administration (FDA) approved the in-flight use of portable defibrillators that emit up to 12 powerful shocks to restart the heart. Despite public pleas, media pressure, and encouraging reports from foreign airlines that use defibrillators, U.S. airlines have resisted incorporating the small, easy-to-use devices (about the size of this book) into their onboard medical kits. American Airlines became the first—and so far the only—U.S. airline to do so, and in July 1997 it began carrying them on all its overseas flights.

For some airlines the chief objection to introducing airborne defibrillators is the cost. At about $3,000 per unit, American Airlines spent

Heartstream/Business Wire/AP

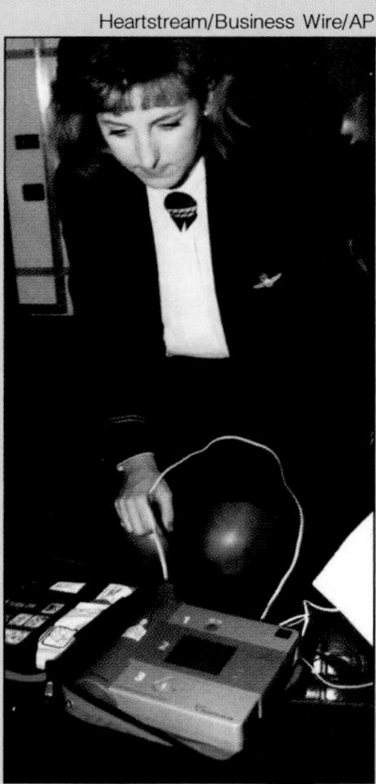

In July 1997 American Airlines became the first U.S. carrier equipped to handle in-flight cardiac arrests.

nearly $1 million for 300 of the devices. Another issue is liability; although the manufacturers make a convincing case that even nonspecialists can correctly use the entirely automated units and that the risk of harming a cardiac arrest victim is negligible, some concern remains that passengers or crew who use the devices incorrectly, or the airlines themselves, may be held legally liable.

Three international carriers—Qantas (of Australia), Virgin Atlantic Airways (of Great Britain), and Air Zimbabwe—have already added defibrillators to the medical kits aboard their aircraft. In a period of four years, six lives were saved on flights of the airlines, a benefit that in the minds of most people would easily offset the cost of installing and maintaining the units. It has also been argued that the few-thousand-dollar price paid for one defibrillator may actually be less than the thousands of dollars incurred by an airline forced to make an unscheduled landing: landing fees, fuel costs, passenger rebookings, and so forth.

The Federal Aviation Administration, the agency that regulates the U.S. airline industry, made onboard medical kits mandatory in 1986, but it has demanded few changes or additions since then. Presently, the medical kits are among the least inclusive of those on all the major airlines worldwide: four drugs—dextrose, epinephrine, diphenhydramine, and nitroglycerin—and a set of basic instruments *(e.g.,* blood pressure cuff, tourniquet, hypodermic syringes). By contrast, Qantas flights are equipped with kits that include 16 injectable drugs, 11 more oral drugs and preparations, and 28 items of medical equipment, *plus* automatic defibrillators.

A special report in the *Chicago Tribune* estimated that the cost of adding portable defibrillators as well as enhanced medical kits like those used by international carriers to every airplane in the U.S. commercial fleet would be about $56 million but could be offset by adding a mere two cents to the price of every airline ticket sold.

—Jackie Orihill

(continued from page 239)

affect the body's synergistic relationships as they compromise the effectiveness of bodily systems individually.

In the case of a patient suffering a chest wound, for example, it is not sufficient that a wilderness medical care provider simply apply bandages as directed by a first aid cue card. A more comprehensive understanding of what is happening in the context of the patient's entire body is necessary. The provider must, for example, ask: What is happening to the respiratory rate? Heart rate? Blood pressure? Is there pressure building in the chest cavity? If so, is it due to internal hemorrhaging, a volume of trapped air, or both?

Although visible symptoms in different emergencies encountered in the backcountry may appear to be quite similar, the physiological implications can be vastly different, so manifestly different forms of treatment may be required in each particular case. A wilderness medical care provider therefore would need to have the skills to be able to make diagnoses and then plan treatment strategies on the basis of a careful consideration of the injured or ill subject's entire body rather than by just addressing point-specific symptoms.

Furthermore, the wilderness medical care provider must be able to communicate and document the progress of a patient's case beyond the obvious signs and symptoms. All prehospital medical care providers are familiar with the SOAP note format. A SOAP note is a collection of observations and documentation about a patient's case that serves both the wilderness medical care provider and physicians who will treat the patient upon his or her return to civilization. The notes are a record of all pertinent medical information acquired about the patient and his or her condition as well as treatment given during the time the patient spent in the wilderness. The acronym stands for the "subjective" observations (those the patient provides him- or herself about what he or she is experiencing), "objective" observations (those recorded by the medical care provider), "assessment" (the diagnosis), and "plan" of action (including treatment strategies and evacuation specifics).

Whatever works. Owing to the logistic challenges wilderness emergency medical care providers face, it is critical that they understand that in the backcountry there is never a form of treatment that is objectively "best." In the wilderness every medical emergency has its own distinct and particular context. Every treatment strategy must be considered from scratch, and methods of treatment must always remain open to creative revision.

Splints for fractured bones, for instance, may be fashioned out of tent poles and ace bandages, sleeping pads and furnace tape, tree branches and T-shirts, or books and bandanas. The training of wilderness medical care providers discourages a dependence on convention, which can be dangerous in an environment that lacks predictability.

The "best" injury. The best injury is, of course, the injury that never happened; the most desirable illness, the one that was not permitted to develop. Wilderness medical care providers must thoroughly understand the concept of consequence to succeed in their work. The amount of time, energy, and suffering that can be saved later by immediately and thoroughly—sometimes even gratuitously—cleaning and disinfecting a minor wound, for instance, can be truly significant in terms of preventing the occurrence later of a massive infection.

Levels of wilderness medical training

As in any branch of medicine, there are various levels of medical training that denote degrees of knowledge and ability in the discipline of wilderness medicine. There are three general categories of wilderness medical certification.

Wilderness first aid and below. This category includes any training in CPR, basic lifesaving, basic wilderness first aid, lifeguard training, and all other levels of training that teach a student only fundamental lifesaving techniques to keep the patient's heart pumping, respiratory system functioning, and circulation flowing at an adequate pressure. Training in this category is generally too basic to include information that would be of great value in extended emergency situations in the backcountry.

Wilderness first responder. This level of wilderness emergency medical training explores more deeply the nature of illness and injuries, with a focus on anatomy, physiology, and pathophysiology. Emphasis is on the knowledge and skills needed to make an accurate diagnosis, provide decisive treatment, and anticipate likely complications. The wilderness first responder (W.F.R.) level of training is the first and more patient-focused half of the standard wilderness emergency medical technician (W.E.M.T.) training. Most backcountry guides, wilderness instructors, and other outdoor recreation professionals are required to hold current W.F.R. certification.

W.E.M.T. and above. This category includes wilderness emergency medical technicians, paramedics, and others with higher levels of medical training, including instruction in wilderness medicine. A large focus of medical training at or above the W.E.M.T. level is on technological support resources, which, as noted above, are typically unavailable in backcountry scenarios; thus, some of the high-level skills learned in W.E.M.T. training are useless in the wilderness.

The future

There are presently no nationally standardized curricula for the certification of students in wilderness medicine. Programs in the U.S. such as SOLO receive approval for their curricula from physician medical directors at both state and local levels. Nonetheless, experts are now working to establish nationally standardized curricula for the next generation of wilderness medical care providers. With this attention have come new training opportunities. Students in traditional medical programs, for example, are discovering course options in wilderness medicine. And students in several wilderness medicine programs in the U.S. are able to spend part of their training assisting medical teams in such remote places as Nepal and El Salvador.

Greater attention has also been given to the design of wilderness medical equipment. As new products become lighter, stronger, and more versatile, backcountry medical kits will have a greater capacity to address a wider range of illnesses and injuries.

Professionals currently working in wilderness emergency medicine are on the cutting edge of the field, as new techniques and innovative ways of providing treatment are continually being developed. It is demanding and rewarding work. Thanks to their efforts, the backcountry has become a less-dire place to experience a medical emergency.

—Dave Kajganich, W.F.R.

NEWS CAP MHA 98

Reality Bites

Are dogs still man's best friend? According to recent reports, the incidence of dog bites serious enough to require medical attention is increasing at an alarming rate. An estimated 4.5 million people in the United States alone (1.8% of the population) sustained a dog bite in 1994, the most recent year for which such statistics are available. The number of dog bites that caused people to seek medical care jumped from 585,000 in 1986 to 800,000 in 1994, an increase of 37% during a period in which the dog population grew less than 2%, to about 55 million. According to Jeffrey Sacks, an epidemiologist at the Centers for Disease Control and Prevention (CDC), those figures mean that "every 40 seconds, somebody is seeing a doctor because of a dog bite."

Indeed, dog attacks are one of the top 10 causes of nonfatal injury in the U.S. In the majority of cases, the victims of attacks are children. An estimated 2.8 million children are bitten by dogs each year, and youngsters aged 10 and under account for well over half of all fatalities from dog bites. Even though dogs were domesticated more than 12,000 years ago, their instinct to chase and catch prey remains intact, which helps explain why canine attacks often involve a running child.

Since dog bites not only may injure tissues but can transmit serious infections such as tetanus and rabies, every bite should be regarded as potentially serious. Even minor bites may require medical attention. Cleansing and sometimes closure of the wound must be done without delay in order to prevent infection. In some cases antibiotics may be appropriate. These steps are particularly important for anyone who suffers from a weakened immune system.

Experts agree that most attacks by dogs are preventable. Many veterinarians advocate better understanding of canines and their behavior as the best way of reducing the number of attacks. Nonneutered male dogs, for example, are more likely to bite than are female dogs and neutered males. It is also thought that the sharp increase in dog bites in the U.S. can be partly attributed to the growing number of ferocious dogs (*e.g.,* rottweilers, pit bulls, German shepherds, Doberman pinschers) bought for protection. Dog owners and potential dog buyers should be aware that certain breeds are more prone to attack humans than are others. According to the CDC, between 1979 and 1996, pit bulls and rottweilers accounted for nearly 45% of the fatal attacks on humans in which the breed of the dog was known.

Along with the CDC, a number of other organizations have begun to sink their teeth into the challenging task of educating the public about canine attacks. In 1997 the American Veterinary Medical Association worked with the State Farm Fire and Casualty Co. to create and distribute brochures aimed at boosting awareness of the problem and encouraging responsible dog ownership.

Springfield News-Leader/Associated Press

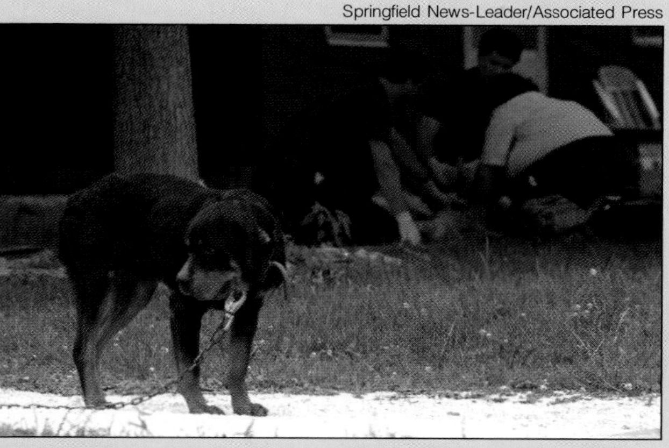

Emergency medical personnel try unsuccessfully to revive a 21-month-old child who was attacked by a rottweiler in Springfield, Mo. The dog had been chained but broke free.

In addition to recommending that dog owners know their pets well, obey leash and licensing laws, and make sure their dogs have had rabies shots, the American Society for the Prevention of Cruelty to Animals (ASPCA) offered the following tips on ways that the public can avoid dog bites:

- Always ask the owner's permission before you approach or pet a strange dog, even one on a leash.
- Before you pet a dog, allow it to see and sniff you.
- Never leave a young child alone with a dog.
- Before entering a stranger's yard, bang on a fence or side of the building to see if a dog responds.
- Be careful when encountering a dog in small or narrow spaces, such as an alley, hallway, or elevator, which can heighten a dog's territorial or protective tendencies.
- Do not approach a mother dog that is nursing pups.
- Outdoor athletes, such as bicyclists, joggers, and inline skaters, should keep a safe distance between themselves and dogs.
- If an unleashed dog approaches, do not try to outrun it. Instead, stand still until something else attracts its interest.
- Do not stare a threatening dog in the eyes. Instead, turn sideways, slowly withdraw, and try to put an object like a tree or a park bench between you and the dog.

When people choose dogs carefully and train and care for them properly, dog-bite tragedies are uncommon.

—Robert Rauch

Report Card on the Environment

Public opinion polls conducted in 1996–97 indicate that Americans overwhelmingly support initiatives for cleaner air and water and safer work sites and consumer products. The public as a whole demands prompt attention to newly recognized environmental hazards. At the same time, however, most people want to see regulatory controls become less costly, less onerous, and less intrusive.

Much has happened since the 1970s, when the Environmental Protection Agency (EPA) and the Occupational Safety and Health Administration (OSHA) were first established and Congress passed the Clean Air, Clean Water, Safe Drinking Water, Occupational Safety and Health, and Toxic Substances Control acts. By just about all measures, the U.S. has made remarkable progress in cleaning up the environment and improving the public's health. As the turn of the century approaches, many wonder whether this progress will continue.

Air quality: room for improvement

The adverse effects of air pollution are by now well documented, from cough and eye irritation to heart and lung disease, cancers, and premature death. Air pollution also has negative effects on the environment itself, upsetting delicate ecosystems and reducing agricultural production. Pollutants in the air come from a variety of sources—stationary sources (factories, smelters, power plants, homes), mobile sources (cars, buses, trucks, trains, airplanes), and natural sources (wildfires, windblown dust, volcanic eruptions).

The Clean Air Act recognizes two categories of air pollutants. The first, called "criteria pollutants," is a group of substances that includes carbon monoxide, lead, nitrogen dioxide, ground-level ozone, particles (soot), and sulfur dioxide. Estimated emissions and monitored concentrations of these six criteria pollutants have been reduced over the past decade. The Acid Rain Program has reduced sulfur dioxide emissions by more than half, from 10.9 million tons in 1980 to 5.3 million tons in 1995. The latter figure was 39% less than the level established as allowable for 1995 (8.7 million tons) by the 1990 amendments to the Clean Air Act. The U.S. has led the world in removing lead from gasoline, paint, and plumbing, and since 1979, when leaded gasoline started being phased out, children's blood lead levels and lead-associated neurological complications and anemia have declined dramatically. Nevertheless, significant exposures to lead still occur from leaded paint in older housing and, primarily in urban areas, soil contaminated by decades of exposure to automobile exhaust.

The EPA has created a Pollutant Standards Index, or PSI, which is used to measure air quality in metropolitan areas. The scale goes from 0 to 500. PSI levels of 0–50 are "good," 50–100 "moderate," 100–200 "unhealthful," 200–300 "very unhealthful"

Wearing gloves, mask, and clothing to protect himself, a worker removes lead-contaminated soil from a residential yard. Although lead is no longer used in gasoline, paint, or plumbing in the U.S., inhabitants of many urban neighborhoods continue to be exposed to hazardous amounts of lead on a daily basis—from paint in old housing and from soil that over many decades became polluted by automobile exhaust.

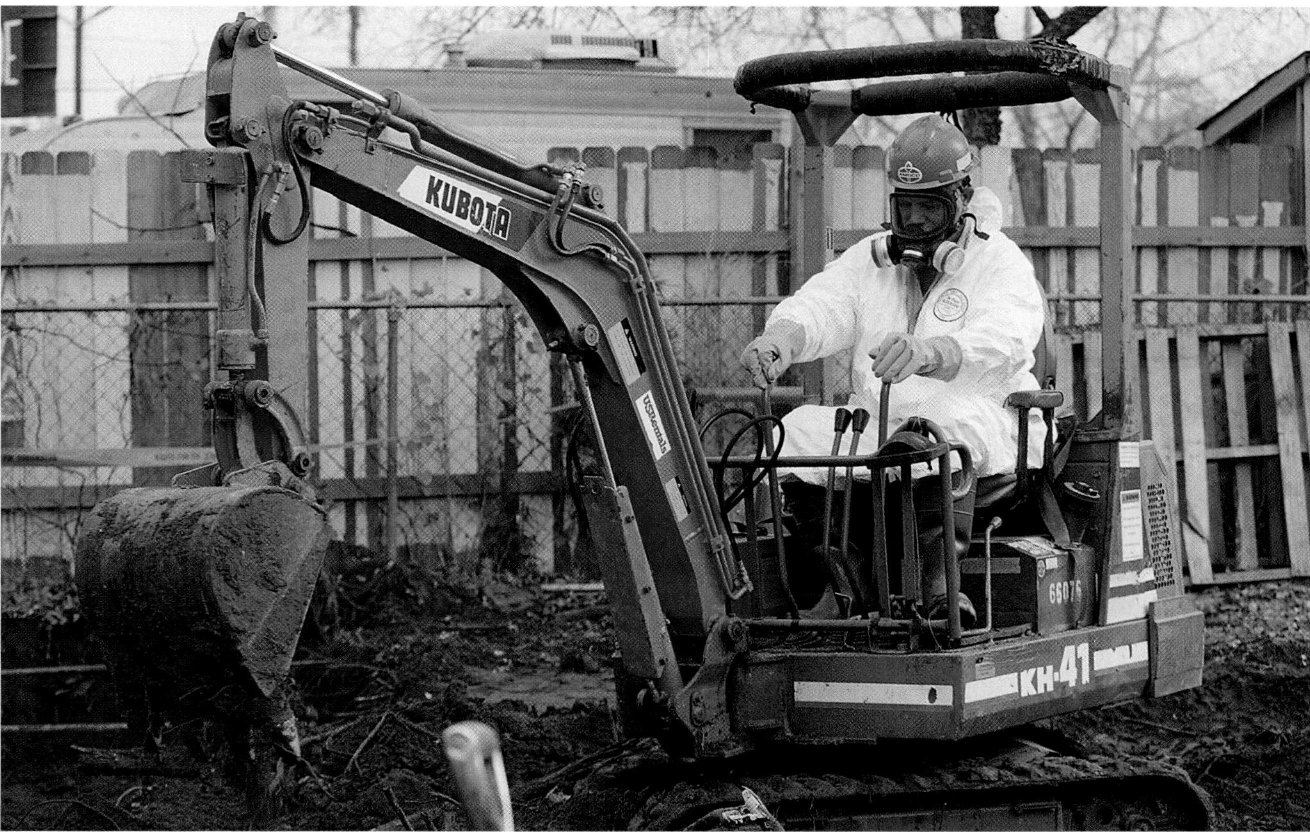

Robert E. Daemmrich—Tony Stone Images

(triggering restrictions on incinerator use and open burning of refuse or leaves), and above 300 "hazardous" (prompting a public health warning and curtailment of electric power and transportation usage).

The second category, called "hazardous pollutants," includes benzene, vinyl chloride, and many other toxic substances known to cause cancers, birth defects, or other serious health effects. In 1991 the EPA asked industries to reduce emissions of 17 especially prominent hazardous air pollutants by 33% initially and 50% by 1996. Several companies further set themselves corporate goals of 75% reductions in emissions of those chemicals they released that were among the more than 300 substances on the EPA's Toxics Release Inventory (an index reported annually since 1987). Data published in 1996 indicated that spectacular progress had been made toward achieving these goals.

Overall, since the passage of the Clean Air Act of 1970, pollutant levels have decreased even while the U.S. economy grew by 100%, population by 28%, and total vehicle miles traveled by 116%. Simultaneous environmental protection and economic growth constitute "sustainable development."

Much remains to be accomplished, however. Nearly 90 million Americans live in counties where air quality in 1995 failed to meet the national ambient air quality standard for at least one of the six criteria pollutants (primarily ozone, followed by particles and carbon monoxide). Moreover, air quality is a moving target. In 1996, under court-ordered deadlines, the EPA issued long-awaited proposals to tighten the standards for ozone and particulates.

Revised ozone standards. The Ground-Level Ozone Air Quality Standard regulates ozone produced by industrial processes (the "bad" ozone; stratospheric "good" ozone protects the Earth from ultraviolet radiation). Control of ozone levels is complicated by the fact that vehicles and factories do not emit ozone per se; they emit volatile organic compounds (VOCs) and nitrogen oxides (NO_x), which undergo numerous chemical reactions in the presence of sunlight to generate molecules of ozone (O_3), while the ozone is being destroyed by other reactions. Furthermore, unfavorable weather conditions—especially stagnant inversions—can wreck a good year's emissions control record. Some ozone production occurs as a result of natural processes.

Repeated exposures to ozone may increase an individual's susceptibility to respiratory infections, inflammatory changes in the lungs, emphysema, and asthma attacks. Children are especially vulnerable to the respiratory effects of ozone in humid summer conditions. Critics of more stringent ozone standards claim, however, that smoking, other chemical pollutants, and biological allergens from pets and roaches are primarily responsible for exacerbating respiratory problems.

At the end of 1996, the EPA proposed revisions to the current standard of 0.12 ppm (parts per million) for ozone, based on an average value measured during the peak hour of a single day. The proposal would change the standard to 0.08 ppm, averaged over eight hours. While the maximum allowable level would be reduced, the longer time period would match extended peak exposures in highly congested metropolitan areas, and areas would not be considered out of compliance unless the three-year average of the annual third highest daily maximum eight-hour value exceeded the standard. Currently, the fourth worst day in three years determines compliance.

After considering extensive public comment on options ranging from 0.07 to 0.12 ppm, the EPA promulgated the new standard at 0.08 ppm, for the annual fourth highest values. Each state will have to revise its ozone implementation plan to comply by further controlling emissions of VOCs and NO_x, especially from vehicles. Of the 98 areas of the country that were designated as having not attained ozone standards in 1990, 55 had achieved "clean air" in 1995. Under the new standard, however, many of these areas will no longer be considered in compliance.

Stricter controls on particles. In 1987, recognizing that the most serious respiratory problems are caused by particles capable of penetrating deep into lung tissues, the EPA moved from an earlier standard based on total mass of suspended particulates to one based on particles smaller than 10 microns in diameter, or PM10 (about one-tenth the thickness of an average human hair). In the meantime, scientific evidence has pointed to particles even smaller than 10 microns as being most harmful. The proposed new regulations on particulate matter therefore add standards for particles as small as 2.5 microns, or PM2.5, for 24-hour and annual averages (50 and 15 μg/cu m [micrograms per cubic meter], respectively), retaining the present annual PM10 standard at 50 μg/cu m.

Monitoring the levels of PM10 and PM2.5 is a complicated business, however. Although numerous studies have documented the harmful respiratory effects of fine particles—one suggested that the stricter standards could save as many as 20,000 lives per year—these findings have been disputed. Even more complicated is the question of how to relate health indicators like death and disease rates to specific sources of pollution in the community and how to track movement of particles across state lines in order that specific polluters may be held responsible for specific violations.

As with the revised ozone standard, the financial consequences of the stricter standards for particulates are enormous. Critics of the proposal favor delaying changes in the regulations until there is better evidence of the precise relationship between health hazards and particle size; proponents of the new standards feel that this approach takes unnecessary chances with the public's health. On July 16, 1997, the EPA issued the final regulation, raising the 24-hour PM2.5 level to 65 μg/cu m and allowing five years for research and development of effective monitoring before actual implementation. By late summer congressional leaders had not yet decided whether to challenge the regulation and try to override a certain veto by Pres. Bill Clinton. (Detailed information on the new regulation is available from the EPA on the Internet at http://www.epa.gov/ttn/).

Where there's smoke.... There is no credible scientific basis for disputing the observation that cigarette smoking causes cancer, heart disease, and lung disease. Now there is compelling evidence that exposure to other people's smoke ("environmental tobacco smoke," or ETS) at work, at home, and elsewhere leads to lung cancer and heart disease in nonsmokers and bronchitis and worsened asthma in children.

ETS is composed of sidestream smoke, which is emitted by the burning cigarette tip, and mainstream smoke, that exhaled by smokers. Sidestream smoke contributes nearly all of the vaporous components and half of the particulate matter of ETS. Because combustion is less complete in sidestream smoke than in mainstream smoke, the former contains higher concentrations of am-

Seth Resnick—Stock Boston/PNI

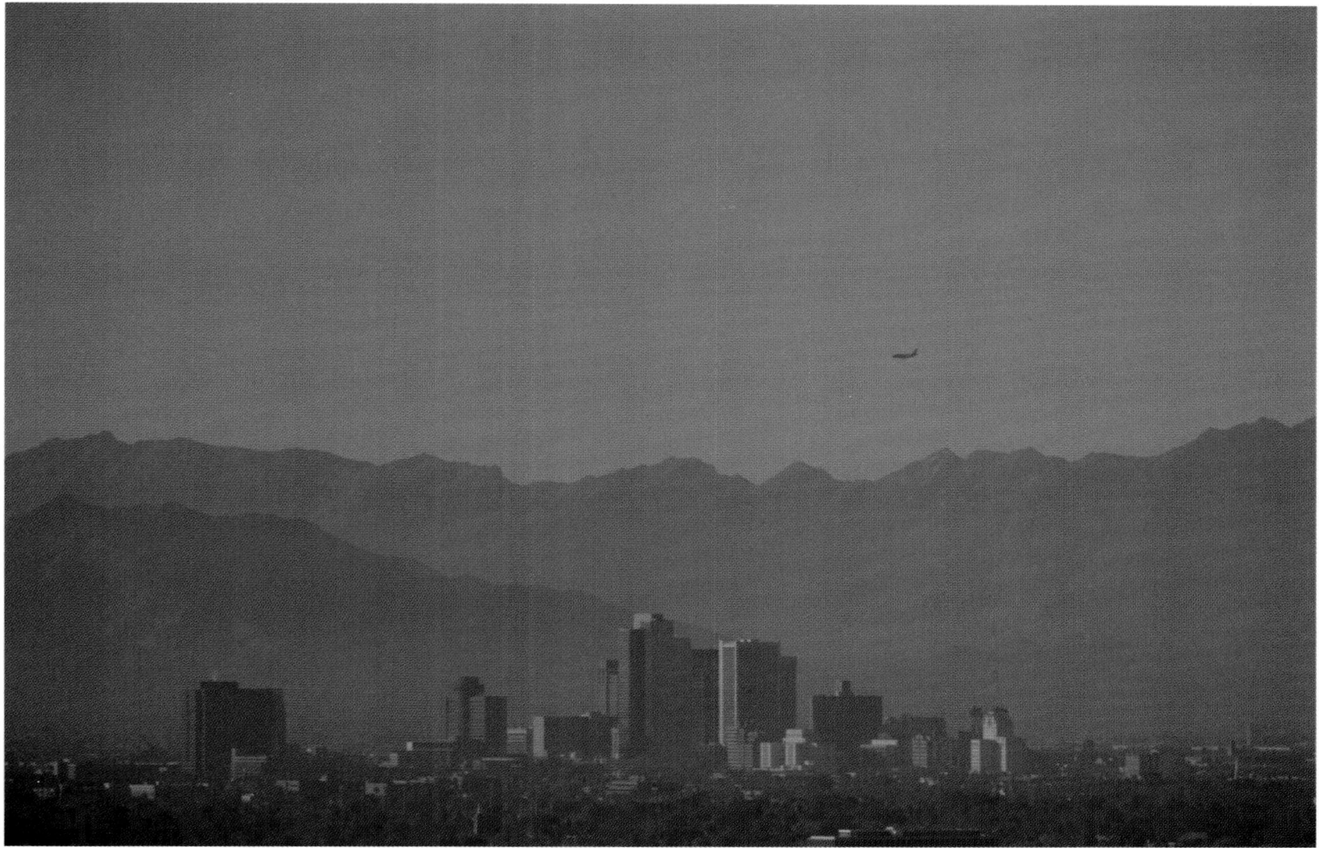

Haze envelops the urban skyline as well as the mountainous terrain beyond Phoenix, Ariz. Air pollutants come from a combination of sources—some mobile (e.g., *planes and trucks), some stationary* (e.g., *factories and homes), and some natural* (e.g., *dust and fires). The most recent statistics on U.S. ambient air quality indicate that some 90 million Americans live in counties that fail to meet established standards for at least one pollutant.*

monia, nicotine, carbon monoxide, and benzene and other carcinogens (cancer-causing substances).

In fact, of the substances classified by the EPA as "known human carcinogens," ETS is the only one for which an increased risk has actually been observed (in female nonsmokers) at *typical* levels of exposure—rather than relying on extrapolation from high-level exposures in experimental animals or situations in which humans have been exposed to unusually high levels. Studies have indicated that hundreds of thousands of children develop bronchitis, pneumonia, or middle-ear disease or experience asthma attacks as a result of exposure to tobacco smoke. Even sudden infant death syndrome has been linked to the presence of smokers in the household.

Restrictions on smoking in the workplace and in public places have measurably reduced the exposure of nonsmokers to ETS. In 1973 Arizona became the first state in the United States to regulate public smoking. Between 1986 and 1992 the percentage of private-sector workplaces with total bans on smoking rose from 2% to 34%. In addition to making the workplace safer for nonsmokers, these restrictions have decreased the extent and amount of smoking by employees who are smokers and may have even helped some to quit. Employers report savings from lower costs for maintenance of mechanical systems and cleaning of workplaces, decreased health insurance expenditures, and increased worker productivity.

Water quality

In August 1996 Congress reauthorized the Safe Drinking Water Act, incorporating important provisions for utilization of the techniques of risk assessment and cost-benefit analysis in making regulatory decisions. Risk assessment is a method of analysis that attempts to answer the question, Does a given contaminant proposed for regulation pose a significant human health risk? Cost-benefit analysis seeks to determine whether the benefits of eliminating a particular contaminant justify the costs of the effort. Special studies were mandated to assess the risks of arsenic, radon, and sulfates in drinking water. And in recognition of the fact that disinfection of drinking water (*i.e.,* removal of disease-causing microorganisms) can produce chemical by-products that may themselves be hazardous to human health, it was decided that the risks of disinfection by-products would have to be weighed against the risks of microbial contamination itself. The 1996 legislation also provided for less-frequent reporting by water systems serving fewer than 10,000 people. Finally, to comply with the spirit of the 1995 Unfunded Mandates Reform Act, Congress authorized loans to help states with the costs of upgrading local water systems.

The 1997 *Annual Review of Public Health,* published by Annual Reviews, Inc., found that the protozoan *Cryptosporidium* had become the most important contaminant found in drinking water.

Twelve waterborne outbreaks have been documented in North America since 1985. About 400,000 people became ill with diarrhea in Milwaukee, Wis., in 1993. Risks are greatest in people with impaired capacity to ward off infections, especially people with HIV/AIDS, transplant recipients, and cancer chemotherapy patients; in Milwaukee and in another major outbreak in Las Vegas, Nev., death rates among immunocompromised individuals were 68% and 52%, respectively. An assay has now been developed to monitor *Cryptosporidium* in sewage, filtered secondary treated wastewater, surface waters, groundwater, and treated drinking water. Studies of the outbreaks over the past decade indicate that a variety of failures in the water-treatment process may have contributed; these include inadequate flocculation (a process by which contaminants are aggregated into fluffy masses that can be removed by filtration), use of filters that were not backwashed, and recycling of waters used to clean the filters. Wells and swimming pools have also been identified as outbreak sources. Chlorination does not kill the organism. For immunocompromised persons, boiling of drinking water is the most reliable method of preventing cryptosporidiosis. Unfortunately, cryptosporidiosis still is not a reportable disease in most states. The contamination of water by *Cryptosporidium* from the feces of livestock is a huge challenge for public health and sanitation authorities in developed countries, just as cholera and typhoid fever remain extremely important fecal-oral waterborne diseases in the less-developed world.

Organochlorine chemicals

Organochlorines are a diverse group of synthetic compounds that can persist in the environment for long periods of time. They are used primarily as pesticides. In the laboratory many of these compounds have been shown to disrupt hormonal equilibrium or cause cancer. Polychlorinated biphenyls, or PCBs, and DDE, a breakdown product of the pesticide DDT, account for most of the organochlorine residues found in the human body (in fat tissues, milk, and blood). High-level exposures can cause skin, liver, and nervous system disorders; in newborns such exposures also may cause impaired muscle tone. PCBs were banned in the mid-1970s but continue to be present in older electrical equipment. DDT likewise was restricted in 1972; average DDE blood levels in Americans are now one-fifth of what they were in the 1960s.

NEWS CAP MHA 98

Something to Wheeze About

Why are children who live in inner-city areas of the United States three times more likely to suffer from asthma than their suburban counterparts? According to a recent study, the answer has a lot to do with a common household pest—the cockroach.

The National Cooperative Inner-City Asthma Study was undertaken to help explain why children from the poorest neighborhoods suffer disproportionately from asthma. Results published in *The New England Journal of Medicine* (May 8, 1997) confirmed what many health experts had long suspected: children who are heavily exposed to cockroach allergen, which is present in the insects' bodies, saliva, and feces and may collect in household dust, are at a high risk for asthma.

Between 1992 and 1993, researchers examined 476 youngsters between the ages of four and nine, each of whom had asthma or showed symptoms consistent with asthma (*e.g.,* coughing, wheezing, shortness of breath) and lived in inner-city neighborhoods where at least 30% of the households had incomes below the 1990 U.S. poverty level. Skin tests revealed that about 37% of the children were allergic to cockroaches, while dust samples taken from their bedrooms showed that more than half of them had high levels of cockroach allergen in their homes. In addition, youngsters who were both allergic to cockroaches and exposed to considerable amounts of cockroach allergen were found to have twice as many unscheduled visits to the doctor, missed days from school, and nights with lost sleep than children who suffered from other types of allergies.

"Now we know that cock-

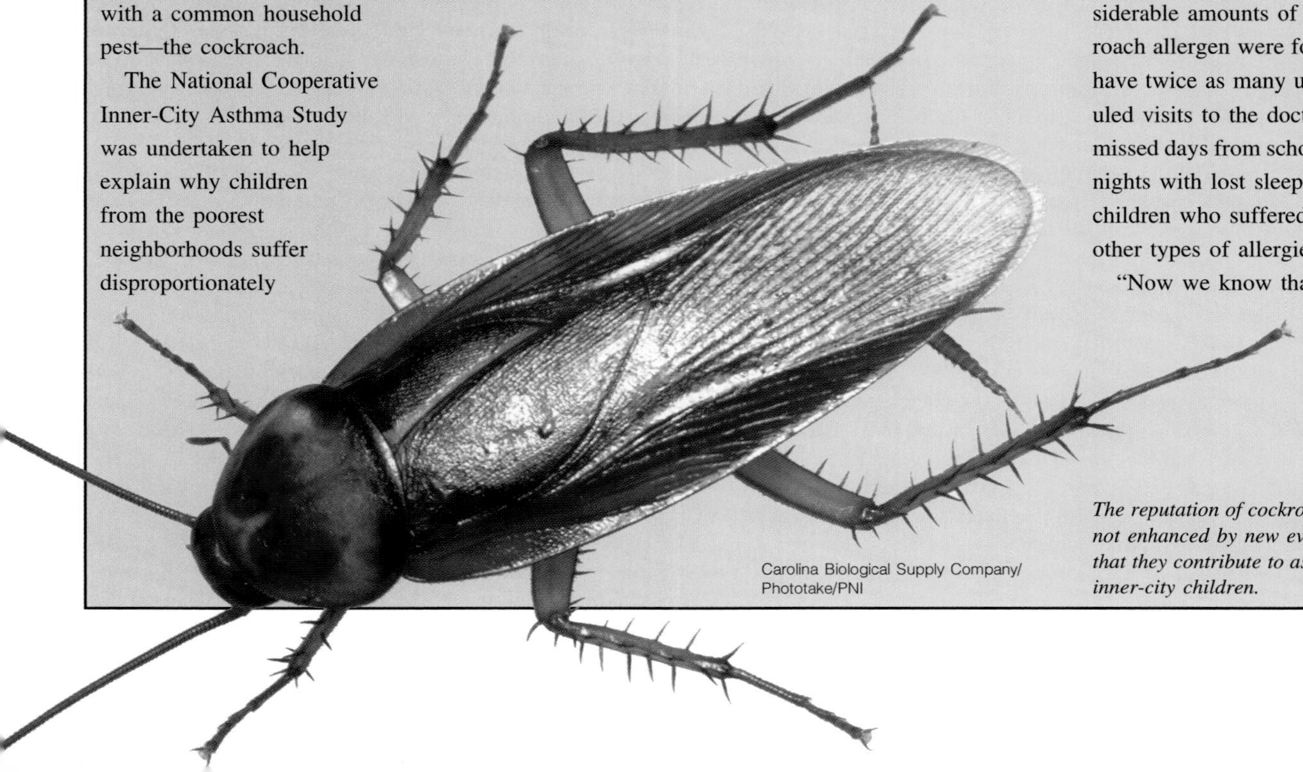

Carolina Biological Supply Company/ Phototake/PNI

The reputation of cockroaches is not enhanced by new evidence that they contribute to asthma in inner-city children.

Dioxins and related compounds are generated when PCBs and other chlorine-containing compounds are subjected to extreme heat in incinerators; dioxin is also a by-product of certain chemical-manufacturing processes and older pulp and paper processing. The EPA's long-awaited reassessment of risks of dioxins is still under review, after the EPA Science Advisory Board ordered a substantial rewrite of the report released in 1994. A major problem for the agency is determining how to evaluate the preliminary evidence suggesting a connection between dioxin accumulation and metabolic and immunologic problems. Another issue is the reliability of dioxin's interaction with cellular receptors, observed in the laboratory, as a predictor of the chemical's effects on the whole body. Finally, scientists are still debating how to regard possible effects at "background" levels already present in the population.

Many organochlorines are known to have the capacity to act like weaker versions of the natural female hormone estrogen. The 1996 amendments to the Safe Drinking Water Act mandated that the EPA and the National Academy of Sciences analyze the potential risks of such hormonal properties of environmental chemicals. Most authorities accept that many chemicals have the ability to mimic or oppose the actions of certain hormones, including thyroid and male and female sex hormones. Determining the net effects of various exposures, however, is a much more complex matter. What effects do exposures to hormonelike compounds in air and water have compared with exposures to much higher levels of estrogenic foods in the diet? What effects do they have compared with the 1,000-times-higher normal levels circulating in the blood and varying with pregnancy and the menstrual cycle in women?

roach allergen contributes to asthmatic severity at high levels of exposure and this provides incentives to reduce that exposure," said Daniel Rotrosen, acting director of the Division of Allergy, Immunology and Transplantation at the National Institute of Allergy and Infectious Diseases (NIAID), which sponsored the study. While it is often difficult or impossible to eliminate cockroaches in apartment buildings, Rotrosen suggested such low-cost methods as putting out roach traps and using child-safe insecticides. There are several additional practical steps parents can take to control roaches.

- Because roaches tend to inhabit dark, damp places, like under-the-sink cabinets and storage areas, these areas should be cleaned periodically.
- All seams or cracks through which cockroaches could travel should be caulked.
- Dishes should be washed promptly and food never left uncovered for long periods.
- Lids should be placed on trash cans and garbage regularly removed from dwellings.
- Mopping floors and vacuuming carpets frequently will help to prevent build-up of cockroach allergen. Reducing or getting rid of upholstered furniture should also be considered.
- To eliminate potential water supplies for cockroaches, all openings leading to a sink or drain should be sealed.

To further explore ways to reduce asthma symptoms and exposure to cockroach allergen, officials at NIAID announced that they would be extending their study to the year 2000.

—Sherman Hollar

Making sound decisions

Risk is the coin of the realm in environmental decision making. Risk is defined as a combination of the probability of exposure to a potentially hazardous substance at various levels and the probability and severity of effects from such exposure. In general, policy makers, environmentalists, and business leaders all seek to reduce the health risks of environmental exposures, especially those considered to be the most serious. In 1990, as part of the amendments to the Clean Air Act, a special Commission on Risk Assessment and Risk Management was mandated. Established in 1994, the commission had 10 members, 6 appointed by Congress, 3 by the president, and 1 by the National Academy of Sciences. The group issued its final report in 1997.

Its proposal for the development of a "framework" for risk management is sure to have far-reaching implications. The framework approach moves beyond the current system—in which substances suspected of causing harm are evaluated one at a time for a single, specific adverse effect (such as cancer) from exposure to a single environmental medium (air, water, soil, food)—to put each environmental problem into public health and ecological contexts. This "putting into context" involves identification of all significant sources contributing to total exposure to a particular substance and all causes of particular health problems (such as lung cancer, heart disease, or birth defects) for which the substance might be partly responsible.

The commission also urged that all "stakeholders"—those individuals and groups having an interest in the particular problem and the risk-management process—be involved from the very start. The goal of such involvement is for policy makers to meet with local people who have firsthand knowledge about specific sources of environmental exposure and cultural practices and behavior patterns that might influence exposure. Such information is generally missed in routine risk analysis. (More information on these risk-management initiatives is available at http://www.riskworld.com.)

The commission made a number of specific recommendations, including the following:

- Congress should coordinate the activities of committees and subcommittees that have overlapping jurisdictional responsibilities for environmental issues.
- Federal regulatory agencies should use their existing discretionary authority to address the most significant sources of total exposure to those hazards still under review and to expand the involvement of stakeholders.
- Congress should reinforce the commission's new framework on a statute-by-statute basis, continuing the process begun in 1996 when the laws governing pesticide residues in foods were overhauled.

- State and local regulatory agencies should not wait for the federal government to take action but should begin immediately to address environmental problems, using methods developed by the commission.

The group endorsed the principle that economic analysis should be a significant—but not an overriding—factor in risk management, bridging a nasty debate in Congress over the value of costly measures to protect the public health. Finally, the commission supported the EPA's proposed new guidelines for cancer-risk assessments using the growing body of data on the mechanisms of action by chemicals at the cellular level, recategorizing chemicals—including agents that cause cancers in test animals by mechanisms thought not to be predictive of risk for humans—and providing explicit information where there is uncertainty about the effects of a particular substance.

Other organizations also were actively seeking new ways to mobilize public support for environmental programs and to bridge the partisan gulf over environmental issues in Congress. Notable among these was Enterprise for the Environment, led by former EPA administrator William Ruckelshaus, and the President's Council on Sustainable Development, led by Jonathan Lash of the World Resources Institute and David Buzzelli of the Dow Chemical Co.

Many groups, public and private, representing disparate interests, are in agreement about goals—namely, that the U.S. be able to achieve solid economic growth without compromising the long-

Chromo Sohm—Tony Stone Images

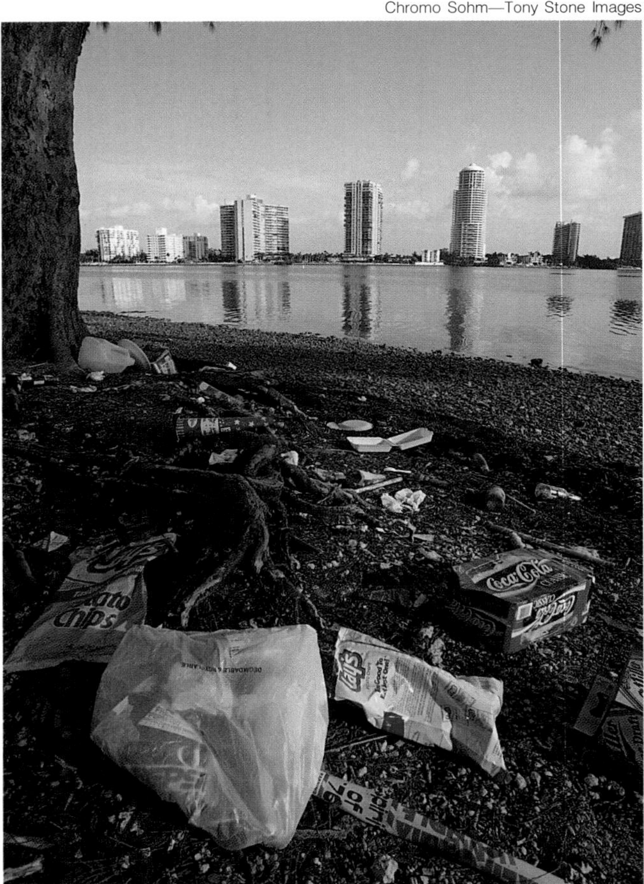

Rubbish strewn along the Miami, Fla., shoreline is both an eyesore and a threat to the public health. Pollution is everyone's problem, and ultimately all segments of society must be engaged in the efforts to protect nature's precious and limited resources.

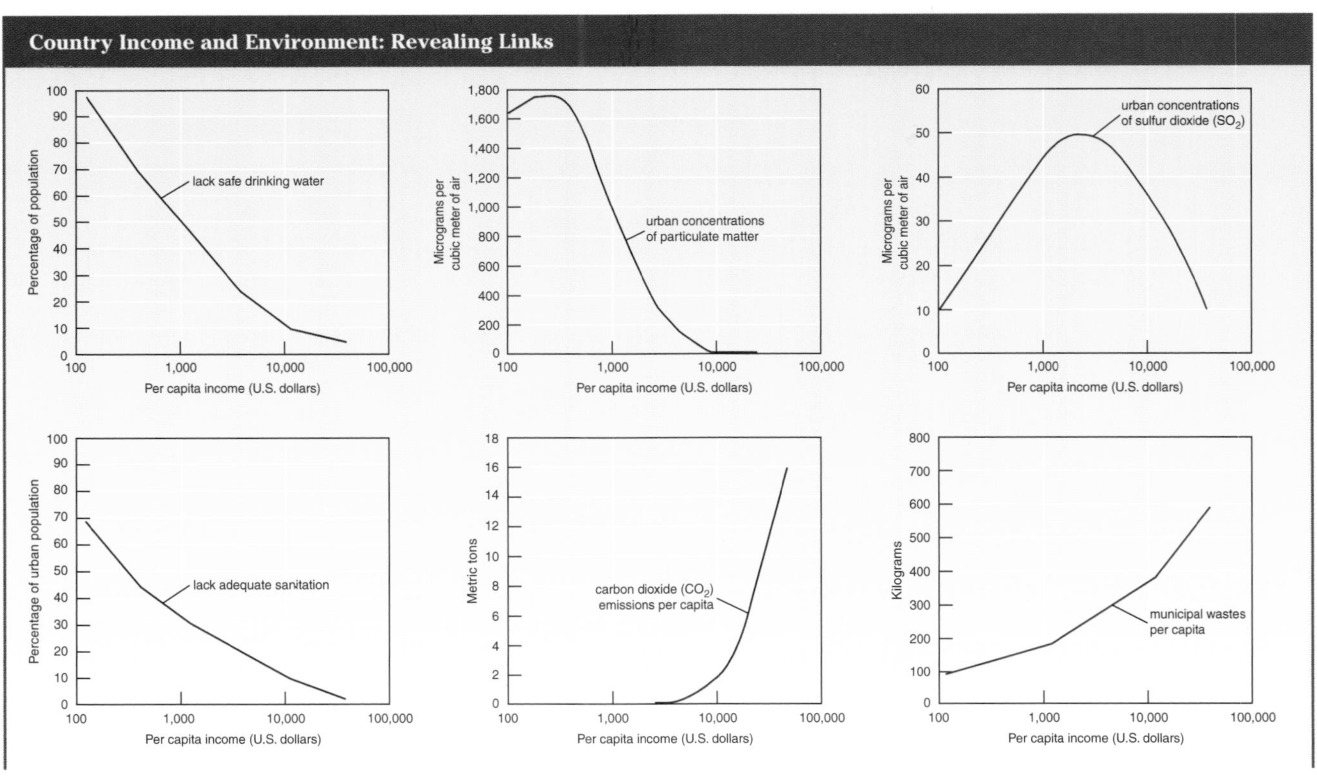

term viability of the environment. What they continue to disagree about are the means for achieving this goal.

Pollution prevention

One of the greatest current challenges facing those concerned with the environment is how to impress upon the U.S. public that everyone, not just a few large corporations, generates pollution. From the home, office, and recreational use of resources to the activities of industry and agriculture, the 6% of the world's population living in the U.S. accounts for 25% of the energy use and pollution on the planet. As is indicated by the graphs on the opposite page, municipal wastes and carbon dioxide emissions are environmental challenges currently facing all developed countries—challenges that will not be met without engaging all segments of society.

One of the most promising—and cost-effective—environmental protection strategies to emerge in recent years is pollution prevention. This approach focuses on reducing the production of pollutants at their source as well as more efficiently recycling materials, water, and other precious resources. Many local organizations are now working to mobilize businesses, government agencies, and community groups and bring them together with academic scientists and engineers who have expertise in the field. Businesses large and small are learning how "environmental accounting" can identify those pollution-reduction strategies with the greatest return on investment. Bankers and insurers, unfortunately, are often skeptical or uninterested. The EPA's environmental leadership programs, the International Organization for Standardization's program for private certification of environmental management systems, the Chemical Manufacturers Association's Responsible Care program, and numerous initiatives from schools, colleges, and community groups represent a clear force for change. Signs of their effectiveness are already apparent in a growing appreciation for the environment and a reduced tolerance for wasteful and polluting activities that put the public health at risk.

—Gilbert S. Omenn, M.D., Ph.D., and Jason M. Omenn

Arsenic-Tainted Drinking Water: Crisis in India and Bangladesh

> *Hundreds of...villages in Bangladesh and neighboring India [have been] hit by a scourge of arsenic poisoning that experts say has no equal in medical history.*
>
> —*Chicago Tribune*, Dec. 15, 1996

During 1996 and 1997, newspapers and journals reported that large portions of the populations in West Bengal, India, and Bangladesh were exposed to elevated levels of arsenic in their drinking water. Indian scientists reported that approximately 200,000 persons in West Bengal alone had developed arsenic-induced skin lesions; if the estimate of 30 million West Bengalis exposed to high levels of arsenic is correct, however, the actual number with adverse skin reactions could be much higher. In Bangladesh at least 23 million persons live in districts where arsenic-contaminated wells have been identified, and by mid-1997 approximately 1,000 cases of arsenic-induced skin lesions had been diagnosed; there were probably thousands more undiagnosed cases. Additionally, some recent cases of skin cancer in West Bengal and Bangladesh are believed to be arsenic-induced. And although reliable statistics are lacking, deaths too have been attributed to arsenic.

Arsenic is an element (with the atomic number 33 and the atomic weight 74.92) that exists throughout the Earth's crust. Arsenic contamination of drinking water results from wells that are located in naturally arsenic-rich layers of rock and soil. In this regard, the current situation in West Bengal and Bangladesh is not unlike the naturally occurring arsenic contamination of drinking water that exists in many other places in the world, most notably, Taiwan, Hungary, Mexico, Chile, China, and Argentina.

For centuries arsenic has been used as a drug and as a poison. Arsenic is thought to exert its toxicity by combining with certain enzymes (organic catalysts) and thereby interfering with cellular metabolism. Individual susceptibility to arsenic, however, varies widely; some persons have developed tolerance to doses that would be lethal to others. Arsenical compounds cause skin lesions (dermatoses) that may be quite painful and in some cases debilitating. Moreover, there is considerable evidence that the lesions can undergo malignant (cancerous) changes. A single large dose of arsenic—much larger than the amount obtained from contaminated drinking water—can result in circulatory collapse, which may be followed by death in a matter of hours. Definitive diagnosis of arsenic poisoning is based on laboratory tests that detect arsenic in urine, skin, hair, or nail samples.

Discovery and unfolding of a calamity

The arsenic-contaminated-water problem in India was first noticed in 1983 when a patient from West Bengal was seen by a physician in Calcutta. The patient had the classic skin manifestations of arsenic exposure: hyperpigmentation (abnormal darkening of the skin, primarily on the palms of the hands, soles of the feet, and the torso) and hyperkeratosis (an overgrowth, or thickening, of the outer layer of skin [epidermis], most often affecting the palms and soles but sometimes occurring on other areas of the limbs). After various possible causes of the patient's specific skin symptoms had been ruled out, water from the village in which he lived was sampled and found to have an unusually high concentration of arsenic. The water had come from a tube well in the village that was not unlike many such wells that were dug in West Bengal and Bangladesh beginning in the early 1960s. The wells were created to provide an additional water supply for a new type of irrigation-intensive rice that was planted as part of the Green Revolution. The intensive irrigation enabled the production of three rice crops a year, which helped feed the population and provided an economic boost for the impoverished region.

Additional patients with dermatologic signs of arsenic poisoning were discovered upon subsequent examination of people living in the patient's village and in nearby villages in West Bengal. Tests demonstrated that these patients also had elevated concentrations of arsenic in their hair, nails, and skin scales (flakes of dead skin). Other individuals in the same villages were considered to be "subclinical cases" because they did not have hyperpigmentation or hyperkeratosis but did have elevated arsenic concentrations that were clearly detected in laboratory tests. Clin-

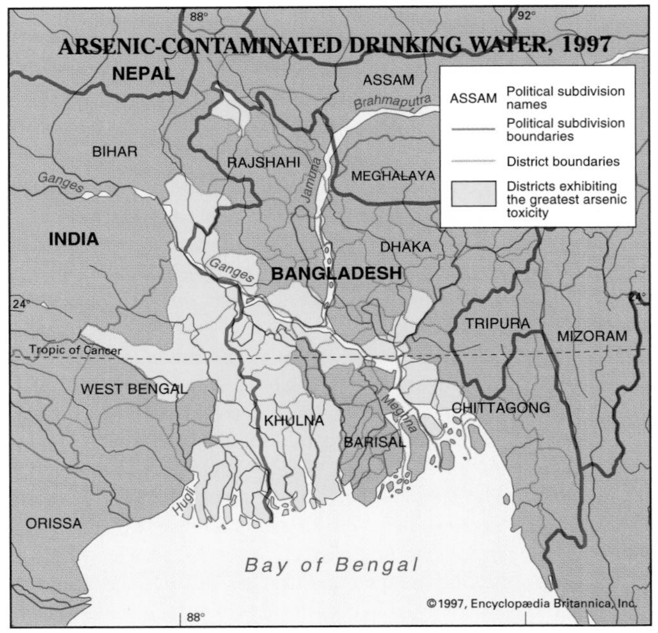

ical surveys conducted after 1983, however, found that there were many further West Bengali patients with the typical hyperpigmentation and hyperkeratosis lesions of arsenic poisoning.

Although the problem of arsenic contamination in West Bengal was first identified in 1983, it was about seven years later, in 1990, that a similar situation became apparent in Bangladesh. A preliminary study carried out by Indian scientists had shown that groundwater on the border between West Bengal and Bangladesh had high levels of arsenic. Further testing showed that a large area of Bangladesh was affected by arsenic-contaminated groundwater. It is particularly ironic that rural Bangladeshis began drinking groundwater from the tube wells for health reasons. A highly successful public health campaign in the 1970s had alerted the population to the dangers of waterborne disease associated with drinking unboiled surface water, so the people in rural areas switched to the allegedly safer well water.

Predicting the health impact

In other arsenic-exposed populations, excess cases of nonmelanoma skin cancers have been well documented. Thus, it is anticipated that many more cases of skin cancer will develop in West Bengal and Bangladesh in the next 5–10 years. The number of cases to date has been low, presumably because of the long latency period—*i.e.,* the time between the initial exposure and the actual development of a malignancy—that is generally associated with chemical carcinogens. The tube wells in West Bengal and Bangladesh have been in existence too short a time for very many excess skin cancers to have become evident; it is also unknown whether the earlier wells were contaminated.

Arsenic-induced health effects, of course, are dependent on the extent of exposure to arsenic. Although there are case reports of arsenic-induced disease and deaths in both West Bengal and Bangladesh, to date there have been no rigorous epidemiological surveys of the population. Such surveys would be immensely helpful in gaining a better public health perspective of the current situation. Presently, there is divergence of opinion about the scope of the problem and what can and should be done about it.

Experiences in the arsenic-endemic areas of Taiwan and Mexico have provided some information about the latency period and prevalence of skin cancers associated with arsenic exposure. A survey of the arsenic-exposed population in Taiwan conducted in the mid-1960s currently provides the best data for estimating the number of skin cancer cases that might develop in India and Bangladesh. Most of the population in the endemic area of Taiwan had been exposed to arsenic-contaminated drinking water all of their lives; their water came from wells that were established around 1910. Over 40,000 exposed and 7,500 nonexposed individuals were examined. The two groups were similar in age and occupation (fishing, farming, and recovery of sea salt). No skin cancers were found in the nonexposed persons. Thus, all of the cases in the exposed population were assumed to be the result of arsenic exposure.

The prevalence of skin cancer increased with increasing concentrations of arsenic in the drinking water. (A study of 296 residents of a town in Mexico where the arsenic concentration of

Skin Cancer and Arsenic Exposure in Taiwan[1]

	Age group (years)									
	0–19		20–39		40–59		≥ 60		Total	
Arsenic concentration in well water (parts per million)	Female	Male	Female	Male	Female	Male	Female	Male	Female	Male
Low (0–0.30)	2,651 (0)	2,714 (0)	1,306 (0)	935 (1)	792 (3)	653 (4)	239 (2)	236 (11)	4,988 (5)	4,538 (16)
Medium (0.30–0.60)	1,507 (0)	1,542 (0)	742 (1)	531 (2)	450 (9)	371 (18)	136 (8)	134 (22)	2,835 (18)	2,578 (42)
High (> 0.60)	2,296 (0)	2,351 (0)	1,131 (4)	810 (18)	686 (33)	566 (56)	207 (22)	204 (52)	4,320 (59)	3,931 (126)
Unknown	4,819 (0)	4,933 (0)	2,373 (2)	1,699 (3)	1,440 (13)	1,188 (61)	435 (27)	429 (64)	9,067 (42)	8,249 (128)
Total	11,273 (0)	11,540 (0)	5,552 (7)	3,975 (24)	3,368 (58)	2,778 (139)	1,017 (59)	1,003 (149)	21,210 (124)	19,296 (312)

[1]The most thoroughgoing studies of the link between skin cancer and arsenic in well water were done in Taiwan in the 1960s; top number=estimated number of persons at risk; (bottom number)=estimated number of skin cancer cases.

Source: U.S. Environmental Protection Agency, *Special Report on Ingested Inorganic Arsenic* (1988).

the drinking water supply was known found a skin cancer prevalence consistent with the Taiwanese findings.)

A dose response for hyperpigmentation and hyperkeratosis by concentration of arsenic has not been reported for the Taiwanese—or any other—arsenic-exposed populations. Data from Taiwan, however, suggest that both types of skin lesions are much more prevalent than skin cancers and occur at a much earlier age. The prevalence rates of hyperkeratosis, hyperpigmentation, and skin cancer, respectively, in the arsenic-exposed population in Taiwan were 183.5 per 1,000, 71 per 1,000, and 10.6 per 1,000. The youngest persons with hyperpigmentation and hyperkeratosis were aged 3 and 4, respectively, while the youngest person seen with skin cancer was 24 years old. Prevalence rates for skin lesions increased with age—the rate for hyperpigmentation rising more steeply than that for hyperkeratosis.

Arsenic skin lesions are unsightly; not surprisingly, people who have them have suffered social as well as physical consequences. Reportedly, in both India and Bangladesh, people have been denied jobs owing to skin manifestations of arsenic toxicity. In both countries marriages are frequently arranged. Wives and mothers who have developed arsenic lesions have been sent back to their parents, sometimes with their children. Some villagers, out of ignorance, have mistaken arsenic lesions for leprosy and have shunned patients socially or forced them to maintain an isolated life. Many people in the arsenic-affected villages apparently believe the arsenic poisoning to be an expression of divine wrath.

Lots of unknowns

The World Health Organization (WHO) has set a "guidance value" for arsenic in water at 0.01 mg/l (milligrams per liter). The U.S. had established a "maximum contaminant level" (MCL) for arsenic in 1942, before the world had ever heard of the problems in Taiwan, Chile, Argentina, or China. The 1996 amendments to the Safe Drinking Water Act mandate that the Environmental Protection Agency propose a new MCL by Jan. 1, 2000, to be finalized by Jan. 1, 2001.

The median concentrations of arsenic found in West Bengal wells with concentrations above 0.05 mg/l have been between 0.1 and 0.5 mg/l. The highest concentration reported thus far is 3.7 mg/l. In Bangladesh the median concentration in above-0.05-mg/l wells is between 0.1 and 0.3 mg/l, and the highest concentration reported to date is 2.9 mg/l. From the information available at present, it is not possible to determine the number of people exposed to various arsenic concentrations; therefore, it is impossible to estimate health risks for the population.

In other countries where arsenic contamination of water supplies occurs, increased risks of various cancers other than skin cancer (including cancers of the lung, bladder, kidney, liver, and prostate) have been reported. Thus far, such an increased cancer risk has not been observed in the arsenic-endemic areas of West Bengal or Bangladesh. Given that there are no "tumor registries" for the area and the reliability of the mortality statistics is questionable, the ability to discern an excess cancer risk other than by a survey employing actual diagnostic tests is quite limited. Still, in view of experiences in other arsenic-endemic areas, it appears likely that an increased prevalence of internal organ cancers will be seen in the arsenic-exposed population in future years.

Other adverse effects of arsenic ingestion have been reported in other countries. These include cardiovascular disease, neuropathy (degeneration of the nervous system, often marked by a loss of sensation in the extremities), birth defects, and peripheral arterial disease. Again, these effects have not yet been reported in either West Bengal or Bangladesh, but their occurrence in the population may be only a matter of time. Other symptoms or health effects that have been reported in West Bengal include hepatomegaly (enlargement of the liver), noncirrhotic portal fibrosis of the liver, and respiratory abnormalities.

Some Indian scientists have speculated that persons with inadequate diets and/or very low socioeconomic status have a greater predisposition to the adverse effects of arsenic; however, not all Indian data are consistent. Investigators have noted that in some villages in West Bengal and Bangladesh, entire households may be adversely affected, yet none of the people living next door show evidence of poisoning, even when both households take their water from the same well. Whether this phenomenon is due to genetic and/or lifestyle differences or to some other factor is unclear.

The soles of these feet bear the classic dermatologic signs of arsenic poisoning—abnormal darkening (hyperpigmentation) and overgrowth of the skin's outer layer (hyperkeratosis). Arsenic-induced lesions are not only unsightly, painful, and debilitating; there is good evidence that they can eventually undergo malignant (cancerous) changes.

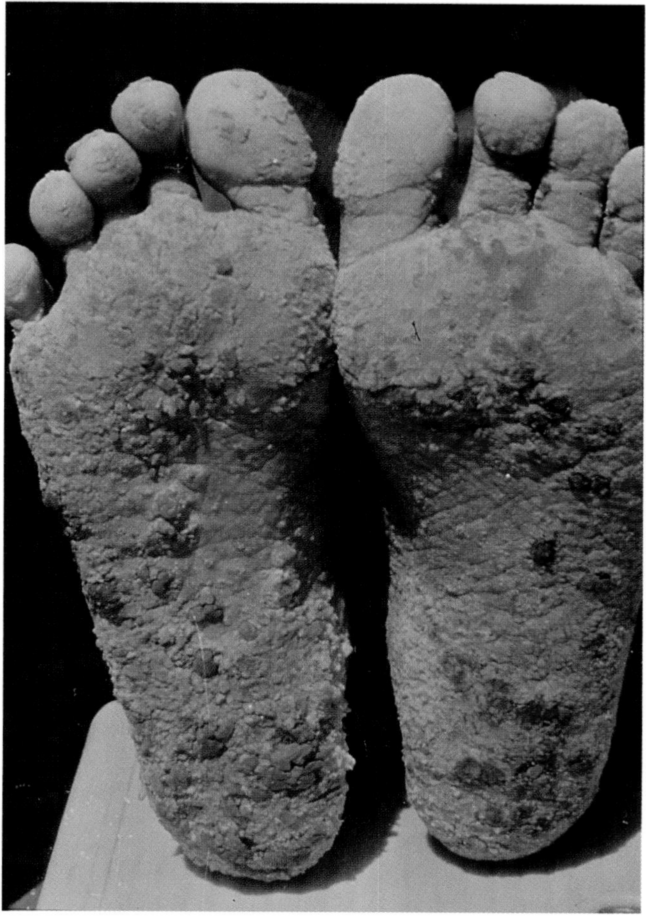

SOES, Jadavpur University, Calcutta

Herman J. Gibb

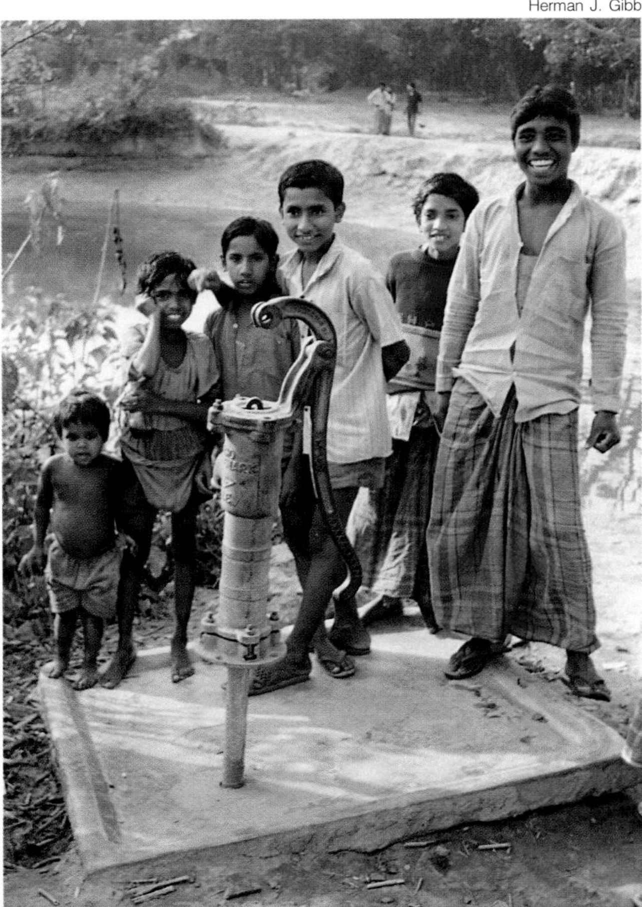

Residents of West Bengal stand at the site of the now-dysfunctional well from which they used to draw their water. The well was shut down by local authorities when it was found to have high levels of arsenic.

Indian scientists are also evaluating the possible role of a selenium deficiency as a predisposing factor for susceptibility to arsenic toxicity. Tests have shown that no selenium was present in the tissue of five patients suffering from arsenic toxicity, but in patients *not* suffering from arsenic toxicity, selenium presence was high while arsenic presence was low.

There are several theories about how the drinking water in Bangladesh and West Bengal came to be contaminated. The most popular theory is that the increased frequency of removal of water from the ground due to the proliferation of tube wells increases the aerated portion of soil. Presumably, the oxidation of the arsenopyrite in the subsoils then results in a release of soluble arsenic into the groundwater. Another theory is that arsenic may be released from iron oxide coatings on grains of sand; thus, the increasing prevalence of flooded fields due to intensive irrigation may speed up the process whereby arsenic leaches into groundwater by hindering the diffusion of oxygen into the ground, which thereby promotes a reduction reaction rather than an oxidation reaction. A third theory is that phosphorus, an ion that is similar to arsenic, may displace arsenic from the pyrite in which it is encased. High levels of phosphorus are reported to be found in the groundwater of the arsenic-affected areas in West Bengal and Bangladesh, possibly as a result of the use of fertilizers.

Response to the crisis

Providing arsenic-free water to the immense populations in West Bengal and Bangladesh that now rely on contaminated water is the most pressing public health need. One problem is the lack of central water-distribution systems in the area. Treatment of water at the sites of the wells or home-treatment methods may be logistically pragmatic, but they are not as satisfactory as central treatment systems. They are also expensive; for many families water-treatment kits may cost nearly a month's earnings. Furthermore, there are problems associated with the disposal of the arsenic once it has been removed from the water.

Arsenic contamination of water is primarily found in wells of 15–150 m (50–500 ft) in depth. It has been suggested by some scientists that deeper wells are not likely to be contaminated. Others, however, contend that no wells in the arsenic-endemic areas of the two countries can be considered free of arsenic.

Some possible alternative sources of water exist. There are some large lakes in West Bengal and Bangladesh, and there is reported to be as much as 4,000 sq km (2,400 sq mi) of wetlands in West Bengal alone. There is also a considerable amount of rainfall in the area. Thus far, however, the potential to make use of these other sources has not been well assessed.

Continuing to drink the contaminated water will only increase an individual's risk of further disease. There is some evidence that patients who have arsenic lesions and who switch to drinking arsenic-free water experience a reduction in the number of lesions. As noted above, people who have inadequate diets may be at a higher risk of developing arsenic-induced disease. Thus, vitamin supplements may be helpful in reducing their susceptibility.

One approach to treating patients has been the use of chelating agents. In medical practice these agents, particularly salts of editic acid (EDTA), are widely used for the direct treatment of metal poisoning. Their purpose is to provide a substance to which the arsenic will attach and be excreted in the urine. Although such treatment causes large arsenic stores to be rapidly eliminated from the body in a matter of hours, most arsenic is rapidly removed by the body even without the use of the agents. Chelating agents may help to remove ingested arsenic more efficiently than the body could normally, but their efficacy in this regard has not yet been well demonstrated. Trials in India, however, are presently being conducted. Of course, the use of chelating agents would be of little benefit if the patient continued to drink arsenic-contaminated water.

The situation in India and Bangladesh has finally attracted worldwide attention. Several conferences addressing the problem were conducted in 1997. Another conference will be conducted in Bangladesh in early 1998. WHO, the World Bank, and several countries are trying to find solutions to the public health crisis—first, by gaining a better understanding of the problem. Among the remedial measures that have been considered are launching large public health awareness campaigns and training medical personnel to detect and treat arsenic-poisoned people. Kunnath Subramanian, a Canadian member of the WHO team that is addressing the problem, has noted that it will take "concerted efforts on the part of many organizations, scientists, and physicians...to efficiently, effectively, expeditiously, and economically tackle this silent epidemic."

—*Herman J. Gibb, Ph.D., M.P.H.*

Taking the Pulse of the U.S. Population

A continuing survey of the United States to obtain information about health conditions of the general population was authorized by legislation signed by the President in July 1956. The new law...launched a program to produce statistics on disease, injury, impairment, disability, and related topics on a uniform basis for the Nation. This marked a significant step in the efforts of the Federal Government to provide tools for improving the health of the American people.

Comprehensive health statistics are needed in this country because a healthy people is perhaps the Nation's greatest resource. The high position of health in the national scene is justified whether the evaluation of it is strictly in monetary terms or in terms of less well-defined but more appropriate scales of national vitality, morale, individual well-being, and other human values. The measurement of this important factor—the people's health—is found in the statistical measurement of well-being.

—*Vital and Health Statistics* (Series 1, number 1)

The National Health Interview Survey (NHIS) described above was initiated in July 1957 during the administration of Pres. Dwight D. Eisenhower and has been collecting data on Americans' health on a continuous basis ever since. The NHIS remains the principal source of information about the health and well-being of the U.S. population and the functioning of the U.S. health care system. NHIS data are widely used inside and outside the government to monitor trends in disease and disability, track progress toward the achievement of national health objectives, assess ongoing and new public health initiatives, determine barriers to appropriate care, target deficiencies in care, and analyze and sometimes revise existing health policies. The year 1997 marked not only the 40th anniversary of the survey but the debut of a virtually all-new version.

Nuts and bolts of a significant survey

When the NHIS began, some of its key defining characteristics were as follows.

- Some 40,000 households in the United States were interviewed each year (that number was increased to close to 50,000 households annually in 1985).
- Interviews were conducted with a responsible adult about his or her own health and that of related children living in the household. All adults at home at the time of the interview participated in the interview. Answers for adults not at home were given by proxy.
- A basic "core" questionnaire collected data about all family members—adults and children—covering four main areas: (1) hospitalizations; (2) use of services provided by or under the supervision of physicians; (3) the effects of poor health on functioning, such as the extent to which illness causes work absence or limits activities; and (4) the presence of chronic conditions.
- This core set of questions about family members was asked each year. In addition, in any particular year supplements were added to collect timely data on topics not covered in the core form. In recent years roughly 6–10 such "Current Health Topic" supplements have been utilized each year; subjects have included AIDS Knowledge and Attitudes, Teenage Attitudes and Practices, Immunization, Drug and Alcohol Use, Family Resources, Environmental Health, and Pregnancy and Smoking.

Despite the fact that over 50,000 U.S. households are interviewed each year, most people are not aware of this vital survey or of the important ways it contributes to health research and policy. Each occupied house or apartment in the United States has a chance to be selected. For logistic reasons certain groups are excluded from the samples—namely, institutionalized patients in long-term-care facilities, armed forces personnel on active duty, and U.S. nationals living in foreign countries. The survey design is such that in any two-week period the households that are selected and interviewed are considered representative of the entire population. Once a household has been selected, a letter is sent explaining the background and purposes of the survey and indicating that an interviewer will be visiting the household soon. Interviewing for the NHIS is done by a staff of about 400 thoroughly trained professional interviewers who work for the U.S. Bureau of the Census. Interviewers visit each household and arrange to conduct an interview with a responsible adult. It is routine to pay several visits in order to arrange to interview people who are hard to find at home.

There are several features of the NHIS that have made it an invaluable source of health information over the years. First, the data are of the highest quality. Because the survey is composed of person-to-person interviews, homes that lack telephone service are included. The rapport between the interviewer and the household members is almost always superior in face-to-face interviews to what it would be over the phone. The rate of cooperation with the survey is extraordinarily high. Over 90% of selected households actually participate (*i.e.,* interviews are completed, and the data become part of the official NHIS results). What accounts for this high response rate? Two factors are considered key: one is the skill, persistence, and patience of the interviewers; the other is the participants' sense that they are contributing vital information to an important national database. In addition, all respondents are given assurance that their answers will be kept confidential.

Not only do NHIS data provide very widely used annual statistics on personal and demographic characteristics, illnesses, injuries, impairments, and chronic and short-term conditions, but owing to the continuous nature of data collection, the size of the samples interviewed each year, and the overall quality of the data, the NHIS lends itself especially well to special-purpose studies. Because a new representative sample is interviewed every two weeks, accurate tracking of changes in acute conditions is possible. This feature was used to track the rise and fall of swine influenza outbreaks in the 1950s, the mid-'60s, and the late '70s. More recently, researchers took advantage of the large size of the NHIS sample to identify a representative sample of adults who had experienced polio in childhood to find out about the limitations and health problems they experienced as adults. That information contributed to the understanding and diagnosis of what is now called postpolio syndrome.

Over time, certain deficiencies in the survey became apparent, and revisions were made. In the 1980s, for example, the sampling method was redesigned to strengthen the ability to make estimates about African-American and Latino populations. Also, as noted above, the basic sample was expanded to include 50,000 households. As important as these changes may have been to ensuring

Kent Knudson—Southern Stock/PNI

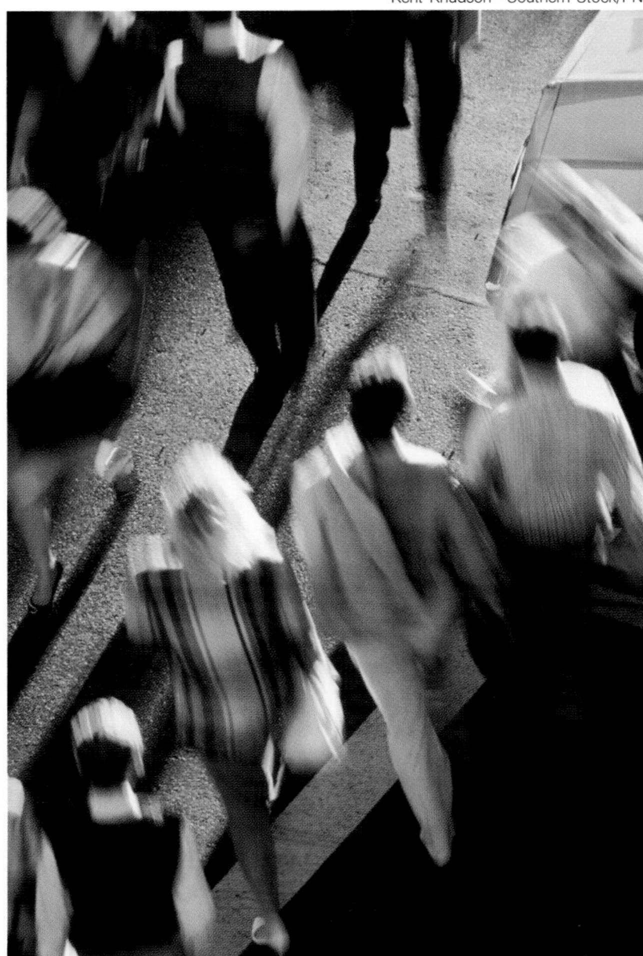

Since 1957 data on Americans' health have been collected on a continuous basis. Among other things, health statistics are needed to monitor trends in disease and disability, target deficiencies in care, and establish or revise national health objectives.

the quality of data, the basic conception of the NHIS remained relatively unchanged for 40 years.

Starting in 1997, however, a radically redesigned survey was put in place. Because of the importance of the NHIS as a source of vital health information and the extent to which the data are used, the changes will be far-reaching. The inauguration of the new NHIS thus can be considered one of the important U.S. health-related events of the year.

Impetus for an overhaul

The original stimulus for reviewing the design of the NHIS was a practical one. By the mid-1980s, the need to collect data *not covered* in the annual core questionnaire had grown substantially. Consequently, the National Center for Health Statistics (the NHIS's sponsor) was finding it increasingly necessary to include supplemental questionnaires in most years. This had the effect of pushing the average length of household interviews to more than two hours. Concerns were raised about the impact of the increased time length on the quality of the data collected. The longer an interview takes, the more likely it is that the participants' ability to concentrate and remember accurately is reduced and that interviewers' concentration and skill are compromised. Therefore, there was clearly a need to streamline the survey. Yet as the content of the core was reviewed, in each area good reasons were found to *expand,* not contract, the basic data that were being collected. It seemed impossible to achieve such an expansion without *increasing* the length of the overall interview. It became apparent that the time had come for a major makeover. A careful review of the survey design revealed five major areas that needed fundamental revision:

1. By the mid-1990s two of the basic NHIS premises were no longer valid. First, in the 1950s when the survey was conceived, surgery and other major treatments required hospitalization. Today a high percentage of surgery is done on a day, or outpatient, basis—patients are not admitted for overnight stays—and many procedures are done not in hospitals but in offices and clinics. Second, when the NHIS was originally designed, physicians were assumed to deliver almost all medical care, primarily during patient visits to their offices. Now many nonphysicians deliver important medical services, and often this is done in health care settings other than doctors' offices. Physical therapists, nurse practitioners, visiting nurses and other home-care providers, physicians' assistants, optometrists, and psychologists are some of the more obvious nonphysician providers.
2. The NHIS essentially collected no information about mental health status and Americans' use of mental health services. Psychological distress was not included as either an acute or a chronic condition. Services to treat mental conditions were counted only if they resulted in visits to medical doctors.
3. While the NHIS was instrumental in developing one particularly useful measure of health status—looking at the ways health conditions affect people's lives by limiting their activities—the survey had not incorporated many other innovative health measures that are now widely used by epidemiologists and statisticians.
4. The NHIS relied upon "condition lists"—*i.e.,* interviewers would read a long list of conditions (arthritis, cataracts, diabetes, eczema, glaucoma, sciatica, etc.), and respondents would answer "yes" if they had them. Methodological studies, however, had shown that such responses often did not correspond with information available from medical records. In recent years it has become clear that clinically important aspects of many conditions are better reflected when people report specific symptoms instead of merely acknowledging the presence of a condition.
5. The NHIS was devised to characterize individuals. Thus, data were coded individual by individual and were not tabulated or organized to characterize the family as a unit. Yet having family-level data is of critical importance for many analytic purposes.

Full-scale face-lift

The need to collect more detailed data in a shortened interview period was clear. But how could the dual goals of sharpening and streamlining the survey be met? The solution was the development of a survey with rotating content. Beginning in 1997 the NHIS included a core set of questions that will be asked in about 50,000 households each year. In addition, each year's survey will feature new and detailed questions in one particular area (*e.g.,* utilization of health services, personal health status, and disease prevention/health promotion). By having rotating emphases, the survey will cover a broader array of pertinent health issues. Among the topics that will now be addressed in considerable detail every third year are the services provided by nonphysicians and health care delivered outside hospitals and doctors' offices.

There is a new emphasis on self-reporting. In the past any knowledgeable adult could be the household respondent. The adults were not statistically representative of all adults. Now and in the future, one household adult will be designated to be the respondent, and a good portion of the data will be collected only about that person. The reason for this change is that methodological studies have shown that self-reporting is superior to proxy reporting on most topics. While proxy reporting may be appropriate for collecting information about certain effects of health conditions, such as a disability that prevents a household member from working, other measures of health status are more meaningful when the individual in question speaks for herself or himself. Functional limitations, pain, fatigue, and psychological distress are examples of illness effects that would not necessarily be reported accurately by another household member. Measures related to mental health will particularly benefit from this change. Another advantage of having a single person as the main focus is that it will simplify the interview process. The NHIS had been extraordinarily cumbersome as an instrument because it involved the collection of parallel data on all family (or household) members. Obviously, it takes less time to collect data on one person than to collect them on several. This is especially true when the individual being interviewed is the one who has ready answers to the questions. Finally, epidemiologists are especially pleased with the new design because having more information about one individual rather than less about several increases the analytic potential of the survey.

In a manner parallel to the selection of a representative adult from each family, one child from each family that includes minor children will be designated a sample child. Detailed questions will be asked about the health and health care of that sample child. Taken together, the children so selected will be a representative sample of all the children in U.S. households.

Previously the NHIS data were collected by means of paper and pencil; the interviewer filled out pages and pages of forms. The revised survey is now computer-assisted. The interviewer enters responses directly into a laptop computer during the interview. Such automation speeds the processing of data and should make survey results available more quickly than in the past.

The content of the NHIS is set on an annual basis. During 1996 two early versions of the redesigned form of the NHIS were tested. The version that began in January 1997 is based on those redesigned protocols and incorporates the best features of both trial surveys.

Of course, some of these changes come at a price. Collecting a wider array of data through the rotating-topic approach means that some estimates that used to be available annually will now be available only every three or four years. The change to increased reliance on self-respondents may lower the response rates. When interviewers were free to interview any person in the household who was knowledgeable, data could be collected about reluctant or difficult-to-find persons. Now the selected individual must provide the answers (or decline to do so). When data are collected about only one adult, the number of cases available for some analyses will be reduced. Finally, annual data will be available about many fewer chronic conditions. Some of the less-common conditions, such as glaucoma, sciatica, colitis, varicose veins, goiter or thyroid problems, which were recorded when the lengthy condition lists of the past were used, will be measured only when health status is the topic of emphasis for a given year.

Some policy makers, researchers, businesspeople, students, and others who depended on annual NHIS statistics in the past may grumble a bit about not having access to as many figures each year. All in all, however, the new face of the NHIS will give most users of the data more and better information about health in the U.S. than ever before.

—*Floyd J. Fowler, Jr., Ph.D.*

Link...No Link

"New study links birth control pills to blood clots...." "Pesticide linked to unusual cluster of pancreatic cancers...." "No link between aluminum cookware and Alzheimer's disease, leading scientists report...." "Salt safe after all...."

Warnings about unhealthy behaviors or dangerous substances in the environment reach millions every day through the news media. Yet because this advice so frequently contradicts earlier, equally dire warnings, the public may be tempted to disbelieve everything they hear. It is not surprising, then, that after nearly two decades of scientific debate about leukemia incidence among children living near high-voltage power lines, the recent news that researchers at the National Cancer Institute (NCI) had found no significant connection between electromagnetic fields and cancer failed to fully quell public anxieties.

In fact, the public's skepticism toward news stories about health risks may be one of the healthiest behaviors of all. While it is always important to keep in mind that spectacular gains in public health and longevity have come about because the experts were right more often than they were wrong, every finding must be taken with a proverbial grain of salt. Of all the sciences, epidemiology—the study of possible links between disease and risk factors in people's lifestyles and surroundings—is among the most error-prone, and the findings of epidemiological studies are certainly among the most difficult to convey accurately in a 30-second TV news report or a few lines of newspaper text.

The gold standard of reliability in biomedical research is the randomized, double-blind, controlled trial. In pharmaceutical trials, for example, participants are randomly assigned to a group that will be exposed to the substance being tested or a group that will receive a placebo. Researchers then track the health of both groups over time, and to protect against observational bias, neither the participants nor the researchers find out who received the actual drug until all the data have been gathered. Almost all new medicines are tested in this rigorous way, and the result is usually a dependable "yes" or "no" about a substance's safety and efficacy.

Epidemiologists, however, can rarely carry out randomized trials, since medical ethics prohibit deliberately exposing people to suspected risks, and in most cases the condition whose cause is being sought has already appeared in the population. Instead, a common strategy in epidemiology is to conduct a "case-control" study (sometimes called a "retrospective" study), in which researchers compare a group of patients suffering from a particular condition with a group of healthy controls, in hopes of isolating differences in nutrition or living conditions that might account for the illness. Another common epidemiological approach is the "cohort," or "prospective," study, in which scientists gather health and environmental data on a large population and then watch over a period of time to see who gets sick.

Both investigational methods can highlight associations between disease and exposure to common risk factors, but both are subject to biases. One type of bias is "selection bias," which may occur in a case-control study if the control group is not strictly comparable to the case group but instead differs in some way that the study designers have overlooked. Several major studies conducted by prominent investigators have been criticized, for example, because control subjects were contacted through random-digit telephone dialing, a method that excludes people of low socioeconomic status, who may not have a telephone or an answering machine. "Recall bias" can also skew results. For example, there is often a greater likelihood that cancer patients in an epidemiological study will remember past exposures to risk factors than will healthy interviewees.

So-called confounders, real but hidden connections that generate spurious epidemiological associations, are a third major type of pitfall in epidemiological studies. The well-documented observation that elderly churchgoers live longer than their less-devout peers, for example, could suggest that believing in God is good for one's health—or it could simply reflect the fact that church congregations provide health-promoting social and emotional support and that church members are less likely than nonmembers to engage in harmful behaviors such as drinking and smoking. In other words, as the crusty but correct scientific axiom goes, "Correlation is not causation."

Few print or broadcast journalists have the expertise, and few members of the general public have the time or the desire, to interpret the latest epidemiological findings in the context of these essential caveats. Indeed, if reporters, readers, and viewers regarded epidemiological findings with the same skepticism as many health experts do, there would be a lot less health news to talk about. Before accepting the findings of an epidemiological study, many physicians insist that there be both a plausible biological explanation for the association between disease and risk factor and a high "relative risk" of illness in those exposed to the risk factor. (Relative risk is the ratio of disease incidence in study participants who were exposed to a suspected risk factor to the incidence in those who were not exposed; one study, for example, found that the relative risk of mouth cancer among people who regularly used high-alcohol mouthwash was 1.50, meaning that mouthwash users were 50% more likely to develop mouth cancer than nonusers.) Robert Temple, director of drug evaluation at the Food and Drug Administration (FDA), told the journal *Science* in 1995, "My basic rule is if the relative risk isn't at least three or four, forget it." Yet in many studies that attract intense public attention, the relative risk is far smaller.

What follows is a brief roundup of some of the most absorbing—but often ambiguous—epidemiological findings reported in 1996 and early 1997, with cautious "verdicts" either linking or failing to link one substance, type of environmental exposure, physiological condition, etc., to a particular human malady.

Abortion and breast cancer

Breast cells proliferate during pregnancy, and women who terminate their pregnancies may be left with many immature breast cells that are more susceptible than other cells to carcinogens. Yet dozens of studies conducted since 1980 have come to conflicting conclusions about whether women who have had abortions are actually at greater risk of developing breast cancer than those whose pregnancies proceed to term. Many of the studies that found a positive association may have been marred by recall bias, since cancer patients are probably more likely to admit having had an abortion than healthy study participants. A team of Danish researchers, reporting in the Jan. 9, 1997, issue of *The New England Journal of Medicine,* sidestepped the problem of recall bias by examining the health records of more than 1.5 million women born in Denmark between 1935 and 1978. The researchers found that the relative risk of breast cancer in women who had had induced abortions was exactly 1.00—*i.e.,* they had no increased risk.

Verdict: No link.

Aspartame and brain tumors

John Olney, a researcher at Washington University, St. Louis, Mo., published a report in November 1996 suggesting that the low-calorie sweetener NutraSweet (aspartame), introduced by Monsanto in 1981, was to blame for a subsequent 10% increase in the incidence of brain tumors in the United States. Scientists at the FDA and the Mayo Clinic, Rochester, Minn., agreed that there has been an increase in the diagnosis of brain tumors in the U.S., but they pointed out that the rise began in the 1970s, well before the FDA approved NutraSweet for marketing. They also noted that brain tumor incidence has not kept pace with the vastly increased use of NutraSweet since the 1980s; if there were a real cause-and-effect link, researchers would expect to see a consistent "dose-response curve."

Verdict: No link.

Sleep apnea and cardiovascular disease

Between 2% and 4% of people suffer from a condition that is as common as asthma or diabetes—namely, obstructive sleep apnea, the involuntary and highly inconvenient closure of the airways during sleep. Several studies in the U.S. have indicated that these interruptions in breathing lower the level of oxygen and raise the level of carbon dioxide in the blood and thereby contribute to hypertension (high blood pressure) and its assault on blood vessels and the heart. To prevent these complications, American physicians often prescribe a treatment called continuous positive airway pressure (CPAP), in which patients are connected via a face mask and tube to a machine that delivers pressurized air to their airways. But in the March 22, 1997, issue of the *British Medical Journal,* a group of researchers who reviewed 54 sleep apnea studies published between 1966 and 1995 concluded that there is no consistent evidence that sleep apnea leads to high blood

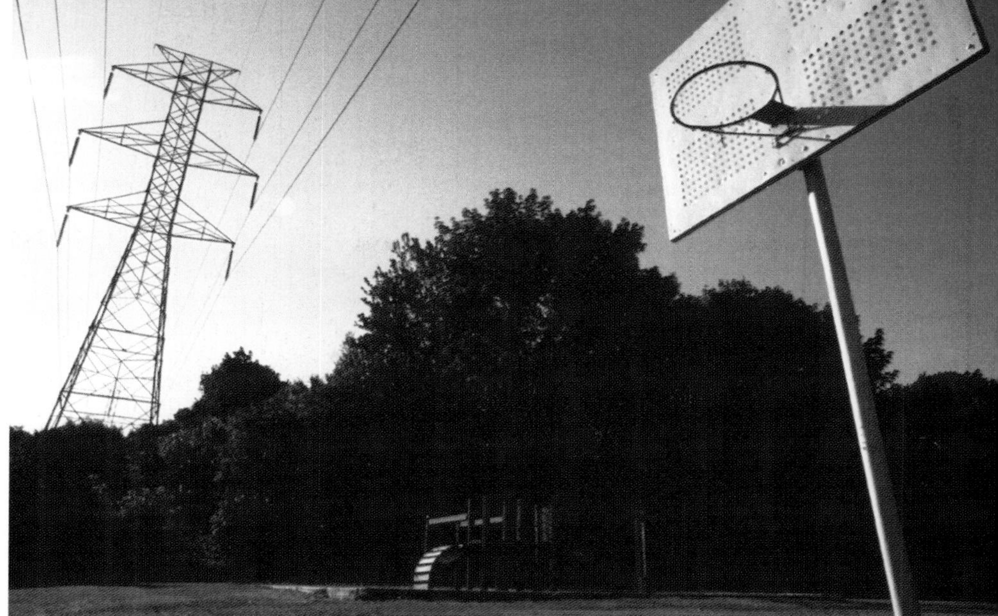

Lori Grinker—Contact Press Images/PNI

Are children who live or play in close proximity to high-voltage power lines at increased risk of leukemia? Recent studies attempting to answer this question have produced no clear answers. If anything, the latest data have added to the confusion. Particularly puzzling to reseachers has been the lack of a clear dose-response relationship.

pressure, heart disease, or stroke or that CPAP is beneficial. Because sleep apnea is most common among the elderly and obese, the researchers questioned whether the condition "is a separate disease entity or [simply] a marker or a symptom of obesity and aging." Few previous studies, they concluded, had adequately sorted out these confounding factors.

Verdict: Tentatively, no link.

Electromagnetic fields and childhood leukemia

A 1979 study indicating that children who lived near high-voltage power lines in Colorado had an increased risk of leukemia sparked public outcry and an extended scientific dispute. A panel of experts convened by the National Research Council recently carried out a meta-analysis of data gathered in more than 500 separate scientific studies. In October 1996 they reported that the literature consistently indicates a relative risk of leukemia of about 1.50 among children who live near high concentrations of electric power lines. The panel concluded that this level of risk, while statistically significant, is so low that no firm link can be inferred.

The following year researchers at the NCI made another attempt to put this issue to rest. Troubled by the fact that in most earlier studies years or decades had passed between the diagnosis of leukemia and measurements of magnetic fields, these investigators designed and carried out a large case-control study in which technicians measured magnetic fields at the homes of 638 leukemia patients under age 15 and those of 620 healthy children. (The technicians were unaware of the children's health status.) In the July 3, 1997, issue of *The New England Journal of Medicine,* the researchers reported that the risk of leukemia significantly exceeded 1.00 in only one group: children exposed to magnetic fields 0.4–0.499 microteslas in intensity, who had a relative risk of 3.28. (A microtesla is, generally speaking, a measurement of the strength of a magnetic field.) But the fact that no known mechanism can explain how magnetic fields cause cancer, together with the fact that the study did not show a dose-response curve—children who were exposed to fields 0.5 microteslas or greater had a relative risk of only 1.41—convinced the NCI investigators that there is "little support" for the leukemia–high-power-line link.

Verdict: Jury still out; link still not clear.

Prozac in pregnancy and child development

Pregnant women are as much at risk for depression as anyone else, if not more so. Commonly prescribed tricyclic antidepressants such as nortriptyline (Pamelor) and selective serotonin reuptake inhibitors such as fluoxetine (Prozac) are known to cross the placental barrier between the maternal and fetal bloodstreams. The medications have not been associated with increased numbers of miscarriages or major birth defects, but a study reported in the Oct. 3, 1996, issue of *The New England Journal of Medicine* found that the relative risk of premature delivery for children born to women who took fluoxetine during the third trimester was 4.80, while the relative risk of poor adaptation to neonatal intensive care, including experiencing respiratory difficulty and jitteriness, was 8.70.

Writing in the Jan. 23, 1997, issue of the same journal, a group of Canadian researchers criticized this study and its implicit condemnation of fluoxetine use late in pregnancy. The Canadian group pointed out that the earlier study had not taken into account confounding factors such as coexisting diseases or the more severe nature of depression in women who had needed fluoxetine throughout pregnancy. The Canadian researchers tested cognitive development and language skills in the children of 80 mothers who had received tricyclic antidepressants at some point during pregnancy, 55 children whose mothers took fluoxetine during pregnancy, and 84 youngsters whose mothers took no antidepressant drugs. The mean test scores of the three groups were similar.

Verdict: Mixed. Fetal exposure to antidepressants appears to be linked to an increased risk of complications at or around the time of birth but may not be linked to retarded neurodevelopment.

Fertility and ovarian cancer

Women who choose fertility over surgical sterilization pay a curious price: a greater chance of developing ovarian cancer. Researchers at the American Cancer Society, reporting in the Feb. 15, 1997, *American Journal of Epidemiology,* followed 400,000 initially cancer-free women over an average of nine years and found that those sterilized by tubal ligation were one-third less likely than the others to die from ovarian cancer. Scientists speculate that either women who have their tubes surgically tied get better gynecological follow-up care than others, so their tumors tend to be caught and treated earlier, or cutting the fallopian tubes somehow prevents carcinogenic substances from reaching the ovaries.

Verdict: Link. Having intact fallopian tubes is a risk factor for cancer—but few women are likely to undergo sterilization simply to reduce that risk.

Red meat and lymphoma in older women

In a prospective study of cancer incidence, researchers at the University of Iowa College of Medicine questioned 35,156 women residing in the state of Iowa about their diets in 1986 and assessed their health status in 1993. All participants were aged 55 to 69 at the start of the study, and none had a prior history of cancer. After adjusting for age, residence, and other possible confounding factors, the investigators compared the relative risk of developing non-Hodgkin's lymphoma (a cancer of the lymphatic system) among the one-third of the group who consumed the most animal fat with that of the one-third who had the lowest animal-fat intake. The former group's relative risk was 2.00. Various types of fat were evaluated, as were various foods per se. The relative risk for saturated fat was 1.69; for monounsaturated fat, 1.90. The risk associated with hamburger in particular was comparatively high, at 2.35, while greater fruit consumption was associated with a risk of 0.64, which means it was protective against non-Hodgkin's lymphoma.

Verdict: A weak link; nonetheless, eating fewer burgers and more fruits and vegetables probably cannot hurt.

Fish and heart disease

Five cohort studies and two case-control studies conducted prior to 1997 had indicated that fish consumption confers protection against coronary heart disease, but four other studies had found no such effect. A team of researchers at Northwestern University Medical School revisited the question, studying health and nutrition records of 1,822 Chicago-area men who, in the baseline year of 1957, were between 40 and 55 years of age and manufactured telephones for the Western Electric Co. They found that for men who ate 35 g of fish (a child-sized portion) or more daily, the relative risk of death from coronary heart disease was 0.62, the risk of death from a sudden heart attack was 0.56, and the risk of death from a nonsudden heart attack was 0.33. The researchers found that these comparatively low levels of risk were specifically correlated with fish consumption—not simply with avoidance of red meat.

Verdict: Link. Eating fish lowers the risk of dying from heart disease.

Joel Rogers—Allstock/PNI

Depression and osteoporosis

Studies have shown that major depression in women is often accompanied by physiological problems such as decreased appetite (anorexia), increased secretion of the hormone cortisol, and decreased levels of growth and sex hormones. Since these nutritional and hormonal changes can affect the development of body tissues such as bone, women with depression may be at increased risk of osteoporosis, a loss of bone mineral density that heightens the risk of fractures. In the Oct. 17, 1996, issue of *The New England Journal of Medicine,* a research team from the National Institutes of Health reported that it had used X-ray absorptiometry to measure bone mineral density in 24 women with a history of major depression and 24 normal women matched for age, body-mass index, menopausal status, and race. They found that in women with past or current depression, bone mineral density was 6.5% lower in the spine, 13.6% lower at the neck of the femur (thighbone), and 10.8% lower at the trochanter (a notch at the top of the femur).

Verdict: A link, though not a striking one. Women with depression, like other women at risk for bone loss, should take steps to guard against osteoporosis (*e.g.,* making sure they get plenty of calcium and exercise).

Bone density and breast cancer

Women, it would seem, just cannot win. Boston University School of Medicine researchers reported in the Feb. 27, 1997, issue of *The New England Journal of Medicine* that postmenopausal women with the highest bone density also have a greater risk of developing breast cancer than their peers with lower bone mass. As part of the well-known Framingham Study, 1,373 women with no history of breast cancer were first evaluated between 1967 and 1970; 91 of the women developed postmenopausal breast cancer. After adjusting for age and other potential confounders, the researchers found that the relative risk of breast cancer in women whose bone mass placed them between the 25th and 75th percentiles was 1.30 compared with women below the 25th percentile. Women between the 75th and 100th percentile had a relative risk of 3.50. It is highly unlikely that greater bone mass *causes* breast cancer; in this case bone mass is probably a marker for cumulative exposure to estrogen, which has been linked to breast cancer.

Verdict: Link, but not an especially meaningful one.

Exercise and breast cancer

A dozen relatively small studies had suggested that exercise lowers a woman's risk of breast cancer, but a large Norwegian study, reported in *The New England Journal of Medicine* on May 1, 1997, nailed down the association more firmly. In a group of 25,624 women, the relative risk of breast cancer among women who exercised regularly compared with their sedentary peers was 0.63—after adjustments for age, body-mass index, height, county of residence, and number of children and the age when they had their first child. The protective effect was even more pronounced in premenopausal women. Researchers speculate that the mechanisms behind this protection may be genetic (a propensity to exercise may be heritable, as is breast cancer risk) or hormonal (exercise decreases levels of estrogen, estradiol, and progesterone, high levels of which have been associated with the development of breast cancer).

Verdict: Link.

Talc and ovarian cancer

Talc (as in talcum powder) has a chemical similarity to asbestos, which raises suspicions about its safety. A report in the March 1, 1997, issue of the *American Journal of Epidemiology* warned that women who dust their genital areas with powder daily have a relative risk of ovarian cancer of 1.60. Daily use of feminine deodorant sprays was associated with a risk of 1.90. The study did not record the types of powders or deodorants the women used, and the results may have been influenced by recall bias on the part of the women who were questioned, but a number of previous studies had reached similar conclusions.

Verdict: A weak link but an easily circumvented one, as powders, deodorants, and similar products that do not contain talc are available.

Calcium supplements and kidney stones

Data on over 90,000 participants in the Nurses' Health Study, a long-term investigation conducted by Harvard researchers, showed that nurses who consumed high levels of fluids, potassium, and dietary calcium had a relative risk of developing kidney stones of between 0.61 and 0.65. Curiously, women who took calcium supplements were more likely to develop kidney stones than women who ate a diet rich in calcium, but their relative risk—1.20—was too low to cause alarm.

Verdict: Weak link.

Cow's milk and diabetes

Finnish scientists found in the early 1990s that infants switched from breast-feeding to cow's milk very early in life were at greater risk of developing Type 1 (insulin-dependent) diabetes, perhaps as the result of an immune reaction against beta casein, the major protein in cow's milk. But a case-control study reported in the *Journal of the American Medical Association* (Aug. 28, 1996) indicated that children in Denver, Colo., who were above the 99th percentile for B-cell autoimmunity—which is thought to be a marker of future diabetes risk—were no more likely than other children to have been exposed to cow's milk in the first three to six months of life. Some researchers objected to this conclusion, claiming that the study was too small to be conclusive and that B-cell autoimmunity is not necessarily a good predictor of who will get diabetes. Then a study by Italian researchers published in *The Lancet* (Oct. 5, 1996) found that 24 of 47 people with diabetes, but only one of 36 healthy volunteers, had immune-system cells primed to attack beta casein—an indication that the immune system can mount a reaction against cow's milk.

Verdict: A questionable link.

Cow's milk and breast cancer

Milk from the mammary glands of cows may pose a health risk for newborns, but it may protect their mothers' breasts against cancer. A 25-year study of 4,000 women in Finland showed that those who habitually drank the most milk—whole milk, at that—had a relative risk of contracting breast cancer of 0.50. The study controlled for other breast cancer risk factors such as smoking, weight, number of pregnancies, and occupation. Scientists speculate that galactose (the sugar found in all types of milk) slows estrogen production and thus reduces cancers.

Verdict: Suggestive but still inconclusive link. Drinking milk may offer women some protection against the development of breast cancer.

—Wade Roush, Ph.D.

Genetics Update

The understanding of human genetics has increased exponentially since scientists first isolated a human gene in 1980. Hundreds of genes have now been identified, and the roles of many, in both health and disease, are well understood. On the basis of these data, tests for a number of genetic diseases have been developed, and innovative treatments are under investigation. As knowledge about the human genome accumulates, however, so do the social, ethical, and legal implications of such knowledge, and new questions are raised for science and society.

In the past year or so, a number of significant events occurred in the field, including the discovery of human genes linked to skin cancer, Parkinson's disease, and hemochromatosis; the completion of the project to sequence the genome of the yeast *Saccharomyces cerevisiae;* and the publication of new recommendations for the use of genetic screening for cystic fibrosis. These topics and others are discussed below.

Progress report on the genome project

How do genes regulate growth and development? This is one of the most fundamental questions in biology, and it lies at the heart of the Human Genome Project, the effort to identify, analyze, and catalog every human gene. Once the chemical structure of the genes is known, investigators will be able to begin elucidating how they work together to make normal functioning possible, as well as how changes in the structure ultimately can cause disease.

The genetic information of living organisms is encoded in DNA, the complex molecule that forms the long threadlike strands known as chromosomes. The genes themselves are distinctive linear arrangements, or sequences, of nucleotide bases (the chemical units that constitute the "building blocks" of DNA) that lie along the length of the chromosome, much like beads on a string. Each gene encodes a specific protein—that is, it contains instructions for the synthesis of the protein. Proteins, in turn, are the agents that carry out chemical processes at the cellular level and help to determine the structure and function of an organism.

Since the genome project began in 1990, the progress toward its initial goals has been even faster than expected. The first goal of the project is to determine the precise chromosomal location of each of the 50,000–100,000 human genes. A map showing the locations of 16,000 genes was published in *Science* in October 1996. (It can be viewed on the World Wide Web at http://www.ncbi.nlm.nih.gov/SCIENCE96.) Investigators estimate that by the end of 1997 the location of more than half of all human genes will be known.

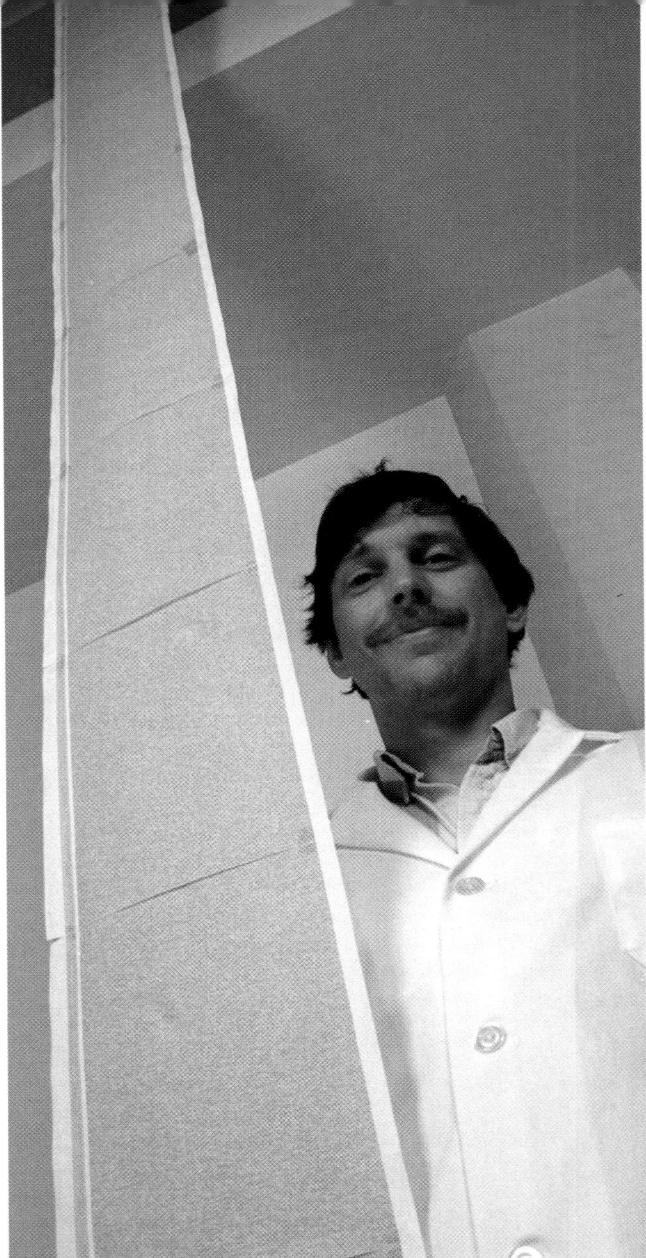

A researcher at the Stanford (Calif.) Human Genome Center proudly displays a computer printout of the genetic sequence of the yeast Saccharomyces cerevisiae. *The sequence of the yeast genome was completed in 1996.*

Determining the location of the genes is only one objective, however. Equally important is the "sequencing" of each gene—that is, elucidating the linear sequence of the four nucleotide bases, adenine (A), guanine (G), cytosine (C), and thymine (T), that make up DNA. Once investigators know the base sequence of a gene, they can determine the gene's protein product and study the protein's function in the body.

Although the human genome contains about three billion bases, only a very small percentage—fewer than 5%—are believed to encode proteins. The function of the remaining, noncoding, sequences of DNA is not yet known. Nevertheless, investigators are working to determine the entire sequence of the human genome. The complete nucleotide sequence, the ultimate genetic map of the entire human genome, is expected to be finished by the year 2005.

Stuart Brinin—KRT

Nonhuman genomes. An important component of the genome project is the study of the genetic material of a variety of nonhuman organisms, including many that are much less genetically complex than humans. Researchers are examining these simpler genomes not only to understand the creatures themselves but also to provide insight into the human genome. The genomic sequences of more than 140 viruses, a number of bacteria, and the yeast *S. cerevisiae* have been determined to date.

The yeast genome, completed in April 1996, is the largest sequenced so far. It is 12 million bases long and contains around 6,000 genes. Information about the sequence of the yeast genome should prove useful in studying human genetic diseases, since more than 40% of disease-related human genes have counterparts in the yeast.

In January 1997 investigators announced yet another milestone: the completion of the sequence of *Escherichia coli,* a common and widely studied bacterium. The microbe was found to have some 4.6 million bases, constituting close to 4,300 genes. These data are a powerful complement to biological information about the organism that had already been accumulated over years of laboratory research.

Another organism whose genome is being studied as part of the Human Genome Project is the nematode (roundworm) *Caenorhabditis elegans.* Like the yeast and *E. coli,* this worm has been studied in the laboratory for decades, so a great deal is already known about its biology. Moreover, a number of the worm's genes also have homologues, or counterparts, in the human genome. Of particular interest is a gene called *clk-1.* (By scientific convention, the names of genes are italicized.) Worms with an altered form of the gene have life spans that are about 50% longer than average. In February 1997 scientists at McGill University, Montreal, announced that they had cloned (*i.e.,* duplicated) and sequenced *clk-1.* Their work confirmed the speculation that the protein encoded by this gene is a metabolic regulator that affects the aging process of cells. They also found that proteins similar to the one encoded by *clk-1* are present in yeasts, rats, mice, and humans and may thus be associated with the aging process in a variety of organisms.

Regulating use of genetic data. As information about the human genome mounts, so too does concern that these data be used only in accordance with internationally accepted medical, scientific, and ethical standards. Toward this end, for the past five years the International Bar Association has been working on a treaty that sets minimum legal standards for the use of human genetic information. The purpose of the treaty is to provide legal protection to people around the world, including those whose legal systems lack laws on these issues. The treaty bans eugenics practices, gives individuals the right to choose whether to learn the results of genetic tests, and prohibits governments from requiring anyone to undergo surgery that would alter his or her genetic makeup. It also states that no human gene or chromosomal segment is patentable, although inventions arising from it could be.

"Disease genes": growing list

One of the immediate benefits of the Human Genome Project has been an increase in the rapidity with which disease-related genes are being identified. Strictly speaking, there are no "disease genes" but rather mutated, or altered, versions of normal genes, each of which has a specific and necessary protein product. A genetic mutation may cause harm in any of a variety of ways. It may, for example, render the gene incapable of instructing a cell to make a particular protein required for initiating a particular cellular function. Or, conversely, a mutation may disrupt the production of a protein whose function is to cause a certain cellular activity to cease at the appropriate time. Another type of mutation can muddle the genetic instructions and thus cause the cell to make a faulty protein that accumulates in an abnormal fashion. Regardless of the underlying mutation, missing or defective proteins can disrupt normal cellular mechanisms, which leads to malfunction of an organ system and, finally, to illness.

The discovery that a particular genetic mutation is linked to a particular disease is useful to scientists because it can ultimately enable them to develop ways to treat—or even prevent—the disorder. In the past year researchers isolated a number of new genes linked to various disorders and elucidated the roles of several other, previously identified genes.

Links to cancer. The most common form of human cancer is basal cell carcinoma, a type of skin cancer that is usually curable but, if not caught early, can cause disfigurement. In June 1996 two different groups of investigators announced that they had isolated a gene called *patched,* or *PTC,* on chromosome 9, which, when mutated, causes this cancer. The normal version of the gene is involved in embryonic development. A mutated form of the *patched* gene also is believed to be responsible for a rare inherited disorder called basal cell nevus syndrome, which can result in multiple cancers.

A team of scientists from the U.S. and Sweden announced late in 1996 that they were close to pinpointing the location of a gene linked to prostate cancer, the most common tumor in men and the second most deadly form of cancer (after lung cancer) in males. The gene, found on chromosome 1, is known as *HPC1* (hereditary prostate cancer 1). Men who inherit a mutated form of *HPC1* have a much higher than average risk of developing prostate cancer. The inherited mutation is thought to be involved in about one-third of all familial cases of prostate cancer and would therefore account for only 3% of all cases; scientists believe, however, that the mutation could underlie some sporadic (noninherited) instances of the disease as well.

The study of the genetics of breast cancer continues to answer questions that have plagued scientists for years, but it also raises completely new quandaries. Since the identification of two genes linked to hereditary forms of breast and ovarian cancer—*BRCA1* in 1994 and *BRCA2* in 1995—researchers have been working to elucidate the mechanisms by which these mutations cause disease. A major step toward this goal came in April 1997 with the discovery of the normal function of *BRCA1* and *BRCA2.* Although their base sequences are quite different, both genes perform a similar role in the cell, namely, that of "caretaker" of the genome. Specifically, they are involved in repairing major breaks in chromosomes. Properly functioning chromosomal repair mechanisms are critical because breaks can lead to genetic instability, which eventually may result in uncontrolled cell growth.

A major question researchers continue to ponder concerns the degree of risk conferred by the inheritance of mutated forms of these genes. Four studies published in May 1997 addressed this issue. One found that only 16% of breast cancer patients with a family history of breast cancer had a mutation in *BRCA1,* much lower than the 45% generally estimated. Another survey showed that mutations in *BRCA1* were more likely than those in *BRCA2* to cause breast cancer in young women. A third study found that women who had inherited one of the mutations could reduce their risk of cancer by having either their breasts or their ovaries removed, a radical treatment that does not completely eliminate the possibility of cancer.

A fourth study, perhaps the most controversial, was one devised to assess the accuracy of risk estimates based on data from high-risk families (those with a large number of members with breast or ovarian cancer). Previous estimates had indicated that mutations in *BRCA1* and *BRCA2* cause about an 85% risk of breast cancer and a 60% risk of ovarian cancer by age 70. (The average risks for U.S. women are about 8% and 2%, respectively.) The new investigation focused on a large group of Ashkenazi Jewish women and men, a population chosen because of its comparatively high incidence of these two mutations. The study found the risks to this group to be somewhat lower than previously calculated—56% for breast cancer and 16% for ovarian cancer—but still much higher than the average for the population as a whole. These results were considered preliminary, and more research will be needed to confirm them.

Candace Barbot—KRT

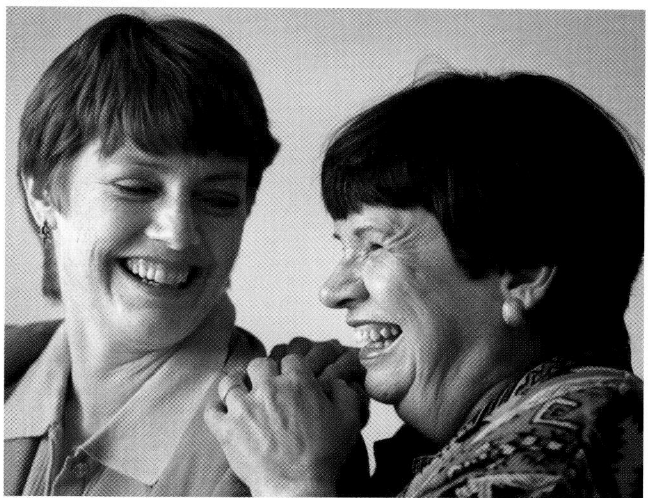

These two women, mother and daughter, both of whom have undergone mastectomies for breast cancer, are among the millions worldwide hoping that genetics research will provide some definitive answers for women from families with a history of the disease.

While those who carry mutations in *BRCA1* or *BRCA2* are unquestionably at increased risk, the fact remains that only about 5% to 10% of all breast cancer cases can be attributed to heredity. Moreover, these two mutations are linked to only about two-thirds of familial cases of breast cancer. The search, therefore, continues for other breast cancer genes. One gene that might fit this description is *CYP17,* a gene that controls the production of the hormone estrogen and appears to influence the timing of puberty in girls. In March 1997 investigators at the University of Southern California announced that a common variant of *CYP17,* found in about 40% of women, may be involved in 30% of all breast cancer cases.

Other disorders. In August 1996 researchers at the firm Mercator Genetics, Menlo Park, Calif., reported that they had identified a mutant form of the gene *HLA-H,* located on chromosome 6, believed to be involved in hemochromatosis (also called iron-overload disease). The disorder is one of the most common hereditary ailments in people of European descent. In subsequent months the finding, considered speculative at first, was confirmed by studies in France and Australia. Untreated, hemochromatosis causes deposits of iron to accumulate in the heart, liver, and other organs, which leads to the development of diabetes, heart disease, and cirrhosis. The mutated gene may disrupt the ability of the intestine to regulate iron absorption.

In what was hailed as a major breakthrough, scientists at the National Human Genome Research Institute in Bethesda, Md., and colleagues reported in November 1996 that they had mapped the general location of the first gene ever to be linked to Parkinson's disease, a neurodegenerative disorder marked by a progressive loss of control over movement and caused by the unexplained death of the brain cells responsible for producing the neurotransmitter dopamine. The new gene was identified in members of a large Italian and Italian-American family in which an early-onset form of the illness is widespread. It encodes a brain protein, called alpha-synuclein, whose normal function is unknown. Although the protein's involvement in the disease mechanism is also unclear, one hypothesis is that mutant forms of alpha-synuclein collect in clumps in brain cells and ultimately cause the death of those cells. The brain tissue of patients with Parkinson's disease is riddled with abnormal structures called Lewy bodies, and a next step for researchers is to determine whether Lewy bodies contain alpha-synuclein. Although the familial form of Parkinson's disease

NEWS CAP MHA 98

Unforgettable Ewe: A Breakthrough in Cloning

With the announcement in 1997 that researchers in Scotland had created the first clone of an adult animal, science began, perhaps more than ever before, to resemble science fiction. In a report published in the British journal *Nature* (February 27), embryologist Ian Wilmut and his colleagues at the Roslin Institute in Edinburgh described having taken a cell from the udder of a six-year-old Finn Dorset ewe to create a genetic duplicate of the animal, a lamb they named Dolly. Because biologists had all but ruled out the possibility that a cell from a mature animal could be manipulated to generate an exact replica of the donor, the achievement by Wilmut and his team was regarded as a major scientific milestone.

The birth of Dolly marked the culmination of a decade of painstaking research by the Roslin Institute scientists. It also validated the theory put forward in 1935 by Hans Spemann, a German embryologist, that an organism could be reproduced by transplanting the nucleus of a cell from one adult animal into an egg produced by another. Most geneticists doubted that this could be done, since experiments had indicated that eggs would reject the differentiated, or specialized, cells found in mature animals. Members of the Roslin team theorized, however, that an egg might bond with a differentiated cell if they could induce the cell to abandon its normal cycle of growth and division and enter a quiescent stage.

To do this, the researchers deliberately withheld nutrients from cells extracted from the udder of the ewe they planned to clone. Egg cells then were removed from a second sheep, a Scottish blackface ewe, and electrical charges were used to fuse the egg cells and the differentiated cells into 277 separate two-celled units. Of the embryos that developed from these fused pairs, only one survived. It was transferred to the uterus of yet another Scottish blackface, and five months later, in July 1996, Dolly was born.

"The point," explained Wilmut in an interview that appeared in *Salon Magazine* (February 24), "is that what we thought happens in all life is that you have a single fertilized egg and as it divides, it progressively differentiates and you get brain and muscle and all of the different kinds of cells that we have. People assumed until now that this was an irreversible process. And what we have shown is that it's not."

News of a successful attempt at cloning a sheep immediately prompted speculation about the possibility—and potential pitfalls—of cloning human beings and fears that technology of this kind could one day be abused. Although Wilmut acknowledged that it is indeed "quite likely" that humans could be cloned, he could not see any practical use in applying this technology to people and emphasized that finding a way to clone humans was not the impetus behind his group's research. Their eventual goal is, rather, to develop genetically engineered animals that will, among other things, produce therapeutic proteins in their milk and provide organs—especially hearts and kidneys—for human patients in need of transplants.

In an address in March to a U.S. Senate panel deliberating on the social and ethical implications of cloning, Wilmut expressed his opposition to any type of research involving the manipulation of human embryos. "I personally have still not heard of a potential use of this technique to produce a new person that I would find ethically acceptable," Wilmut stated, adding, "I hope...we do not see human cloning in our lifetimes."

Sharing Wilmut's hope were a number of medical experts. The director general of the World Health Organization, Hiroshi Nakajima, is-

accounts for only a small percentage of cases, discovering how the defective protein leads to the destruction of brain cells may provide clues to the disease mechanism in patients with the more common, sporadic form of the disease.

Progress was made during the year in the study of a number of genes linked to eye diseases. Two of these were genes responsible for two different forms of glaucoma, a condition in which elevated pressure within the eye leads to the loss of peripheral vision. The first, a gene called *TIGR,* found on chromosome 1, is linked to juvenile-onset open-angle glaucoma, an aggressive hereditary form of the disorder that may begin as early as the teenage years. The disease can be successfully treated if it is diagnosed before the optic nerve has sustained irreversible damage. Thus, the discovery of the gene, which should allow early diagnosis of the condition, could save the sight of affected individuals. The second glaucoma gene, *CYP1B1,* located on chromosome 2, is thought to play a part in 80–90% of cases of primary congenital glaucoma, a leading cause of blindness in infants. In April 1997 investigators at the University of Connecticut Health Center announced that they had found three mutations that affect the functioning of the normal protein encoded by this gene. Still another gene linked to early vision loss was also found on chromosome 1. A mutation in this gene is responsible for Stargardt disease, a rare genetic form of progressive degeneration of the retina that strikes children and young adults.

In August 1996 an international research team announced that it had found a gene that provides the first biological evidence of a relationship between the skin disease epidermolysis bullosa, which is characterized by blisterlike lesions, and the muscle-wasting disorder muscular dystrophy. The discovery came from

sued a statement declaring that cloning humans "would violate some of the basic principles which govern medically assisted procreation." In the U.S. the National Bioethics Advisory Commission (NBAC), which consists of 18 leaders in the medical and legal fields, concluded in a report to Pres. Bill Clinton in June that it would be "morally unacceptable for anyone in the public or private sector...to attempt to create a child" by implanting cloned embryos in a woman. The NBAC also urged Congress to prohibit experiments aimed at cloning humans for a period of three to five years. Earlier, on March 4, President Clinton had announced a ban on the use of federal funds for any experiments in human cloning.

Najlah Feanny—Saba

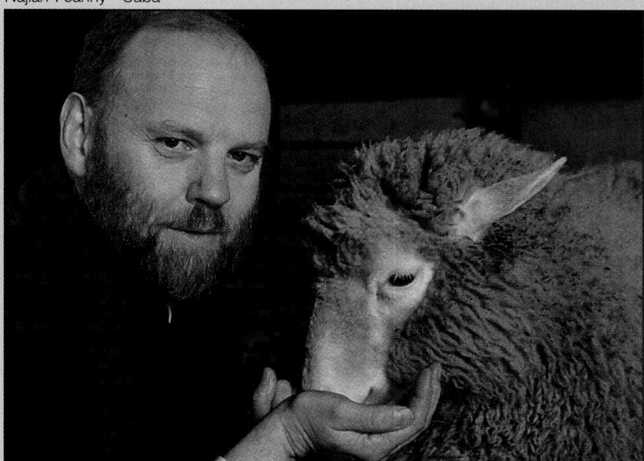

In February 1997 Scottish embryologist Ian Wilmut introduced the world to Dolly, the first clone of an adult animal.

These measures alarmed some scientists, however. They worried that legislation prohibiting or restricting cloning might prevent many medical advances and hinder other areas of genetic research. "Unless a bill is written in a way that places a very tight fence around that which the public and the Congress want to forbid," said Harold Varmus, director of the National Institutes of Health, a cloning ban could effectively "cut off research intended to advance toward a wanted goal."

While the debate raged, researchers proved they were not sheepish about continuing experiments with cloning. Just days after Dolly's existence became public, Donald Wolf, a scientist at the Oregon Regional Primate Research Center, Beaverton, announced that he and his colleagues had produced two monkeys by means of a procedure similar to the one used by the Roslin scientists, though the cells used by Wolf's team were taken from embryos, not from a mature animal. In July the Roslin team announced the creation of a second sheep, Polly, who possessed a human gene. The gene was added to the nucleus of a cell taken from an adult sheep in hopes that it would cause a human protein to be produced in the offspring animal's milk. Once extracted, the protein in question would be valuable to patients who lacked it, such as people with hemophilia and certain types of bone disease. In August an agribusiness research company, ABS Global Inc., in DeForest, Wis., announced that its scientists had produced three genetically identical calves from a cell taken from the tissues of a 30-day-old calf fetus.

In light of these later experiments, which seemed to increase the possibility that humans would someday be cloned, many wondered whether Dolly might turn out to be a wolf in sheep's clothing. Wilmut remained confident that his research would prove beneficial, however, and speculated on the practical prospects for cloning technology in the near future. "Of course there will be a long time for testing the [therapeutic] products before they go into commercial use," he said, "but there will be animals that are able to secrete new proteins, different proteins, in three years."

—*Sherman Hollar*

a study of four families with members who were born with the skin condition and developed muscular dystrophy later in life. Individuals who suffer from epidermolysis bullosa lack a protein called plectin, which is involved in anchoring skin layers. The new evidence suggests that a plectin deficiency may sometimes affect muscle as well as skin and that the presence of epidermolysis bullosa may be a warning sign of the muscle disease. Further research is needed to determine the function of the newly identified gene.

Reports published in the spring of 1997 linked two different genes to two separate forms of mental retardation. The first gene, believed to contribute to mental retardation in individuals with Down syndrome, was found on chromosome 21. Scientists have long known that individuals with Down syndrome have an extra version of chromosome 21; that is, instead of having the normal pair of chromosomes, they have three (hence the alternate name trisomy 21). Until now, however, no particular gene on chromosome 21 had been implicated in the condition. The mechanism by which the newly identified gene causes retardation is still unknown and, the researchers say, other genes are likely to be involved as well. The second gene, called *UBE3A,* is linked to Angelman syndrome, an inherited disorder that affects roughly one in 30,000 infants. The syndrome is characterized by moderate to severe mental retardation, seizures, absence of speech, inappropriate laughter, and an unsteady gait. *UBE3A* codes for an enzyme that marks proteins for processing or degradation. A counterpart gene in the fruit fly codes for a protein that plays a major role in neural development, a fact that may point the way to the function of the human protein.

Other noteworthy discoveries of the past year included: a gene involved in bone development and implicated in the rare human skeletal disorder cleidocranial dysplasia syndrome; a brain receptor that plays a part in the ability to filter out extraneous sounds and that, in its defective form, may be linked to the auditory hallucinations of schizophrenia; and a new cholesterol-metabolism gene, mutations in which are responsible for a rare fatal genetic disorder called Niemann-Pick type C disease.

Genes and behavior

Behavior is believed to stem from complex interactions between genes and environmental factors rather than from genes alone, as reports in the popular media often imply. Thus, headlines that proclaim the discovery of a gene for such and such a behavior are invariably misleading. Nevertheless, evidence is accumulating to support the notion that there is a biological basis for some aspects of behavior. In the past year there have been exciting new findings of genes linked to behavior—and a report disputing earlier claims of one such association.

The identification of a gene that contributes to anxious behavior was reported in November 1996. The gene, *5-HTT,* which is located on chromosome 17, codes for a protein called the serotonin transporter. The protein regulates the brain's ability to use the neurotransmitter serotonin, a chemical involved in numerous brain functions, including mood control. The gene is found in two forms, or variants—one containing a long sequence of bases and one a short sequence. Data showed that people who inherited the shorter variant of the gene scored higher on personality tests that measure neurotic behaviors such as worry, fear, and pessimism—which led some commentators to refer to it as the "Woody Allen gene." The investigators were quick to point out that (1) the short form of the gene is extremely common in the general population and (2) some 10–15 other genes may be involved in these behaviors.

In a report in the June 12, 1997, *Nature,* a team led by scientists at the Institute of Child Health in London concluded that there is a clear genetic basis for the difference in social skills between men and women. The researchers found that the parental origin of the X chromosome—*i.e.,* whether it is inherited from the mother or from the father—is closely correlated with the ability to cope with social situations. (As noted earlier, human chromosomes exist in pairs; females normally have two X chromosomes, and males normally have an X and a Y.) Developmental disorders that affect language and social functioning—autism, for example—are known to be more common in males than in females. Scientists have conjectured that a more general male-female difference in reactions to social situations may have a genetic component. To examine this hypothesis, researchers studied a group of 80 girls with Turner's syndrome, a chromosomal disorder in which the affected individual has only a single complete X chromosome. This X chromosome can be inherited from either the father or the mother. The girls who inherited the X chromosome from their fathers had much better social skills than those with a maternally derived X chromosome. The investigators concluded that social functioning is influenced by a gene on the X chromosome and that this gene is "switched off," or deactivated, when it is inherited from the mother, a phenomenon called genomic imprinting. This finding may explain why men, whose X chromosomes are always maternally derived (since they necessarily receive the Y chromosome from their fathers), are more vulnerable to developmental disorders involving social functioning.

Finally, researchers from the U.S. and Finland announced in November 1996 that they had been unable to duplicate data published in the January *Nature Genetics* that linked a specific dopamine receptor gene to thrill-seeking behavior. One of the authors of the earlier report defended his group's work, saying that the gene they had studied was probably only one of several that affect the behavior.

Genetic testing

Once a disease-linked gene has been isolated, researchers try to determine which mutations in the gene's sequence disrupt normal cellular functioning and cause the disorder. When the disease-related mutations have been identified, samples of DNA can be tested to see if the mutations are present. DNA analysis may be used for a variety of purposes, including diagnosing the disease in question in a person who is at risk, testing a fetus for the genetic defect, and detecting whether an individual planning to conceive carries the mutated gene. Although at the present time the applications of genetic testing are limited, its uses are growing.

In April 1997 an advisory panel convened by the National Institutes of Health (NIH) recommended that the genetic test for cystic fibrosis—the most common inherited disorder among U.S. Caucasians—be made available to all couples planning to have children and that insurance cover the cost. It was the first time that a genetic test had ever been recommended for individuals other than those known to be at risk for a particular disorder. The panel also recommended that extensive education and counseling be provided to couples undergoing testing, informing them of the nature of the disease, the limitations of the test, and their reproductive options.

The gene associated with cystic fibrosis was identified in 1989. Since then, there has been much debate surrounding genetic testing for the disease. Although the disorder is caused by a mutation in a single gene, investigators have identified more than 600 different possible mutations. Some mutations result in milder forms of the disease than others; the effects of some mutations are unknown. A major problem with the available test is that it is not sensitive enough to detect all possible mutations. This lack of test sensitivity was part of the reason the American Society of Human Genetics had come out against general population screening in 1990 and 1992. Poll results also show that there is limited public interest in such screening. The decision of the NIH panel seems to represent the coming-of-age of genetic testing.

A simple, noninvasive prenatal test may eventually provide a risk-free way to screen for disorders caused by single-gene mutations. The technique relies on the analysis of fetal DNA derived from a sample of the expectant mother's blood. Fetal cells, which carry the entire genetic complement of the unborn fetus, are shed into the maternal bloodstream beginning early in pregnancy. The new procedure can be carried out as early as 10 weeks after conception. It is less dangerous than the invasive prenatal diagnostic techniques currently in use, amniocentesis and chorionic villus sampling, both of which are associated with a slight risk of miscarriage. The new test is still experimental.

—*M.J. Friedrich*

The Genetics of Alcoholism

Beverages containing alcohol are an important feature of many cultures. For millennia the relationship between alcohol consumption and various aspects of life have been investigated. Genes have long been suspected of playing a role in the development of alcoholism. Ancient Greek scholars—including Aristotle and Plutarch—observed that "alcoholism runs in families." In the last two decades, well-conducted studies have confirmed this seminal observation. N.S. Cotton's comprehensive review of familial alcoholism studies published in 1979 estimated that one of every three persons who abuse alcohol is likely to have at least one parent who is alcohol-dependent. (It is important to note that "familial" does not necessarily imply "hereditary.")

Learning from twins

Studying twins has been a particularly useful way to assess the relative strength of genetic and environmental components of alcoholism. Since monozygotic (MZ) twins are genetically identical and dizygotic (DZ), or fraternal, twins share only part of their genes (on the average 50%), a greater concordance (similarity of characteristics) between MZ twins than between DZ twins is expected if a trait is under genetic control. An estimate of heritability can be calculated from the exact difference between MZ and DZ concordances. Heritability estimates range from zero to one; zero implies no genetic source of variation of an observed characteristic, whereas one implies that all of the variation is genetic.

The data on alcohol dependence and alcoholism reported in twin studies also point to the existence of a genetic factor. A recent and especially well-designed twin study supported the hypothesis that genetic factors play a major role in the development of alcoholism in women. The concordance was consistently higher in MZ female twins than in DZ twins. From this and other twin studies, it has been fairly well established that the likelihood for a woman to inherit a predisposition toward alcoholism is between 50% and 60%. The data from twin studies certainly confirm the significance of genetic factors in determining individual differences in alcoholism. But while twin studies are a powerful tool for estimating heritability, they do not completely exclude environmental effects.

Alcoholism among adoptees

Adoption studies allow genetic and environmental factors to be assessed independently. Interest in the study of adopted children of alcoholics was initiated by researchers Marc A. Schuckit, Donald W. Goodwin, and George Winokur in the early 1970s. These investigators observed that half-siblings of alcoholic subjects who had an alcoholic biological parent but were raised by nonalcoholics became alcoholics more frequently than those whose biological parents were moderate drinkers. This emphasizes the role of heritable factors, especially because alcoholism in a surrogate (adoptive parent) did not increase the risk in the children. Subsequent extensive studies conducted in Denmark, Sweden, and the United States showed that sons of alcoholics had a nearly fourfold higher alcoholism rate than adoptees whose biological parents were nonalcoholics, whether they were raised by nonalcoholic foster parents or by their own biological parents. Moreover, adopted sons of alcoholics were more likely to be alcoholic at a relatively early age than were their peers. Further extended analysis of large adoption studies from Sweden provided substantial data on at least two types of genetically influenced alcoholism: types I and II.

Genetically influenced alcoholism

Type I alcoholism is the more common of the two types and occurs in both men and women. Its acquisition requires both genetic predisposition and environmental provocation, and it generally does not start until after age 25. Type I alcoholism is the least severe type, associated with relatively mild alcoholism in either biological parent. Type I alcoholics infrequently have alcohol-related encounters with the legal system.

Type II alcoholism is less common and is usually limited to males. It is particularly heritable, with the risk of developing alcohol-abuse problems being nine times greater in predisposed sons than in the general population. Environmental factors appear to play a rather minor role. The time of onset of type II alcoholism is very early adolescence. Typically, the father is a severe alcoholic, but alcoholism in the mother is uncommon. Type II alcoholism is usually quite severe and difficult to treat. The affected individual often encounters legal problems as a result of his use of alcohol. Although it is widely acknowledged that type II is heavily influenced by genetic factors, alcoholism is a clinically heterogeneous disorder, which in all cases is the result of genetic and environmental factors.

The extensive heterogeneous nature of alcoholism explains the difficulties in determining the specific genetic influence. The transmissible component in alcoholism undoubtedly involves multiple genes that may be more or less specific in precipitating alcoholism. Despite the fact that it is a genetically influenced disorder, alcoholism is in many respects different from other disorders that follow a more traditional Mendelian mode of inheritance—*i.e.,* those governed by the basic laws of inheritance for physical traits that are determined by single genes. In contrast to a number of disorders such as Huntington's disease and sickle-cell disease, alcoholism develops in some individuals only when genetically influenced predisposing factors interact with environmentally determined precipitating factors. The search for potential causative genes is complicated because alcoholism is a common and complex non-Mendelian disorder with a number of features characteristic of complex diseases:

1. Alcoholism is a clinically heterogeneous disorder with variable age of onset.
2. The disorder may not be caused by any single gene but may develop from the additive effects of multiple genes (known as *multigenic,* or *polygenic, inheritance*).
3. Single mutations at different genetic loci may result in indistinguishable disease states (*genetic heterogeneity*).
4. Not every individual who inherits the genes will develop the disorder.
5. The disorder may reflect the complex interactions between alleles (any of the alternative forms of a gene that may occur at several loci).
6. A substantial number of individuals without an inherited predisposition manifest alcoholism resulting from nongenetic causes.

Colin Wheeler

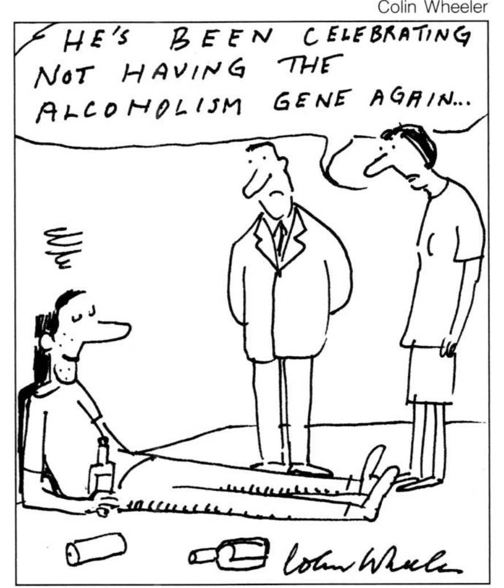

HE'S BEEN CELEBRATING NOT HAVING THE ALCOHOLISM GENE AGAIN...

Landmark research initiative

While the above limitations make the quest to uncover particular genes involved in alcoholism a daunting task, the presence of genetic factors predisposing individuals to the development of alcoholism offers scientific researchers a unique opportunity to learn how and why alcoholism occurs. The pursuit of this challenging research became possible in 1989 when the National Institute of Alcohol Abuse and Alcoholism of the U.S. National Institutes of Health established the Collaborative Study on the Genetics of Alcoholism (COGA). The COGA project is a unique and comprehensive research effort whose goal is to elucidate the genetic mechanisms that contribute to a person's susceptibility to alcohol abuse and dependence. Not only will various types of alcoholism be defined by COGA, but the findings should enable clinicians to develop preventive interventions for high-risk individuals. It is also expected that the research will lead to new treatments. Many scientists are collaborating to ultimately assess some 2,400 individuals from about 325 families over a period of 10 years. To achieve their goal, investigators have designed a comprehensive research protocol that is divided into several stages.

Selection of study subjects. The initial study subjects (the "probands") are randomly selected clients in outpatient and inpatient alcohol treatment facilities. These subjects must not be intravenous drug users, infected with HIV, or terminally ill. They must be able to participate in the interview process and provide written informed consent for their own and their families' participation in the study.

In addition, the subject's family must be large and complete enough to enable a detailed genetic study, and at least two first-degree relatives must live in the area covered by one of the six COGA centers. To be classified as "alcoholic," probands and other affected relatives must meet the criteria for *alcohol dependence* set forth in the *Diagnostic and Statistical Manual of Mental Disorders, Third Edition, Revised (DSM-III-R;* 1987): (1) regular daily intake of large amounts of alcohol, (2) regular heavy drinking limited to weekends, or (3) long periods of sobriety interspersed with binges of daily heavy drinking lasting for weeks or months. Other definitive criteria for alcoholism, established by John P. Feighner and colleagues in 1972, are also used. These include: manifestations of alcohol withdrawal, such as tremulousness or hallucinations; drinking before breakfast; drinking nonbeverage forms of alcohol—*e.g.,* hair oil, mouthwash, Sterno; and arrests or trouble at work associated with drinking behavior.

The control families (two parents and three or more offspring over the age of 14) are selected randomly from the community. Because the control subjects are supposed to reflect the "baseline" for alcohol-related parameters in the general population, alcoholics or people with other illnesses (with the exception of HIV/AIDS) are included. All control subjects participate in a personal interview, personality tests, neuropsychological assessment, and a series of neurophysiological tests, including an electroencephalogram, or EEG, measuring spontaneous electrical activity in the brain and evoked response potentials, showing brain activity in response to sensory stimuli. Researchers also obtain blood samples from the controls, which are used for studying biochemical markers, distinguishing substances in the blood or on genes—such as proteins or enzymes—that are reliably associated with dependence or nondependence on alcohol.

After extensive interviews with nuclear family members (*i.e.,* the proband and his or her spouse and first-degree relatives), extensively affected families are selected for genetic study; such families provide especially useful information when it comes to doing complex "linkage" and "association" analyses (discussed below).

Stage I—assessing subjects and families. All probands, their spouses, and their first-degree relatives who meet the protocol's admission criteria are interviewed, using a questionnaire—the Semi-Structured Assessment for the Genetics of Alcoholism

(SSAGA)—that was developed specifically for use in COGA. This state-of-the-art set of diagnostic questions assesses behavior, personality factors, and traits such as alcohol cravings, morning drinking, obsessive-compulsive personality, and depression. The interviews include children and adolescents (those aged seven and older), for whom age-appropriate questionnaires have been designed. An additional questionnaire enables investigators to interview parents about their children's psychiatric status.

The data derived from these interviews constitute the stage I sample. Because the data are generated by means of a single, well-defined ascertainment scheme, they allow COGA researchers to study the familial transmission of alcoholism in a scientifically refined manner.

Stage II—in-depth analyses. More detailed studies of genotype and phenotype are carried out on families with three or more alcohol-dependent members. (The *genotype* is the genetic constitution of an individual, which determines hereditary potentials and limitations from the time of embryonic formation through adulthood. *Phenotype* comprises all the observable characteristics of an individual that result from the interaction of his or her genotype with the environment.)

In addition to evaluating these personal characteristics, researchers also establish the family history of alcohol dependence and general psychopathology for all family members. This family history complements and validates personal interview data and allows researchers to assess family members who are unavailable for interviews. Whenever possible, the researchers obtain medical and psychiatric records to supplement these data. Assessment of juvenile participants includes looking at school records as well as other appropriate socioenvironmental variables.

Blood samples are obtained from all family members to prepare their DNA for genetic linkage and association studies. Researchers generate tissue-culture cell lines from the blood of adult subjects. These cell lines can be used to produce high-quality DNA that can be frozen and stored (*i.e.,* cryopreserved) for later analyses. DNA derived from the blood of children is also cryopreserved because it may not be known until many years later whether they will develop alcoholism.

Stage III—extending the family tree. These detailed phenotypic and initial genetic analyses of a core group of family members allow researchers to identify subsets of families for additional genetic studies. Thus, for some of the initial probands, the stage II sample is extended by administering the complete assessment protocol to the nuclear families of second- and third-degree relatives. This is done if the proband's family history suggests that these extended families include two or more alcohol-dependent members, even if the connecting relative is unaffected. Similarly, if one of the proband's first-degree relatives is alcoholic, the study will include the nuclear families of second-degree relatives of this family branch. The goal of these extensions is to establish large, densely affected, multigenerational family trees. At this stage, however, researchers try to avoid including nuclear families with two alcohol-dependent parents in the analyses; their exclusion facilitates the tracing of alcohol-related behavioral and genetic traits.

Stage IV—genotyping. By mid-1997 DNA samples from about 990 subjects from 106 families constituted the first wave of COGA's genotyping effort—*i.e.,* the use of sophisticated tools of biotechnology to determine specific genetic constitution. An important focus of the stage-IV analysis is the evaluation of sibling pairs in which both siblings are alcohol-dependent. Because siblings share 50% of their genetic material with each other and with their parents, the similarities and differences in genotype and behavior that exist between them are particularly informative. Under the diagnostic criteria for alcohol dependence described previously, 385 sibling pairs fall into this category. For more than 90% of these pairs, DNA samples also are available from at least one parent. The considerable size of this sample will enable scientists to detect genes contributing to the susceptibility for alcoholism, even if several genes interact to produce the phenotype.

Many of the sibling pairs also have undergone neurophysiological evaluation. These data will allow researchers to detect genes that influence heritable EEG and other brain wave characteristics. Thus far, neurophysiological analyses have focused on families with at least three alcohol-dependent first-degree relatives. Accordingly, quantitative differences between members of the test families and the general population provide a measure of the subjects' susceptibility to alcoholism. This correlation enhances researchers' ability to identify the underlying genes through linkage analyses.

Auspicious start!

Linkage analyses assess the relationship between genes located on the same chromosome that causes them to be inherited together. Association analyses look at the occurrence together of two or more phenotypic traits more frequently than would be expected by chance. Thus far, COGA has concluded the first linkage analyses (using 291 biochemical markers in 382 sibling pairs in which both are alcohol-dependent, 182 affected-unaffected pairs, and 47 pairs in which both are unaffected by alcoholism). Preliminary results indicate three genetic loci of significance. Two of the loci appear to increase the risk for the development of alcoholism, while one genetic locus appears to significantly reduce the risk of developing alcoholism. This locus is located in the general region of the ADH2 and ADH3 isozymes, a type of complex chemical protein that speeds up the metabolism of acetaldehyde (a by-product of alcohol produced by the liver that is extremely noxious, often causing tremendous flushing and malaise). This important observation had already been well established in Asian populations but had not been seen before in Caucasian samples. It should be noted that this novel protective locus was found only in Caucasian individuals in the COGA sample who were unaffected by alcoholism, which implies that some other, as-yet-unknown chemical substances may be operative in nonalcohol-dependent individuals.

This provocative finding means that the COGA initiative already has uncovered not only new loci that are the likely sites of genes that predispose individuals toward alcoholism but a potential protective factor as well—a most auspicious scientific beginning. The actual search for genes that predispose to or protect against alcoholism will, of necessity, be time-consuming and challenging. Nevertheless, the tools and methods for undertaking such a daunting search are all in place, and future research will contribute greatly to the understanding—if not get to the very root—of a common and devastating disease.

—Henri Begleiter, M.D.

Deconstructing Managed Care

Employers got nervous with just fee for service,
their medical bills were too high
So they gave up their voice and physician choice
to give HMOs a try.
But how we now cringe that this rationing binge
has sidetracked good care and health
Which today is replaced by a shiny new face,
the accumulation of wealth....

—Deborah Smith Park

That excerpt from the poem "With HMOs—Well, Who Really Knows?," published in the Oct. 2, 1996, issue of the *Journal of the American Medical Association (JAMA),* is just one expression of the mounting concern that is being voiced by many parties about the state of health care delivery in the United States and particularly about the quality and management of "managed care."

Perceptions of managed care

The March 15, 1997, *Congressional Quarterly* ran a cover story that stated: "The managed care industry is under siege. Consumers, unhappy with their health care, are pressuring lawmakers to regulate health maintenance organizations and other so-called managed care insurance plans. The accusation: These companies are putting profits before patients." Concerns about profits before people were certainly evident in the responses of Americans to a recent poll conducted for the National Coalition on Health Care (NCHC), an organization that has as its honorary cochairpersons former presidents Gerald R. Ford and Jimmy Carter. Almost 80% of respondents said that something is "seriously wrong" with the U.S. health care system; 87% said the quality of care needs to be improved; and 80% blamed the profit motive for compromised quality in health care. The health care expert Paul M. Ellwood (who coined the term *health maintenance organization [HMO]* in the 1970s) recently pointed out that managed care is now the largest single industry in the world; in the U.S. alone it is a trillion-dollar-a-year enterprise.

Writing in the Jan. 15, 1997, issue of *JAMA,* health policy analyst Peter P. Budetti of Northwestern University, Evanston, Ill., noted that in just a few years Congress and the White House had gone from being "strong proponents of managed care to being overtly ambivalent" about it. Budetti attributed that growing disillusionment and change in attitude to "a perception that there is a genuine backlash...on the part of constituents"—a public that is "not happy with managed care." He specified two particular emerging areas of concern—consumers' worries about managed care's impact on the quality of care and doubts about whether managed care will, in fact, deliver the long-term cost savings it promises.

Pres. Bill Clinton recently spoke about the "many Americans [who] worry that lower costs mean lower quality and less attention to their rights." He expressed his concern that "whether they have traditional care or managed care, none of our people should ever have inferior care." At the same time, the president appointed a 34-member advisory committee to draft a bill of rights that ensures that patients will get the information and care they need "when they need it." He reaffirmed his support of the managed-care concept, saying that when "managed well [it] can be the best deal for our families."

When managed care first emerged, it was supposed to provide less-expensive care to people who could not afford conventional insurance. But as Sen. Edward M. Kennedy recently charged, "Too many managed-care firms and other insurance companies have decided that the shortest route to higher profits and a competitive edge is by denying patients the care they need and deserve."

Laying blame

Managed-care plans are frequently used by the public, politicians, and the mass media as a "whipping boy"; at least some of that criticism is misdirected. Managed-care plans are not, for example, responsible for such unwelcome realities as health care delivery having become largely a business, third-party case managers being the ones who determine how much and what kind of care patients get, and treatment decisions being influenced more by bottom-line issues than by concerns about the welfare of the patient.

Managed-care organizations (MCOs) behave the way they do because they must respond to an incentive system created primarily by employers and the government. MCOs have found themselves pulled into an increasingly competitive marketplace in which purchasers are searching for low bidders. Not only are the plans operating in a competitive marketplace, but they cannot continue to survive as businesses if they attempt to provide more services than those for which they are adequately reimbursed. While it is true that a number of managed-care plans have been greedily withholding care and deserve to be chastised for their actions, from a public policy perspective, the public's overall health care wants and needs can be provided only at a level and quality commensurate with the level of resources it is willing to expend.

Working definitions

The reader expecting to find a succinct, widely agreed-upon definition of *managed care* will be disappointed. Still, because so many terms and acronyms are bandied about in discussions of managed care, it helps to have some very basic working definitions. The Health Insurance Association of America (HIAA) defines managed-care plans as those that integrate the financing and delivery of appropriate services to covered individuals. To meet this definition a plan must have each of the following:

- arrangements with selected providers to furnish a comprehensive set of health care services to members
- explicit standards for the selection of health care providers
- formal programs for monitoring quality of care and utilization of services
- significant financial incentives for members to use providers and procedures associated with the plan

Another criterion that probably should be added to the above is that a plan must have financial incentives for providers to limit unnecessary procedures and procedures of questionable benefit; ideally, those incentives should not result in limitations on needed or appropriate care.

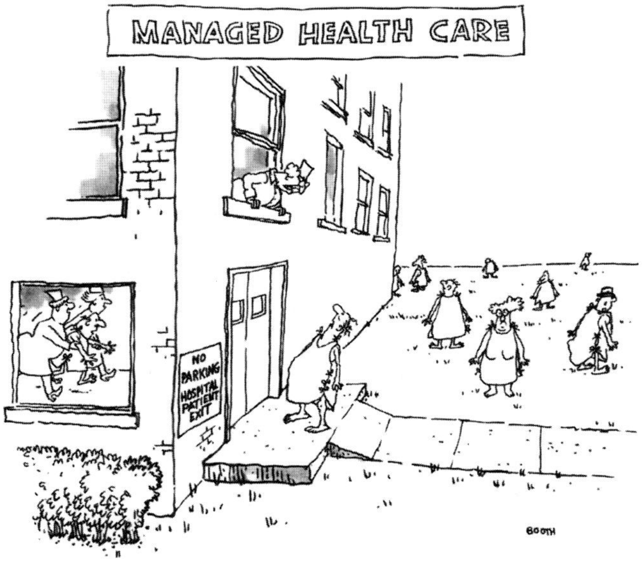

"You don't get a room, Mr. Rheinschreiber, because you don't pay for a room! That's the whole idea of same-day surgery."

An important distinction in managed care has to do with the designated form of payment. In *capitation,* one of the most widely used financing mechanisms, a health plan pays a provider a specified per-patient monthly fee to provide a set of specifically contracted health care services to enrollees. This payment mechanism contrasts with traditional *fee-for-service,* under which doctors are paid by the visit or for specific services rendered. The most important distinction that should be made in regard to capitation and fee-for-service is the inherent difference in their respective financial incentives. In capitation the provider or plan is financially rewarded for limiting the amount of provided services. In fee-for-service the provider is financially rewarded for providing more services. Managed-care consultant Allan Baumgarten has observed that some view capitation as the best way of preserving physician autonomy while at the same time aligning the financial concerns of purchasers, the health plan, and providers, while others view capitation as a terrible evil that undermines a physician's duty to provide the best-possible care to a patient.

People often use the terms *managed care* and *HMO* as if they were equivalent; they are not. An HMO is one type of managed-care plan, but not all managed-care plans are HMOs. Rather, managed care is a large umbrella category, under which HMOs, as well as at least a dozen other types of health care plans, fall.

In its simplest form, managed care is nothing more than health care with cost controls. There are various ways, however, that MCOs can control costs: by (1) operating efficiently, (2) restricting the amount of care provided, (3) limiting payments to providers, (4) limiting enrollees' access to lower-cost providers, and (5) emphasizing the prevention of illness or disability so that expensive treatments are not required. While some MCOs have implemented prevention programs, the large majority of plans have not. Instead, they focus on the first four means of controlling costs.

Ironically, just as Americans are getting used to *managed care,* the term seems to be falling from use. As Baumgarten has pointed out, "Managed care [has acquired] some negative baggage in recent years; HIAA rarely uses the term anymore, preferring terms like 'comprehensive' or 'coordinated care.'" In addition, two national managed-care associations merged in 1995 to form the American Association of Health Plans (AAHP), which chose not to use "managed care" in its name.

Though the term may be phased out in the future, what is now called a managed-care organization is an enterprise that provides and/or finances health care, using provider-payment mechanisms that encourage cost containment, selective contracting with networks of providers, and controls on the utilization of health services. An HMO is a prepaid plan that provides comprehensive care and an agreed-upon set of benefits to a group of enrollees for whom a monthly premium is paid to the plan. The premium covers the provision of all the needed care for the enrollees as long as that care is included within the contracted set of benefits. The HMO accepts financial risk for its enrollees' care. In an HMO a primary care doctor often serves as a "gatekeeper," controlling access to specialists, tests, and procedures. In a "pure," or traditional, HMO, enrollees may see only those doctors employed by or under contract with the HMO.

When Ellwood first promoted the idea of the HMO, he hoped that by creating a prepaid system responsible for delivering all needed care, providers would be motivated to help enrollees *maintain* health—by promoting good health practices and preventing disease—since the HMO's costs would be lower the less it was required to treat disease. Unfortunately, the health maintenance expectations of the early HMO days, for the most part, have not been realized.

Lest it seem simple, there are at least five types of HMOs that are distinguished from each other in fairly subtle ways:

1. A *group model* is an HMO that collects premiums and fees but pays a negotiated fee to an organized group (or groups) of doctors to deliver a set of benefits to enrollees. (The doctors work in a dedicated HMO facility and contract with hospitals for patient care. The health plan has an exclusive relationship with one or more of the doctors' groups.)
2. A *network model* is an HMO in which the relationship between the plan and the doctors' groups is not exclusive, and the doctors often work out of their own private offices.
3. A *staff model* directly employs its own doctors at its own facilities.
4. An *individual practice association model (IPA)* contracts with individual doctors or groups of doctors and pays them on either a per capita or a fee-for-service basis.
5. Finally, a *mixed model* has various relationships with providers—for example, it contracts exclusively with medical groups and nonexclusively with solo practice physicians in the same area.

In addition to HMOs, there are two newer types of managed-care plans—*preferred provider organizations (PPOs)* and *point-of-service (POS)* plans—that are growing faster than and differ from traditional HMOs in a variety of ways. A PPO is a plan in which insurance companies and other financing mechanisms contract with a limited network of doctors who agree to provide services to enrollees at discounted fees in anticipation of receiving an increased volume of patients. PPOs are often used by self-funded plans in which the employer, rather than an HMO or insurance company, assumes the financial risk for the cost of

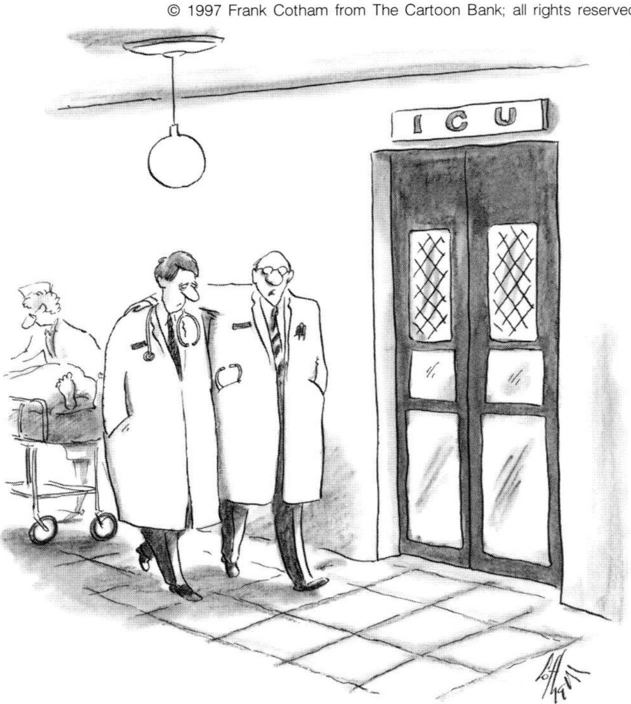

"It's tough losing a patient to a rival HMO."

services; PPOs do not bear financial risk. Enrollees can see doctors outside the PPO, but if they choose to do so, their co-payments are higher. There is a strong financial incentive to utilize doctors on the "approved" list of "in-network" doctors. POS plans offer enrollees financial incentives to use doctors under contract to the plan but, with certain limitations and for an additional cost, allow them to use doctors outside the plan. Within the broader categories of MCOs are many specific types of plans. Among them are *exclusive provider organizations (EPOs), integrated delivery systems (IDSs), provider sponsored organizations (PSOs),* and *independent provider organizations (IPOs).*

Follow the money

What began as a fairly simple concept has evolved into a highly complex alphabet soup of organizations and plans with a plethora of confusing relationships that, more often than not, leave the public bewildered. One way to comprehend some of managed care's complexities is to think of MCOs as businesses with the same drives, needs, and criteria for judging their own success or failure as other businesses. In other words, MCOs can survive only with a healthy bottom line. When reporters Bob Woodward and Carl Bernstein were unraveling the Watergate scandal in the motion picture *All the President's Men* (1976), their covert source, Deep Throat, advised them to "follow the money."

To follow the money of an MCO, one must determine which party or parties—employees, employers, health plans, or care providers—are at financial risk for the care rendered. For example, if a company pays a premium to a health plan that is under contract to provide a specified set of benefits to its employees and then that plan contracts with a physicians' group to provide all the needed care for a set fee, the plan has transferred the financial risk to the physicians' group. In this example the physicians' group now has the financial incentive to provide as little care as possible and a significant disincentive to provide any "extras" in the way of services.

In "the good old days" of indemnity insurance, employers would pay a premium to an insurance company; the insurance company was then at financial risk, since it had agreed to cover the cost of all the needed health services under its contract with the employer. While in many ways this is not really different from the financial risk the health plans now accept, in the old days if the insurance company had miscalculated the risk, it would make up for any loss of income by raising its premiums the following year, and the employers would generally pay. Today, however, employers are unwilling to assume the cost of ever-escalating premiums. Indeed, it was largely the double-digit rises in health spending of the 1980s and early '90s that stimulated the public and private sectors to turn to managed care.

A recent report by the U.S. Department of Health and Human Services showed a major slowdown in national health spending, which was attributed to the growth of managed care. Health spending grew 5.1%, to $937.1 billion, between 1993 and 1994 and 5.5%, to $988.5 billion, from 1994 to 1995—the lowest rates of growth in three decades. Whether such low rates will be maintained in future years is unclear.

Quality in question

A recent public opinion poll commissioned by the American Psychological Association showed that more than four out of every five Americans are worried that managed care will negatively affect either the quality, the cost, or their access to health care, and 55% of the respondents believe that some government oversight is necessary to ensure high-quality care at reasonable prices. On the other hand, a comprehensive review of the medical literature to assess the quality of care and patient satisfaction in HMOs versus indemnity plans (between the years 1980 and 1994) showed that both types of plans provided enrollees with care that was of comparable quality. There was no clear winner in terms of enrollee satisfaction between HMO and indemnity plans. Any generalizations about the superiority of one type of plan as compared with the other, the authors of the review concluded, "must be made with caution."

Several more recent studies have raised concerns regarding the quality of managed-care plans. For example, John E. Ware, Jr., and colleagues at the Health Institute New England Medical Center, Boston, tracked more than 2,200 HMO patients with high blood pressure, diabetes, recent heart attacks, congestive heart failure, or depression over a four-year period (from 1986 through 1990) to see whether they received quality care. They found that younger, primarily healthy HMO members thrived, but the health of the elderly and plan members with chronic illnesses declined. The health of 54% of the chronically ill Medicare patients deteriorated while they were in managed-care plans; by contrast, only 28% of Medicare patients with fee-for-service coverage experienced a similar decline. Ware expressed concern that "we are moving very quickly to try to achieve the same kind of cost containment and quality working with the elderly that we've achieved with the nonelderly under managed care, without making the adjustments for elderly patients that we need to make." He added, "There probably isn't an HMO in the country that has an information system that could tell you the functional outcomes of an elderly patient in the last four years." In response to this study, a panel of experts convened by the National Committee for Quality Assurance (NCQA) agreed to use Ware's techniques nationwide to measure how seniors in managed-care plans were faring. Shortly thereafter, the Health Care Financing Agency proclaimed that all health plans contracting with the federal government had to use the "health of seniors" measure developed by Ware and his research team.

In regard to the relative quality of managed versus fee-for-service care, the health economist Uwe Reinhardt has quipped, "The numbers can be argued either way, and unless somebody paid me to say something different, I would say I do not know what's going on." Ellwood recently spoke out on the quality issue: "Professional black boxes and undocumented claims of superior

NEWS CAP

Canadian Health Care: In Critical Condition?

For years Canada's national health care system, popularly known as "medicare," has been viewed as an exemplary one by advocates of health care reform in other countries. Under the Canada Health Act of 1984, every Canadian resident is entitled to free comprehensive medical care and hospital treatment, the cost of which is paid through a combination of federal and provincial taxes. In addition, Canadians may also choose their own health care providers, and physicians themselves are given considerable leeway in their decisions to prescribe treatments and admit patients to hospitals.

Recently, however, the glowing reputation of Canadian health care has begun to fade as financial pressures have threatened the system. Medical costs have risen sharply, while cuts in federal spending have reduced provincial health care budgets. Complaints about hospital understaffing, long waits for nonemergency surgery, and a countrywide scarcity of state-of-the-art technology have increased. Another telltale sign that medicare is in trouble, according to critics of the system, is the growing number of Canadians seeking medical treatment in the U.S.

Although many Canadians are convinced that their system is in a state of crisis, the National Forum on Health, a panel of 24 academics, physicians, and community leaders responsible for advising the federal government on ways to improve health care, dismissed that view in a report, *Canada Health Action: Building on the Legacy,* published in February 1997. The report attributed the widely held belief that government underfunding had jeopardized medicare to "unplanned or inconsistent action, fear mongering and misinformation." The forum suggested that the solution to the system's problems lay in identifying ways to manage medicare more effectively and insisted that the amount of money Canadians were paying for health care was sufficient.

The forum also addressed the question of whether Canada should implement a two-tiered system, which would permit patients who could afford it to pay for private health care. In response to those who had argued that offering private care as an alternative to medicare would relieve much of the pressure on the public system, the forum averred that the two-tiered option would prove both inequitable and costly. Not only would such a system violate Canadians' long-standing commitment to the principle of equal access to medical services, but it would erode medicare's base of support by drawing away both patients and physicians. The panel members instead called for an expansion of the public system to cover home care and pharmaceuticals, arguing in their report that "it makes little sense to guarantee public coverage when services are provided in hospitals, yet provide partial or no coverage at all for the same services out of hospital."

Suggestions as to how to improve medicare were made by other groups as well. After conducting a three-year national study, a team of scholars from Queen's University, Kingston, Ont., and the University of Ottawa declared that Canada could reduce public health care expenditures by 15%, without compromising the quality of medical service, by "shifting to less costly modes of delivery," such as same-day surgery and home care. Introducing U.S.-style health maintenance organizations into Canada was also seen as a possible—but controversial—solution by some health policy analysts.

So, what is the prognosis for Canadian medicare? Despite the many proposed remedies, it does not look bright. Although the federal government announced in August 1997 that it would be allocating Can$100 million to long-term-care institutions, a report by the Canadian Union of Public Employees and the Service Employees International Union called this "nothing more than catchup money for a sector that has been losing resources for years while it tries to absorb greater numbers of sicker patients." Federal cash transfers to the provinces were scheduled to decline to Can$11.1 billion per year by the year 2000, far below the optimal Can$12.5 billion per year recommended by the National Forum on Health. David Dingwall, Canada's health minister, indicated there was little chance that the federal government would abandon its plans for the reduction.

—*Jeff Wallenfeldt*

individual credentials and results are no longer enough!" He stressed that "now we are ready for the next phase [of managed care] that will measure and produce better quality health care." In a recent editorial published in *JAMA,* called "Managed Care—a Work in Progress," Ellwood proposed new "principles of accountability to the public for health quality"—rules that emphasize patients before profits.

The initial hope on the part of the promoters of HMOs was that capitation would encourage the plans and providers to keep their enrollees healthy by implementing prevention programs, since a healthy population would need fewer services, and fewer services would mean lower expenditures. It takes a number of years, however, before most prevention programs produce results. This is especially true in regard to chronic diseases. Thus, from a financial perspective, unless enrollees remain in the same health plan long enough for it to reap profits from having prevented diseases that would have been costly to treat, the implementation of prevention efforts and "wellness programs" can actually add to the provider group's costs rather than produce a savings.

Gagging on restrictions

It may not be an exaggeration to say that in the past 10 years a revolution has been occurring in the United States in the fundamental relationships that patients have with their physicians. This revolution has been waged primarily in the name of more efficient care, but many of the battles that have been fought have not considered the consequent "casualties." Overt evidence is offered in the continuing "horror stories" that appear in the mass media, as well as in professional medical journals—stories about outpatient mastectomies, one-day hospital stays for appendectomies and births, physicians who earn more by treating patients less, patients' inability to receive needed care due to denial of coverage by managed-care plans, and the impact of confidentiality clauses, better known as "gag rules" or "gag clauses."

Gag rules are clauses in contracts between MCOs and contracting physicians that limit the physician's freedom to communicate openly with his or her patients. For example, doctors are prohibited from discussing more costly treatment options even if these might be in the patient's best interest. As already noted, some HMO payment policies provide direct financial incentives to physicians for withholding care.

Gag rules have placed physicians—who were once expected to dispense honest information and comfort and to put the health and well-being of their patients first—in an acutely uncomfortable if not untenable position. An editorial that appeared in *The New England Journal of Medicine,* written by its editor, Jerome P. Kassirer, looked at the public's dilemma: "Patients are vulnerable and dependent...and need to know that their physicians are not only at their side but on their side."

As physicians have become increasingly dependent on one type of managed-care organization or another for their livelihood, they are increasingly having to choose between the tenets of the Hippocratic Oath, "I will follow that system or regimen which, according to my ability and judgment, I consider for the benefit of my patients, and abstain from whatever is deleterious and mischievous," and those of what might be dubbed the "Hypocritic Oath," which would state something along these lines: "I will do no harm to the corporate bottom line, and I will follow that system or regimen which, according to my ability and judgment, I consider for the benefit of my employer."

The following are examples of clauses contained in contracts between HMOs and physicians that either prohibit or restrict physicians from communicating openly with patients:

- "This agreement may be terminated without cause by either party, upon written notice by the terminating party to the other party, of the intent to terminate at least 90 days in advance of the intended termination date."
- "This contract may be immediately terminated for provider's direct contact of [HMO] members in regard to matters pertaining to the plan without plan's prior written approval, or provider's making any repeated disparaging remarks or expressing opinions regarding plan or any of its affiliates that are negative in nature."
- "Provider shall use its best efforts to insure that no employee of the provider or subcontractor of the provider makes any derogatory remarks regarding [the HMO] to any member."
- "Do not discuss proposed treatment with Kaiser Permanente members prior to receiving authorization."
- "Physician shall take no action nor make any communication which undermines or could undermine the confidence of enrollees, potential enrollees, their employers, plan sponsors or the public in Choice Care, or in the quality of care which Choice Care enrollees receive."

A study undertaken by the American Medical Association looked at the contracts of some 200 HMO physicians and found "gag language" in almost every one. In response to the rash of negative publicity about gag clauses, a number of such organizations announced that they were dropping gag rules from their contracts. One of the largest managed-care companies, Humana, said it wanted to eliminate "confusing contract language" between managed-care organizations and doctors, insisting that "these clauses were never intended to hinder communications."

By late fall 1996 some 16 states had passed legislation to limit gag rules in health plan contracts, while similar bills had been drafted and introduced in at least 13 additional states. On Jan. 1, 1997, the federal government adopted a new policy limiting the types of bonuses that can be paid to doctors as a reward for controlling the cost of services to Medicare and Medicaid patients. The stated purpose of the policy was "to protect patients against improper clinical decisions made under influence of strong financial incentives." On the other hand, after holding hearings on gag rules, Congress did not pass the grandly titled legislation known as the Hippocratic Oath and Patient Protection Act, which would have banned gag rules altogether.

The initial spate of congressional measures aimed at stopping various abuses allegedly committed by managed-care companies has fueled a highly charged debate about the role of government in regulating managed care. Companion bills sponsored by Senator Kennedy and Rep. John D. Dingell would ban gag clauses, require health plans to pay for emergency care, prohibit plans from setting "arbitrary" limits on medically necessary care, and require all plans to have quality-assurance programs.

Commentary from Koop

In a special fall 1996 issue of *Time* magazine, "The Frontiers of Medicine," former U.S. surgeon general C. Everett Koop speculated on the future of U.S. health care. In an article entitled "Manage with Care," Koop posed these key questions: "Will HMO patients of the future find sensitive doctors free...from the financial pressure to order more tests and procedures, free to do the best...for their patients? Or will HMO patients find themselves in long lines for short visits, confronting bureaucratic 'gatekeepers' who shunt them to a small number of overworked doctors who are paid extra to skimp on tests and operations?" While Koop believed that it could be five years or even as long as a decade before it was known which one of these scenerios would be played out, he suspected that it would be the latter. He voiced his concern that with insurance companies, HMOs, physicians in private practice, hospitals, drug companies, and a host of other vested interests fighting furiously to come out on top, "the patient may end up on the bottom."

In raising a red flag about managed care, Koop, who is certainly among the most respected and trusted physicians in the U.S., has probably accelerated and validated the public's growing negative view of managed-care plans. An even more pressing problem, in Koop's view, is the 40 million Americans currently uninsured—a number that may reach 60 million by the year 2000. The urgent need, he says, is to reform the overall health care system rather than just "squabbling about managed care." Currently, health care reform "poses the greatest political challenge to a democratic republic, because each of us is being asked to do something for all of us, and many of us feel that what might be best for all of us is not best for each of us. It's that simple."

Though highly critical of the current direction of managed care, Koop also acknowledged the flaws in traditional fee-for-service medicine. The positive attribute of the latter type of care, however, is that physicians can act as advocates for their patients. Managed-care plans have not yet assured the public that they are either allowing or encouraging physicians to do the same. As the aforementioned NCHC poll indicated, the current public perception is that managed-care plans, especially investor-owned, for-profit ones, are primarily interested in managing costs and secondarily in maintaining health.

Choosing carefully

One of the most difficult decisions many individuals have to make these days is which managed-care plan to enroll in, assuming one still has that choice. Some people turn to "patient satisfaction" surveys conducted by individual plans or accrediting organizations, and many choose on the basis of HMO rankings published in popular magazines. Others play Russian roulette. The following are some important points that the wise consumer will look into before making a selection:

- how participating physicians are paid
- how treatment decisions are made and reviewed
- whether needed medications are covered by the plan
- how a plan determines whether a treatment is "experimental"
- the "medical-loss ratio"—*i.e.,* the ratio between what a health plan spends on medical care provided to its enrollees and what the plan receives in premiums (the lower the ratio, the more profit the plan can make)
- whether there are gag clauses in the MCO's contracts with physicians
- whether physicians can be terminated at will by the MCO
- what percentage of claims the plan denies
- whether unanticipated emergency room visits are covered
- what appeals procedures exist for members whose claims are turned down
- how chronically ill persons (who tend to be the most frequent health care users) rate the plan
- whether the plan is registered with the AAHP and accredited by the NCQA

Current trends, future prospects

Despite the well-publicized horror stories about gag clauses, drive-through deliveries, outpatient mastectomies, and denial of needed treatment, managed care appears to have a secure foothold. "The change [from the old days]," said John Erb, a principal with A. Foster Higgins, a major employee benefits consulting firm, "is permanent. Once you become a pickle, you can never become a cucumber again."

The extent of this accelerating movement is demonstrated by the almost doubling of the U.S. population enrolled in managed-care plans between 1992 and today. In 1992, 36% of the population was enrolled in managed-care plans; by 1996 enrollment was up to 61% (160 million people). In 1993 about half the Americans insured through employers were in managed-care plans; by 1996 three-quarters were. Meanwhile, traditional fee-for-service plans served just over a quarter of American workers in 1995, which was down from one-half of employed people in 1993. As already noted, the trend is away from the more restrictive type of MCOs that had dominated the market since the early 1980s and toward plans that offer enrollees new options, including more open networks of physicians, hospitals, and other categories of health care providers. In January 1997 the group InterStudy reported that "pure" HMOs accounted for only 17% of existing managed-care plans.

Ever since the federal and state governments discovered that managed care could lower the cost of care, there has been a continued effort to encourage Medicare and Medicaid beneficiaries to join HMOs. Membership in Medicaid HMOs grew 140% between 1993 and 1996, and Medicare HMOs experienced an 81% rise in enrollment during the same period. Nearly one-third of all Americans covered by Medicaid are currently in an HMO, as compared with 12% of Medicare beneficiaries.

Given the fluidity of the current health care marketplace, it is difficult to predict the future. Nonetheless, in its publication *Tracking the System: American Health Care* (1996), the National Committee for Quality Health Care attempted to do so. It specu-

Forecast for Managed Care

Type of plan	1990 (percentage of U.S. population)	2000 (projected percentage of population)
Unmanaged fee for service	5	5
Managed fee for service	55	15
HMO	20	35
Preferred provider organization	15	15
Point of service	5	30

Source: National Committee for Quality Assurance.

lated that in 2000 only 5% of the U.S. population would be covered by "unmanaged" fee-for-service plans and 15% would be in managed fee-for-service plans, while the rest would be enrolled in one of the three dominant types of managed-care plans (HMOs, PPOs, or POS plans). According to Alan G. Raymond, author of a consumers guide to managed care, the two most frequently voiced perceptions of managed care are (1) that such plans "have excellent caring doctors, offer the best coverage imaginable, keep you healthy and cost a lot less than traditional health insurance" and (2) that they are "impersonal and bureaucratic, deny needed care in order to save money and you can't even choose your doctor." Not surprisingly, however, he suggests that "the truth lies somewhere in between."

—Lester E. Block, D.D.S., M.P.H.

Britain's Health Service Pushes 50

"For British Health System, Bleak Prognosis." Few Britons would dissent from the stark January 1997 *New York Times* headline. Along with anxieties about education and unemployment, concerns about the future of the National Health Service (NHS), 50 years old in July 1998, are prominent in the minds of the British people. Many observers think that national worries about the NHS, more than any other issue, lost the Conservatives the 1997 election.

Reporter Sarah Lyall's front-page article painted a gloomy picture indeed. On occasion during the winter of 1996–97, one university hospital in London had as many as 30 patients lined up on gurneys outside the emergency room waiting for treatment for serious conditions such as heart attacks and pneumonia. Lyall points to other cracks in the NHS: waiting lists for operations that may include over one million of the population, dangerously ill psychiatric patients having to be kept in the community because of a lack of suitable facilities, and the rationing of services, which has recently been introduced by many health authorities. Lyall concludes by quoting Rodney Walker, former chair of the NHS Trust Federation, which represents British hospitals. The NHS, said Walker, must change its mission from serving everybody to serving "those people who need it most. It has got to become a safety-net service looking after the old and the weak."

Pioneering health care in postwar Britain

The National Health Service was one of several brave new enterprises pioneered after World War II by Great Britain's new socialist government. The principles of this tax-funded health service that promised to be free at the time of delivery were set out in a leaflet sent to every home in the country. "It will provide you with all medical, dental, and nursing care," Health Minister Aneurin Bevan told Britons in the summer of 1948. "Everyone—rich or poor—can use it," he asserted. From its beginning the NHS was very popular, especially with a population accustomed to both wartime rationing and a system of health care that did not include everybody. Naturally enough, doctors grumbled about the bureaucracy of the new system, but they recognized that overnight one of their bugbears had been abolished: bad debts. After a decade of working with the NHS, some two-thirds of physicians would probably have voted in favor of maintaining it. One shrewd observer, political scientist Harry Eckstein of the University of

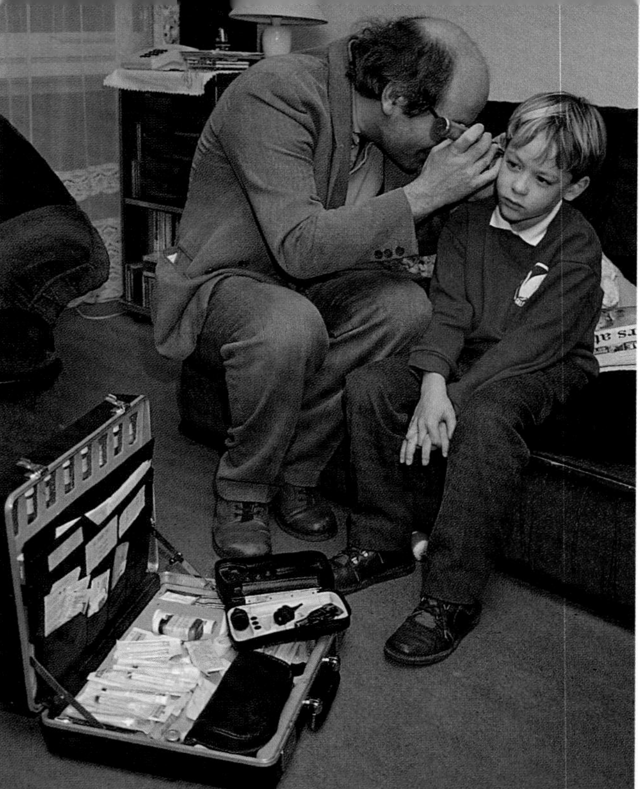

A general practitioner makes a house call in Abingdon, Eng. Since its inception, the National Health Service has depended on GPs to deliver the vast majority of care and to be the health system's "gatekeepers."

California, Irvine, concluded in his book *Pressure Group Politics* (1960) that the NHS had become "accepted as an altogether natural feature of the British landscape, almost a part of the Constitution."

The great achievement of the NHS was to ensure that high-quality health care became available all over the country. Initially, the unmet needs and the uneven distribution of care were strikingly evident. Comedians had a great time cracking jokes about the surge in demand for spectacles, dentures, and hearing aids, but many of the elderly in the U.K. had earlier been unable to afford these enhancements to their quality of life. Indeed, between 1948 and 1957 the NHS supplied almost 600,000 hearing aids.

In 1948 large rural counties had little access to specialist care; the 450,000 widely scattered inhabitants of Lincolnshire, for example, had no full-time pediatrician or pathologist. Under the NHS the full range of specialist services was introduced across the country. Crucially, general practitioners were made "gatekeepers" to the specialists; to this day, NHS patients cannot refer themselves to specialists for advice but have to go through their family doctors—a situation that results in lean, efficient administration of services. In 1979, for example, GPs dealt with 90% of all illnesses at a cost of only 23% of the total NHS budget. This heavy emphasis on family medicine has continued, with GPs encouraged to form associations with nurses and other health care practitioners in specially built, dedicated facilities.

The downside to centrally managed health care was also evident from the beginning. There were inevitable compromises made in order to persuade doctors to enter the NHS, and the three main elements of health care—general practice, hospital care, and social services—to this day have never been properly coordinated. A succession of economic crises in Britain since the war have delayed an ambitious decade-long hospital-building plan. Thus,

Nigel Barklie—Impact Photos

doctors have had to practice late-20th-century medicine in mid-19th-century buildings. The creature-comfort aspects of the NHS have always been neglected, with patient accommodations being unattractive, if not frankly grubby, and staff being casual, if not sometimes rude, in their treatment of patients. Such infelicities have led to frequent complaints, even by a population already resigned to dirty streets and long queues for public transportation.

More seriously, there has always been rationing in the NHS, particularly in the form of long waiting lists for hospital admission. Nonemergency procedures—those that are necessary to enhance the quality of life, such as hip replacement or cataract surgery—are performed relatively infrequently. Of even greater concern has been the long-standing covert rationing of lifesaving procedures, particularly hemodialysis; British patients aged over 65 with kidney failure have always been less likely to be treated than their counterparts elsewhere in the West, merely on the grounds of age. Yet patients were not told that the grounds for rejection were economic rather than medical in nature. The NHS makes little accommodation for "Cinderella" specialties, which continue to suffer from undeserved neglect. In 1961, for instance, the government spent more on compensating farmers for losses due to fowl pest (an economically important disease of chickens) than it did on community mental health care. Community mental health services are *still* seriously neglected—treatments for substance abuse being one prime example. Recently, large multicenter cancer-treatment trials have had to be curtailed owing to the lack of funds.

Faced with the obvious shortcomings of the NHS—as indicated by the widespread publicity about long waiting lists, delayed operations, and even deaths—the central and local governments reacted not by increasing the proportion of expenditures on health but by trying to increase the efficiency of the system. It would be surprising if in a complex organization like the NHS, which employs more people than any other enterprise in Europe, considerable efficiencies were not possible, and there have been several attempts at improving the organization. Since the beginning there have been no fewer than four major management reorganizations in the NHS, culminating in the changes introduced by the Margaret Thatcher government in 1989. That latest round of reforms depended upon creating a competitive internal health care market, in which GPs were viewed as "fundholders" responsible for their own budgets and for purchasing care for patients from various providers, and where independent trusts were established to run the hospitals.

Maturing gracefully or showing its age?

Recent surveys have shown that for the first time in a decade, more patients are satisfied than are dissatisfied with their treatment under the NHS. Moreover, 60% of today's NHS managers believe that the reforms have made things better. It is claimed that the "throughput" of patients has been increased and hospital waiting lists have been reduced. Nonetheless, the queues for health care in Britain would barely be tolerated in any other industrialized country—in mid-1997 there was still a backlog of some 31,600 patients, for instance, who had been waiting for hospital treatment for more than a year. It seems that the definition of a "hospital wait" used to arrive at these totals was altered, which possibly resulted in a lower figure than would have been

Link/Impact Visuals

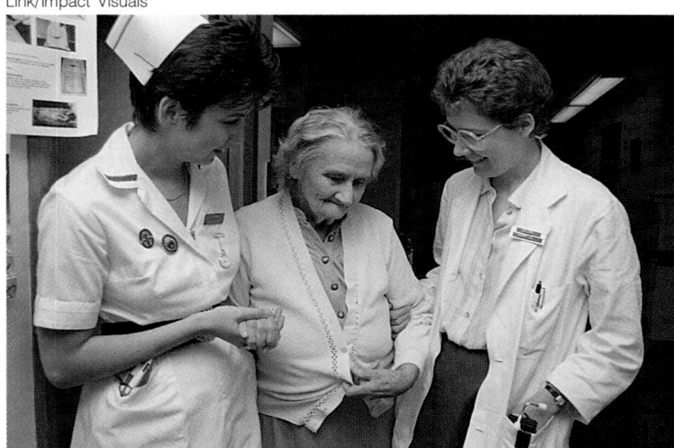

A geriatric patient in a hospital in Stafford, Eng., is attended by caring staff members. It seems likely that in the near future Britain's elderly will get little help from the government in paying for long-term care.

expected. Hence, many outside observers conclude that the improvements have been little but cosmetic. Opinion polls through early 1997 indicated that voters overwhelmingly believed the NHS would fare better under a Labour government. Whatever the truth, the reality is that the changes under Thatcher almost doubled NHS administrative costs from 6% before the Conservatives came to power to 11% today.

Then, too, rather than voicing the usual complaints about conditions and then getting on with their work as usual (and probably enjoying it), many physicians now seem genuinely anxious about the future. Some health care facilities have announced a list of procedures that they will no longer undertake, such as cosmetic surgery, removal of tattoos and impacted wisdom teeth, and in vitro fertilization.

More worrisome is the tendency for the health care system to relapse into the patchiness of service that was the situation before the start of the NHS, when a particular treatment may have been available in one locale but not in another a few kilometers away. A good example of this "treatment by postcode" is that for the blood-clotting disorder hemophilia. A genetically engineered and highly purified clotting factor concentrate is available for priority patients and has revolutionized patient care in the south of England as well as in Scotland and Northern Ireland. Elsewhere, some health directors have stated that this concentrate should not be prescribed and that patients will have to rely on the traditional—less safe but cheaper—preparation derived from human plasma, which carries the risk of transmitting viral infection, such as hepatitis. "To leave the decision [about the choice of treatment] to the vagaries of local purchasers," the U.K. Haemophilia Centre directors wrote to the *British Medical Journal,* "is to abrogate [the health department's] responsibility for an important aspect of health care."

Politicians consistently fail to address one point that most physicians make about the decline of the NHS. Britain's expenditures on health care have always been among the lowest in Western countries. The highest of all is the U.S., which spends 14.5% of gross domestic product (GDP), followed by France (9.9%) and Germany (9.6%). Britain spends only 6.9%, and given that its GDP is moderate, the actual expenditure per inhabitant is low: $1,300 a head annually, compared with $3,830 for the U.S.

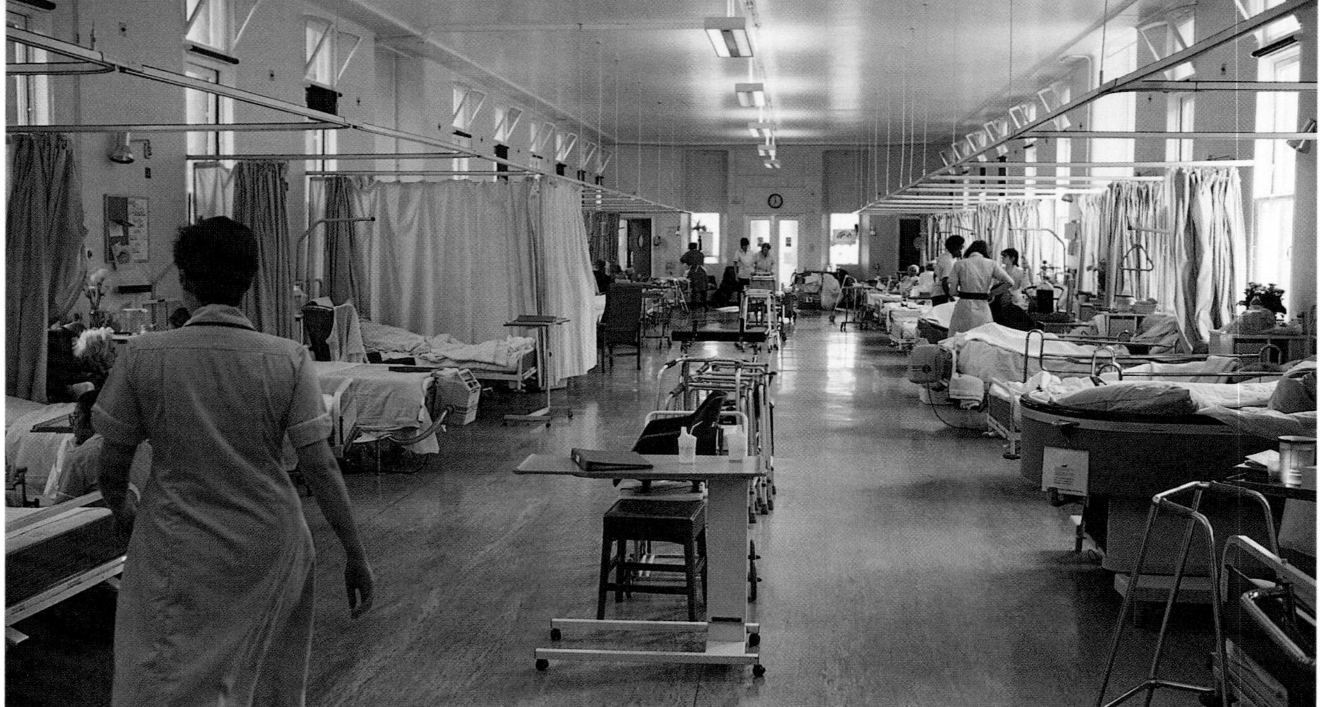

A large ward at King's College Hospital, London, offers little in the way of amenities. English hospitals are presently functioning at a bare-bones level. Owing to drastic cuts in NHS spending, Great Britain now has the lowest proportion of hospital beds of any country within the European Union.

Still, the United Kingdom is faced with exactly the same problems as most other Western industrial countries. The population is graying, and nearly half the health care budget is already being spent on those over the age of 65, whose proportion among the population is rising. New complex and expensive treatments are coming on the market at an ever-increasing rate. The expectations of the population for health care are continually rising; patience is wearing thin with a system in which surgical procedures are canceled at the last minute and mixed-sex hospital wards are common.

Just to maintain national health care in Britain at its bare-bones level has since 1979 required a 3% increase in funding every year. For the next three years, real spending is set to rise by a figure that has varied in official statements from 0.3% to 0.5% but that is, in any case, inadequate. The problem has been brought into focus by drastic cuts in one expensive item: hospital beds. In 25 years England and Wales lost half of their hospital beds, from 450,000 in 1970 (9 beds per 1,000 population) to 222,000 in 1995 (4.3 per 1,000). England now has the lowest proportion of hospital beds in the European Union, and the cuts are still being made. Many experts think that the right number should be about 300,000 and that if this level is not achieved, crises such as those described in the *New York Times* will continue.

The decades ahead

What, then, of the future? Many see "creeping privatization" of the NHS—with physicians and other health care providers defecting and setting up private fee-for-service practices—as one likely scenario. Already it is difficult to find a dentist who will provide treatment under the NHS rather than privately, and it seems likely that in the future the elderly will have to pay for their own long-term residential care, with little help from the state. Private medical services have quadrupled in the past 25 years and now cover 12% of the population. Yet even now such services are valued more for their quality and convenience than for their sophistication and ability to treat serious conditions such as myocardial infarction (heart attack) or to perform lifesaving surgery such as organ transplantation (which they tend to leave to the NHS). Many Britons, however, could never afford the fees for private care.

Other suggestions for mending the NHS that have been explored in public debates on rationing include establishing priorities in the use of medical resources (as has been done in the state of Oregon and in New Zealand), yet such measures are unlikely to produce dramatically large savings in the near future. Imposing charges for nonessential operations like elective plastic surgery and extraction of impacted wisdom teeth and for the personal comfort elements such as single-bedded hospital rooms has also been proposed, as has a special tax earmarked for improving standards in the NHS.

The reluctant conclusion of many medical professionals is that the downward slide of the NHS will continue, although general practice may well remain the popular first-class, cost-effective service it is. Conversely, the NHS hospital system may end up merely as a safety net for the indigent and the disadvantaged, with the remainder of the population having to find its own solutions for hospital care through private insurance. As a whole, Western countries stoutly resist raising taxes, and Britain is no exception. Without adequate revenue, the sort of utopian NHS that Britons like to talk about is pie in the sky.

Persistent and effective popular pressure on the British government to improve the NHS seems unlikely, since the public comes into contact with the stark realities of hospital medicine too rarely to be motivated to lobby consistently. Britain also has many other calls on its government funds—for education, housing, and infrastructure improvements—while it retains some extraordinarily costly delusions of imperial grandeur, as is shown by its relatively heavy military expenditures. It would be a brave person indeed who would predict what the NHS will look like 10 years hence, when it is pushing 60.

—Stephen Lock, M.D.

John Cole—Impact Photos

Assisted Suicide: No Constitutional Right

American physicians and their patients have always been uncomfortable talking about death and the dying process. This is somewhat ironic, given that most people readily admit that they worry about pain and suffering at the end of life and fear losing control or being dependent on others for their every need. In many opinion polls, a majority of Americans have indicated that they think dying people should have more control over decisions at the end of life and that physicians should be able to prescribe lethal doses of drugs for dying patients who wish to end their lives. Two U.S. circuit courts have ruled on the issue, both finding language in the Constitution that can be interpreted as affording a right to physician-assisted suicide. In June 1997, however, in two stunning unanimous opinions, the U.S. Supreme Court reversed the opinions of these lower courts, ruling that citizens of the U.S. have no constitutionally protected right to physician-assisted suicide.

Challenges to state laws

In the spring of 1996, within a month of each other, two U.S. Circuit Courts of Appeals struck down two state laws prohibiting assisted suicide. In the 9th Circuit, which includes Alaska, Arizona, California, Hawaii, Idaho, Montana, Nevada, Oregon, and Washington, three terminally ill patients (all of whom have since died) and four physicians challenged a Washington state law that makes it a crime for a doctor to aid a patient in committing suicide. In the 2nd Circuit, which includes New York, Connecticut, and Vermont, three dying patients (none still living in 1997) and three physicians challenged a similar New York state law, under which physician-assisted suicide is punishable as second-degree manslaughter. None of the patients was suicidal at the time the legal action was initiated, but all wanted to be able to obtain prescription drugs that they could take to end their lives if their suffering became unbearable. The physicians in the two cases said that they felt unable to comply with their patients' requests because of the laws on the books in their respective states. Each case presented the same two issues: (1) Is there a constitutional right to the assistance of a physician in committing suicide? (2) If so, does the state nonetheless have a sufficient interest in prohibiting the exercise of this right?

In the first case, *Washington* v. *Glucksberg,* the Court of Appeals for the 9th Circuit Court found that the due process clause of the 14th Amendment to the Constitution ("No State shall...deprive any person of life, liberty, or property, without due process of law") could be interpreted to include the right to assisted suicide. The court ruled that the constitutionally guaranteed exercise of "liberty" includes the liberty of competent, terminally ill patients near the end of life to determine the "time and manner" of their death. In arriving at this decision, the court referred to constitutional precedents on the right to abortion and the right to refuse treatment. It noted that just as a woman's right to make a decision about abortion is protected by her right to privacy, so is the dying patient's decision to request help in ending his or her life. The court also concluded that the right to refuse medical treatment is the same as the "right to hasten death"

(continued on page 279)

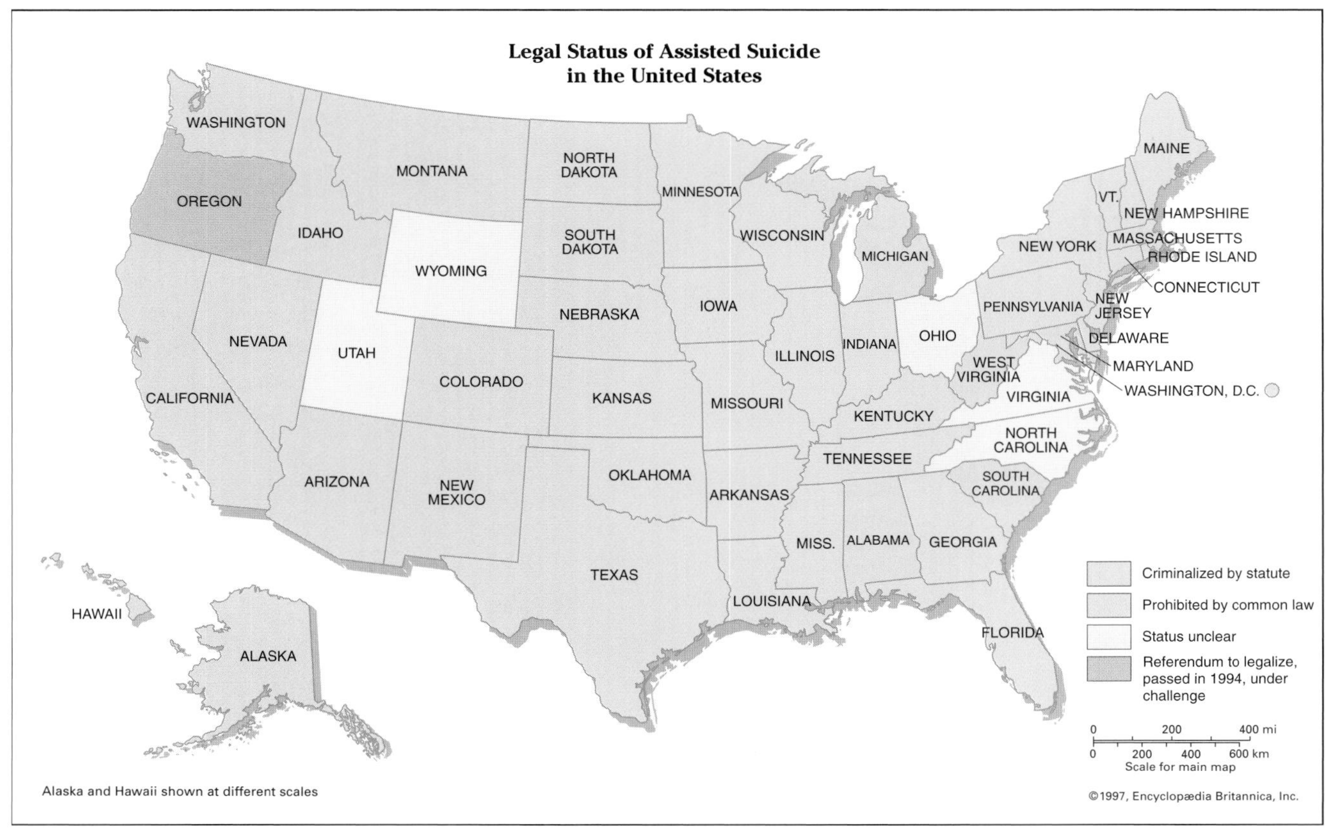

NEWS CAP MHA 98

Dr. Death's Very Still Lives

Is Jack Kevorkian obsessed with death? Certainly the 13 paintings shown in the spring 1997 exhibit "The Double Cross of Justice," at the Ariana Gallery, Royal Oak, Mich., would suggest so. Some would argue that the pictures offered dramatic proof that the pathologist, who, in late summer 1997, acknowledged having helped 46 people die (the unofficial number was closer to 100)—as an alternative to suffering ongoing pain or increasing debilitation—is bent on provoking controversy. At the very least, his work—on canvas and at bedside—provokes thought. Kevorkian, who neither considers himself an artist nor particularly enjoys the process of painting (his artistic training is limited to adult-education classes), calls his paintings "political cartoons," the meanings of which are straightforward.

Stanley Rosenthal, associate professor of art at Wayne State University, Detroit, Mich., characterized Kevorkian's technique as "amateurish" and dubbed the style "melodramatic surrealism." Another critic found the works "garish" and "profoundly disturbing." However one chooses to describe Kevorkian's largely death-oriented paintings, they present the world view of an iconoclast who has long railed against the medical establishment, the health care industry, the U.S. justice system, and organized religion. Six of the recently exhibited works were new; the others (some of them re-creations of lost works from the 1960s) were part of a previous exhibit, "Very Still Life," at the same gallery. (The paintings are not for sale, but reproductions of them are; the proceeds support Kevorkian's efforts on behalf of physician-assisted suicide.)

Among the most intriguing of the new works is "Genocide"; within a barbed-wire-embedded frame, two hands hold a severed head by the hair. One hand extends from a sleeve marked with a Nazi swastika and the date 1945; on the other sleeve an insignia and the date 1915 link its wearer to the annihilation of hundreds of thousands of Armenians by the Ottoman Turks. Kevorkian, who is of Armenian descent, stained the frame with his own blood. Another painting that depicts humanity's inhumanity is "The Gourmet (War)," in which Mars, the Roman god of war, coaxes a bleeding decapitated body to feast upon its own head. "War," wrote Kevorkian of the painting, "is worse than evil. It is mind-boggling suicide—mass suicide—with humankind devouring or trying to devour itself." Kevorkian's description of "For He Is Raised" is perhaps even more controversial than the painting itself, which depicts rabbits pulling a marionette Jesus from a rainbow-colored Easter egg: "The annual resurrection by dumb bunnies of a pathetic, despairing, almost scorned image of purported divinity is hardly noticeable amid the tawdry paraphernalia of irresistible paganism."

"Genocide," painting by Jack Kevorkian.

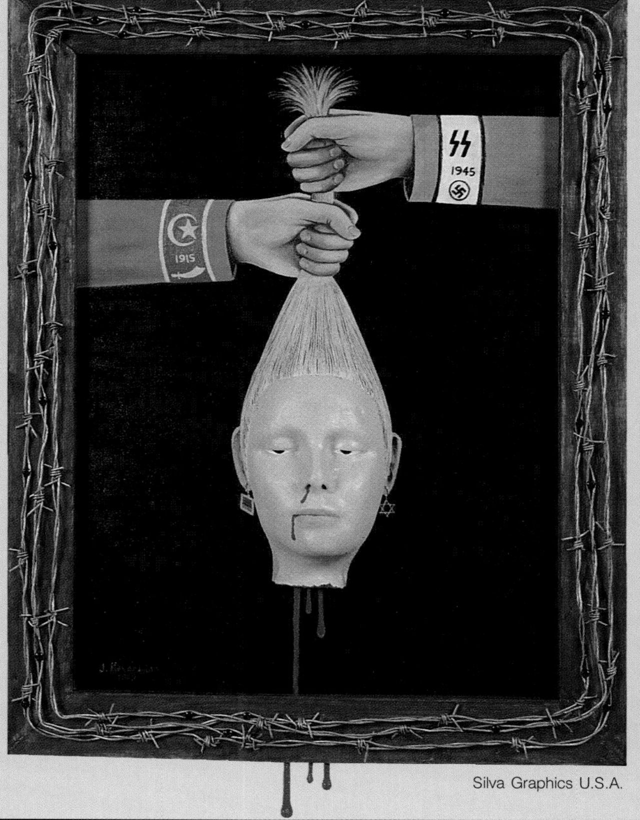

Silva Graphics U.S.A.

In "Nearer My God to Thee (In the Shadowy Valley)," the pathologist-painter's existential dismissal of the fear of death ("After all," he asks, "how excruciating can nothingness be?") is represented by a frantic subject's hopeless clawing at the abyss. On the other hand, Kevorkian's keen awareness of the trauma of life lived in pain is conveyed in "Fever," one of a series of paintings (now lost) illustrating individual symptoms of illness.

In contrast to the emotional intensity of his other works is his quite conventional portrait of the composer Johann Sebastian Bach. A self-taught musician who plays Baroque-style organ music and jazz flute, the "suicide doctor" was also slated to release a compact disc in the spring of 1997—about the same time that a legal suit against him was declared a mistrial. (In three previous trials for his assistance in suicides, he was acquitted.)

—*Jeff Wallenfeldt*

(continued from page 277)
and therefore includes the right to a physician's assistance in ending one's life.

In the New York state case, *Vacco* v. *Quill,* the Court of Appeals for the 2nd Circuit disagreed with the above analysis but nonetheless found a right to physician-assisted suicide in another provision of the 14th Amendment, the clause that guarantees all citizens equal protection under the law. Using logic substantially identical to that of the 9th Circuit, the 2nd Circuit also equated suicide with the refusal of life-sustaining treatment. It concluded that if the law permits patients who are dependent on life-support systems to demand that such treatment be discontinued—in essence, in the court's view, to commit suicide—then the law also must permit terminally ill patients who are not dependent on machines to have access to a physician's help in committing suicide. Both courts agreed that physician-assisted suicide could be heavily regulated by the states and that it was possible for the states and physicians to distinguish between good and bad suicides and to assist only those patients who were terminally ill, enduring terrible pain, and very near the end of their life.

Michelle Gabel—KRT

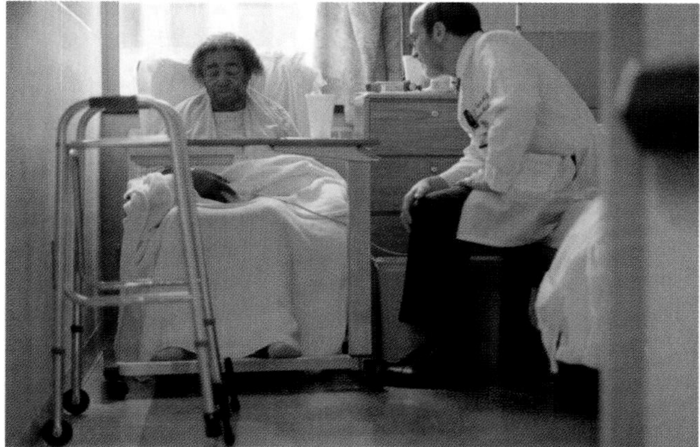

Rochester, N.Y., physician Timothy Quill, an outspoken advocate of assisted suicide, visits with a patient. Quill was the lead plaintiff in a suit to strike down the New York state law that makes it a crime for a physician to help a dying patient end his or her life.

Unanimity on the highest court

The U.S. Supreme Court agreed to review both of these cases in September 1996 and issued its rulings on June 26, 1997. The high court's rulings are discussed in detail below.

Washington* v. *Glucksberg. Chief Justice William Rehnquist, writing the opinion of the court, summed up the issue as follows: "The question before us is whether the 'liberty' specially protected by the Due Process Clause [of the 14th Amendment] includes a right to commit suicide which itself includes a right to assistance in doing so." Rehnquist enumerated two necessary conditions that had to be met by any fundamental constitutional right: (1) the fundamental right must be "deeply rooted in this nation's history and tradition" or fundamental to ordered liberty; and (2) the fundamental right must have a "careful description."

The court concluded that there is no historic tradition of treating suicide as a fundamental right, noting that to find such a right it would instead have to "reverse centuries of legal doctrine and practice, and strike down the...policy choice of almost every state." In a review of the history of laws against suicide and assisted suicide, the court noted that suicide was decriminalized in the U.S. not because the states approved of it or wanted to encourage it but rather to reflect the growing consensus that it was unfair to punish the suicide's family for his wrongdoing. Though no longer punishable by law, suicide nevertheless remains "a grievous, though nonfelonious, wrong." Nor, said the court, was any exception ever made for those who were "near to death."

Because the court found that no fundamental constitutional right to assisted suicide could be discovered in either the history of the U.S. or the concept of ordered liberty, the state of Washington needed only to demonstrate that its ban on assisted suicide was rationally related to legitimate government interests. The court concluded that this requirement had unquestionably been met. The court went on to list the following legitimate governmental interests in outlawing assisted suicide: (1) preserving human life; (2) preventing suicide; (3) protecting the integrity and ethics of the medical profession; (4) protecting vulnerable groups from abuse, neglect, and mistakes; and (5) preventing the first step "down the path to voluntary and perhaps even involuntary euthanasia." Noting that the 9th Circuit's decision seemed to permit surrogate decision making and, in some instances, lethal injection by a physician or family member, the court concluded, "It turns out that what is couched as a limited right to 'physician-assisted suicide' is likely, in effect, a much broader license, which could prove extremely difficult to police and contain. Washington's ban on assisting suicide prevents such erosion."

Ultimately, the court held simply that the state of Washington's law against assisted suicide "does not violate the Fourteenth Amendment, either on its face or as applied to competent, terminally ill adults who wish to hasten their deaths by obtaining medication prescribed by their doctors."

Vacco* v. *Quill. The chief justice, again writing for the court and reversing the 2nd Circuit's opinion, stated the question as whether the state of New York, by making it a crime for one person to aid another in committing or attempting suicide while at the same time permitting patients to refuse lifesaving treatment, thereby violates the equal protection clause of the 14th Amendment. The court held that it does not.

Unless a state law infringes upon a fundamental right, the court said, or singles out a particular group of people for unequal treatment, it will be upheld as long as it bears a rational relation to some legitimate end. The court had already concluded in *Washington* v. *Glucksberg* that statutes outlawing assisted suicide do not infringe upon fundamental rights. It had also concluded that state laws banning assisted suicide are reasonably related to legitimate state interests. Thus, the only real question in *Vacco* v. *Quill* was whether there is a rational difference between assisting a patient in committing suicide and withdrawing life-sustaining treatment. The court answered this question at the outset, stating that on its face the New York law draws no distinctions between people but treats all citizens of the state the same: "Everyone, regardless of physical condition, is entitled, if competent, to refuse unwanted lifesaving medical treatment; no one is permitted to assist a suicide."

The 2nd Circuit had overlooked this point, probably because it took into account only the universe of terminally ill people near the end of life and tried to find a new constitutional right by characterizing the right to refuse treatment as a right to commit suicide in this context. Having determined that ending or refusing lifesaving medical treatment is "nothing more nor less than assisting suicide," the 2nd Circuit had concluded that those terminally ill people who are not dependent on life-support technologies are effectively denied equal protection by the prohibition of assisted suicide. The Supreme Court emphatically disagreed and specifically upheld as rational the historic legal distinction between refusing treatment and committing suicide:

> *Unlike the Court of Appeals, we think the distinction between assisting suicide and withdrawing life-sustaining treatment, a distinction widely recognized and endorsed in the medical profession and in our legal traditions, is both important and logical; it is certainly rational.*

The high court noted that the principles of causation and intent are critical in determining culpability in criminal law. With regard to causation in this case, the court noted that when a critically ill patient refuses life-sustaining treatment, the cause of death is an underlying fatal disease or pathology; if, on the other hand, a patient ingests lethal medication prescribed by a physician, the cause of death is the medication. With regard to intent, when a physician provides aggressive palliative care, pain-killing drugs may sometimes hasten patients' deaths, but, said the court, "the physician's purpose and intent is, or may be, only to ease his patients' pain." On the other hand, a doctor who assists a suicide necessarily intends that the patient die. Similarly, a patient who commits suicide with a doctor's aid "necessarily has the specific intent to end his or her own life," whereas a patient who refuses or discontinues treatment might not have such intent. The court noted that the law has historically distinguished between actions done "because of" a given end and actions done "in spite of" their unintended but foreseen consequences and used the example of Gen. Dwight D. Eisenhower's ordering U.S. soldiers into battle in World War II, knowing that many would certainly die because

NEWS CAP MHA 98

Presidential Apology for the Study at Tuskegee

On May 16, 1997, in the East Room of the White House, Pres. Bill Clinton issued a formal apology for the Tuskegee Study of Untreated Syphilis in the Negro Male, the "longest nontherapeutic experiment on human beings" in the history of medicine and public health. That study, conducted under the auspices of the U.S. Public Health Service (PHS), was originally projected to last six months but spanned 40 years—from 1932 to 1972. The purpose of the study was to determine the effect of untreated syphilis in black men. The men in the study were never told that they had syphilis, a sexually transmitted disease. Instead, government doctors told the men they had "bad blood," a term that was commonly used to describe a wide range of unspecified maladies.

The study, in Macon county, Ala., included 600 black men, 399 with syphilis and a control group of 201 who did not have the disease. The men in the study were the sons and grandsons of slaves. Most had never been seen by a doctor. When announcements were made in churches and in the cotton fields about a way to receive free medical care, the men showed up in droves. Little did they know the high price that would be paid over the next four decades as they were poked and prodded by an endless array of government medical personnel. In the mid-1940s, when penicillin became the standard cure for syphilis, the Tuskegee subjects were not treated with the drug. Even as some men went blind and insane from advanced (tertiary) syphilis, the government doctors withheld treatment, remaining committed to observing their subjects through to the study's predetermined "end point"—autopsy. To ensure that the families would agree to this final procedure, the government offered them burial insurance—at most \$50—to cover the cost of a casket and grave.

The research project was finally stopped after Peter Buxtun, a former venereal disease investigator with the PHS, shared the truth about the study's unethical methods with a reporter from the Associated Press. On July 25, 1972, news accounts sparked a public outcry that ultimately brought the notorious experiment to an end. Congressional hearings were conducted, which led to federal legislation strengthening guidelines for protection of human subjects in research. Fred Gray, a civil rights attorney, filed a class-action lawsuit on behalf of the men that resulted in a \$10 million out-of-court settlement for the victims, their families, and their heirs. Almost a quarter of a century after the study ended, however, there remains among many African-Americans a legacy of deep mistrust that hampers efforts to promote health and prevent disease in this population group.

During the White House ceremony, the president directed his words to Carter Howard, Frederick Moss, Charlie Pollard, Herman Shaw, Fred Simmons, Sam Doner, Ernest Hendon, and George Key, the study's sole survivors, all of whom are over 90 years of age and the first five of whom were present for the occasion:

> *[They] are a living link to a time not so very long ago that many Americans would prefer not to remember but we dare not forget. It was a time when our nation failed to live up to its ideals, when our nation broke the trust...that is the very foundation of our de-*

of his order. His intent was to defeat Germany, not to have U.S. soldiers killed, and this is what made his orders lawful.

Implications of the decisions

There were five votes for each of the opinions written by the chief justice. All nine justices agreed that state laws prohibiting assisted suicide violate neither the due process nor the equal protection clause of the 14th Amendment, even as applied to physicians who prescribe overdoses of medications to competent, terminally ill patients who want to commit suicide. Nonetheless, five justices wrote concurring opinions to express additional or different reasons for this conclusion.

In retrospect it is not difficult to see how the "right" to physician assistance in suicide failed to gain constitutional recognition. To find such a right, the court would have had to find a constitutional right to suicide itself, and there is no historical or legal support for this. Moreover, the precedents the proponents relied on—the right to choose abortion and the right to refuse treatment—were easily distinguishable from the right to assistance in ending life. The court itself remains deeply divided on abortion and, if anything, has moved toward limiting rather than expanding the abortion rights articulated in 1973 in *Roe* v. *Wade*. The right to refuse treatment is deeply rooted in American law, and so are the principles of intent and causation in the criminal law—principles that distinguish suicide from refusing treatment and assisted suicide from withdrawing treatment. This latter distinction is one that has been made by every court since the landmark 1976 decision in the case of Karen Ann Quinlan (a young woman who was in a persistent vegetative state and whose parents sued for—and won—the right to discontinue life-sustaining treatment).

It would have been more comforting for U.S. health care professionals had the court more explicitly ruled that what the physicians wanted to do in these cases was not, by definition, assisted suicide (since the patients were not suicidal and the drugs that would have been used had another medical use), and thus the

mocracy. The United States government did something that was wrong, deeply, profoundly, morally wrong. To the survivors, to the wives and family members, the children and the grandchildren, I say what you know: No power on Earth can give you back the lives lost, the pain suffered, the years of internal torment and anguish. What was done cannot be undone. But we can end the silence. We can stop turning our heads away. We can look at you in the eye and finally say on behalf of the American people, what the United States government did was shameful, and I am sorry.

In that emotional statement, Clinton apologized on behalf of the American people—something his five predecessors in the White House had not done; he and the other persons present experienced the power of forgiveness from men who suffered at the hands of doctors in the PHS. The president placed the burden of responsibility for the abuse on the medical research establishment when he stated, "The people who ran the study at Tuskegee diminished the stature of man by abandoning the most basic ethical precepts. They forgot their pledge to heal and repair." The government, Clinton announced, was providing a $200,000 grant to help establish a center for bioethics in research and health care at Tuskegee University as part of a lasting "memorial" to the study's victims.

Shaw, aged 94, expressed gratitude to Clinton "for doing your best to right this wrong tragedy and to resolve that Americans should never again allow such an event to occur." The legacy of Tuskegee goes well beyond the syphilis study—it is part of the history of racism and discrimination in the United States. The presidential apology may be the crucial first step in addressing the fear and mistrust that shapes the behavior and attitudes of many African-Americans not only toward participating in medical research but also toward receiving health care that they need and deserve.

—Stephen B. Thomas, Ph.D., and Sandra Crouse Quinn, Ph.D.

Close of a tragic chapter: Just short of his 95th birthday, Herman Shaw, a survivor of the Tuskegee Study of Untreated Syphilis in the Negro Male, receives a warm embrace after a formal governmental apology from Pres. Bill Clinton as Vice Pres. Al Gore applauds.

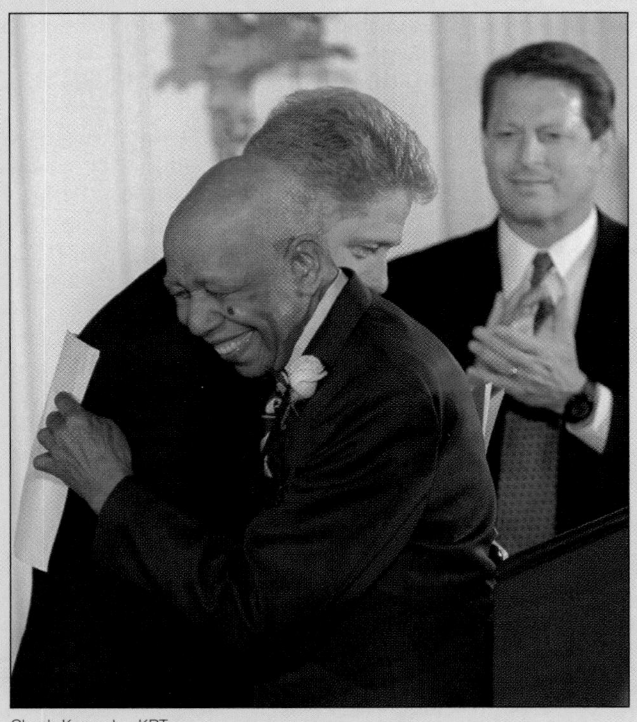

Chuck Kennedy—KRT

Rick Rickman—Matrix

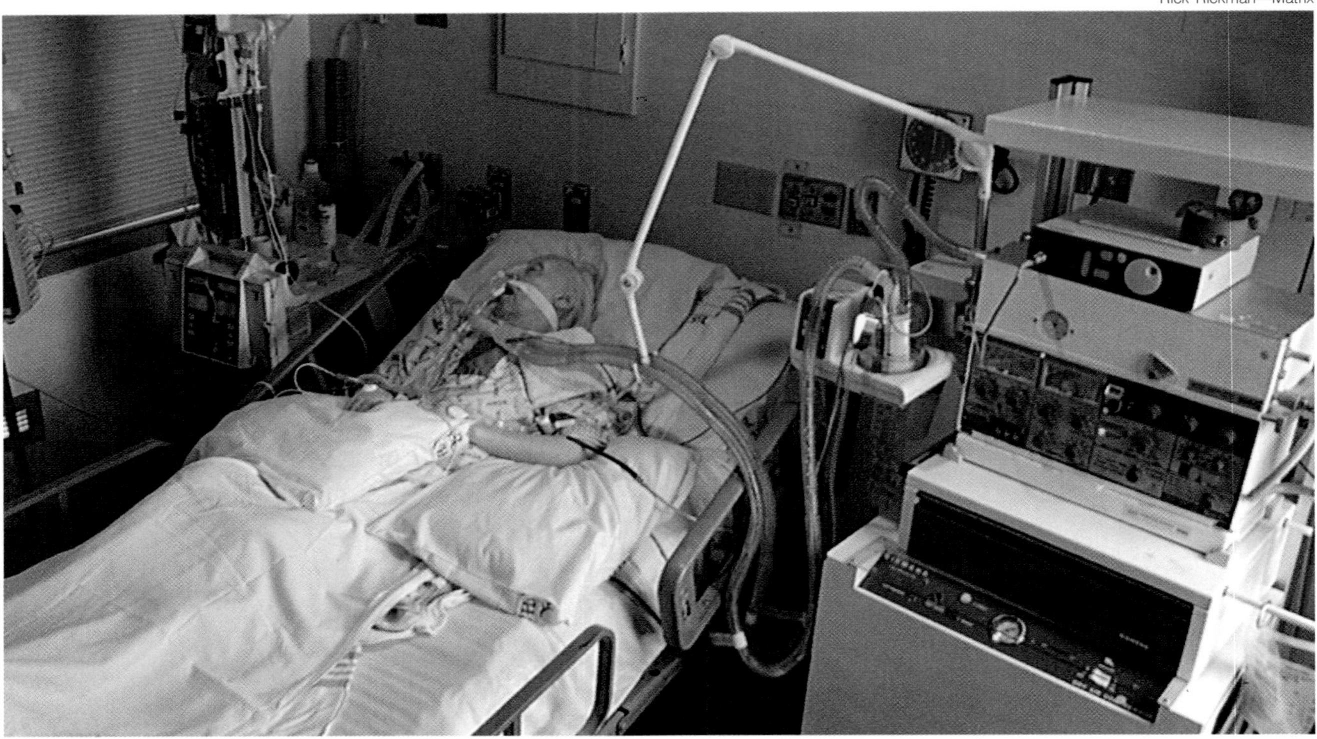

constitutionality of the statutes as applied to the physicians did not even have to be adjudicated. The avoidance of this central question and the emotional nature of the court's deliberations indicate that the justices—like all Americans—have a very difficult time coming to grips with the dying process. The abstract nature of the opinions in these cases can also be explained by the fact that there had been no trial in either of the lower court cases, and thus there were before the Supreme Court only physician affidavits attesting to fear of legal redress and the stories of patients who were already deceased.

Physicians who aggressively treat pain need not change their treatment of the terminally ill as a result of the court's opinion. Doctors who provide palliative care with the primary intent of relieving pain and suffering, and with the patient's consent, were strongly encouraged by the court to continue to do so. Indeed, at least five of the justices suggested that there may be something akin to a "right not to suffer," at least for those near death, and that states have no constitutional authority to prohibit or inhibit physicians from doing all in their medical power to prevent such suffering. Thus, the decision should provide an impetus to the efforts to improve care for the dying. If terminally ill individuals could be assured of receiving adequate pain relief and dying with dignity, there would be little need for assisted suicide.

The movement to find a constitutional right to physician-assisted suicide is dead. The states remain free, as they were before these opinions, to change their laws banning suicide. But the problems surrounding how Americans die have little to do with the suicide laws and everything to do with the reluctance to face and discuss death. The opening of some real discussion of these issues may be the most enduring consequence of these Supreme Court opinions.

—*George J. Annas, J.D., M.P.H.*

The 1997 Supreme Court decisions upholding state laws against assisted suicide are sure to focus public opinion more squarely on the real issue—how Americans die. (Above) It is the worst fear of many that they will end their days dependent on machines and isolated from human contact, like this elderly patient in a California hospital intensive care unit. (Below) To be cared for at home and provided with adequate pain relief is the "last wish" of increasing numbers of the terminally ill.

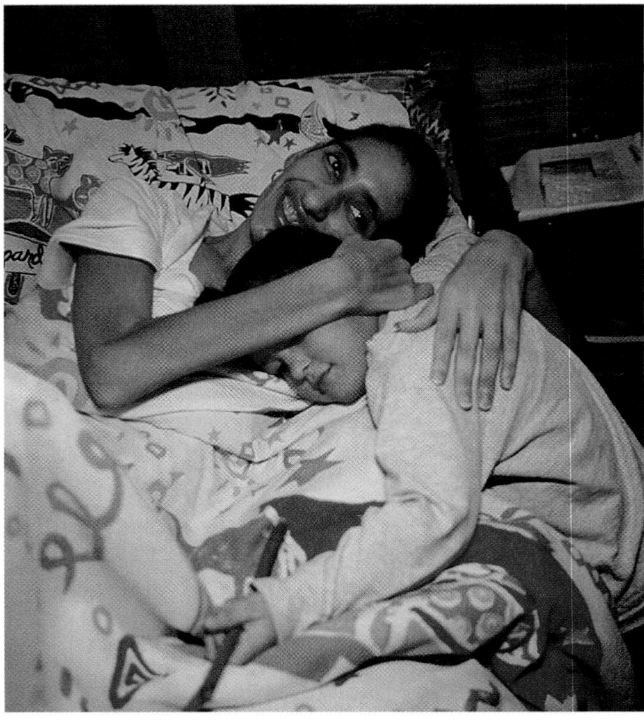

"Amalia and Amanda, New York City" (1994), ©Nan Goldin from the exhibition and book *Hospice: A Photographic Inquiry;* courtesy of Matthew Marks Gallery, New York City

Leprosy at Century's End

Two events seem almost certain by the year 2000. First, in the United States the country's only leprosy hospital, located at Carville, La., will close its doors. Second, internationally, the World Health Organization (WHO) will announce that leprosy has been eliminated. While these developments would seem to indicate that this ancient scourge is on the verge of disappearing, it is debatable whether such a conclusion is justified.

Some 10 million–12 million people alive today have, or have had, leprosy, and around 888,000 currently require drug treatment. India has the largest number of cases, with more than 7 million overall, of whom 554,000 still need treatment. Brazil is second, with 320,000 total and 106,000 needing treatment, followed by Indonesia, with 217,000 and 34,000, respectively. In some areas of the world—parts of China, for example—leprosy incidence (the rate of new cases being reported) is declining, while in others—*e.g.,* parts of Brazil—it continues to rise.

Kari Lounatmaa--Science Source/Photo Researchers

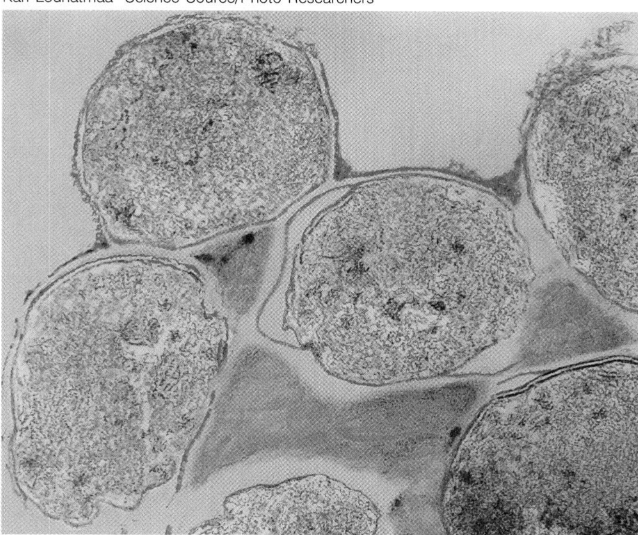

The rod-shaped Mycobacterium leprae *(which appears round in cross-section in this electron micrograph), identified as the cause of leprosy in 1873, continues to baffle scientists in many ways.*

Many mysteries

Leprosy is a chronic infectious disease that affects the skin, the peripheral nerves (those outside the brain and spinal cord), and the mucous membranes of the face. It is caused by the leprosy bacillus, *Mycobacterium leprae,* a relative of *M. tuberculosis,* the organism responsible for tuberculosis (TB). (A bacillus is a rod-shaped bacterium.) Scientists theorize that the leprosy bacillus enters the body through a break in the skin or through the mucous membranes of the nose. The disease can be transmitted from person to person by prolonged close contact, but even today scientists are uncertain exactly how it spreads. In fact, much remains mysterious about leprosy. At least in part this is because the bacillus has never been grown in a test tube, and the only tools for studying its transmission have been a limited number of animal models, chiefly armadillos and mice.

The geographic distribution of the bacillus is another mystery. Some scientists suspect that the organism exists in the soil in many parts of the world, but again, because it cannot be grown in a laboratory culture, the only evidence of its presence in a given region is the appearance of the disease itself. Besides humans, the only animals known to develop leprosy in nature are New World armadillos and African primates. For experimental purposes scientists have been able to grow the bacillus in mice.

Historically, the physical deformities of leprosy—and ignorance about its mode of spread—caused those affected by the disease to be regarded with fear and dread. In a 14th-century manuscript illumination, lepers begging for alms carry a noisemaker to warn villagers of their approach.

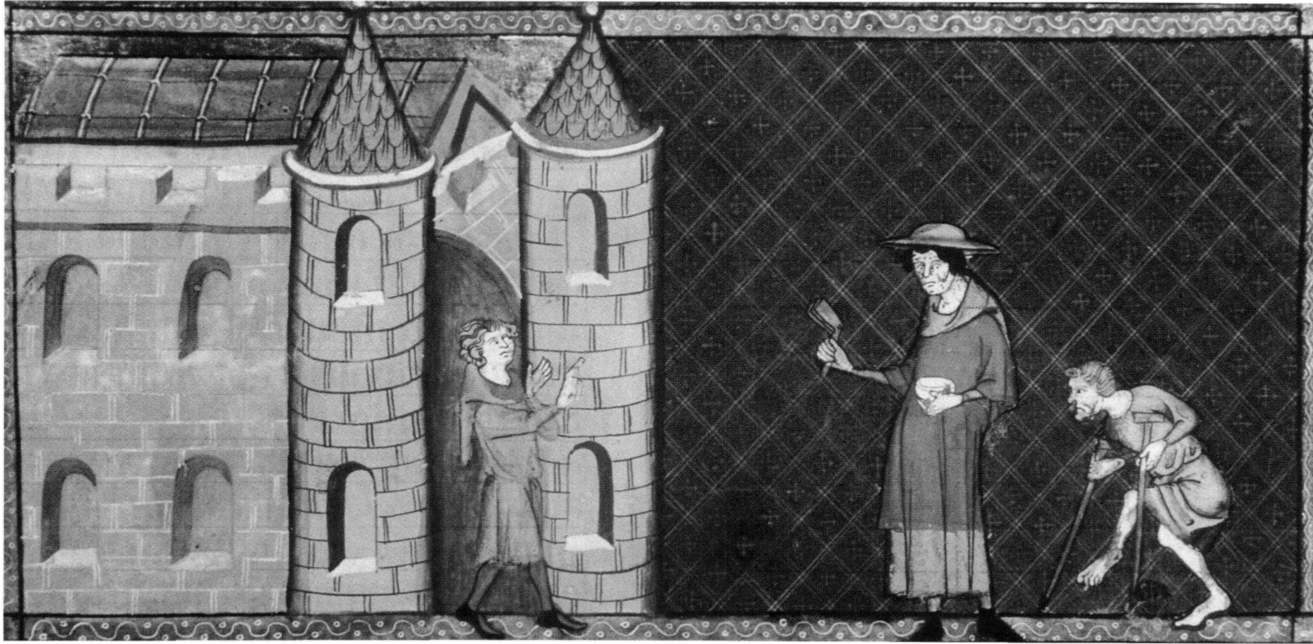

The Granger Collection, New York

(Below) Sean Sprague—Panos Pictures; (bottom) Ben Edwards—Impact Photos

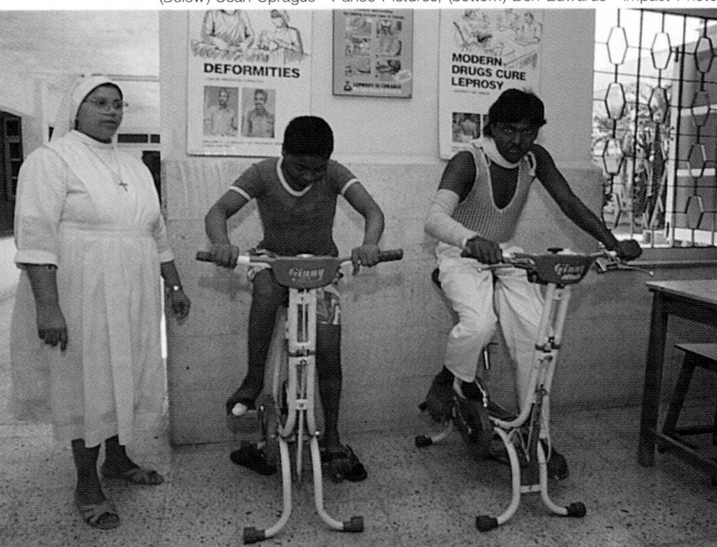

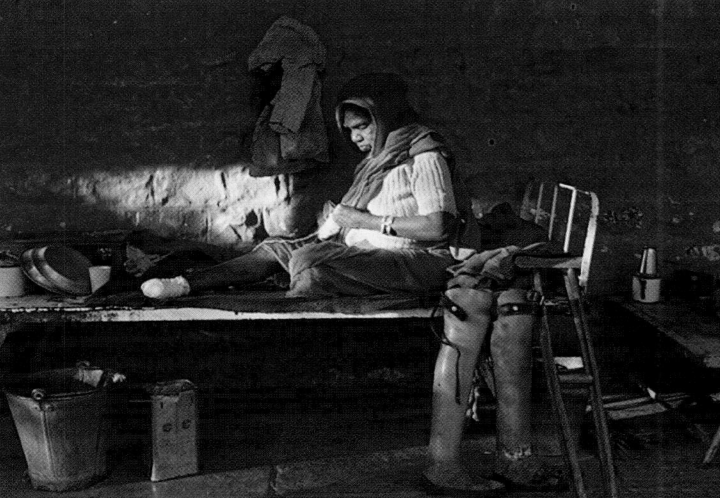

(Top) Two men who are currently being treated for leprosy undergo rehabilitation therapy in a hospital in Bombay (Mumbai). (Above) A patient in another Indian leprosy hospital has lost limbs as a result of the disease. India now leads the world in leprosy cases, with more than half a million people who still require drug treatment.

If the organism that causes leprosy is widely distributed and the disease is contagious, it seems logical to ask why leprosy is not a great deal more prevalent than it is. The answer is that the infection apparently is quite difficult to contract. The vast majority (95% or so) of people simply are not susceptible to the bacillus and, despite repeated exposure, will never develop leprosy. Among the few individuals who do contract the disease, it will be self-limiting and will disappear before any symptoms have become evident. Even in cases where early symptoms of leprosy develop, most patients will self-heal. This rather unusual pattern of infection, along with the three- to five-year incubation period (the time that elapses between contact with the bacillus and the onset of symptoms), makes the epidemiology of leprosy particularly difficult to study.

A tropical disease—in Norway?

People tend to think of leprosy as a tropical malady because most cases today are found in less-developed countries, which are mainly in the tropics. This has not always been the case. In 1200 AD an estimated 19,000 leprosy hospitals existed all over Europe. The disease is much older than that, however. An illness that fits the description of leprosy appears in documents from India that date to about 600 BC. A similar ailment was described in a Chinese medical text from 400 BC. Tradition has it that members of the army of Alexander the Great contracted the illness when they invaded India in the 4th century BC. Returning home, they carried it into the Middle East and then throughout the eastern Mediterranean. Leprosy was introduced into western Europe by crusaders returning between the 11th and the 13th century AD.

Rather abruptly and for unknown reasons, the incidence of leprosy began to decline in Europe—with the exception of Scandinavia—between AD 1200 and 1300. In Norway the disease persisted until the 20th century but has now disappeared. It was first introduced into what is now the United States by African slaves and/or the French Canadians (Acadians) who were expelled from the area of present-day Nova Scotia and New Brunswick by the British in 1755 and who migrated to Louisiana. Another immigrant group known to include people with leprosy moved to the U.S. from Scandinavia, mainly Norway, in the middle of the 19th century, settling principally in Minnesota. The disease was transmitted and has persisted in Louisiana, where occasional new cases appear even today among people of Acadian descent. Curiously, leprosy was not transmitted in Minnesota, and the disease had completely disappeared there by the early 20th century. New cases continue to be diagnosed in the U.S. in immigrants from countries where leprosy remains prevalent.

Transmission: another puzzle

In the many centuries since leprosy was first described, a number of theories have been proposed to explain how the bacillus is transmitted. In the 19th century leprosy was believed to be a hereditary ailment. This made sense, as it frequently occurred in households among individuals who were members of a single family. In 1873, however, G.H. Armauer Hansen, a physician working in a leprosy hospital in Bergen, Nor., discovered the leprosy bacillus in a sample of tissue from one of his patients. (About 2.5% of the population of Bergen was affected by leprosy at that time.) Hansen was able to identify the organism under the microscope because its propensity to collect iron caused it to appear brownish in color compared with the tissue itself. His discovery was momentous; not only did it demonstrate that leprosy was infectious, but it was the first association of a microorganism with an infectious disease.

The route of transmission of leprosy remained a matter of debate. The prevailing opinion for many years was that the illness spread via prolonged skin-to-skin contact. Then the theory of respiratory transmission became popular; it posited that the bacillus entered the human body through the lining of the nose. For a time, scientists even entertained the possibility of transmission by insect bites. In the past few years, experiments with a mouse model of the disease have shown that transmission is indeed possible through the intact lining of the nose and breaks in the skin but not via the mouth, lungs, or digestive tract or through unbroken skin. And although leprosy can be produced in mice by exposing them to the bacillus, the disease cannot be transmitted from an infected to an uninfected mouse.

About one thing scientists are in agreement: human leprosy epidemics start with an infected individual. This proposition was convincingly demonstrated in some Pacific Island populations early in the 20th century. What is not clear is whether transmission requires direct contact with an infected person or simply contact with something in the environment (presumably wet soil) that has itself been contaminated by an infected person. Some authorities suggest that sturdy footwear and modern sanitation would do more to prevent leprosy than all the sophisticated biomedical approaches put together.

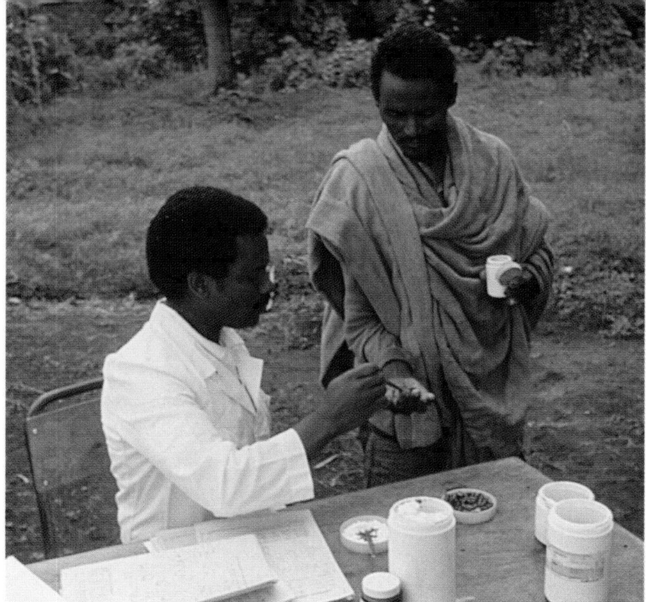

A man in Ethiopia receives multidrug therapy as part of the World Health Organization's campaign to eliminate leprosy. Depending on the extent of the disease, treatment takes from six months to two years.

Course of the disease

In the beginning the leprosy bacillus attacks the skin. The skin lesions are not painful; rather, because the bacillus begins immediately to destroy small nerve endings in the skin, these spots are often numb. As the disease progresses, the lesions may spread to all areas of the skin surface that are cool enough for the bacillus to persist and multiply—ideally, a temperature between 26.7° and 29.4° C (80° and 85° F). Typically, the first areas to become involved are the earlobes (which are cooler than the rest of the body) and the legs and forearms. Eventually, in the most disseminated form of the disease, the whole body surface may be affected, with the exception of the scalp, arm pits, groin, and areas usually covered by bra straps, watchbands, and the like, which are too warm to provide a hospitable environment for the bacillus.

The bacilli gradually migrate up the small nerve endings in the skin, ultimately destroying nerve trunks that supply sensation to large body areas. The result is loss of sensation in these areas. Destruction of the posterior tibial nerve in the ankle results, for example, in anesthesia of the soles of the feet. Involvement of the nasal passages results in chronic nasal stuffiness and nosebleeds. Involvement of the mucous membranes of the throat produces chronic hoarseness. Eye involvement leads to impaired vision.

In addition to destroying nerves, leprosy also causes destruction and loss of tissue. Three mechanisms contribute to the process. First, lesions can grow into nodules, which may eventually ulcerate. Second, immune responses trigger inflammation of tissues containing the bacilli; these tissues can then break down and ulcerate. Third, the loss of sensation leads patients to overuse sore or painful extremities that they would normally (*i.e.,* when warned by pain) spare.

Therapy: current state of the art

The current treatment of leprosy is extremely effective, halting the progress of the disease. The bacilli can be killed rapidly, and multidrug therapy—the use of two or more antileprosy drugs in combination—prevents the development of drug-resistant strains. Indeed, multidrug therapy—a practice now widely accepted in the treatment of TB and AIDS—was first proposed after scientists observed that some cases of leprosy were becoming resistant to

The dramatic impact of multidrug therapy is evident in the "before" and "after" photos below. Currently available antileprosy drugs are extremely effective in halting the progress of the disease, although they cannot restore nerve function once damage to nerves has proceeded beyond a certain point.

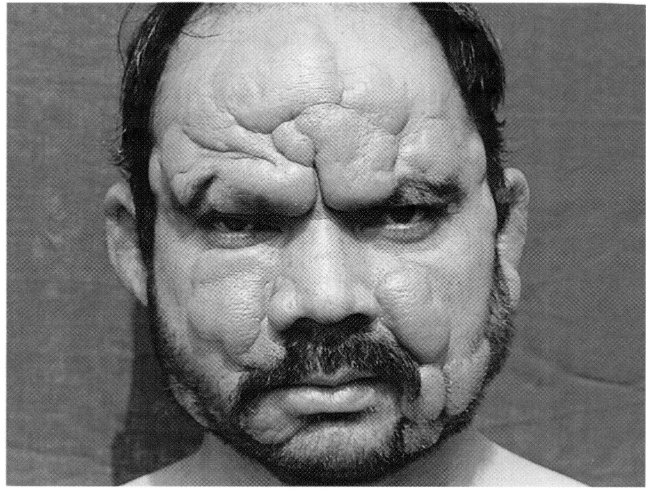

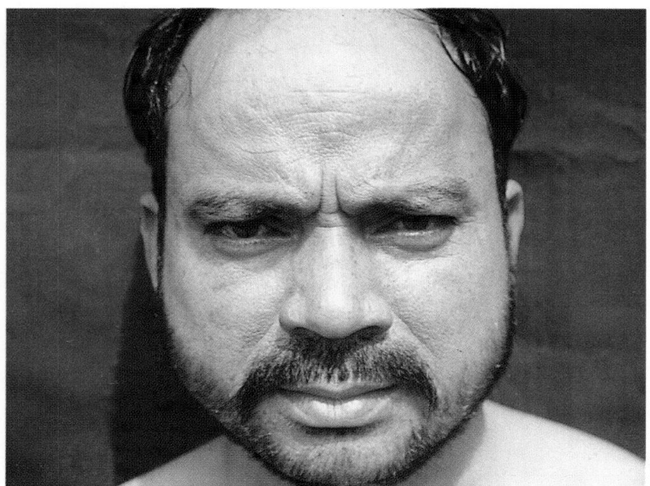

Photographs, WHO; (top) H. Anenden; (above) LEP

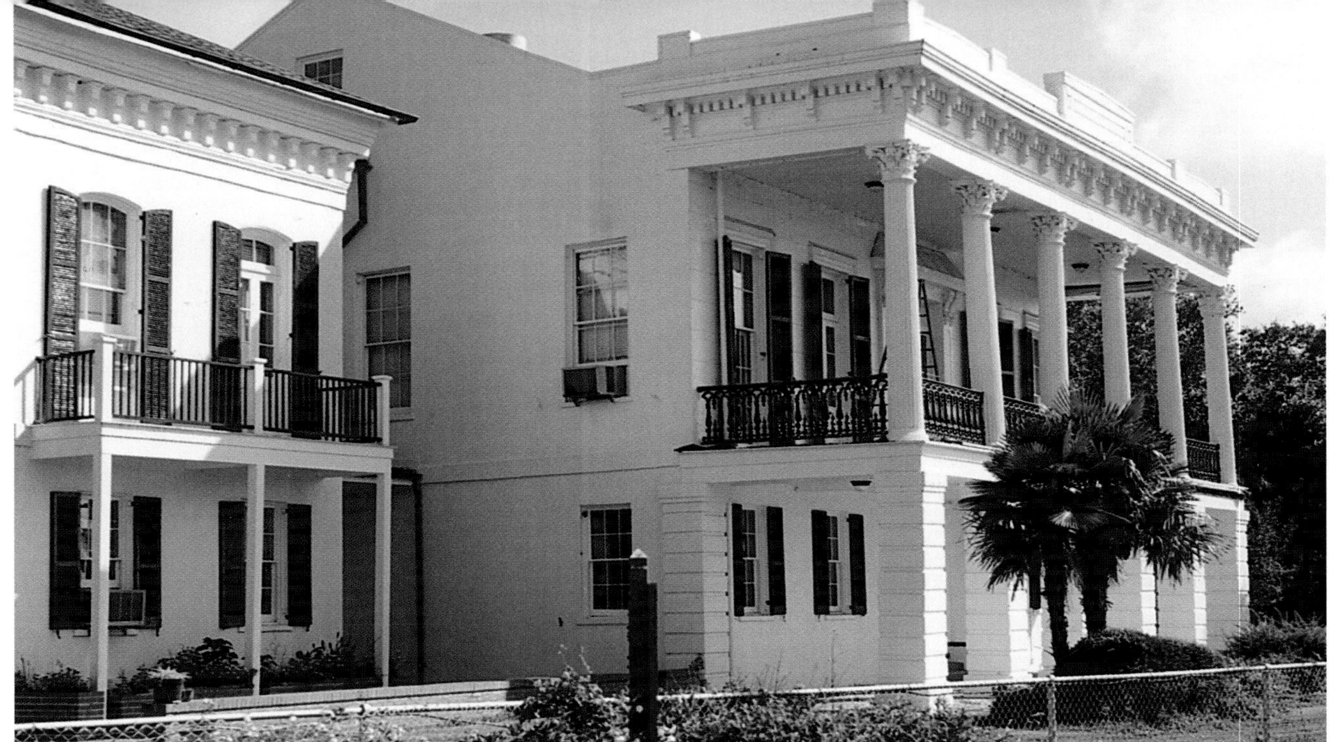

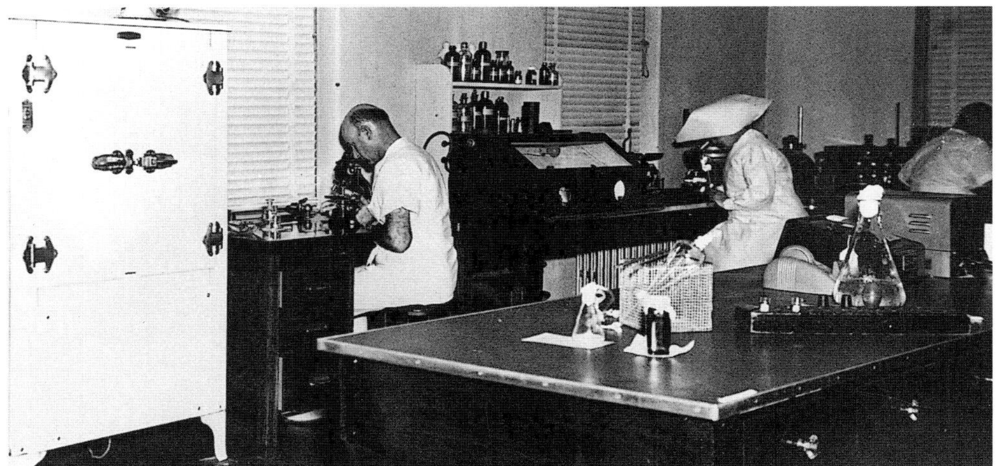

(Above) The administration building at the Gillis W. Long Hansen's Disease Center, Carville, La., was once a plantation house. Established in 1894 by the state of Louisiana, the center became a national leprosy hospital, under the auspices of the Public Health Service, in 1921. (Left) Sister Hilary Ross, of the Daughters of Charity, and her staff work in the Carville laboratory in the 1950s. (Below) Several generations of residents are buried in the Carville cemetery.

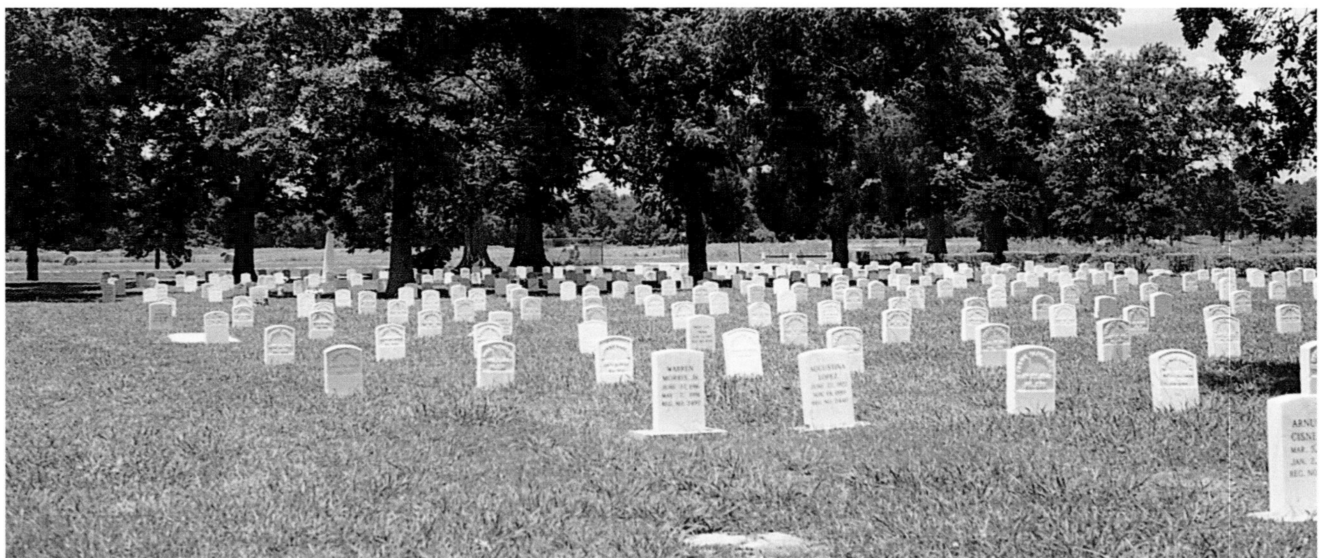

Photographs, Gillis W. Long Hansen's Disease Center; (top and above) Tanya Thomassie

Photographs, Gillis W. Long Hansen's Disease Center; (bottom) Tanya Thomassie

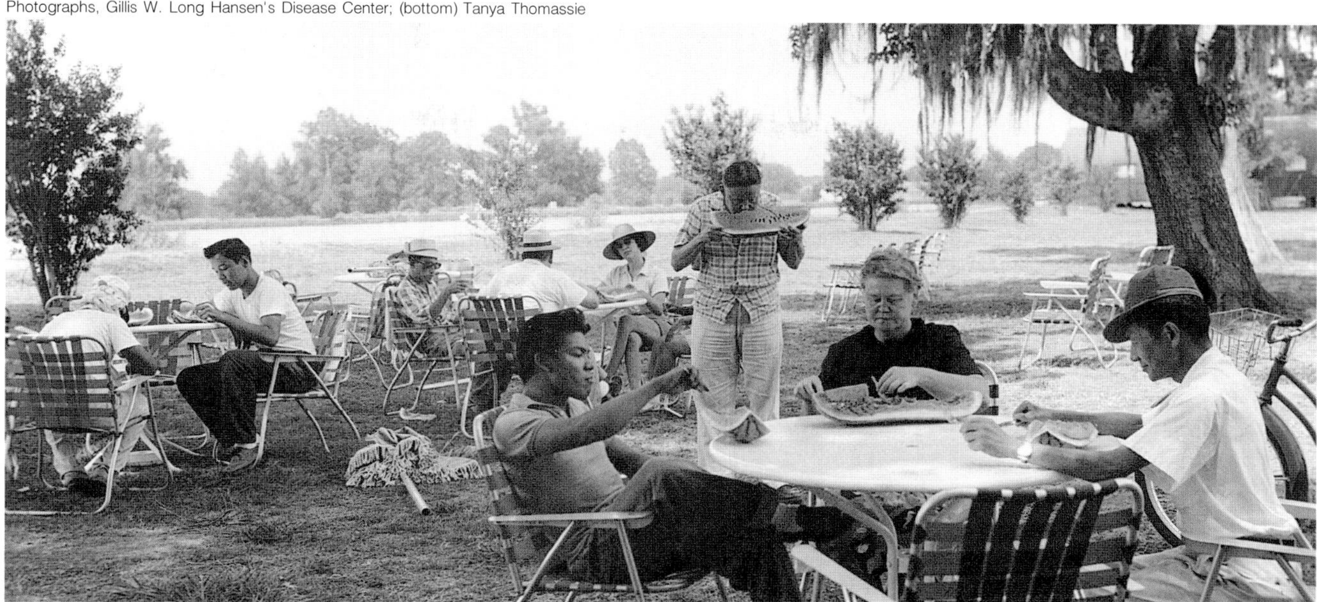

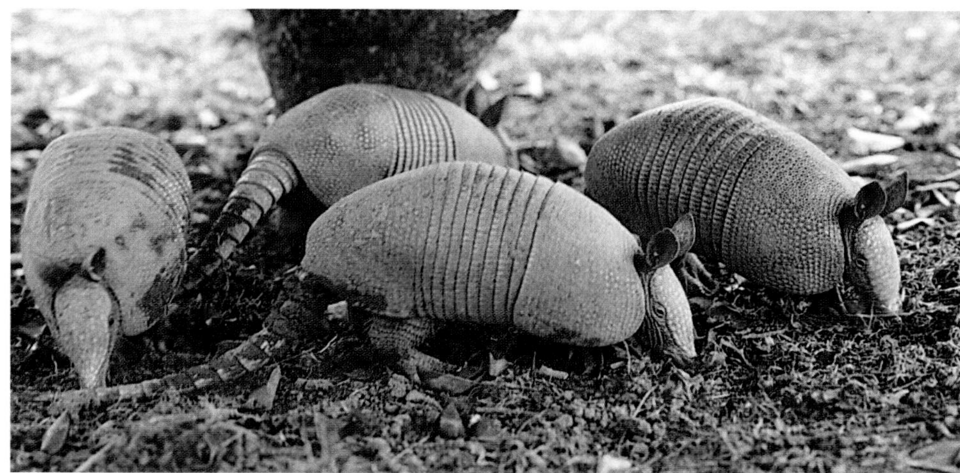

(Above) Life at Carville, where the patient population numbered nearly 500 at its peak, was much like life in any small town. The shores of the center's 8.1-ha (20-ac) man-made lake have seen many a picnic. (Right) The armadillo, one of the few animals that is naturally susceptible to leprosy, has been used widely as an animal model for the human disease. The animals pictured here were part of a group inoculated with the leprosy bacillus by Carville scientists in the 1970s.

the sulfones, the earliest antileprosy drugs. A multidrug regimen developed by WHO is the current standard of treatment.

For patients with localized forms of leprosy and relatively few leprosy bacilli in their bodies, two drugs, dapsone and rifampin, are given for a total of six months. For patients with more widespread disease and relatively large numbers of bacilli, three drugs—dapsone, clofazimine, and rifampin—are given for 24 months. Most patients are able to tolerate the drugs well, and relapses, in general, are rare, occurring in less than one per 1,000 treated patients. Effective treatment has made leprosy curable for decades—in the sense that the disease-causing organisms can be killed and the infection eradicated.

Leprosy is much more than an infection, however. It is a disease that can result in significant disfigurement and disability. Killing the bacillus has no effect on body tissues that have already been damaged or destroyed. Up to a point, nerve function can be restored by antileprosy drugs, but once the disease process has progressed beyond that point, the loss of function is permanent. Nerve impairment—of which leprosy is the leading cause worldwide—leads to paralysis, loss of sensation, and changes in the individual's physical appearance. About 7% of newly diagnosed leprosy patients today have visible deformity or damage to their hands or feet or impaired vision. These disabilities can interfere with the patient's ability to earn a living and otherwise lead a normal life. If the damage is unsightly, and it frequently is, then the patient also must cope with loss of social acceptance.

Carville: first—and last—U.S. leprosarium

In the late 19th century, a 17-year-old cub reporter for the *New Orleans Daily Picayune* and a young professor of dermatology at Tulane Medical School were moved by the plight of 10 leprosy patients living together in a squalid cottage in New Orleans. They set about establishing a proper hospital for leprosy patients in Louisiana. A major consideration in choosing a location for the facility was that it be close enough to New Orleans that Tulane medical school faculty members could conveniently study the disease. This provision for research was a major innovation;

previous leprosy hospitals had existed mainly to isolate patients from the general population and to provide them with care.

After several false starts, the Louisiana Leper Home was established at the site of an abandoned plantation near Carville, La., some 120 km (75 mi) upriver from New Orleans. The first small group of patients arrived via coal barge from New Orleans in November 1894. Within a couple of years, nuns from the Daughters of Charity arrived to care for the patients, a service the religious order continues to this day.

By the early 20th century, a sufficient number of cases had been diagnosed among immigrants to the U.S., primarily in New York, Texas, Florida, and Louisiana, to create concern on a national level, and in 1919 it was proposed that the country establish a national leprosy hospital. Public pressure restricted the possible sites; Angel Island in San Francisco Bay and one of the Florida keys were seriously considered. Eventually the Louisiana facility was chosen, largely because it was already established as a leprosy hospital. In 1921 the operation of the hospital was transferred from the state of Louisiana to the U.S. Public Health Service. From the beginning, the mission of the national hospital was threefold: patient care, teaching, and research.

The federal government largely rebuilt the facility during the 1930s. It was designed to house as many as 600 patients. The new buildings were state-of-the-art for their day. Patients resided in dozens of individual dormitories, all connected by covered walkways. Housing was built to accommodate about two dozen professional staff and their families. The new hospital had physicians' offices, an infirmary, an operating room, a pharmacy, an X-ray department, and a cafeteria and was able to provide physical, occupational, and recreational therapy. It had a patient canteen, library, recreation area, post office, golf course, school (accredited through grade 12), cemetery, jail, and 400-seat movie theater, as well as Catholic and Protestant chapels. For a time the center at Carville maintained its own internal telephone system, a power plant to generate its own electricity, and even a sizable dairy. It still operates its own water and sewerage systems. In short, it was designed to be a self-contained village, which, in many important respects, is exactly what it became.

Before the development of any effective treatment for leprosy, states had their own laws for the reporting and isolation of leprosy patients. Although not as harsh as the laws enforced in medieval Europe, they were nonetheless onerous. Individuals who were diagnosed with leprosy were removed from their homes, by force if necessary, and transported to Carville. Patients were advised to adopt an alias to protect their families from the stigma of the disease. It was routine for a married patient to be divorced by his or her healthy spouse. (Remarriage to a fellow Carville patient also was common.) In growing isolation from their families, patients frequently lost contact with life outside the institution, and their world shrank to the confines of the Carville community. Yet the stories told by patients who lived at Carville in the early decades of the 20th century do not paint a picture of isolation and despair. They tell instead of a close-knit community, friendships formed, and the kindness of the nuns.

Human trials of new remedies were the only method of research at the time, and Carville patients participated willingly. In the beginning virtually all attempts to improve treatment failed or were impractical. In 1941, however, this situation changed. One of the new remedies worked—and worked dramatically. The new treatment was called glucosulfone sodium, or Promin. Promin had drawbacks—it had to be given intravenously, on a regular schedule, and for a long period of time—but it was effective.

The next step was to develop an oral antileprosy drug, which would enable people with leprosy to be treated as outpatients. This goal was accomplished in the 1950s with the creation of sulfoxone sodium (Diasone), which was followed by dapsone, the parent chemical compound of Promin and Diasone. (Collectively these compounds are known as the sulfones.) Later came clofazimine, thalidomide (discovered to be useful in leprosy only after it had been found to cause birth defects), and rifampin.

By the 1960s newly diagnosed patients were no longer being forcibly removed from their families, jobs, and communities. An outpatient clinic was set up in San Francisco, and several private physicians were caring for leprosy patients in Texas. Some patients elected to go to Carville for treatment of complications or suspected drug-resistant disease or for reconstructive surgery. Some went for an initial examination and tests and to begin treatment. Carville doctors were available for telephone consultations as needed. Physicians trained at Carville seminars were identified as regional consultants. The trend toward decentralization of services and outpatient treatment grew steadily.

By the 1970s it had been shown that within a few days of starting drug treatment, leprosy patients were no longer infectious—thus, the rationale for isolation was removed. By the 1980s all newly diagnosed patients were encouraged to remain at home. Even the experimental drugs at that time, clofazimine and thalidomide, were made available to patients outside Carville through their private physicians or a national system of outpatient leprosy clinics set up, funded, and directed through Carville. By the early 1990s Carville had ceased to accept long-term admissions.

The village has now shrunk from a peak of some 500 patients in the 1950s to about 130 long-time residents, most in their 70s or older, who are free to come and go as they please. Although many have deformities and disabilities, the vast majority have been technically cured for decades. The research laboratory has moved from Carville to the campus of the Louisiana State University School of Veterinary Medicine in nearby Baton Rouge. New drugs and diagnostic tests and potential vaccines are now tested on experimental animals, and some research, using leprosy bacilli isolated from animals, is carried out entirely in test tubes.

Multidrug therapy: the standard

Resistance to the sulfones was first described in the mid-1960s, after these drugs had been in use for some 20 years. The discovery of resistant strains of *M. leprae* was made possible by what was then a new technology, a method of culturing (growing) bacilli from humans in the footpads of mice. As this procedure was adopted by leprosy-research laboratories around the world, reports of sulfone resistance grew. By that time other drugs were available, and it became the practice to switch a patient who developed sulfone-resistant disease to one of the other agents. When resistance to rifampin was described at Carville in the early 1970s in patients receiving it because they already had sulfone-resistant disease, the bacilli were shown in the laboratory to be resistant to both the sulfones and rifampin. The specter of a return to untreatable leprosy prompted the development of multidrug therapy. In 1971 at Carville the standard treatment regimen for advanced cases was changed from dapsone alone to dapsone plus rifampin for three years, followed by dapsone alone for life.

In the early 1980s, faced with many reports of sulfone resistance in patients treated with sulfones as a single drug, along with data suggesting that drug-resistant bacilli were being spread to new patients who might not respond to sulfones at all, WHO officials decided that the time had come for global action. After careful deliberation, experts assembled by WHO recommended that all leprosy patients receive multidrug therapy.

Ben Edwards—Impact Photos

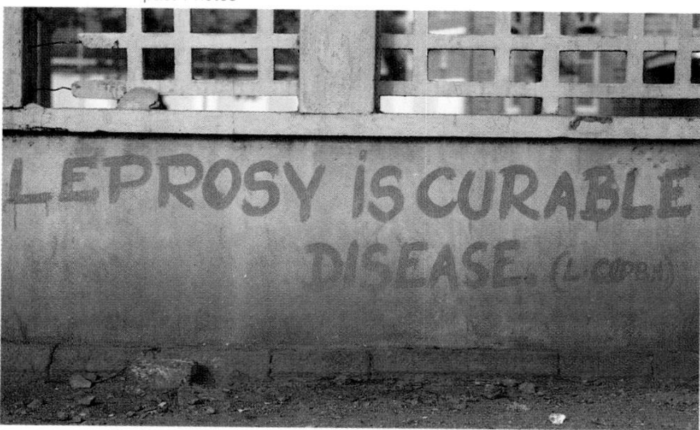

Slogan on a wall in Pune, India. Few authorities dispute the efficacy of modern combination drug therapy, but some take issue with the way the World Health Organization is going about "eliminating" the disease.

One of the measures suggested by this group was something that had never been systematically tried before: all leprosy treatment was to be strictly limited in duration. Patients with localized leprosy would be treated for only six months, and the most advanced cases would receive treatment for only two years. Initially these recommendations were highly controversial, but as experience with these regimens accumulated and as they were shown to be successful, they became the standard of treatment.

With the prospect of improved treatment and at the urging of groups long interested in combating the stigma of leprosy, public health authorities embraced the slogan "Leprosy is curable." It became popular in these circles to allude to the cumulative number of patients treated with these regimens as the number of patients "cured." Logically, these cured patients were taken off the lists of those with leprosy, which in turn led to reductions in the total number of patients receiving services in a given area of a country, in the country as a whole, and indeed in the world.

These quite reasonable practices had a reasonable, but to some surprising, consequence. Contributions to voluntary antileprosy organizations and support for government-funded antileprosy programs began to drop. The reasoning was that if leprosy was easily curable and dramatically fewer people had the disease than just a few years ago, then support for leprosy could be diverted to other worthy, but more pressing, programs. This notion was undoubtedly bolstered by the mushrooming AIDS epidemic.

Such was the situation when WHO, in partnership with voluntary and government antileprosy programs, launched its ambitious campaign to eliminate leprosy worldwide by the year 2000. It was believed that if support could continue to the year 2000, leprosy "as a public health problem" could be eliminated.

WHO's strategy: success by definition?

The WHO initiative to eliminate leprosy by 2000 will probably succeed. Skeptics would say, however, that this success is more a matter of semantics than of medical progress. In formulating its antileprosy program, WHO has changed the definition of two key epidemiological terms, *case* and *elimination*. Thus, a "case," which formerly was defined as a person with leprosy, is now defined as a person with leprosy who requires WHO multidrug therapy. According to this definition, once a patient has completed drug therapy, he or she is no longer included in the statistics. Since the recommended course of therapy is as short as six months for most patients, only half of those diagnosed and started on treatment in any given year are counted as "cases" for that year. As noted above, prior to the advent of multidrug therapy, it was advised that patients with the most advanced type of disease continue treatment for life. In those days the official number of leprosy cases in the world included all those still living who had ever been diagnosed with advanced disease, or some 10 million to 12 million cases. By changing the definition, WHO authorities have reduced that number to around 888,000. The natural history of the disease, however, is unchanged.

The term *elimination* has traditionally been defined by epidemiologists as the absence of new cases. Now it is defined by WHO as a prevalence of leprosy patients (*i.e.,* those requiring multidrug therapy) of less than one per 10,000 population. By this definition, Bangladesh, seventh in the world in leprosy prevalence, had virtually eliminated the disease by the end of 1995—a year when 8,800 new cases were detected there.

Finally, the expectation that leprosy will be eliminated by the year 2000 is likely to be self-fulfilling to a certain extent. With the perception that the disease has been eliminated, there will be reduced funding for the finding of new cases. Consequently, the number of new cases being reported will decrease.

Consigned to history?

Since the elimination program started, many concerned authorities have watched closely for evidence that combination drug treatment is interrupting the transmission of leprosy. The number of new cases detected each year continues to be around 550,000.

The accuracy of this detection rate is yet another subject of debate. On one side are those who feel that the long incubation period of leprosy necessarily means that the clear impact of combination drug treatment will be slow in coming. The current high rate of new cases, these authorities speculate, may be due to overdiagnosis on the part of career leprosy workers fearful of losing their jobs if the disease is declared eliminated. On the other side are those who claim that any observed reduction in leprosy incidence is the result of reduced program support and its inevitable consequence, reduced efforts to identify new cases. Moreover, they feel that there has already been ample time for multidrug therapy to reduce transmission if it was indeed capable of doing so. Whichever group is correct, support for antileprosy efforts will fall dramatically after the year 2000. As for the future of the disease and of those needing drug treatment or rehabilitative services, only time will tell.

—*Robert C. Hastings, M.D., Ph.D.*

Spotlight on Brief Therapy

In 1997 the mental health profession continued to evolve new and innovative ways to address mental health concerns. Approaches developed over the past several decades have replaced older, less effective methods of treatment, and fresh approaches will undoubtedly continue to be introduced into the therapeutic armamentarium. Despite the common misconception that therapy is almost always a long-term process that deals primarily with an individual's past, *brief therapy* methods represent the *mainstream* practice of psychotherapy today.

A concept comes of age

In the late 1960s the social climate encouraged a break with long-held traditions and orthodoxy. This extended to the mental health profession, where psychotherapists were increasingly challenged to go beyond merely explaining people's problems to actually resolving them. Traditional psychotherapy was typically a long-term affair; this was most apparent in its in-depth explorations of past influences on current symptoms. Therapies were usually bound to particular schools of thought (such as Freudian or Jungian analysis) that tended to be elaborate in their theorizing about abstract personality issues but often were not effective in providing relief from specific symptoms. Furthermore, professional help was often too expensive to be available to all who might benefit from it.

A demand for increased clinical services was propelled by the public's desire to obtain relief from a wide variety of problems. Researchers and clinicians were exhorted to come up with methods that would meet the diverse needs of patients at large—and that would do so in a timely manner. As a result, new types of therapy evolved. These approaches are briefer in duration than traditional methods, and they are more results-oriented for specific clinical problems.

In many industrialized countries profound changes are occurring in the way health care services are delivered, largely for economic reasons. In the United States for well over a decade, there has been a health care cost crisis, which has resulted in a need to streamline the delivery of care and make services cost-effective. This dynamic tension between providing health care that is profitable (for insurers) and at the same time beneficial (for consumers) is now more compelling than ever. Third-party payers understandably do not want to pay the costs of excessive or inefficient services for their subscribers in any health care arena—including mental health care. Consequently, insurers impose definitions that are used to determine which mental health problems are eligible for coverage and how long a prescribed therapy may take to resolve those problems—a system now quite familiar to most Americans and known as "managed care."

Psychotherapists in the U.S. (*i.e.,* state-licensed providers of mental health services, such as psychiatrists, psychologists, clinical social workers, and marital and family therapists) have had to adapt their treatment methods in order to meet the growing mandate for achieving measurable results in a limited number of therapy sessions. The onus is on therapists to use only treatments of proven value. These are known as "empirically validated treatments," or EVTs. Except in cases where the insured has a particularly serious condition, such as a psychotic disorder that requires hospitalization, there are time-limited constraints on outpatient treatment. Most insurers will cover their subscribers for only 6 to 20 psychotherapy sessions. Thus, in the age of managed care, brief therapy approaches have become important for reasons beyond the original desire to get the broadest possible results in the least amount of time.

Another reason for the increasing appreciation of briefer therapies is the mounting evidence that despite the "blueprints" that more traditional forms of psychotherapy were supposed to provide, patients often did not follow the "long-term plan." The clinical research indicates that the average patient attends fewer than 10 sessions no matter what treatment model the clinician adheres to. In fact, the most common duration of treatment is a single session, with no further contact. There are many reasons why an individual might see a psychotherapist only once; these range from not liking the clinician to simply desiring a single opportunity to "get things off one's chest." The key point is that for most people therapy tends to be brief, regardless of the clinician's philosophy or treatment plan.

Drawing by Bruce Eric Kaplan; © 1994 The New Yorker Magazine, Inc.

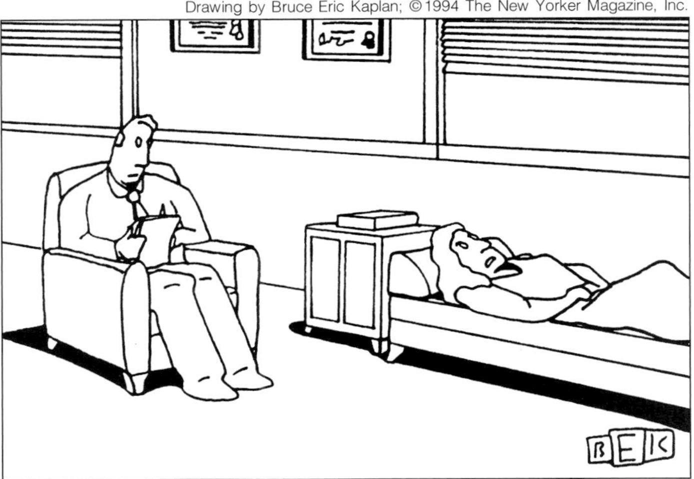

"Well, I do have this recurring dream that one day I might see some results."

From this perspective, brief therapy is not new. What is new, however, is the profession's greater willingness to "catch up" to the reality that consumers know what they want; moreover, they use therapeutic services in certain ways that may have little to do with a therapist's allegiance to a particular philosophy or treatment model. This is yet a further reason for the proliferation of shorter-term therapies. People have come to expect individual consideration in their health care rather than formulaic approaches whose "one-size-fits-all" methods may, in fact, *not* fit.

Variations on a (brief) theme

"Brief therapy" is not one specific modality. It is a generic label for a broad array of psychotherapeutic methods that may differ markedly from one another in terms of how clients' problems are conceptualized and treated. A number of methods that emphasize brevity have been developed by individual therapists and go by such names as *directive therapy, strategic therapy, solution-*

oriented therapy, short-term anxiety-provoking psychotherapy, time-limited psychotherapy, intensive short-term dynamic psychotherapy, and *interactional, developmental, and existential therapy.* On the whole, however, most brief therapies are eclectic, or *multimodal,* in their approach, and they share the key defining characteristics of being short-term and results-oriented. Other common denominators that further characterize brief therapy approaches include:

- an emphasis on the **context** of psychotherapy as a special relationship involving empathy, support, education, and gradual progress toward well-defined goals
- an emphasis on **action,** with minimal focus on intellectual analysis of past influences and traumas but a strong focus on the acquisition of specific problem-solving skills (treatment may include "homework" assignments between sessions that provide structured learning situations for the patient)
- an emphasis on **results supported by research** along with the recognition that the amount of time spent in treatment should not be equated with the depth or breadth of the results—in other words, *brief* does not mean *shallow* or *superficial*
- an emphasis on **resolving current symptoms,** which are seen as the product of ineffective attempts by an individual to cope with some stressor or life challenge, rather than an underlying problem that must first be identified and then "worked through" (such presumably underlying issues—*e.g.,* unconscious conflicts—are often abstract, theoretical formulations that cannot be defined clearly, nor can their precise role in generating specific symptoms be determined)

The above characteristics, all typical of brief therapy approaches, may be embedded in various practical frameworks. Practitioners of brief therapy have no illusion that in the course of treatment they can (or should) attempt to "reconstruct" entire personalities. Rather, specific problems and symptoms are methodically identified, as are specific resources for resolving them. On the other hand, it is not wise to rush the client through treatment, since it is well recognized that his or her need to be heard, understood, and empathized with is crucial to the success of *any* therapy. The key, then, is staying focused on what is central and relevant to resolving specific problems as quickly and efficiently as possible.

Amenable problems

What sorts of problems are most amenable to brief therapy? Fortunately, many of the most common mental health problems are resolvable in a limited time. A good example is the most common problem for which people seek psychotherapy: depression. Several brief therapy methods have proved highly effective in treating depression. These include cognitive, behavioral, and interpersonal psychotherapies that address common errors in thinking, ineffective behaviors, and difficulties in relationships, respectively. Problems in any or all of these areas may either cause or contribute to depression. Each of these approaches can effectively resolve depression for most people in about a dozen sessions.

Anxiety disorders are another common reason for people to seek professional help. These include:

- **panic attacks,** the sudden onset of unwarranted fear so intense that the sufferer may even believe death is imminent
- **social phobias,** in which people are so fearful of being scrutinized or judged harshly that they may involuntarily tremble, stammer, sweat, or become physically ill in the presence of others
- **specific phobias,** intense and irrational fears—*e.g.,* of heights (in general) or elevators (in particular); snakes, spiders, or sharks; being run over by a train; fire; water; and a vast variety of other particular objects, situations, or circumstances
- **obsessive-compulsive disorders,** persistent and intrusive thoughts and/or the need to engage in some ritualistic behavior over and

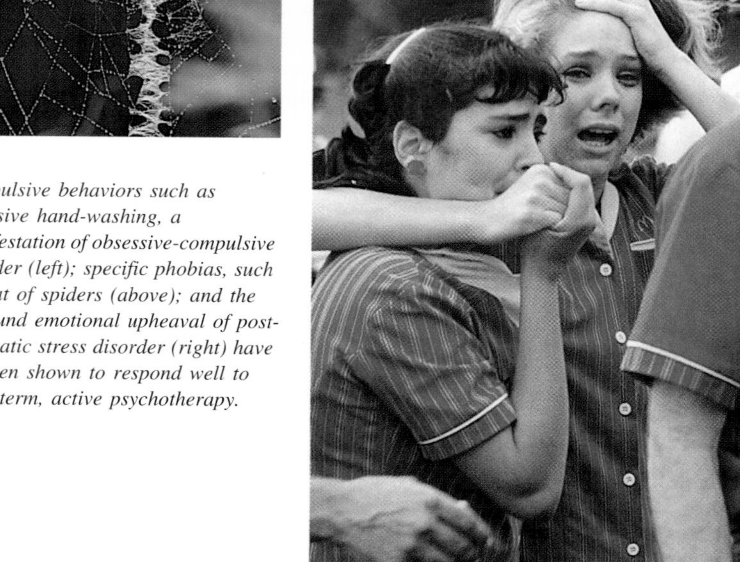

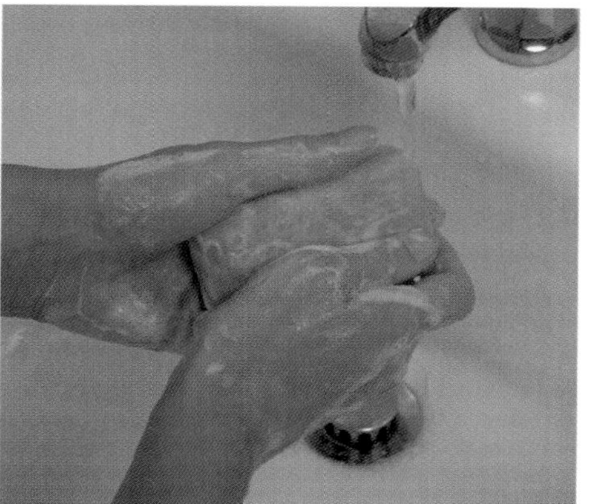

Compulsive behaviors such as excessive hand-washing, a manifestation of obsessive-compulsive disorder (left); specific phobias, such as that of spiders (above); and the profound emotional upheaval of post-traumatic stress disorder (right) have all been shown to respond well to short-term, active psychotherapy.

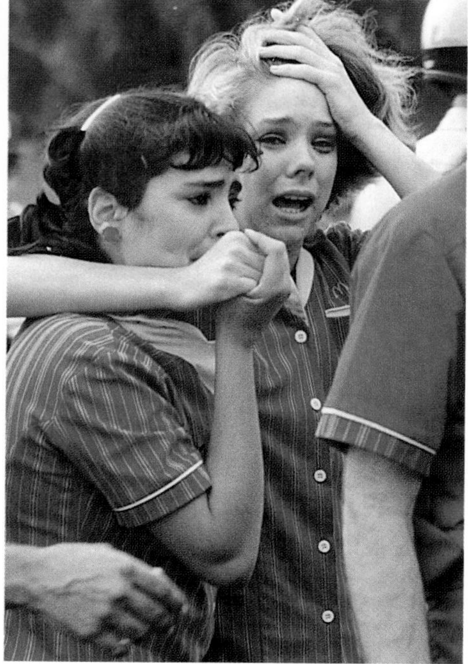

(Left) Peter L. Chapman—Stock, Boston/PNI; (center) Stephen Krasemann—Tony Stone Images; (right) Barry Fitzsimmons—San Diego Union-Tribune

over again, such as washing hands or checking to see whether a door is locked or the stove turned off
- **post-traumatic stress disorders,** the anxiety, depression, and flashbacks associated with a previous profoundly disturbing experience, such as being raped, being in an automobile crash, or experiencing a brutal crime

A variety of brief therapy methods are helpful in treating anxiety disorders. Cognitive therapy can help the sufferer come to terms with the irrationality of his or her reactions to certain stimuli. Other commonly successful approaches to treating anxiety conditions are exposure treatments (slowly increased exposure to an anxiety-producing stimulus under carefully constructed, safe conditions) and systematic desensitization (the use of relaxation techniques during exposure to imagined or actual events that provoke anxiety).

Still other conditions that have been shown to be responsive to brief interventions include eating disorders, pain, headaches, irritable bowel syndrome, certain forms of sexual dysfunction, and marital distress. The lack of mention here does not mean that a disorder will not be responsive to brief therapy. When a patient takes a particular problem to a qualified therapist, that practitioner is likely to be able to judge what type of treatment will be most effective.

Combining medication with brief therapy

Brief therapy interventions in the problem areas cited above may be offered independently of or in conjunction with medication. In many cases psychotherapy alone is as effective as or more effective than medication alone. Fortunately, it is not an "either-or" choice. Mental health professionals are mandated to offer all realistic treatment options with which they are familiar and for which they have been trained. Although a psychologist or social worker may not be able to actually prescribe drugs, he or she can refer the patient to an M.D. who can.

In some cases medication can be a wonderful ally in the treatment process, and so the appropriate use of medication in conjunction with brief therapy approaches is quite common. A compulsive hand-washer, for example, may fare well with behavioral treatment that focuses on refraining from acting on the urge to wash, reducing both the length of time and number of times a day spent performing the behavior, replacing the washing with another activity that occupies the hands, etc. That patient may benefit even more—completely overcoming the desire and need to wash hands that are not dirty—with appropriate response-prevention treatment plus a medication such as clomipramine (Anafranil) or one of the selective serotonin reuptake inhibitors—*e.g.,* fluoxetine (Prozac) or paroxetine (Paxil).

How long is "brief"?

Each client has unique needs and circumstances, of course, so what matters most is that whatever treatment is chosen, it is effective as well as efficient. What does the scientific literature indicate in regard to "usual" treatment duration for problems considered amenable to brief therapy? Definitions of brief therapy tend to specify anywhere from one to 20 sessions. Some recent research found that patients typically anticipate 6 to 10 sessions of therapy and that they report the greatest amount of change occurring in 6 to 8 sessions. These findings support earlier data gathered on about 2,400 patients over a period of 30 years; after 8 sessions approximately 50% of patients experienced measurable improvement, and by 26 sessions approximately 75% were demonstrably better. A meta-analysis (comprehensive review) of nearly 400 psychotherapy outcome studies involving more than 25,000 subjects—patients and controls (people receiving no treatment)—showed that psychotherapy was effective and that 17 sessions was an average treatment length.

Brief versus long: is one "better"?

If the main criterion for determining superiority of one treatment approach over another is simply the cost, then clearly short-term intervention is better for the patient. If the criterion is the resolution of specific symptoms, then brief therapy also fares quite well. If, on the other hand, the crucial criterion is patient satisfaction, there is considerable evidence that patients in longer-term therapy report a more enhanced quality of life than those who receive shorter-term therapy. Some patients desire an ongoing relationship with a clinician who knows them well and in whom they have developed deep trust. They value the opportunity to master important skills over longer periods of time and broader life experiences. These patients may want long-term care and not just the remission of current symptoms.

Most often, people have multiple problems, not just one, and therapists may enhance, diminish, or change approaches altogether as they receive relevant feedback from the patient. In general, the evidence strongly suggests that patients do best when they have the freedom to choose their own therapist and therapy modality and when they actively participate in that chosen treatment. This point has significant implications today, as managed care typically imposes artificial constraints on treatment (*i.e.,* it strictly limits patients' choices).

Scientific studies are invaluable for identifying the specific variables that influence the success of psychotherapy. The American Psychological Association (APA) has recently formed a Task Force on Psychological Interventions to help clinicians become familiar with those treatments that are best supported by data from controlled research. In controlled studies the therapeutic procedures are well defined, so it is generally possible to determine whether a therapy produces a specific effect. Patients are selected for a narrow range of symptoms and a specific diagnosis. It is fortunate for consumers that brief therapies can be studied under controlled conditions. The net result is a greater appreciation for all that shorter-term therapies can yield: positive, significant results that last. Longer-term therapies, given their broader focus and indeterminate length, cannot be studied as efficiently as briefer ones.

Another APA working group, the Task Force on Promotion and Dissemination of Psychological Procedures, has as its goal the dissemination of information from researchers to clinicians about EVTs. A list of EVTs was first published in 1995, then updated in 1996 and 1997. The task force has identified approximately two dozen therapies that it considers "effective" and another two dozen considered "likely to be effective" but still requiring further validation. To qualify as an EVT, a treatment must be time-limited, highly structured, and successful at resolving the patient's primary presenting problem.

A meeting of minds

In December 1996 in San Francisco, the Milton H. Erickson Foundation, Phoenix, Ariz., sponsored a five-day congress on brief therapy, at which dozens of short-term treatment modalities were represented. The meeting drew nearly 2,000 practicing psychotherapists from around the world. A number of scientific sessions looked at potential new applications for brief therapy. These included enhancing sports performance and treating substance abusers and victims of domestic violence. Innovations in treating problems already known to respond to brief therapy, such as marital distress, anxiety, and depression, were also introduced during the congress.

Getting into therapy: tips and caveats for consumers

Listed below are some factors to consider in seeking treatment.

- A consumer needs to know that a clinician is familiar with and has been trained in brief therapy methods that are known to be effective. Prospective patients can and should ask about the specific training of the clinician in question.
- Clinicians are ethically bound to discuss the efficacy of the treatment they intend to provide to new patients. They must also inform patients of valid alternatives.
- Consumers should know that there is almost never a "best treatment" for the problem because most problems are multifaceted.

It can be reasonably argued that alleviation of symptoms is not the sole criterion for "successful treatment." Considering these and other factors, it is clear that there is still no substitute for good clinical judgment derived from experience and training. Moreover, it should not be forgotten that shorter- and longer-term therapies each have their advantages, and "cost effective" may not necessarily be "best."

There are no national organizations devoted solely to brief therapy from which consumers can obtain referrals. It is always wise for a consumer to ask a trusted professional, such as one's family physician or primary care provider, for the names of qualified, reputable psychotherapists. Individual therapists will usually provide basic information over the phone, such as their fees, hours, and availability; whether they accept particular types of insurance; and whether they have special training or experience relevant to particular problems.

During a first appointment a client can expect to be asked to describe current problems, symptoms, and what efforts, if any, have already been made to resolve matters. The client can also use the first session to get an idea of the clinician's style—*e.g.,* his or her ability to listen well and provide empathy, support, and feedback and willingness to offer specific advice or other concrete information. During a first (or second) session the clinician should outline a sensible treatment plan and begin to structure active learning and skill-building opportunities. He or she should also indicate how progress in therapy will be measured. Above all, the consumer should feel that the relationship has the potential to be a positive and caring one focused on progress.

The mental health profession takes its mission—to help people in distress—seriously. The good news that emerges from the growing emphasis on briefer and more results-oriented therapies is that the great majority of people needing help can get it.

—*Michael D. Yapko, Ph.D.*

Making Headway Against Migraine

Headache has long been considered an inevitable part of the human condition. To the ancients, headache was a form of retribution visited upon them by the gods as punishment for blasphemy and other religious or worldly transgressions. Other early theories postulated that headaches were a sign of demonic possession. In the 1st century AD, the great Roman physician Aulus Cornelius Celsus described headache as: "much torpor, heaviness of the head, anxiety, and weakness." Of headache sufferers, he wrote, "For they flee the light; the darkness soothes their disease; nor can they bear readily to look upon or hear anything disagreeable." This very apt description of one particular kind of headache—migraine—applies just as well to today's sufferers (migraineurs) as it did to those of ancient Rome. The 2nd-century Greek physician Galen pronounced this type of headache *hemikrania* (*hemi* meaning "half" and *krania* meaning "cranium," or "skull"), describing headaches that frequently occur on one side of the head.

Over the past 10 years, headache has yielded many of its secrets to neuroscientific research. The findings have both underscored the logic of some traditional headache treatments and revealed the limitations of others. New theories on the origin and causes of headache are resulting in pharmacological treatments that directly address the mechanisms that underlie head pain. In particular, the serotonin receptors (cells found on blood vessels and nerve terminals in the brain that receive stimuli and transmit nerve impulses) have been identified as appropriate targets of therapeutic interventions.

A headache is not just a headache

Before discussing headache in any depth, it is important to establish some basics. First, there are many different headache types. Benign *primary* headaches must be differentiated from *secondary,* or organic, headaches. Primary headaches are those that are not due to other underlying diseases but have their own causes. Secondary headaches are those that result from other medical conditions, some of which may be serious, such as high blood pressure, brain tumor, aneurysm, brain hemorrhage, or meningitis.

Primary headaches can be classified as *tension-type, migraine,* and *cluster.* Tension-type headache occurs in 70% of the population and is characterized by mild to moderate steady pressure-type pain on both sides of the head. It tends to last for only a few hours and is easily treated with over-the-counter pain relievers or, alternatively, relaxation techniques. This kind of headache is termed tension-type because some individuals who get it may have tense muscles in the head, neck, or jaw and/or significant psychological tension (stress) in their lives. Most patients with tension-type headache, however, have biochemical defects that are similar to those of migraineurs.

Migraine may be inherited and usually begins between the ages of 8 and 25; in the United States it affects about 12% of the population (18% of women and 6% of men). The pain of migraine is throbbing or pounding, often occurs on only one side of the head, and may be associated with nausea, vomiting, and sensitivity to light and sound. In some cases a migraine attack is preceded by a visual aberration, or aura (*e.g.,* seeing many dots or zigzag,

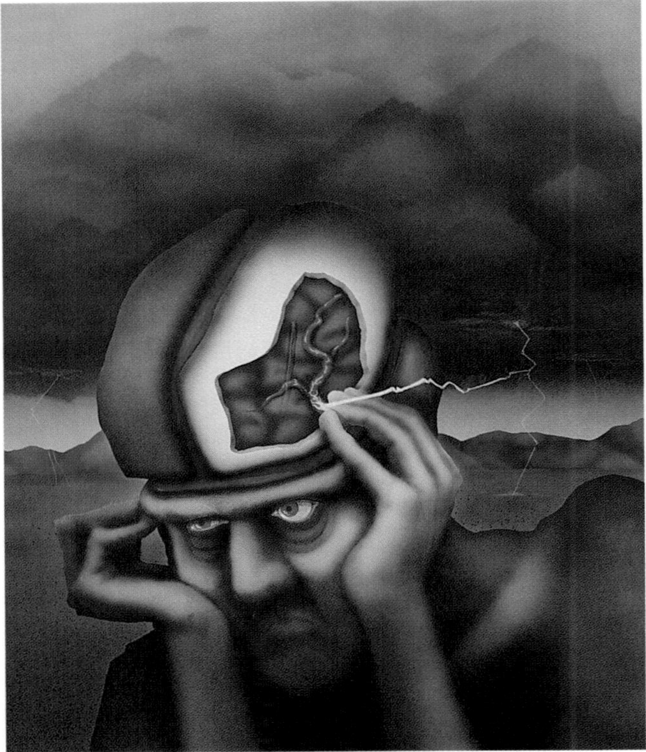

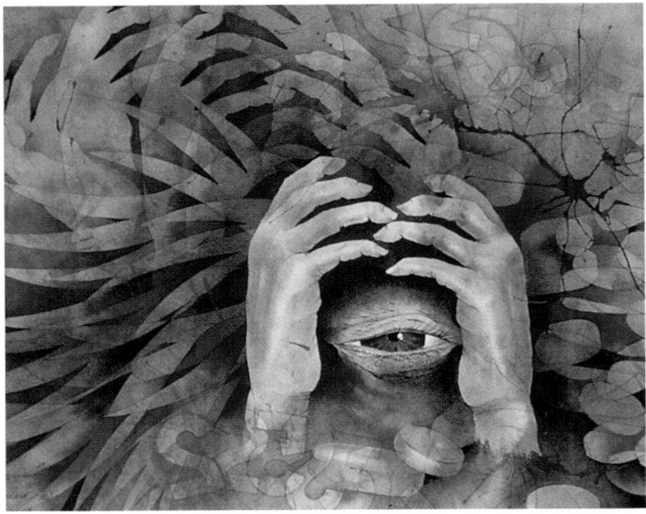

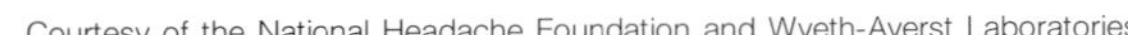

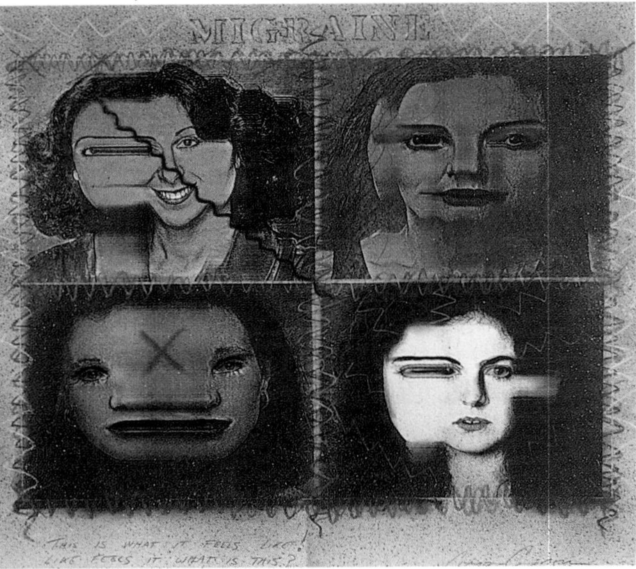

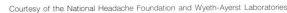

Vivid pictures of pain: three migraine headache sufferers illustrate the migraine experience (counterclockwise from above): "This Is How It Feels" by Clayton Campbell, "The Storm Returns" by Tom Wood, and "Violent Passages" by Louise Woodard.

colored, or shimmering lines), which lasts for 20 to 30 minutes. Migraine headaches vary from mild and annoying to disabling. For most patients attacks occur on average one to four times per month and last 12–48 hours. Often they cause disability severe enough to require patients to retreat to a dark, quiet room, refrain from moving, be absent from work, and miss out on usual home and leisure activities.

Cluster headache affects only about 0.1% of the population and occurs in middle-aged men five times more frequently than in women. In only about 3% to 15% of patients does it appear to be strongly inherited. Cluster headache is characterized by severe, painful attacks that occur in "clusters," periods that last four to six weeks, during which patients have one to three attacks each day and often awaken from sleep with a headache. Cluster pain, typically described as "steady," "boring," and "excruciating," is located in or around the eye and is frequently associated with redness and tearing of one eye and a stuffed or runny nostril on the same side of the head as the pain. Each attack lasts 45 to 90 minutes and is so severe that the patient often cannot stay still and must rock or pace. Patients tend to feel fine between attacks but anticipate the next attack with understandable dread.

Though secondary, or organic, headaches are uncommon, certain "red flags" should be regarded as potential signals of a serious condition. Headaches of this sort should be promptly evaluated by a physician. Signals include:

- any headache described as the "first severe headache" or the "worst headache ever"
- a headache associated with fever and stiff neck
- a headache associated with slurred speech, altered gait, or other neurological symptoms
- a progressive headache that follows head injury or trauma

Since migraine is common and tends to be so disabling, it has been the focus of intensive research and has received more attention than have other types of headache.

Headache's causes: cumulative insights

Because most headaches are not caused by brain tumors, hemorrhage, allergies, sinus problems, or dental problems, neurologists have had to look elsewhere for answers. Currently not all the mechanisms of headache (in general) and migraine (in particular) are understood. Most headaches, however, can be attributed to biological mechanisms in the brain, blood vessels, muscles, and occasionally the neck, rather than to psychological factors. Although social and emotional factors may play an important role

From R.P. Woods, M. Iacoboni, and J.C. Mazziotta,"Bilateral Spreading Cerebral Hypoperfusion During Spontaneous Migraine Headache," *The New England Journal of Medicine*, vol. 331, no. 25 (Dec. 22, 1994), pp. 1689–92; ©1994 Massachusetts Medical Society

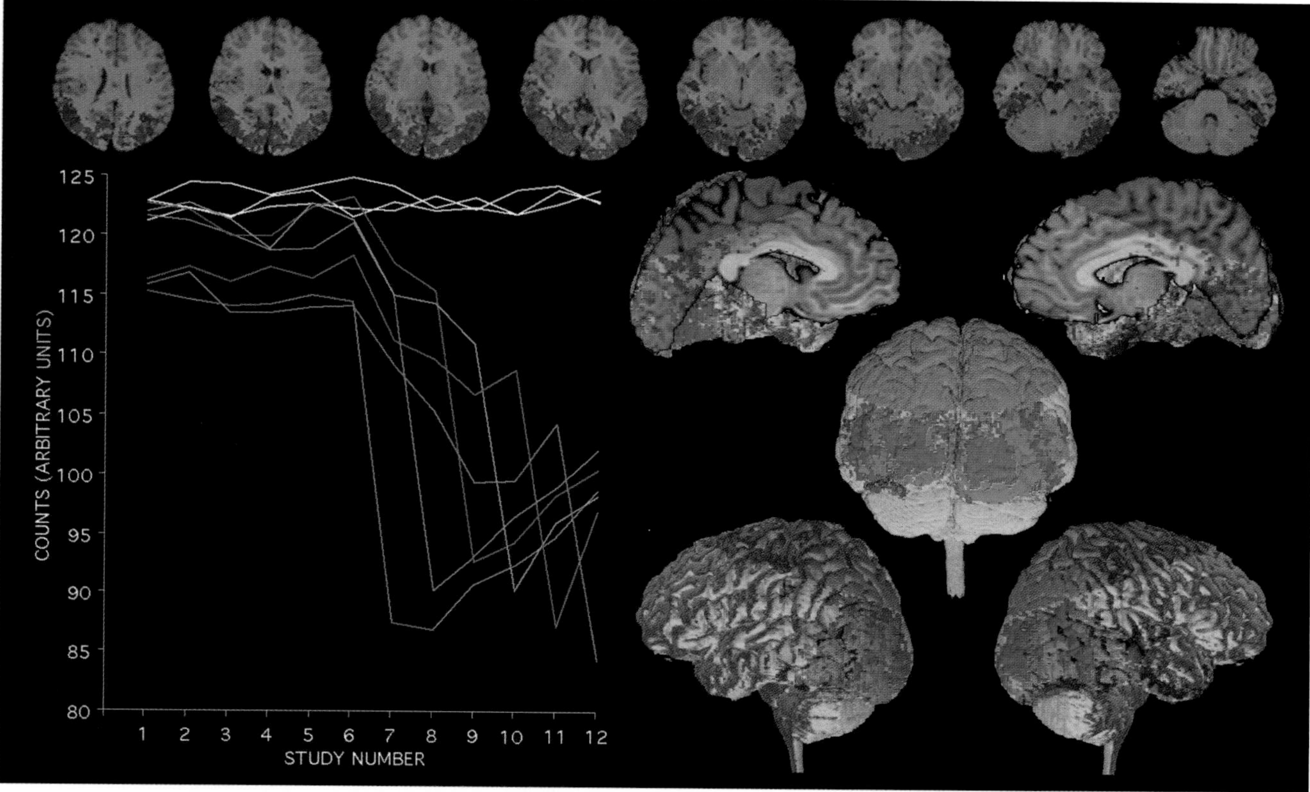

These complex brain images delineate alterations in the brain's blood flow during the migraine headache of a 21-year-old female subject. The top eight two-dimensional images show various planes of the brain in which blood flow was measured ("counts"on the graph) in a series of studies. The five three-dimensional images were obtained by positron emission tomography scanning; the six colors, to which the colors on the graph correspond, depict brain areas of interest in which blood flow altered during the progress of the headache. The grey areas were outside the field of the PET scanner.

in headache, they usually act as triggers rather than as underlying causes. Diet; assorted sights, sounds, and smells; weather; atmospheric pressure; lack of sleep; physical exertion; and various medications may also act as triggers. The specific stimuli will vary widely among patients.

Some researchers believe that headache pain is due to the release of chemical substances that affect the brain's outermost (peripheral) blood vessels—those in the meninges, membranes that cover the brain. Others maintain that all clinical manifestations of migraine, including the pain, are the result of central nervous system processes that take place deep within the brain and in the brain stem. A unifying theory that encompasses many hypotheses has been proposed.

The latter holds that prior to a migraine attack, the platelets (the small disk-shaped components of the blood) become rich in the neurotransmitter serotonin (5-HT). (Neurotransmitters are naturally occurring brain chemicals that transmit nerve impulses.) Serotonin levels in the blood increase just before a headache begins and decrease during and after the headache itself. In 1967 a platelet-releasing factor was found to be present in the blood during a typical migraine attack. Once 5-HT has been released from the platelets, it acts as a potent vasoconstrictor, narrowing the blood vessels; 5-HT is thought to be one of a number of naturally occurring substances that work together to sensitize the blood vessel walls to painful distention (vasodilation).

Early theories suggested that migraine began with a tightening of the arteries carrying blood to the occipital lobes in the back of the brain—specifically to the visual cortex. This, in turn, led to dilation of the arteries on the surface of the scalp, putting pressure on the pain-conducting nerves in the walls of these arteries, which resulted in a headache. These changes were accompanied by a decrease in cerebral blood flow and spreading electrical activity across the cerebral cortex.

This excitation of neurons across the cerebral cortex, so-called cortical spreading depression, was first described in 1944 by A.A. Leão at Harvard Medical School, whose experimental studies were carried out in rabbits. Leão theorized that after a sudden increase in electrical activity in the rear of the rabbit's brain, an electrical wave begins at the back of the brain and slowly spreads forward. Rabbit brains provided an excellent model for studying electrical events in the brains of migraineurs. In the late 1980s K.M.A. Welch and co-workers at the Henry Ford Hospital in Detroit used the procedure known as magnetoencephalography to measure both electrical potentials (patterns of electrical discharge) and magnetic waves given off by the brains of patients early in an attack. They noted temporary decreases in the patients' electrical cortical potentials, which suggested a mechanism in human brains that correlated with the spreading depression proposed by Leão. Welch and other researchers also noted low levels of magnesium within the brain cells, which they thought might lead to the electrical irritability of the cortex and the spreading electrical charges.

In 1981 Jes Olesen and associates in Copenhagen demonstrated that migraineurs with a visual aura preceding the headache have a decrease in cerebral blood flow that begins in the occipital region and extends forward in a wavelike fashion across the cortex at a speed of two to three millimeters per minute. Interestingly, this wave, which lasts for several hours, does not follow the vascular pathways. The visual warning symptoms of a migraine aura begin while the cerebral blood flow is diminished, after which the flow increases to above normal and then returns to baseline. This pattern apparently does not occur in patients who have migraine without aura.

In 1994 Roger P. Woods, Marco Iacoboni, and John C. Mazziotta of the University of California, Los Angeles, were able to delineate the alterations in the brain's blood flow in relation to migraine headache. They happened to be measuring a patient's cerebral blood flow, using the imaging technique known as positron emission tomography (PET), when the patient unexpectedly developed a migraine headache. The ensuing scans showed

NEWS MHA 98 CAP

Exercising Caution: Concussions and Athletes

During a high school football game, a wide receiver strikes his head on the ground as he is being tackled. He remains conscious, but for 20 minutes he feels dizzy and has trouble focusing his attention. His symptoms clear at halftime, and he asks to return to the game. Should the player be allowed to take the field again?

Definitely not, according to guidelines for the management of sports-related concussions released by the American Academy of Neurology (AAN) in 1997. In a report published in the March issue of *Neurology,* a committee of AAN experts stressed that athletes who have their "bell rung" during a game may be more seriously affected than coaches or the athletes themselves often realize at the time. Repeated concussions occurring within a short period of time—a phenomenon known as "second-impact syndrome"—may result in cumulative brain damage and even the athlete's death in some cases.

"People throw around the phrase 'minor concussion,' but there is no such thing," said James P. Kelly, director of the Brain Injury Program at the Rehabilitation Institute of Chicago and one of the chief authors of the AAN report. Kelly and his fellow researchers defined a concussion as an alteration in mental status that results from a head trauma but that may or may not involve the loss of consciousness. An estimated 300,000 sports-related concussions occur in the U.S. every year. Second-impact syndrome has been reported in football, ice hockey, boxing, and snow skiing but could occur in many other sports, recreational or competitive.

In their report, AAN members used a grading scale to categorize concussions and made treatment recommendations for each of the three grades:

- Grade 1: The athlete suffers momentary confusion (frequently observed symptoms include vertigo, inattention, befuddled facial expression, delayed verbal or motor responses) but does not lose consciousness. The athlete should be examined immediately and at five-minute intervals thereafter but may return to the sports activity if the concussive symptoms last less than 15 minutes. A second Grade 1 concussion in the same contest, however, would eliminate the player from competition that day.
- Grade 2: Again, the athlete is temporarily confused but is not rendered unconscious; the concussive symptoms in this case last longer than 15 minutes. The player should be removed from the contest for immediate examination and not be allowed to return. Computed tomography (CT) or magnetic resonance imaging (MRI) scanning is recommended in all instances where symptoms worsen or persist more than one week.
- Grade 3: The athlete is rendered unconscious. If the loss of consciousness is prolonged, the athlete should be transported by ambulance to the nearest emergency room and should be withheld from play until asymptomatic for two weeks. If unconscious for only a few seconds, the athlete should not play until asymptomatic for one week. A player who suffers a second Grade 3 concussion should be withheld from the sports activity until asymptomatic for one month. Any athlete with an abnormality on CT or MRI scans that is consistent with brain swelling, contusion, or other intracranial pathology should be withheld from play for the season and discouraged from future participation in contact sports.

If followed, the AAN guidelines should effectively prevent second-impact syndrome. The Centers for Disease Control and Prevention emphasized in an article published in *Morbidity and Mortality Weekly Report* (March 14, 1997) that doctors, physical education instructors, coaches, trainers, parents, and the general public should become familiar with the new recommendations. One organization, the Washington, D.C.-based Brain Injury Association, has begun distributing the guidelines in public schools through its Head Smart program.

—*Sherman Hollar*

not only reduced blood flow on both sides of the brain but that the reduced flow originated in the occipital lobes and spread forward into the temporal and parietal lobes (*see* illustration, page 295).

In 1995 Cornelius Weiller, H.C. Diener, and others at the University of Essen, Ger., identified the so-called migraine generator in the brain stem in nine patients during one-sided migraine headaches without aura. They, too, utilized high-resolution PET scanning to define changes in regional cerebral blood flow within specified cortical and brain-stem regions and found that migraine was accompanied by consistent activation within the upper brain stem (specifically, in the midbrain and pons), as well as in the cingulate, auditory, and visual cortices. After being given an effective migraine medication, sumatriptan (*see* below), these patients no longer had head pain, but increased blood flow within the brain stem persisted for more than 24 hours. This suggested a prominent role for two areas of the brain stem not previously associated with migraine—the dorsal raphe nucleus in the midbrain (containing 5-HT) and the norepinephrine-containing locus coeruleus in the pons. (Norepinephrine is another neurotransmitter.) It was these areas that acted as the migraine generator, and they were active long after the headache had disappeared.

The so-called trigeminal nerves and blood vessels in the meninges are connected to the brain stem by a system that relays sensory information to the thalamus deep within the brain and then on to the cortex, where the pain is registered. It is at this interface between nerve endings and blood vessels in the meninges that the typically throbbing or pounding pain of migraine is thought to be generated.

A variety of neurotransmitters may be involved in this process, and it is likely that other brain chemicals mediate the dilation of the blood vessels and/or the plasma leakage from blood vessels, causing a cascade of biochemical reactions that leads to synthesis of pain-promoting chemicals such as prostaglandins and histamine, which are associated with inflammation. Brain blood vessels have specific receptors that react to these chemicals, which may explain why headache but not other pain of vascular origin develops in response to some stimuli. The release of these neurotransmitters is blocked by medications such as sumatriptan, zolmitriptan, and dihydroergotamine (*see* below).

A recent hypothesis about vascular headache pain focuses on nitric oxide (NO), a gas that diffuses freely across membranes. This theory postulates that NO may be in part responsible for headache-associated vasodilation. Medications such as calcium channel blockers, tricyclic antidepressants, and others that block 5-HT prevent the formation of NO and are often helpful in treatment of headache.

Enlightened treatment

Each type of headache has its own set of treatment protocols. Most primary headaches are self-limited—that is, they go away on their own; nonetheless, it is usually appropriate to administer medication to relieve pain and abort the headache process before it progresses into a full-blown attack, which may lead to significant disability. In the case of migraine, preventive medications can be given daily to decrease the frequency and possibly the severity and duration of attacks. Most tension-type headaches respond well to over-the-counter pain relievers—analgesics, such as aspirin and acetaminophen, and nonsteroidal anti-inflammatory drugs (NSAIDs), such as ibuprofen and naproxen. Combination agents that contain aspirin, acetaminophen, and the vasoconstrictor caffeine may be even more effective for tension-type headache. Caution must be used, however, when taking nonprescription drugs for pain, because chronic overuse may lead to the "rebound" headache phenomenon, sometimes called "withdrawal" headache, in which headaches become more constant and severe, as well as harder to treat.

Isometheptene, an antispasmodic agent that constricts blood vessels, is combined with the analgesic acetaminophen and dichloralphenazone, a mild sedative, in an effective prescription medication that treats both tension-type and migraine headache. The NSAIDs and stronger opiates, *e.g.,* codeine, can also be used within appropriate limits to relieve almost any acute headache. Some patients do well with occasional use of a combination product that contains aspirin, caffeine, and butalbital (a potent sedative).

Medications that hold promise as agents that may help prevent migraine are ones that in some way block serotonin from binding to the serotonin receptor subtype 5-HT$_2$, lower the reactive potential of the receptor, or modulate the discharge of neurons that are activated by serotonin. Several migraine-specific agents taken regularly for a minimum of three to four weeks have proved useful in decreasing the frequency of migraine. These include beta-adrenergic blockers (also called beta-blockers) such as propranolol and atenolol; calcium channel blockers such as verapamil; tricyclic antidepressants such as amitriptyline and nortriptyline; another type of antidepressant medication, monoamine oxidase inhibitors, such as phenelzine and tranylcypromine; some anticonvulsant agents such as divalproex sodium and possibly gabapentin; and serotonin antagonists such as methysergide and cyproheptadine.

Migraine and cluster headaches present great therapeutic challenges. Early treatment of these types of headache included nonspecific drugs (tablets and suppositories). Today patients may take tablets or administer headache medications by self-injection and nasal spray (*see* below), which, like suppositories, may be more appropriate for those with nausea and vomiting.

Ergotamine tartrate has been used extensively for more than half a century to abort migraine attacks. The substance was initially believed to act only as a vasoconstrictor. Now, however, it appears that ergotamine stimulates 5-HT$_1$ receptors, which accounts for its effectiveness in interrupting the migraine process before the headache has become advanced and resistant to treatment. Excessive use of ergotamine, however, is associated with so-called ergot rebound headache (recurrent headaches that are increasingly tolerant to ergot). Therefore, in most cases ergotamine should be taken only one day per week. The exception to this rule is during "menstrual migraine," when women may be advised to take ergot medication as many as three days in one week. Ergotamine tartrate is available in both suppository and tablet forms.

A derivative of ergotamine—dihydroergotamine (DHE)—has been available since 1945 and offers relatively prompt relief of migraine symptoms, generally with less nausea than other ergot preparations. This form of the medication, too, is believed to act on the 5-HT$_1$ receptor. DHE's advantage over ergotamine tartrate is that it can abort an acute migraine attack that has already progressed to severe headache, generally without inducing nausea and vomiting.

Whereas ergotamine causes nausea as a side effect, sumatriptan, a vasoconstrictor and a powerful and highly selective 5-HT_1 agonist that became available in 1993, rapidly relieves both head pain and migraine-associated nausea. (An agonist is a chemical capable of initiating a reaction or an activity by combining with a receptor on a cell.) Although both sumatriptan and DHE are available by injection, only sumatriptan is supplied in a convenient, easy-to-administer, self-injectable form.

A tablet form of sumitriptan is now available as well. Sumatriptan has a shorter duration of activity than DHE, as well as a more rapid onset of activity. Sumatriptan seems to work more rapidly than DHE during the first 2 hours, but the effects of both agents are roughly equal at 24 hours following injection. DHE results in a lower incidence of recurrent headache than sumatriptan, perhaps as a result of its longer persistence in the body.

Medications in the nose: nothing to sniff at

Intranasal delivery of medications such as sumatriptan and DHE has been demonstrated to be safe and effective in migraine, although neither of these medications is currently available commercially in such a formulation. Nasal administration promises convenient, rapid therapy without the inherent limitations imposed by self-injection and suppository methods. It also has an advantage over oral medications such as tablets or capsules, which have considerably slower onset of activity. As might be expected, injectable forms of these agents provide the most rapid relief; intranasally administered agents, however, are right behind, producing earlier relief than oral forms.

Clinical studies suggest that in the coming years intranasal delivery may become a method of choice for delivering headache medications. A number of agents appear to have potential.

- Butorphanol nasal spray is a strong, easy-to-use opiate that may block pain within 15 minutes in many patients; it is especially useful in that it may obviate the need for a visit to the emergency room for treatment of acute pain. Butorphanol often provides an alternative for management of severe headache pain when the more migraine-specific medications are contraindicated or have failed; moreover, butorphanol may have a slightly lower abuse potential than other opiates, but it still must be prescribed cautiously.
- A 4% solution of lidocaine, a type of painkiller that has been around for a long time and that dentists often use as an anesthetic, has been used in drop form in one recent randomized, double-blind, controlled trial. It was found to provide prompt but usually unsustained relief of migraine pain. An earlier trial had shown that lidocaine sometimes works in the treatments of cluster headache. Not yet adequately tested, intranasal lidocaine has been associated with rapid headache recurrence, which appears to be an important drawback that may limit its clinical utility.
- Intranasal capsaicin (red pepper extract) seems most likely to be of benefit for cluster headache sufferers; it appears to provide both pain relief and prevention of headache during the cluster period. Capsaicin desensitizes the sensory neurons by depleting the nerve terminals of substance P, a neurotransmitter that is believed to contribute significantly to the transmission of the "pain message."

In the pipeline

There are other promising pharmaceuticals in the pipeline for migraine. One of these, zolmitriptan (called 311C90 during early investigational studies), is a centrally and peripherally acting serotonin agonist that may directly interfere with inflammation. Zolmitriptan should soon be approved by the U.S. Food and Drug Administration to treat acute migraine. It is hoped that its use will decrease headache recurrence and that it may provide slightly faster onset of relief than some currently available agents.

Still other experimental agents, including rizatriptan, naratriptan, eletriptan, and VML 251 (a compound as yet unnamed), work only peripherally. Each of these agents is roughly similar in action and side-effect profile to sumatriptan, but as a group they may give clinicians more options for matching therapeutic agents to specific patients' requirements.

If any one of these newer drugs has characteristics that offer even slight improvement over sumatriptan, it could capture a significant share of the market for drugs used in the acute treatment of migraine. The characteristics under study are efficacy, speed (the time to meaningful headache relief), duration of effectiveness, likelihood of recurrent headaches, and, of course, safety and tolerability.

Outlook bright

This is an undeniably exciting time in neuroscientific research in general and in headache research in particular. The next five years promise to bring many new oral and intranasally delivered agents for the specific treatment of migraine headaches. The search for medications with a novel mechanism of action is ongoing; researchers are looking for agents that will stop a migraine attack more quickly, more completely, or more consistently than is currently possible or one that could be given daily to prevent such attacks entirely. It is also realistic to expect breakthroughs in understanding of the genetics of migraine, which may lead to more accurate diagnostic tests for migraine and more effective treatments.

—Alan M. Rapoport, M.D.

HEADACHE HELP

- Duckro, P.N., Richardson, W.D., and Marshall, J.E. *Taking Control of Your Headaches: How to Get the Treatment You Need.* New York: Guilford Press, 1995.
- Lipton, R.B., Newman, L.C., MacLean, H., and Mark, M. *Migraine: Beating the Odds; The Doctor's Guide to Reducing Your Risk.* Reading, Mass.: Addison-Wesley Publishing Co., 1992.
- Rapoport, A.M., and Sheftell, F.D. *Headache Relief.* New York: Simon & Schuster, 1990.
- Rapoport, A.M., and Sheftell, F.D. *Headache Relief for Women: How You Can Manage and Prevent Pain.* Boston: Little, Brown and Co., 1995.
- Robbins, L.D., and Lang, S.S. *Headache Help: A Complete Guide to Understanding Headaches and the Medicines That Relieve Them.* Boston: Houghton Mifflin Co., 1995.
- Saper, J.R., Silberstein, S.D., Gordon, C.D., and Hamel, R.L. *Handbook of Headache Management.* Baltimore, Md.: Williams & Wilkins, 1993.

(Opposite page) Mike Guastella—Associated Press

Alzheimer's Disease Update

In the past few years the news media have paid an enormous amount of attention to Alzheimer's disease, a fact that reflects both the accelerated pace of research and the growing public awareness of this age-related neurodegenerative disorder. Also in the past few years, the first drugs for the specific treatment of Alzheimer's disease were approved for use in the U.S., a development that has raised the hopes of both patients and families.

Of particular importance to the relatives of those with Alzheimer's disease, and especially to their children, have been advances in the understanding of the genetics of the disease; the prospect of genetic testing has stirred understandable anxiety among those who may be at increased risk. For the scientists involved in the research, recent years have been exciting and marked by real progress on several fronts. The following strives to put recent developments into perspective, examining the expectations that have been raised by the new findings and perhaps alleviating some of the confusion and concern that have surrounded them.

Facts and figures

Although dementia is typically defined as a decline in intellectual or cognitive abilities sufficient to interfere with a person's work or social life, it nearly always has other features. Prominent among these are problems with memory for recent events and impairment of other higher functions such as spatial orientation and ability to perform mathematical calculations. Dementia has many causes, from stroke to severe vitamin deficiencies, and evaluation of the patient by a physician, preferably a neurologist or psychiatrist, is essential to the diagnosis.

Alzheimer's disease is the largest single cause of dementia in persons over the age of 65. The percentage of this age group who are affected varies widely from study to study, but the most reliable figures place it at about 8%. The percentage of those affected increases with the age of the population, however; thus, estimates of the prevalence of Alzheimer's disease in the over-80 age group range from 20% in some surveys to an astonishing 50% in others.

For the industrial countries of the Western world, where life expectancy is now over 80, the growing number of persons at risk for Alzheimer's disease is a public health problem of potentially major proportions. Presumably, the same issues will confront less-developed countries as life expectancies increase with improved standards of living. In general, however, the incidence and prevalence of Alzheimer's disease do not appear to vary substantially from country to country.

Disease hallmarks: plaques and tangles

Two different kinds of abnormal structures, or lesions, are typically seen in the brains of individuals with Alzheimer's: neuritic plaques and neurofibrillary tangles. When these two are present

The candor of former U.S. president Ronald Reagan (shown in July 1997 greeting visitors to the Reagan library) and his family when he was diagnosed with Alzheimer's disease contributed enormously to the public awareness of the disease. The prevalence of this age-associated disorder is fairly certainly destined to increase in the near future.

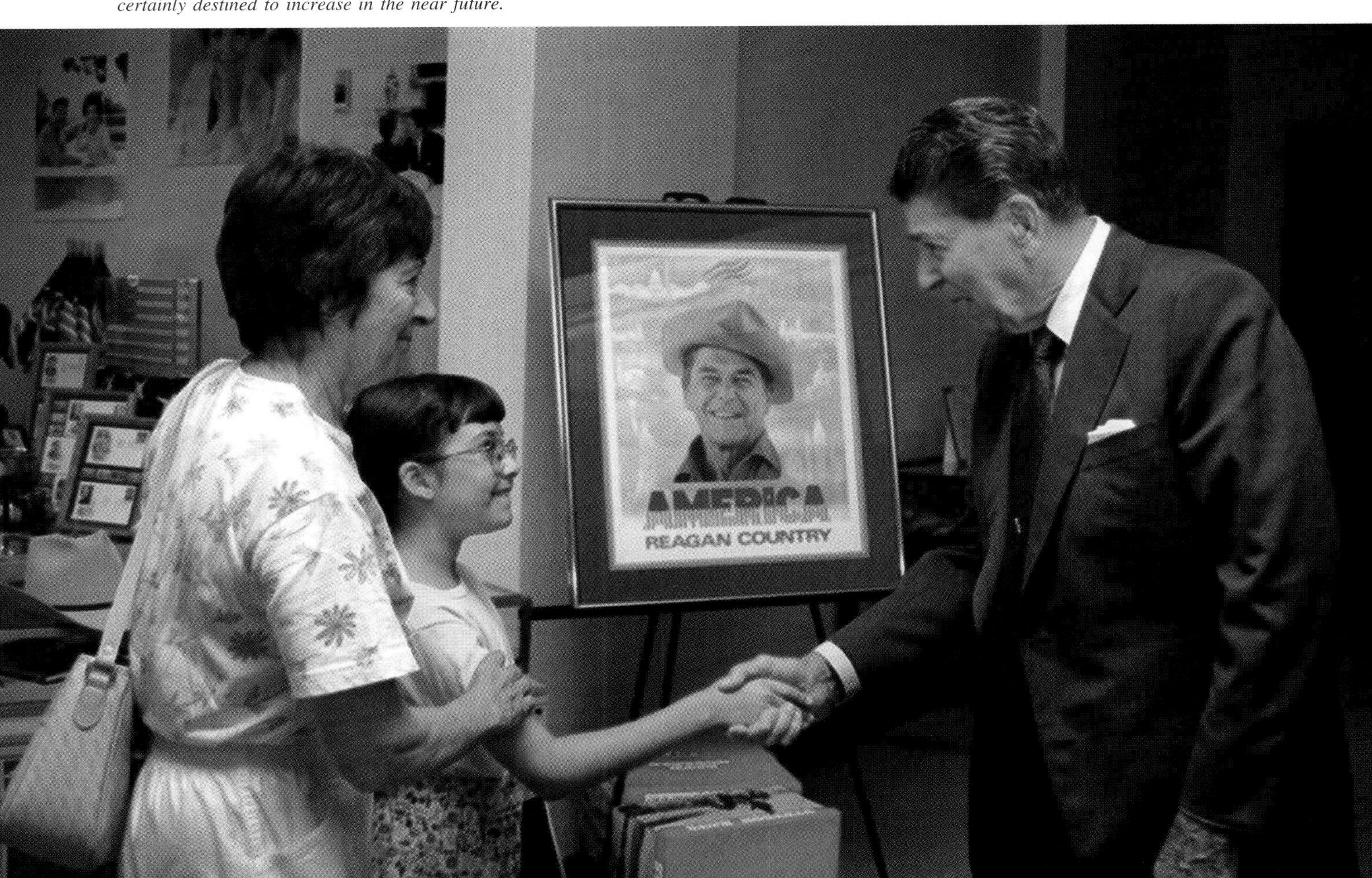

in large numbers in tissue taken from the cerebral cortex of a deceased patient, the diagnosis of Alzheimer's disease can be made with certainty. Despite widely publicized recent reports of innovative tests for detecting Alzheimer's disease during life (discussed in detail below), autopsy of the brain remains the sole reliable method for confirming the diagnosis.

The neuritic plaque is a complex structure consisting of a central core of protein material called amyloid, surrounded by degenerating neuronal processes (structures that project from nerve cells and normally connect them to each other). In apparent response to the degeneration, two of the major types of supporting cells in the brain, astrocytes and microglial cells, increase in size—and perhaps in number—and cluster around the plaque.

The neurofibrillary tangle is a mass of filaments, usually within a neuron (nerve cell) but also sometimes seen as a "ghost" after the neuron has degenerated. Plaques and tangles are not found in all regions of the brain; for the most part, they are present in the cerebral cortex, including the hippocampus. These are areas believed to be important in the higher intellectual functions such as memory and abstract thinking, which are so often impaired early in the course of Alzheimer's disease.

(Top) Robert D. Terry; (below) Peter Davies

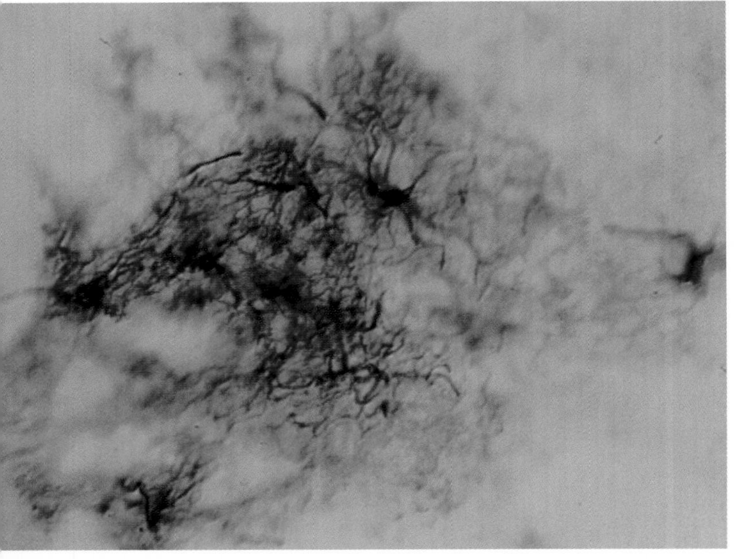

(Above) Seen under the microscope, a neuritic plaque from the brain of an Alzheimer's disease patient is surrounded and infiltrated by astrocytes (stained brown), one of the brain's major types of supporting cells. (Top) While many of the pathological features of Alzheimer's disease are visible only when brain tissue is examined under the microscope, the characteristic shrinkage of the brain is immediately apparent at autopsy.

In very general terms, the more plaques and tangles the neuropathologist finds in the brain on autopsy, the more severely demented the patient at the time of his or her death. The development of these lesions therefore appears to be an important part of the disease process. Over the last few years, scientists have gained greater understanding of the nature and formation of the lesions, but they still do not agree exactly which features are the most important for disease progression—and thus should be the prime target for drug development. For now, multiple lines of research are under way.

Amyloid accumulation: a central puzzle

A huge amount of research over the past 10 years has focused on the amyloid protein. The chemist George Glenner and his colleagues at the University of California, San Diego, first isolated and sequenced a portion of the amyloid protein from the brains of Alzheimer's patients in 1986. Several groups of investigators used the published protein sequence to identify the gene that encodes, or directs the synthesis of, the protein. Scientists now know that this protein, which is called beta-amyloid, is a peptide (a small protein) consisting of a linear sequence of from 40 to 42 amino acids. (Amino acids are the building blocks of protein.)

The gene that encodes the beta-amyloid sequence is large and complex and has the capacity to direct the production of at least five amyloid precursor proteins (APP). The simplest of these, and the major protein produced from the *APP* gene in the brain, is APP695, a molecule consisting of 695 amino acids. (By scientific convention, the names of genes are italicized.) The precise amino acid sequence of the material found in the deposits in the brains of Alzheimer's patients is located in a region toward one end of this long protein. The normal function of the APP still is not known, nor do scientists yet understand the function of the peptides produced when special enzymes, acting like a "chemical scissors," cleave, or cut, the larger protein molecule into smaller units.

It is clear that deposition of beta-amyloid in Alzheimer's disease must take place as a result of cleavage of APP695 at two sites, one at either end of the 40–42-amino-acid peptide. Early biochemical studies showed that in the healthy brain APP is indeed cleaved, but at a site *within* the peptide sequence rather than at either end of it. If the beta-amyloid sequence is normally interrupted, scientists reasoned, it would be impossible for molecules of the material to accumulate in the brain. This supposition proved incorrect, however. While it is true that most of the APP in the brains of normal individuals is cleaved within the amyloid peptide, scientists found that a small amount of the 40–42-amino-acid peptide is being produced continuously. It appears, therefore, that while all individuals make some beta-amyloid protein, it is deposited in large quantities only in persons with Alzheimer's disease.

Photographs, Peter Davies

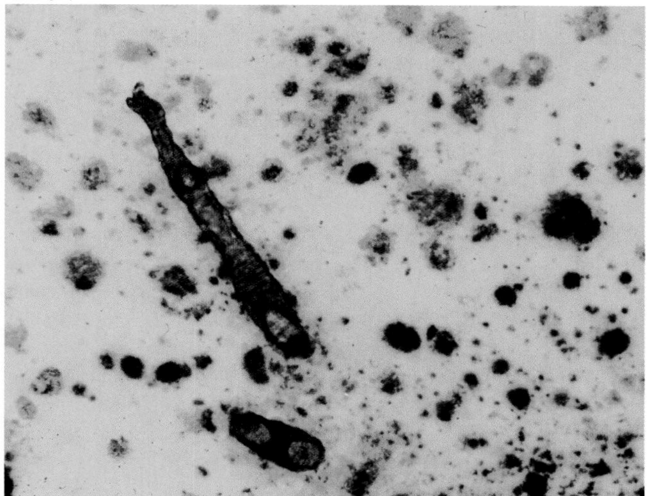

Although the accumulation in the brain of amyloid (brown) has long been recognized as a characteristic feature of Alzheimer's disease, the protein's precise role in the disease is still a mystery.

If accumulation of beta-amyloid is now acknowledged as a characteristic feature of Alzheimer's disease, its precise role in the disease process is not yet understood. The "amyloid hypothesis," or "amyloid cascade hypothesis," proposes that amyloid production and/or deposition is a critical event, triggering the other pathological features and clinical symptoms of the disease. A great deal of work on this hypothesis has led to several alternative theories. Some investigators believe that the level of production of beta-amyloid is critical and that if this level could be lowered, development of the disease would be slowed. One strategy, then, might be to inhibit the enzymes that snip the APP molecule at either end of the beta-amyloid sequence. (Presumably, a different enzyme is active when the molecule is cleaved within the sequence.) Although these enzymes are not yet well defined, several groups of investigators are pursuing this approach.

Other authorities reason that since beta-amyloid is universal in the normal human brain, what is presumably abnormal in Alzheimer's disease is the accumulation of this material. Laboratory studies suggest that high concentrations of beta-amyloid are toxic to nerve cells. Several research teams are trying to find out how this substance builds up in the brain tissues and how to prevent this from happening.

Still a third group of investigators is focusing on the details of beta-amyloid production. It may be that the length of the peptides—whether they are 40 or 42 amino acids long—is the key. Thus, it has been suggested that both 40- and 42-amino-acid peptides are present in the normal brain but that a change in the relative ratio of the two may cause problems. Disproportionate production of the 42-amino-acid peptide seems to occur in at least some cases of Alzheimer's disease, although the total amount of the peptide remains relatively constant. Clearly, further work will be needed to resolve this issue.

Why anti-inflammatory drugs might help

Microglial cells, or microglia, in the brain may play a part in the formation of the neuritic plaques. Microglia have some similarities to white blood cells in that they share at least some cell-surface proteins related to immune system function. Microglia may serve to monitor the presence of infections or "foreign" proteins in the brain; they are known to respond to brain injuries such as strokes by increasing in size, and perhaps in number, around the damaged area. "Activated" microglia, like those formed following brain injury, are also seen around neuritic plaques, and scientists speculate that they may be responding to the presence of beta-amyloid deposits. This tendency of microglia to collect in the brain has clear similarities to the tendency of white blood cells to cluster at sites of injury or infection elsewhere in the body. Nonetheless, inflammation as it is usually understood does not occur in Alzheimer's disease. There is, for example, no evidence of infiltration of white bloods cells around blood vessels or of fluid accumulation (edema) in the brain, as are present in classical inflammatory diseases of the brain, such as multiple sclerosis. Some researchers believe that the activation of microglia may play a role in the neuronal degeneration in Alzheimer's disease. It has been suggested that microglia may actually participate in amyloid deposition by inappropriate degradation of the APP molecule to yield the 40–42-amino-acid peptide.

On the basis of the observed parallels with the process of inflammation, some scientists have proposed that anti-inflammatory drugs may be useful in treating Alzheimer's disease. This notion has also received support from epidemiological studies in which people who regularly used ibuprofen-containing products were found to have a lower-than-average risk of developing Alzheimer's disease. It is too soon to tell whether this observation will be confirmed in larger populations. Nonetheless, some investigators have become intrigued with the idea that nonsteroidal anti-inflammatory drugs, or NSAIDs (aspirin, ibuprofen, naproxen, and others), may prevent or retard the development of the disease. A few small-scale clinical trials of NSAIDs for this

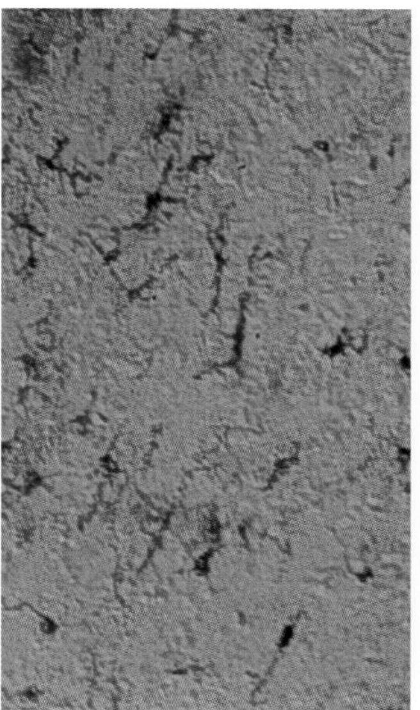

In the normal brain, microglia appear as a delicate network of cells and their projecting processes (left); in the brain tissue of those with Alzheimer's disease and most other neurodegenerative disorders, the microglia are more numerous and larger than normal (right).

purpose are already under way, and others are in the planning stage. Drugs like ibuprofen have side effects, however, notably stomach irritation, and their long-term use may have risks that outweigh the potential benefits.

Neurofibrillary tangles: cause or effect?

For many years scientists assumed that the neurofibrillary tangles of Alzheimer's disease represented residual material remaining after the death of a neuron. The formation of tangles was thus seen as a consequence of the illness rather than as an important early event in the disease process. This perception is changing with improved technology for visualizing early stages of tangle formation and clearer definition of some of the critical biochemical events involved. Tangles are made up of aggregates of filaments that have an extraordinary structure in that they appear as two helically wound strands, which are usually referred to as paired helical filaments. A few researchers have suggested that the microscopic images reveal a "twisted ribbon" configuration, in which a single strand is wound into a spiral. Regardless of their precise structure, these filaments do not occur in the normal brain.

In Alzheimer's disease, however, masses of paired helical filaments collect to form the neurofibrillary tangle. Whereas the filaments in aggregation are insoluble, individual filaments appear to be soluble and are composed primarily of a protein called tau. There is still a great deal of debate regarding how tau, a normal brain protein, is modified and incorporated into these filamentous structures. It has become clear that both structural changes in tau and phosphorylation of the protein molecule (*i.e.,* addition of phosphate) are important for filament formation, but the details of these processes are not clear. Exciting recent work in this area by investigators at the Albert Einstein College of Medicine, Yeshiva University, Bronx, N.Y., has revealed the presence of enzymes that are involved in the process of cell division in nerve cells in early cases of Alzheimer's disease. Normally, nerve cells in the brains of adult humans and other higher mammals do not divide, at least not in significant numbers. The presence in Alzheimer's brains of these cell-division enzymes, most of which are involved in the addition of phosphate to proteins, suggests that the neurons might be receiving a cell-division signal, which results in disruption of the cell's normal function and perhaps in its ultimate death.

Using high concentrations of purified tau produced in the laboratory, scientists have succeeded in making small numbers of paired helical filaments. While interesting, this work does not solve the puzzle of how these structures are formed in the neurons of a person with Alzheimer's disease. To date, in fact, no one has been able to demonstrate filament formation in neurons, either in

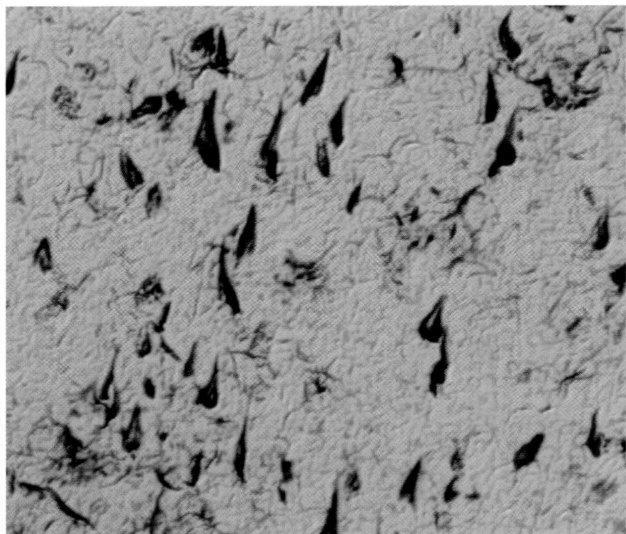

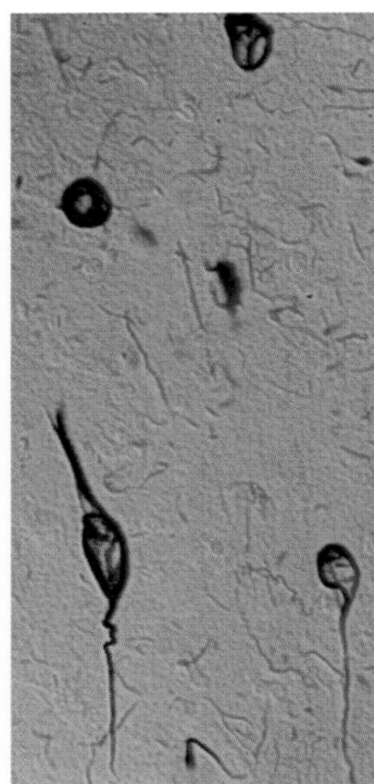

The brain lesions known as neurofibrillary tangles are a hallmark of Alzheimer's disease. Under the microscope tangles may be seen as masses within the cytoplasm of neurons (far left), often appearing to wrap around the nucleus (the unstained "hole" visible in some of the tangles). Sometimes a tangle will remain as a "ghost" after the degeneration of a neuron (left). The tangles themselves are composed of aggregates of filaments. Each filament has a highly regular structure (below) that suggests a pair of helically wound strands—or possibly a single ribbonlike strand twisted around itself to form a spiral.

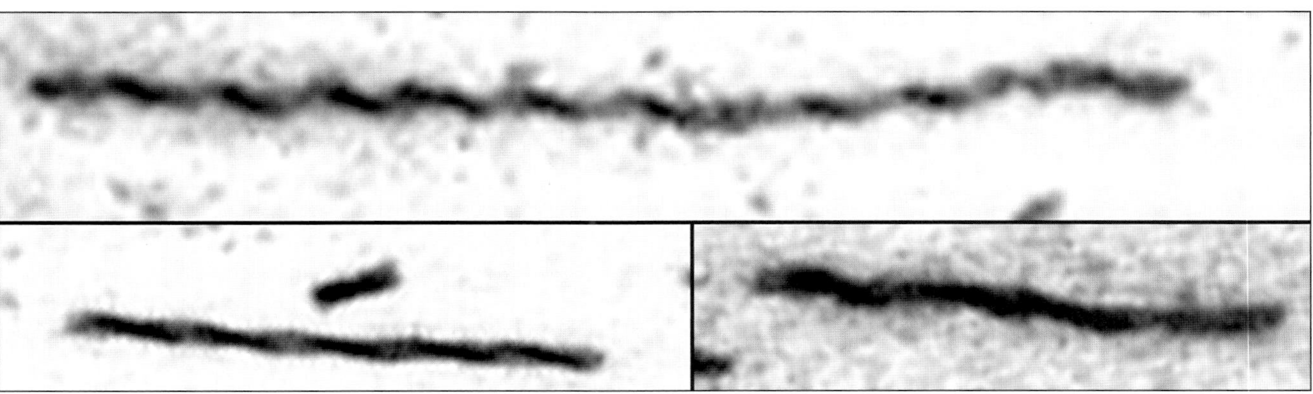

Photographs, Peter Davies

laboratory cultures or in animal experiments. Among a variety of aged animals that have been examined at autopsy, only sheep and grizzly bears have been found to develop small numbers of tangles, but neither animal provides what could be considered a convenient animal model for studies of the mechanism of filament formation.

The development of neurofibrillary tangles, while characteristic of Alzheimer's disease, is not unique to it. Other disorders in which tangles are seen include progressive supranuclear palsy (also called Steele-Richardson-Olszewski syndrome) and the unusual syndrome of Parkinson's disease, amytrophic lateral sclerosis, and dementia that occurs only among the Chamorro Indians of Guam. In both these conditions, tangles are found but very few plaques and little or no evidence of amyloid deposition. In the past two years, neurologists have identified an inherited dementia that is marked by degeneration of neurons in the frontal and temporal regions of the brain, some tangle formation, but few or no plaques. This disorder, found in only a few Caucasian families in the U.S., Italy, and Australia, appears to involve abnormalities of tau that may be somewhat different from those occurring in Alzheimer's disease, but the details are not yet known.

Treatment: no breakthroughs yet

In the late 1970s several research teams found evidence that neurons that use acetylcholine as a neurotransmitter (*i.e.,* a chemical that transmits nerve impulses) are selectively destroyed in the brains of patients with Alzheimer's disease. This work has been confirmed numerous times since then, and it has now been established beyond doubt that the supply of acetylcholine to the cerebral cortex, including the hippocampus, is deficient in these patients. Acetylcholine has long been considered to be important in processes such as memory and higher cognitive function (among others), and this research led to what has been called the "cholinergic hypothesis" of Alzheimer's disease. This hypothesis proposes that the major cognitive problems in Alzheimer's disease can be attributed to a lack of cholinergic neurotransmission (*i.e.,* transmision of those nerve signals that rely on acetylcholine) and that therapies directed at restoring this deficiency should improve patients' cognitive function.

Acetylcholine-based therapies. The cholinergic hypothesis of Alzheimer's disease has proved correct, but only to a very limited extent. Both tacrine (Cognex) and donepezil (Aricept), the two drugs approved in the U.S. for treatment of the cognitive dysfunction of Alzheimer's disease, are inhibitors of acetylcholinesterase, the enzyme that normally degrades acetylcholine in the brain. (By preventing the breakdown of acetylcholine, these substances increase the amount available for nerve-signal transmission.)

Both of these drugs have been shown to produce some improvements in function in Alzheimer's disease patients. The improvements are relatively small, however, and neither drug appears to have any effect on the underlying disease process. While they give the patient a short period of slightly improved functioning (and the family some respite), the drugs should not be expected to do more. Other similar compounds are being tested in clinical trials, including compounds designed to mimic the action of acetylcholine at one or more of its receptors in the brain.

The brain has two major classes of acetylcholine receptor, the muscarinic and the nicotinic receptors. They are named for muscarine and nicotine, the compounds that bind to them. A number of pharmaceutical companies have designed compounds to act at these receptors, and some of these agents are already in the early stages of testing for use in Alzheimer's patients. Although a majority of these compounds act at muscarinic receptors, there is increasing interest in compounds that act like nicotine. This interest has been piqued by some controversial evidence that smokers are at lower risk for Alzheimer's disease than nonsmokers. There are actually quite strong data showing that smoking lowers the risk of developing Parkinson's disease; the data concerning smoking and Alzheimer's disease are less clear. Studies of nicotine-like compounds for treatment of Alzheimer's disease are currently under way.

Although it is too early for any definite conclusions, it appears that acetylcholine-based therapies do produce some small improvements in the symptoms of Alzheimer's disease. While it is undoubtedly true that cholinergic neurons degenerate in Alzheimer's disease, this deterioration seems to be only one of many causes of the clinical features. Other brain changes seen in the disorder, including losses in numbers of other neurons and decreases in the number of synapses (the connections between neurons), indicate that restoration of normal function will require more than just replacement of acetylcholine.

Estrogen: a preventive? After it was established that the cholinergic neurons play a part in Alzheimer's disease, research in rats suggested that estrogen might be an important growth factor for these cells. Estrogen was shown to stimulate the activity of the enzyme responsible for the synthesis of acetylcholine, and this discovery led, in the early 1980s, to the first studies of estrogen treatment in postmenopausal women with Alzheimer's disease. Short-term treatments did not appear to have any beneficial effects. More recently, however, studies have suggested that postmenopausal women who take estrogen have a lower risk of Alzheimer's disease than women who elect not to use hormone replacement therapy.

The findings of these two studies are not necessarily contradictory; estrogen could provide some protection against the development of the disease but have no effect on the course or symptoms once it has developed. In the U.S. a series of very large studies of the risks and benefits of estrogen replacement therapy are under way, although it will be a considerable time before scientists can come to any conclusions about the effect of the treatment on Alzheimer's disease incidence in older women.

Antioxidant treatment. A recent widely publicized clinical trial of vitamin E in Alzheimer's disease highlighted the growing interest in the theory that antioxidants may have a place in treatment of the disorder. The trial followed several hundred patients with moderate-to-severe disease for a period of two years. Patients were placed on one of four regimes: a placebo (an inactive, "dummy" drug), vitamin E alone, vitamin E and selegiline, or selegiline alone. Selegiline, a drug originally developed as an antidepressant, appears to slow deterioration in patients with Parkinson's disease. The results of the trial were somewhat surprising. All three patient groups treated with active drugs did a little better than the one that received placebo. Nonetheless, all four groups showed deterioration in functioning over the two years, and the differences in the extent of the decline were small. Opinion remains divided over whether to recommend vitamin E or selegiline (or both) for people with Alzheimer's disease.

Despite this uncertainty, the vitamin E research has drawn attention to the possible role of free radicals in the neuronal degeneration of Alzheimer's disease. Free radicals are unstable molecules (especially oxygen molecules) that seek to become stable by giving up electrons, a process that can damage cells. One normal function of vitamin E (and vitamin C as well) is to protect cells against this damage. Free radicals are generated by the normal process of metabolism, but increased production may occur in response to small strokes or perhaps even amyloid deposition. Thus, some scientists theorize that vitamin supplementation in Alzheimer's disease may provide additional defense against the formation of free radicals and thereby slow the rate of neuronal death. At the moment, most authorities agree that it is important for Alzheimer's patients to have a balanced diet and/or a multivitamin supplement, but few would go so far as to endorse vitamin supplementation as a preventive.

Unproven therapies. A whole host of compounds either are being tested for the treatment of Alzheimer's disease or have been suggested as treatments by one group or another. Many of these therapies are only loosely based on knowledge of the biology of the disease, and while it is certainly possible that one or more of them may produce some benefit, they lack a compelling scientific rationale. It is unfortunate that the large size of the patient population attracts organizations whose principal concerns are financial gain rather than the well-being of patients. Claims of dramatic benefits for these untested remedies should be regarded with a considerable degree of caution.

Genetic clues: an ambiguous trail

Advances in molecular genetics (the science of the molecular structure of DNA) have allowed scientists to focus on families in which Alzheimer's disease clearly appears to be inherited, and this work has led to some spectacular successes in identification of genes involved in the disease. In the vast majority of cases, however—the so-called sporadic cases—there is no clear-cut evidence that Alzheimer's disease is an inherited illness. The families that are the focus of molecular genetics studies are relatively rare and have somewhat atypical forms of the disorder.

A family that this author and his colleagues have followed will illustrate this point. The investigators' initial contact was with a 47-year-old man who was already quite severely demented, having begun at age 42 to show symptoms of memory loss, disorientation (he could not find his way to the supermarket just four blocks from his house), and calculation skills (he lost his job as a civil engineer at age 43). The patient was the youngest of seven children. Two of his brothers and a sister had died in their early 50s of what had been termed "presenile dementia," and their mother had died at a similar age with a diagnosis of Alzheimer's disease. Closer questioning of the surviving relatives revealed that there had been several similar cases in previous generations. In all of the affected individuals, the disease seemed to begin in the early 40s, and death occurred in the early 50s. Until the patient in question died at age 53, no autopsy had been conducted on any family member. The autopsy revealed numerous neuritic plaques and neurofibrillary tangles in virtually all regions of the cerebral cortex and thus confirmed the diagnosis of Alzheimer's disease.

Analysis of several similar families has led scientists to the conclusion that Alzheimer's disease can indeed be inherited, but a genetic cause for the illness can be determined with some degree of certainty only in families like the one described above. Where the onset of Alzheimer's disease in several family members occurs at an older age—in, say, the 70s—investigators are rarely able to pick out a pattern of inheritance at all. It must also be said that even when patients are diagnosed in their 40s or 50s, a familial pattern is often difficult to discern. It therefore does not appear to be true that all early-onset Alzheimer's disease is inherited. Nonetheless, intensive investigation of the pattern of inheritance in some families has led to the discovery of genes that, when defective, can cause Alzheimer's disease. To date, three different genes have been identified as sites of mutations that can cause the disease, and it is clear that there must be at least one more.

The first such mutation was discovered in 1989. A team of investigators at St. Mary's Hospital in London reported a single alteration in the sequence of the gene that encodes the APP, which gave rise to a single change in the amino acid sequence of the protein and appeared to cause Alzheimer's disease in a large family in which an early-onset form of the disease was clearly inherited. This mutation was just "downstream" of the region of

Disease-Causing Mutations of *APP* Gene

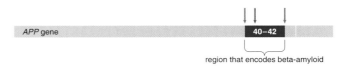

Sites of mutations that cause Alzheimer's disease
Site of mutation that causes hereditary congophilic amyloid angiopathy, Dutch type

the protein where the beta-amyloid sequence is found. Around the same time, another mutation was discovered in the *APP* gene, this time directly affecting the beta-amyloid region of the protein sequence. It turned out that this latter mutation did not cause Alzheimer's disease but was associated with massive amyloid deposition in blood vessels of the brain. Patients with the mutation died of strokes, but their brains showed no signs of plaques and tangles, nor did these patients exhibit the dementia typical of Alzheimer's disease. The disorder is generally called hereditary congophilic amyloid angiopathy, Dutch type (so called because the families with the largest number of affected members are from The Netherlands).

The discovery of the first Alzheimer's disease-associated mutation led quickly to intensive screening of the *APP* gene in other Alzheimer's families, as well as in individuals for whom there was no clear evidence of inherited disease. A few other mutations were found in families, but it quickly became clear that other genes must be involved because the vast majority of people, whether from Alzheimer's families or not, did *not* have mutations in the *APP* gene. One of the mutations identified by this research was of particular interest because it involved a change of two amino acids in the APP molecule just "upstream" of the beta-amyloid sequence. This "Swedish mutation" (so named because it was found in a large Swedish family) appears to cause a large increase in the amount of the 40–42-amino-acid peptide produced from the APP, perhaps six to eight times the normal amount, and this discovery has provided the basis for one of the major hypotheses about the causation of Alzheimer's disease.

Because many of the larger families with inherited Alzheimer's disease did not appear to have mutations in the *APP* gene, researchers continued to screen the DNA of these families for another gene defect. In the early 1990s this same approach had enabled geneticists to locate the Huntington's disease gene, and it has yielded some success in Alzheimer's disease. In July 1995 researchers at the University of Toronto identified a gene on chromosome 14 that is mutated in several large families with a history of Alzheimer's disease. This gene, which was named *presenilin 1* (*PS1*), is the site of several different mutations in a group of families with early-onset Alzheimer's disease. In fact, mutations in this gene appear to be the largest single cause of inherited Alzheimer's disease.

Again, however, it was clear that not all families had mutations in *PS1*, and the following month, August 1995, several research teams announced that they had found a gene on chromosome 1 that was similar in sequence to *PS1*. This gene, which they called *presenilin 2* (*PS2*), is also a site of mutations that cause Alzheimer's disease in a few families. Notable among these are the descendants of some Volga Germans (Germans who immigrated to Russia) who now live in the northwestern United States.

The function of the presenilin genes is not yet known. Researchers speculate that the proteins they encode will prove to be so-called membrane-spanning proteins present on membranes of internal cellular structures. Why or how mutations in these genes cause Alzheimer's disease is not at all obvious, partly because scientists have no idea of the normal function of their proteins. Once again, though, it turns out that several large families with inherited Alzheimer's disease, and all of the sporadic cases so far examined, do *not* have mutations in either of the presenilin genes. At least one more (and most researchers believe more than one) currently unknown gene defect causes inherited Alzheimer's disease. Moreover, there may be no genetic basis in the majority of cases.

The ApoE story

A team of investigators at Duke University, Durham, N.C., were heavily involved in the search for gene defects causing Alzheimer's disease but were focusing for the most part on cases with later onset. This work led them to discover not a gene defect that causes Alzheimer's disease but a version, or variant, of a gene that appears to be associated with an increased risk for development of the disease. To understand this work, a little background is necessary.

Apolipoprotein E, or ApoE, is a protein that binds and transports lipids, including cholesterol, in the blood. It is also present in the brain, where its function is presumably similar. The gene that encodes the ApoE protein occurs in three common forms in the general population—*ApoE2, E3, and E4* (*ApoE1* is extremely rare). Because genes exist in pairs (one gene inherited from the mother, one from the father), a given individual will have one of six possible combinations of *ApoE* genes (*E2/E2, E2/E3, E2/E4, E3/E3, E3/E4, or E4/E4)*. The Duke team noted that the *E4* gene occurred more frequently in patients with Alzheimer's disease than in the general population, an observation that has since been confirmed a number of times.

The majority of Caucasians have the *ApoE3* gene, and only about 20% have an *E4* gene; an even smaller percentage have an *E2* gene. In large groups of Alzheimer's patients, perhaps 40% will have an *E4* gene. The presence of an *ApoE4* gene apparently makes it more likely that Alzheimer's disease will develop. Two points must be made clear, however. Even if 40% of Alzheimer's patients have an *ApoE4* gene, this means that 60% of patients do not. The presence of an *ApoE4* gene thus is not necessary for the development of the disease. Further, about 15% of normal individuals who live to be 100 years old without becoming demented have an *ApoE4* gene, so having the gene does not mean that the development of Alzheimer's disease is inevitable.

The situation in non-Caucasian populations is not as clear at present. In the U.S. the *ApoE4* gene is more common in African-Americans than in Caucasians, but so far no difference has been found in gene frequency between African-Americans with Alzheimer's disease and the rest of the African-American population. In the population of Japan, *ApoE4* is less frequent than in Caucasians but is found more commonly in Japanese Alzheimer's patients than in the rest of the population.

At present it is far from clear why the *ApoE4* gene is associated with Alzheimer's disease. It may be that the ApoE4 protein is less efficient than ApoE3 at transporting lipids in the brain. If a degenerative process such as Alzheimer's disease begins, patients with ApoE4 may be at a disadvantage, being less able to support neurons that are attempting to cope with the insult.

It has also been suggested that ApoE4 binds beta-amyloid less well than ApoE3 and thus allows more accumulation of amyloid in the brain. There does not appear to be any clear relationship between atherosclerosis (the buildup of fatty deposits in the blood vessels) and Alzheimer's disease, but recent work does show quite clearly that having both conditions at the same time causes a more severe intellectual decline than having only one or the other.

Diagnosis: ongoing challenge

Given the vast amount of research that has been conducted over the past few years, it is perhaps surprising that autopsy is still the only way to determine definitively if a patient has Alzheimer's disease. Periodically, reports appear in the news media about potential new tests, usually based in some fashion on the growing understanding of the biology of the disease. Genetic testing has been widely debated, but it is obvious that such tests are essentially meaningless except in members of those very rare families with a strong history of Alzheimer's disease and an identifiable genetic mutation. In these few families, accurate testing of the siblings and children of a patient is possible and is today being carried out with the assistance of trained genetic counselors and psychologists. In no other circumstance is it possible to say who will and who will not suffer from this disease. Given the present state of knowledge, a positive test for the *ApoE4* gene cannot predict when—or if—a person will develop Alzheimer's disease, nor can it determine for certain if a demented individual has the disorder or some other kind of dementia.

The new methods proposed as being diagnostic for Alzheimer's disease include an eye test that measures the speed of pupil dilation, assays of beta-amyloid, ApoE, and tau concentrations in cerebrospinal fluid (fluid taken from the spinal canal by lumbar puncture), measurement of calcium concentrations in skin cells, and a variety of other, even more esoteric measurements. None of these has yet proved reliable.

One of the major problems in determining the validity of such tests when applied to people already diagnosed with dementia is that no one knows for certain which of the individuals really do have Alzheimer's disease and which do not. All of the experimental tests must rely on autopsy for confirmation, and this process usually involves a delay of several years. It will therefore be some time before enough data can be accumulated to determine the accuracy of any proposed new diagnostic technique. As stated above, examination and evaluation of the patient by an experienced clinician, in most cases a neurologist or psychiatrist, remains absolutely essential for the most accurate possible diagnosis.

Of mice, models, and progress

Now that several Alzheimer's disease-related genes have been identified, scientists are attempting, by means of molecular biology techniques, to transfer the mutations into mice. Their hope is to produce a mouse that predictably develops a disease with all the same features as the human illness—an animal model. Several strains of mice with mutant human *APP* genes have already been bred and studied in great detail. So far, although these animals do develop extensive deposition of amyloid in their brains, they show no signs of developing paired helical filaments or neurofibrillary tangles.

A good animal model would be of enormous value in Alzheimer's disease research, especially for the development of drug treatments to slow or halt the course of the disease. At present, the only way to test such drugs is in patients, a procedure that is both expensive and time-consuming. An animal model would also enable researchers to study the mechanisms by which the disorder progresses. In the meantime, the search for treatments to slow or prevent Alzheimer's disease is proceeding along several parallel tracks, which, it is hoped, will converge on a successful therapy in the not-too-distant future.

—*Peter Davies, Ph.D.*

Despite an enormous amount of research and many advances in the understanding of Alzheimer's disease, diagnosing the illness during life remains problematic. Only a thorough evaluation by a qualified clinician can provide a diagnosis with any certainty.

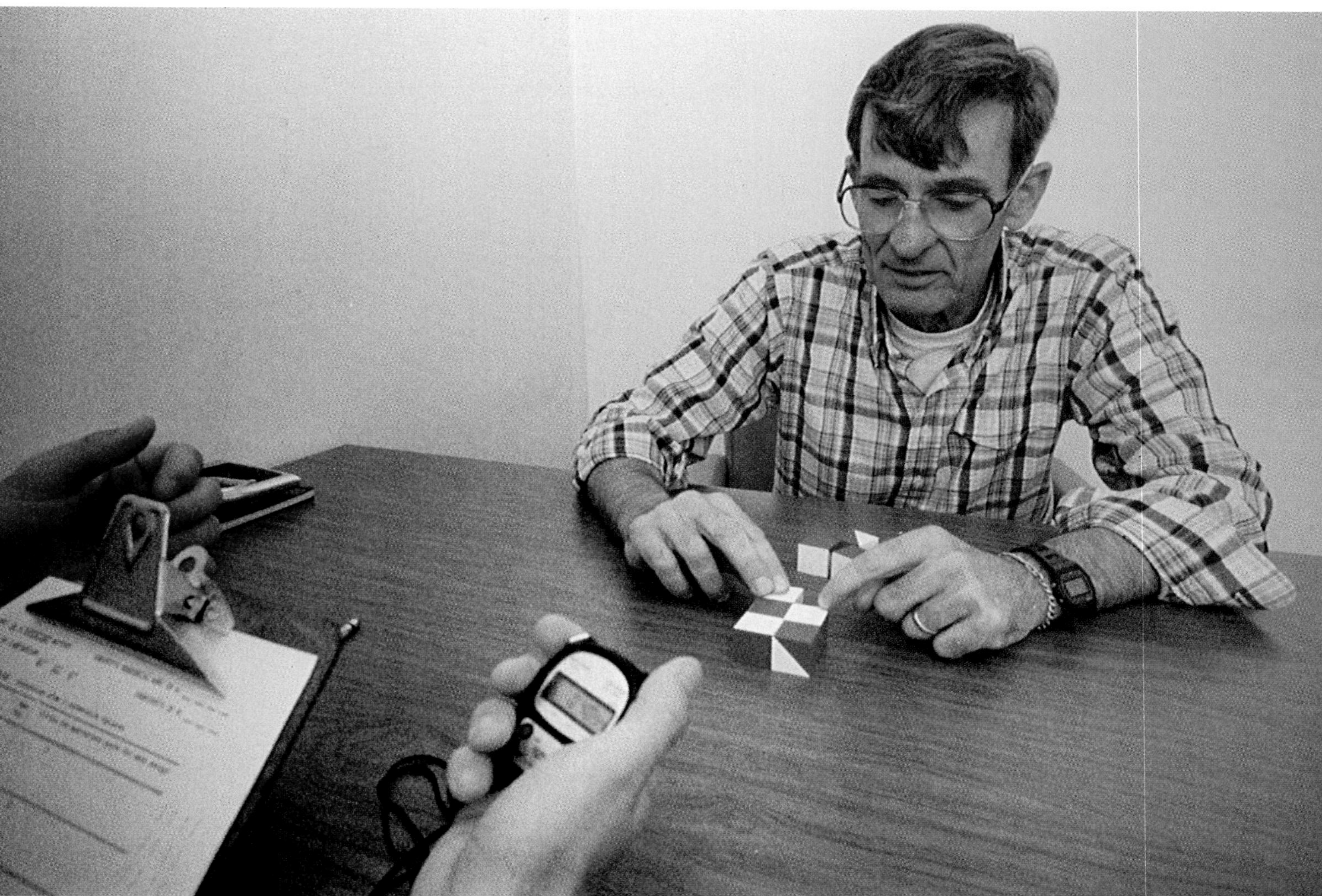

Lynn Johnson—Aurora

Body Weight: Biology, Not Behavior

Obesity, long thought to be largely a psychological or behavioral problem, is now increasingly coming to be regarded as a medical condition. Perhaps most influential in changing the scientific thinking about obesity has been the identification of several genes believed to play a part in regulating the accumulation of body fat. The 1997 report of a human virus capable of inducing obesity in animals raised the intriguing possibility that overweight, in at least some cases, may be infectious and that otherwise "normal" people could be at risk of contracting it.

The growing acceptance of obesity as a biological problem and the availability of moderately successful weight-loss drugs have begun to have an impact on the practice of medicine. At the same time, the seriousness of obesity as a predisposing factor for other health problems is being increasingly recognized. At a World Health Organization meeting in June 1997, nutrition and health authorities from 25 countries declared that obesity should be regarded as one of today's "greatest neglected public health problems," with a health impact that "may well prove to be as great as that of smoking." (Obesity is generally defined as a body weight 20% or more over normal for the individual's height, age, and sex. Severe, or morbid, obesity is 100% over normal.)

Although only a handful of obesity-related genes have been identified, more than 20 are believed to contribute to the condition in humans. Most authorities suspect that the vast majority of overweight individuals probably have defective versions of several of these genes. Nonetheless, most scientists also expect that genetic alterations will ultimately prove only to influence—not to determine—an individual's risk of becoming obese. Lifestyle factors such as diet and activity level will, they believe, be shown to be at least equal in importance to genetic predisposition, if not more important.

Remi Benali—Gamma Liaison

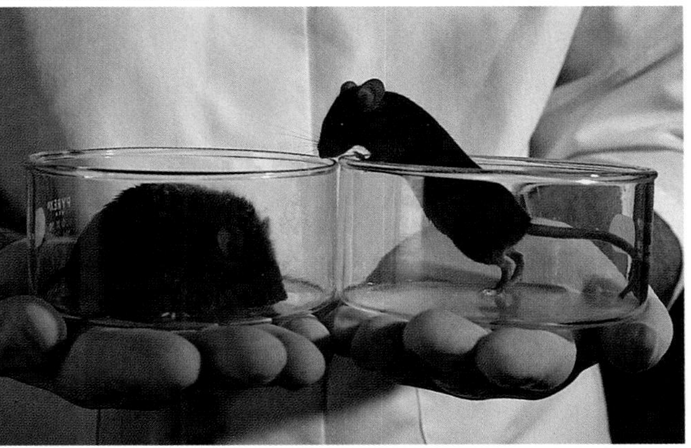

Both of these mice have defective ob *genes, a condition that predisposes them to being overweight. After receiving an injection of the hormone leptin, however, the mouse at right shed 30% of its body fat.*

Fat-related genes

Five single-gene defects have been identified as causes of obesity in animal models of the condition. In each case the gene responsible appears also to be present in humans. Four of the defects involve recessive genes, which means that an individual must inherit two defective genes in order to be affected. (Nearly all genes exist in pairs, with one inherited from the mother and one from the father. A single defective gene, if recessive, will not be expressed.) The fifth known defect, a mutation in the so-called *agouti* gene, is dominant; thus, animals with even one defective gene will become obese. (By scientific convention the names of genes are italicized.) A sixth genetic alteration may help explain why some individuals become fat as a result of eating high-fat or high-calorie diets, while others do not.

The *agouti* gene. The first genetic obesity syndrome to be identified was seen in a breed of mouse called the yellow obese mouse. As the name implies, affected animals are overweight and have bright yellow coats. They are also distinguished by higher-than-normal blood levels of insulin, resistance to the action of insulin, and a tendency to develop tumors. The underlying problem is a defect in a gene called *agouti.* In skin cells the gene encodes a protein that acts by opposing the binding of melanocyte-stimulating hormone (MSH) to melanocytes. Melanocytes, pigment cells that give color to the animal's skin and fur, are stimulated by MSH. Normally, the agouti protein is secreted only transiently, but in the yellow obese mouse the protein is produced continuously. The presence of excessive amounts of agouti protein prevents MSH from binding to the melanocytes, with the result that affected mice have fur that is yellow rather than their normal dark color. In the brain the excess agouti protein increases the activity of fatty acid synthase (FAS), an enzyme that regulates fat synthesis. Increased FAS action causes increased fat synthesis, which contributes to obesity. A gene similar to the *agouti* gene has been discovered in humans. A mutation or defect in this gene may contribute to some cases of human obesity.

The *ob* gene and the role of leptin. In 1994 scientists at Rockefeller University, New York City, discovered the sequence of the *obese,* or *ob,* gene. Mutations in this gene are responsible for the massive obesity that occurs in mice that are homozygous for the altered gene (*i.e.,* they have inherited abnormal versions of the gene from both parents), designated as *ob/ob* mice. The *ob* gene encodes a protein called leptin. In 1995 three separate groups of scientists reported that they had isolated leptin and determined that the substance could reduce obesity in *ob/ob* mice and in some other strains of mice.

Leptin is produced in fat cells and circulates in the blood, providing a means of communication between fat tissue and the brain. When stores of body fat rise, circulating levels of leptin increase. The increase in leptin levels may signal the brain to decrease food intake and increase energy (*i.e.,* calorie) expenditure in order to limit the accumulation of fat. Conversely, when food supplies are limited and body weight and fat stores begin to decrease, leptin concentrations decline. The lower leptin concentrations may signal the brain to increase food intake or food-seeking behavior. Low leptin levels also may result in a lower metabolic rate, which conserves energy.

Leptin is thought to function by suppressing neuropeptide Y (NPY), a protein that acts in the brain as a potent stimulator of food intake. When leptin levels are low, NPY levels rise, which leads to increased intake. If a defect occurs in the production of leptin or in the action of leptin receptors in the brain, NPY levels may persist at a high level, and obesity results.

Bob Kramer—Stock, Boston

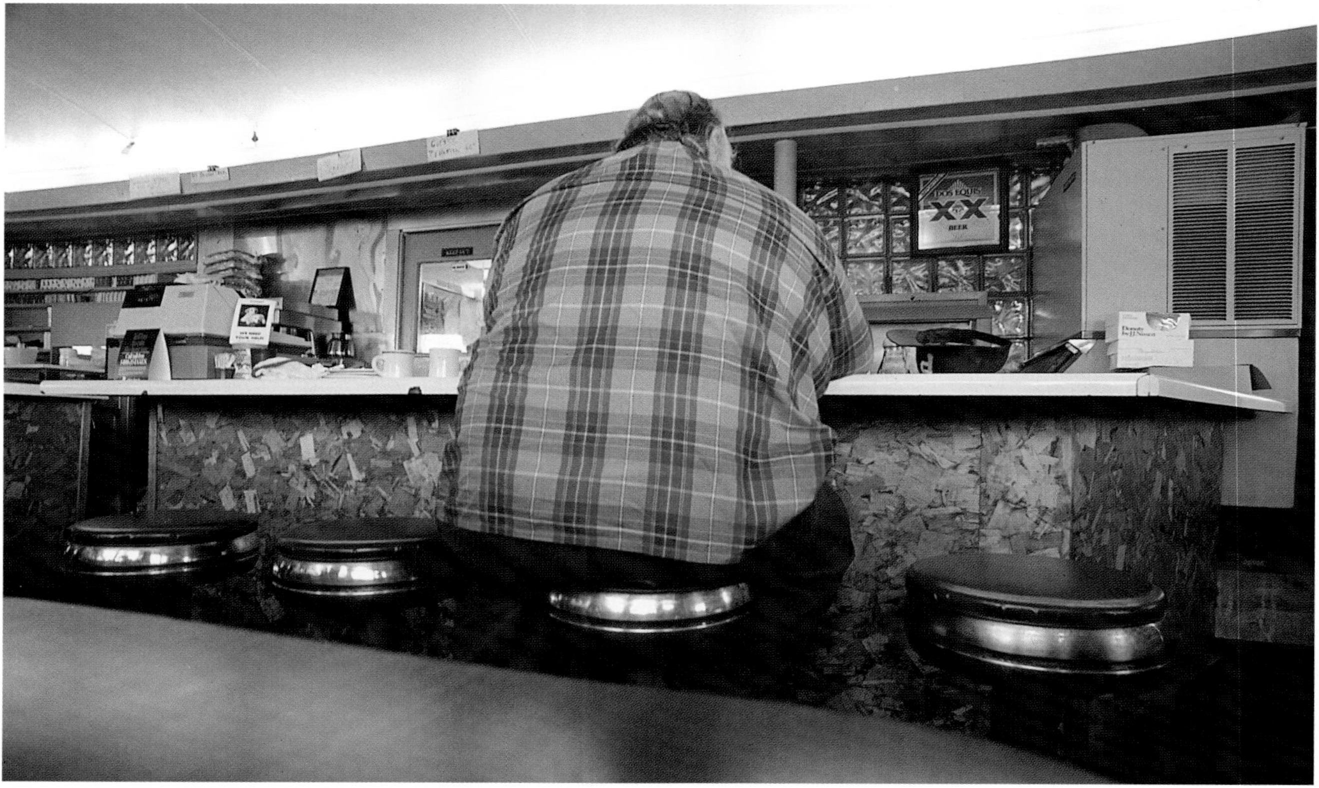

Although once widely viewed as a behavioral problem, obesity is now accepted by most medical professionals as having a biological basis. The prevalence of obesity in the U.S. has increased in recent decades; today some 30% of all American adults are overweight.

From an evolutionary perspective, scientists believe that the adaptive advantage of leptin was not in preventing obesity but rather in protecting against starvation. For most of the time that life has existed on Earth, food supplies have been limited. Thus, starvation, not obesity, was the greater threat to survival. In a starving person, fat stores dwindle. Leptin levels decrease, which leads to increased levels of NPY in the brain and the stimulation of feeding. In addition, during starvation the interaction of leptin and other hormones produces reductions in metabolic rate to conserve energy. Some scientists postulate that in females leptin has still another function: to signal the brain that fat stores are large enough to support pregnancy.

Abnormalities in leptin production or function may produce obesity in two ways. First, as noted above, the lack of functional leptin due to a mutation in the *ob* gene produces obesity in mice that are homozygous for the mutation. Second, the availability or activity of leptin may be altered by a defect in the gene that codes for leptin receptors in the brain. This condition is described below in the section on the *db* gene.

In 1995 scientists found that when leptin is injected into *ob/ob* mice, the animals' food intake decreases and body weight and body fat decline. These early observations raised hopes that defects in the protein or its receptor would prove to be common in overweight humans and that leptin might be a useful treatment for obesity. In the meantime, however, several studies have shown that the vast majority of obese individuals have normal or high leptin levels. In most people leptin levels correlate with body fat; thus, the greater a person's fat stores, the higher the leptin level. These findings suggest that the problem in most obese people is not a defect in production of leptin but rather a defect in the body's response to the protein. The situation is similar to that observed with insulin in obese humans and other animals. Although overweight people tend to have high levels of insulin, the insulin does not function properly in their bodies; as a result, the rate of diabetes mellitus in overweight persons is unusually high. Nonetheless, even very obese individuals experience a drop in blood sugar in response to sufficiently large doses of insulin. It is hoped that leptin will act in a similar fashion and that obese individuals, despite their already elevated blood levels of the protein, will experience weight loss and reduction of body fat in response to greatly increased leptin levels.

In fact, researchers have shown that mice made fat by a high-fat diet have higher-than-normal leptin levels in their blood. Moreover, when injected with leptin, these animals lose weight. Leptin levels after injection are quite high. Human trials are now under way to test the effects of leptin as a treatment for obesity.

The *db* gene. Animals with a defect in a gene called *db* (for diabetes) become obese and, relatively early in life, diabetic. Two different defects in the *db* gene have been described in rodents, and the human counterpart of the gene has been identified.

The *db* gene encodes a protein that is a receptor for leptin. As noted above, leptin is produced by fat cells, circulates to the brain, binds to specific leptin receptors, and signals the brain regarding the levels of fat stores in the body. The leptin receptors are located on certain cells in the hypothalamus, an area of the brain that regulates many bodily functions, including food intake and energy metabolism. Defects in the leptin receptor or defects in the cellular response once leptin has bound to the receptor produce a syndrome similar to leptin deficiency. Mutations in the *db* gene result in defective or inactive leptin receptors. Consequently, despite increases in leptin levels, leptin cannot bind to its receptors and thus is ineffective. Lacking feedback from the body on the state of fat stores, the brain stimulates increased food intake and reduced energy expenditure, and the result is obesity.

The *fat* gene. In mice, mutation of a recessive gene dubbed *fat* causes obesity and high insulin levels. The *fat* gene codes for the enzyme carboxypeptidase E, which is responsible for converting insulin from an inactive form (proinsulin) to an active form. Mice with this gene defect have increased levels of glucose (sugar) and proinsulin in the blood and a high ratio of proinsulin to insulin. The defect does not hamper the ability of insulin to lower blood glucose, and diabetes associated with defects in the *fat* gene responds to insulin injections.

The *tub* gene. Mutation of the *tubby,* or *tub,* gene in mice causes obesity in later life, along with insulin resistance (but not diabetes), degeneration of the retina of the eye, and hearing impairment. This mutation apparently affects one form of phosphodiesterase, an enzyme important in the regulation of energy metabolism. With age these mice develop abnormalities in the hypothalamus. Compared with mice that have normal *tub* genes, animals with defective genes demonstrate decreased satiety after a meal and thus are more likely to overeat. At the same time, they show lower levels of energy expenditure, which means that they burn fewer calories and store more as fat.

Energy production and UCP-2. Alterations in a gene that codes for uncoupling protein-2 (UCP-2) may help explain why some animals and people are thin, while others, who may eat no more than many lean individuals, have difficulty controlling their weight. To appreciate the role of UCP-2, it is necessary to understand the ways the body stores and utilizes fat. Fat stored in the body is classified as either "white" or "brown." White fat is responsible for the storage of fat for energy reserves. The main function of brown fat is to generate heat for the regulation of body temperature and/or energy balance. White fat is present in humans and all other animals. Brown fat is present in many animals and in human infants but exists only in limited quantities in adult humans. The role of brown fat in energy balance and tolerance to cold in adult humans is not yet clear. Most of the knowledge about brown fat comes from animal studies. When animals, particularly rodents, are exposed to cold temperatures, their bodies increase heat production in order to maintain the body temperature. Similarly, overfeeding of rodents results in increased heat production to dissipate the excess energy. In both instances the site of the increased heat production is brown fat.

The mechanism for this increased heat production is a protein called uncoupling protein-1 (UCP-1). UCP-1 is present in the mitochondria (the energy-producing compartments of cells) of brown fat cells but not white fat cells. UCP-1 acts by dissociating the utilization of body fuels, specifically fatty acids from food, from the production of adenosine triphosphate (ATP), the body's chief energy-storage compound. Normally, when fatty acids are burned in the mitochondria, ATP is formed as an energy reserve for the cell. When UCP-1 is present, the energy that normally would go into ATP is released as heat, which radiates from the body, rather than being stored. This increased heat may serve to keep the animal warm when it is exposed to the cold or to dissipate energy when it is overfed.

For many years scientists have been puzzled by the observation that most humans appear to be able to increase energy expenditure when they overeat, yet adult humans have little brown fat, and the amount present does not appear sufficient to account for the increased energy expenditure with overeating. It was scientists at the University of California, Davis, who recently identified UCP-2, another form of UCP. These investigators demonstrated that UCP-2 is present in many human tissues, including white fat. When a high-fat, high-calorie meal is eaten, the activity of the gene that encodes UCP-2 increases in some people more than others. The resultant increase in heat production may allow some people to eat a higher-fat or higher-calorie diet yet not get fat. Conversely, a person with insufficient activity of the gene, and thus insufficient levels of UCP-2, may be unable to dissipate the excess energy and may gain weight. UCP-2 does not increase in humans exposed to cold, which suggests that there may be still other forms of UCP or other mechanisms regulating the ability of humans to adapt to the cold.

Fat and viruses: intriguing links

The first evidence that a virus could produce obesity was published in 1982. Investigators at the Rockefeller Institute (now Rockefeller University) found that the virus that causes distemper in dogs could produce severe obesity in mice. Since that initial announcement, three more animal viruses have been shown to produce obesity in animals, including a lethal avian virus that causes infected chickens to gain weight rapidly before they die.

In 1996 researchers from the University of Wisconsin-Madison Medical School, including these authors, showed for the first time that a human virus related to the suspect avian virus was also capable of producing obesity in chickens. The investigators found that Ad-36, a member of the adenovirus group (which includes agents responsible for common respiratory infections), caused a peculiar syndrome: birds injected with the virus became obese but, paradoxically, had lower levels of cholesterol and triglycerides than uninfected controls.

Having discovered the effect of Ad-36 on chickens, the Wisconsin researchers decided to screen both overweight and lean human subjects for antibodies to the virus (which would indicate previous infection). None of the lean subjects had antibodies to Ad-36. Among the obese individuals, however, about 15% had the antibodies; significantly, these same people also had lower cholesterol and triglyceride levels than obese subjects without Ad-36 antibodies. The finding in humans of a similar syndrome (obesity with low cholesterol and triglyceride levels) as that seen in animals experimentally infected with Ad-36 is strong circumstantial evidence of an association between this virus and human obesity. Much additional research will be needed to determine if the virus truly causes obesity in humans and to establish the mechanisms responsible.

The drug "revolution"

Obesity treatments that rely on diet, exercise, and behavior modification techniques have been notoriously unsuccessful in producing lasting results. Surgical treatment is reserved for those people who have very severe obesity. Because early weight-loss drugs were found in the 1950s and '60s to be addictive, medication has not been considered by most physicians as a reasonable alternative for obesity treatment.

"Phen-fen." The negative attitude toward drugs changed in 1992 when it was shown that two second-generation obesity drugs, phentermine and fenfluramine, often prescribed in combination, produced weight loss that persisted over a period of three and a half years. (Like many other drugs taken concurrently, phentermine and fenfluramine have been approved for use separately but not together.) This marked the beginning of the "phen-fen" revolution. By mid-1997 millions of Americans had taken these drugs, and it had become clear that they produced modest long-term weight loss.

In July 1997, however, a report from the Mayo Clinic described the development of heart valve problems in a series of patients taking "phen-fen," which prompted the U.S. Food and Drug Administration (FDA) to require a warning on the drug labels. From the reported data, it is impossible to determine if the heart valve lesions are due to "phen-fen" or to obesity itself, which can produce heart abnormalities. More research is needed, but the Mayo Clinic data serve as a warning to physicians to use this drug combination very carefully and only in patients for whom there is a clear potential health benefit.

Dexfenfluramine. Recognition that obesity may have a genetic component, combined with the rapid increase in the prevalence of overweight individuals, has prompted drug companies to search for new, more effective treatments. Dexfenfluramine (Redux), approved by the FDA in April 1996, was the first new obesity drug on the market in the U.S. in nearly 25 years. The drug, which has been used in Europe for some time, has been shown to reduce body weight and maintain the loss during study periods of up to 12 months; thus, it is the only obesity drug available in the U.S. that has been approved for use for periods of up to one year.

In general, the side effects of dexfenfluramine are modest, but two major concerns have been raised in past year. First, dexfenfluramine (along with fenfluramine and other obesity drugs) has been implicated in the development of a serious disorder called primary pulmonary hypertension (PPH). In PPH the walls of blood vessels in the lungs become thickened, which impedes the flow of blood and causes the heart to work harder than usual to keep blood circulating to the lungs; this situation eventually leads to heart failure and, within about five years after onset, a 50% risk of death. PPH is extremely rare in the general population (about one or two cases per million each year), which makes it difficult to study.

If the worst predictions about dexfenfluramine and related compounds were to come true, about one person in 20,000 taking these drugs would develop PPH. The actual effect of the drugs is difficult to predict, however. Some scientists think PPH may be brought on by obesity itself, which would thus confound the association with weight-loss drugs. And because obesity is associated with about 300,000 deaths each year in the U.S. alone, most experts feel that the risk of remaining overweight is greater than the risk posed by the drugs. They also agree that these medications should be used only for the treatment of true obesity and not for loss of a few unwanted pounds.

The second concern is that use of dexfenfluramine could cause neurological damage. Animals treated with doses larger than are

Mark Humphrey—Associated Press

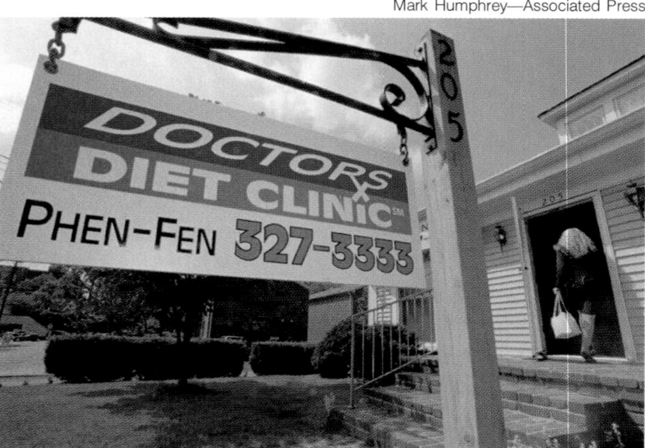

A diet clinic prominently advertises the availability of the "phen-fen" combination. Despite the risks associated with obesity drugs, the modest weight loss they produce may have significant health benefits.

normally used in humans develop changes in certain brain cells. The changes observed in experimental animals did not appear to affect their mental functioning, but many physicians are concerned that humans who take medication for an extended period may be at risk of unknown neurological harm. Clearly, the long-term use of these drugs must be further studied.

Orlistat. Orlistat (Xenical), scheduled to be approved by the FDA in 1997, is unlike other obesity treatments available in the U.S. in that it does not act on the brain. Orlistat inhibits the enzyme lipase in the digestive tract. Since lipase is critical for the digestion of fat, blocking its action reduces the absorption of fat from food. The unabsorbed fat is removed from the body in the stools. Regardless of fat intake, about one-third of the dietary fat consumed by an individual taking orlistat is eliminated from the body. Although the drug produces only modest weight loss, in clinical trials lasting two years, it was shown to be significantly more effective than a placebo medication.

The side effects of orlistat are generally more of a nuisance than a medical concern. If more than about 30 g of fat is eliminated in the stools, unpleasant side effects such as oily stools, diarrhea, abdominal cramping, and flatulence may be noted. Orlistat causes a slight loss of fat-soluble vitamins (A, D, E, and K) in the stools, and people using the drug probably supplement their diets with a multivitamin tablet. PPH is not expected to be a problem with orlistat.

The currently approved obesity drugs produce a weight loss of about 8–10% of initial body weight when used alone. Combinations of obesity drugs produce losses of about 15%. However, for most overweight individuals, these small percentages are not enough to produce dramatic improvements in appearance. Nonetheless, numerous studies show that even modest reductions in weight may be effective in reducing diabetes and hypertension, lowering high blood cholesterol and triglyceride levels, and preventing other complications of obesity. Thus, it appears that people who use these medications may significantly improve their health even if they do not manage to achieve a normal weight. In the meantime, the search for better treatments continues.

—Richard L. Atkinson, M.D.,
and Nikhil V. Dhurandhar, Ph.D.

Help for Halitosis

In 1693 Antonie van Leeuwenhoek, the Dutch creator of the first modern scientific microscope, described a truly debilitating problem that affected many of his friends and acquaintances:

> *There are more animals living in the uncleaned matter in one's mouth than there are men in a whole kingdom, especially in those who never clean their mouths, owing to which such a stench comes from the mouths of many that one can hardly speak to them.*

Offensive breath (halitosis) is an unfortunate, if not socially devastating, condition that has afflicted humankind since the dawn of civilization. Mention of it—often as a "curse"—can be found in the oldest Chinese, Egyptian, Greek, and Roman literatures. The term *halitosis* is derived from the Latin *halitus,* meaning "breath," and *osis,* meaning "abnormal," or "diseased." Historically, halitosis described bad breath emanating from the mouth but originating in some other part of the body. Other terms that describe odors coming from the mouth and sinuses, respectively, are *fetor oris* and *fetor ex ore,* from the Latin *foetor,* "to stink." *Fetor narium* specifically designates odors emanating from the nose. In this report, for the sake of clarity, *halitosis* is used to describe any detectable noxious or disagreeable odor originating in or emanating from the mouth or nose.

Causes and culprits

Today's specialists in halitosis treatment differentiate between *incidental* and *chronic* malodors and those that are *local* (in the mouth) and *systemic* (elsewhere in the body and often disease-related). Incidental bad breath may be caused by the consumption of foods with strong odors, such as garlic and raw onion; drinking alcohol; particles of food trapped in the mouth or between the teeth; tobacco use; neglect of dental hygiene; or improperly cared-for dentures, especially those worn overnight. Another common cause of incidental halitosis is decreased salivary flow during sleep that leads to "morning breath." Less commonly, persons who sing or orate for extended periods of time (*e.g.,* teachers, professional entertainers, and lecturers) develop incidental halitosis due to a dry-mouth syndrome.

About 90% of all halitosis originates in the mouth and not, as many people mistakenly believe, in the stomach or gastrointestinal tract. The actual culprits are gram-negative anaerobic bacteria, microorganisms that live and function in an oxygen-deprived environment; "gram-negative" indicates that they do not hold a purple dye when exposed to a special laboratory stain (Gram's stain). These organisms reside everywhere in the mouth, and each is capable of producing large volumes of volatile sulfur compounds (VSCs). Hydrogen sulfide, methyl mercaptan, and dimethyl sulfide are the primary VSC components that contribute to halitosis.

Periodontal (gum) disease, an infection of the tissues surrounding and supporting the teeth, is caused by plaque (a sticky, white film of bacteria that forms on the teeth). The bacteria create toxins that irritate the gums and can also produce VSCs. Although gum disease may be the local cause of halitosis, recent studies have shown that periodontal treatment, while saving the teeth and restoring the gums, often does not resolve the odor problem—presumably because a bacterial problem persists in the rest of the mouth.

Any slight reduction of moisture in the mouth increases the likelihood of halitosis. *Xerostomia,* the medical term for dry-mouth syndrome, is extremely common. The wide range of conditions that can affect oral moisture include menstruation, menopause, vitamin or mineral deficiencies, radiation therapy, chemotherapy, long periods of not eating, and many commonly used prescription and over-the-counter medications (antihistamines, antidepressants, and antibiotics, to name just a few). A complete list of the factors and conditions that can cause xerostomia would be much too long to present here. What is important is that whenever moisture levels in the mouth drop below optimal—regardless of the reason—anaerobic bacteria proliferate; these very specific microorganisms ferment to produce the distinctly noxious gases that characterize halitosis.

In a small minority of cases, chronic oral malodor is a symptom of a clearly defined disease occurring elsewhere in the body. Obviously, almost any bodily illness that causes a chronic reduction in salivary flow would affect breath odor. Before the advent of today's sophisticated diagnostic instruments, medical and den-

At best, poor Edna might have been able to briefly mask her problem with a swish of the mouthwash touted in this 1920s ad. The public still seems willing to buy virtually any product that promises to banish bad breath.

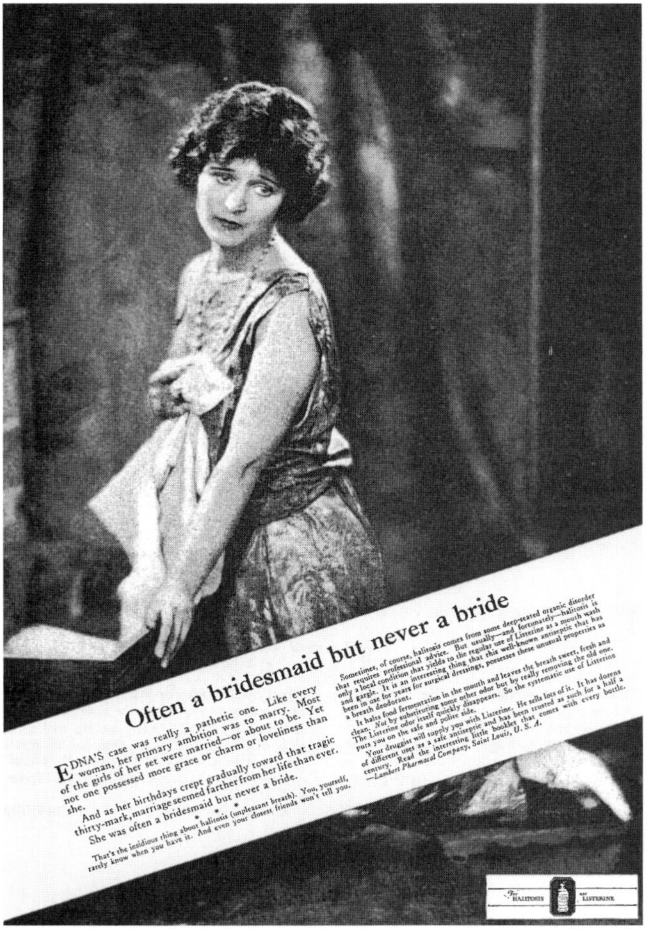

The Granger Collection, New York

Marie-Susanne Langille—The Gazette/Associated Press

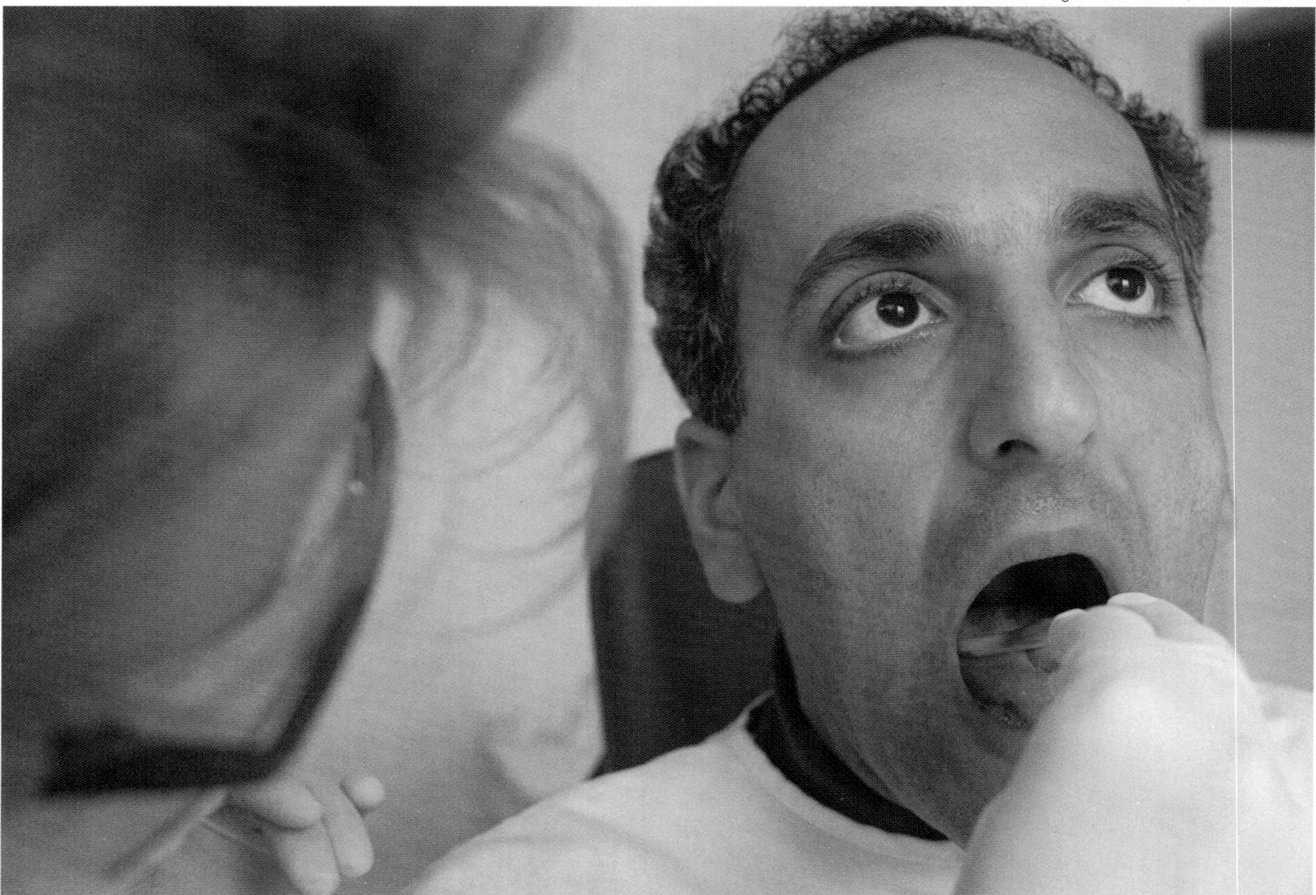

A dental hygienist uses a scraper to remove bacterial debris—a major source of mouth malodor—from the upper back portion of her client's tongue. Effective halitosis-control regimens prescribe thorough daily cleaning of the tongue—and of every other reachable surface in the mouth.

tal practitioners knew that certain odors emanating from the mouth reflected serious systemic disorders. Diabetes, kidney disease, leukemia, liver dysfunction, and endocrine and metabolic disturbances are just a few of the diseases that produce discernible breath odors that experienced clinicians can usually identify. Tumors or infections anywhere in the respiratory system (nose, sinuses, bronchi, trachea, or lungs) also result in some degree of bad breath.

Exaggerated concern?

Dentists generally encounter three categories of halitosis patients: those who have bad breath and know it, those who have bad breath but do not know it or are unsure of their condition, and those who think they have bad breath but in reality do not. Members of the latter group are sometimes referred to as "halitophobics" (*see* below).

Writing in the April 1996 *Journal of the American Dental Association (JADA),* Mel Rosenberg, an Israeli dentist, noted that "self-reports of bad breath are notoriously subjective. For example, among 88 women who complained of bad breath, 25 rated their own breath as a 5 ('the most foul odor imaginable') on a scale of 0 to 5." Interestingly, in one study female subjects rated their own breath as offensive with greater frequency than male subjects. Yet objective measurements revealed that the men had bad breath more often than the women.

Whether people are right or wrong about their own problem, halitosis is widespread. In 1995 a survey of 556 American Dental Association members found that 92% reported seeing patients with chronic bad breath in their regular practice, and more than 41% saw six or more halitosis sufferers in an average week. Incidental halitosis affects most people at some time, and as much as 10% of the population may have chronic halitosis. In the U.S. alone, an estimated 25 million to 27 million people flock to dentists' offices annually seeking help for bad breath.

Tricky diagnosis

Recently developed diagnostic equipment is now available to aid the dentist in evaluating several aspects of the halitosis picture. Portable sulfide monitors can measure VSCs in the oral cavity, nasal passages, and/or lungs. While these monitors have a high degree of accuracy, current models are not standardized, which makes it difficult or impossible for clinicians who use them to compare data. Fortunately, standardized gas analysis machines are being developed and should appear on the market in the near future.

A more sophisticated piece of diagnostic equipment enables the dentist to determine whether periodontal disease is the cause of halitosis. This machine measures both the temperature below the gums and the depth of pockets of inflamed gum tissue, both of which are indicative of disease well before major damage to the gums and teeth has occurred.

Even with the best tools and the most thorough examination and history taking, however, the diagnosis of halitosis can be tricky. One reason is that odors may have more than one origin. Another is the aforementioned condition known as halitophobia, or "phantom halitosis." Patients with this condition are convinced they have a serious foul-breath problem even though none can be measured on the gas analysis meter. The probable explanation is that the patient is responding to a bad taste in the mouth, which he or she mentally translates into an odor problem. This makes sense because the sensory centers for smell and taste in the cortex of the brain are in close proximity, so there may be some degree of "crossover" in sensory messages, which, in the halitophobic patient's mind, only serves to reinforce the halitosis certainty.

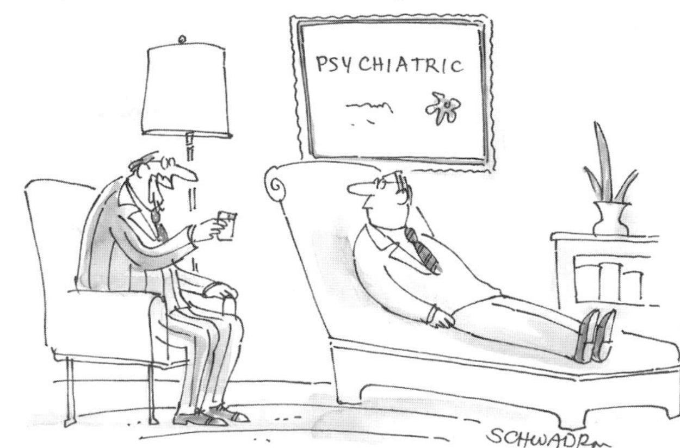

"You know your problem with women, Elliot? You need some breath fresheners. Here, try these."

Enlightened treatment

Traditionally, dental specialists have recommended the cleaning of specific areas of the mouth as the way to eliminate malodors and prevent dental disease, such as decay (caries) or pyorrhea (inflammation of the tooth sockets). Dentists correctly urge all patients to brush and floss their teeth daily. Only recently, however, has it become apparent that complete control of oral malodor requires that every reachable surface in the entire mouth be meticulously cleaned. Odors must be eliminated at the molecular level.

Not only must the teeth and gums be brushed and flossed, but the hard palate (roof of the mouth), the soft palate (the fold at the back of the hard palate that separates the mouth and pharynx), the tongue, and every other soft surface in the oral cavity that is accessible must be scrupulously rid of bacterial debris. A number of studies have shown that the top rear portion of the tongue is the most frequently overlooked source of mouth malodor. Dental hygiene, therefore, should include daily cleaning of the tongue, with a brush and/or a soft "tongue scraper." When a patient uses a tongue-cleaning device for the first time, he or she may gag slightly. But most people quickly get the hang of the procedure so that it easily becomes routine.

To banish bad breath, one must eliminate the underlying cause of the odor. Yet most people attempt to mask rather than remove the odor. In fact, those seeking halitosis cover-ups spend an estimated $1 billion annually on over-the-counter products such as mints, gum, breath sprays and drops, mouthwashes and rinses, "fresh-breath" toothpastes, etc.—none of which has anything more than a temporary effect (lasting at most a few hours). Many widely advertised and commonly used products actually make the problem worse. One group of masking agents, for example, contains alcohol. Not only are these products relatively ineffective, but the alcohol they contain tends to have a drying effect that increases the likelihood of xerostomia, which, as noted above, is one of the basic prerequisites for halitosis. Most commercial mouthwashes contain alcohol and therefore would fall into this group.

Other products contain chlorhexidine, a strong antimicrobial agent that can be extremely effective in controlling bacteria. Unfortunately, however, chlorhexidene rinses have some undesirable characteristics; they have a bitter taste, are costly, and cause temporary discoloration of the teeth. A new group of products contain oxidating agents as the key active ingredient. Because the organisms (bacteria) responsible for VSCs are anaerobic—that is, they thrive in an environment devoid of oxygen—agents that increase oxygen are able to inhibit the production of offensive gases. New and increasingly effective oxidizing agents, in combination with various other agents, are now in various stages of testing and may hold the ultimate solution to this vexing affliction.

Breath of fresh air

In September 1996 the editor of *JADA,* Lawrence H. Meskin, called attention to the vast number of bad-breath "franchises" that "are springing up" across the United States. "Advertisements for these clinics promise cure rates of 98 percent or higher. And for those who are geographically unable to visit a clinic, home treatment programs are available." Meskin noted that "the Internet also has become a venue.... People with a breath problem can now 'talk' with halitosis experts without having to identify themselves." He then proceeded to point out that the scope of treatment for bad breath falls within the normal limits of routine dental services. "There is nothing unique in the treatment approach advocated by fresh breath entrepreneurs," he said. Ultimately, he castigated his dental colleagues for not showing enough concern about their patients' breath problems. Meskin challenged them "to push [the halitosis-clinic entrepreneurs'] hype aside by giving [halitosis treatment] its appropriate place in your treatment armamentarium."

New treatment materials and new analytic tools are being developed that will vastly improve the dentist's ability to treat every aspect of the halitosis problem. Already available are products (*e.g.,* mouth rinses, toothpastes, and gels) that contain a buffered solution of chlorine dioxide, which stimulates an oxidation process, and specially designed tongue cleaners that have the capability of extending odor elimination in the mouth to an entire day rather than merely some part of an hour.

—Marvin Cohen, D.D.S.

NEWS CAP MHA 98

Furor over Fluoride in the U.K.

When sodium fluoride was first added to the public water system of Grand Rapids, Mich., in 1945, some charged that it was a communist plot to undermine the American way of life. In fact, the Grand Rapids Fluoridation Project, aimed at eliminating the epidemic of tooth decay in schoolchildren, proved to be one of the most successful public health undertakings in U.S. history. The 15-year study demonstrated that Grand Rapids youth aged 12–14 years had 50–63% fewer cavities in 1960 than their counterparts in 1945. Today about 62% of the people in the United States—some 155 million Americans—have fluoride in their water, the effects of which are far-reaching. Never has the oral health of children and young adults been better.

That is hardly the case across the Atlantic; in Great Britain rampant tooth decay remains endemic, and public suspicions about fluoridation run high. In 1996 only about 10% of the British population had fluoridated water. Antifluoridation crusaders, including a strong contingent in Parliament, have repeatedly frustrated government attempts to add the chemical to public water supplies. Opponents are convinced that fluoride does more harm than good. They point to a handful of studies that have shown some connection between very high levels of fluoride in water and damage to kidneys and other organs and a rare form of bone cancer.

L.L.T. Rhodes—Tony Stone Images

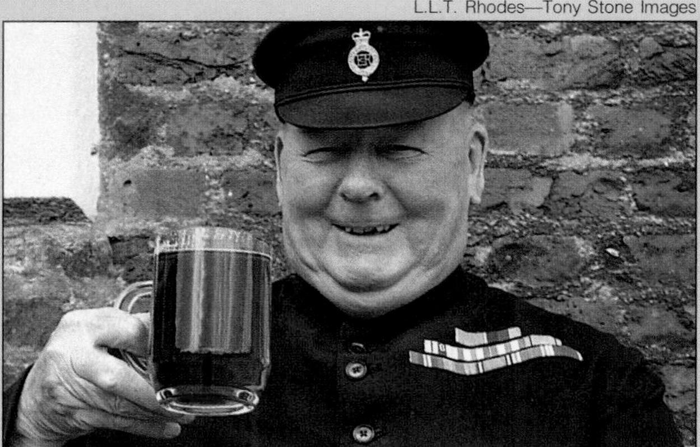

Fluoride? Not in this Englishman's pint of ale.

Even more prevalent—and scientifically justified—are Britons' concerns that fluoridation leads to dental fluorosis, a condition in which teeth become stained, mottled, and sometimes pitted. Such a connection was established in the 1930s, when fluorosis was found to be common in the teeth of people whose water systems had a high level of natural fluoride. At the same time, it was discovered that fluoride also had a cavity-fighting role; children with stained teeth had few cavities. Subsequent studies found that fluoride combines with crystals in the tooth structure to help protect and strengthen the surface enamel of teeth (where caries formation begins).

If it is clear that fluoride helps prevent cavities, it is also clear that too much exposure is undesirable. The optimal fluoride level—the level that prevents cavities but does not lead to fluorosis—has been established at one part fluoride per million parts water (1 ppm). But as fluoridation opponents are quick to point out, people may be getting a lot more fluoride than they know. It is not only added to water supplies; in some places natural fluoride can be found in groundwater in concentrations of up to 14 ppm. In the U.S. more than two million drinkers in about 1,300 mostly rural communities are served by water with natural fluoride levels of 2 ppm or higher. Fluoride is also added to many toothpastes and mouthwashes at concentrations of 1,000–1,500 ppm (an amount that is *not* considered dangerous because such dentifrices are not swallowed).

So, is Sir Ivan Lawrence, a Tory member of Parliament and leader in the fight against tampering with the British water supply, being an alarmist when he calls fluoride "one of the most toxic poisons known to man"? Probably. Nonetheless, antifluoridation sentiments in the U.K. remain strong despite the country's record of poor dental health. Many British opponents simply do not like the "idea" of having a foreign substance added to their drinking water. As the leader of a group that recently defeated a plan to fluoridate the water serving residents of Scarborough, Yorkshire, put it, "I believe very strongly that water is precious and that they shouldn't force us to do something if we don't want it."

Meanwhile, in the U.S. at least a few fluoride challengers have made themselves heard (including an organized group of dentists and the national PTA). This vocal minority believes that the U.S. health care establishment's blanket endorsement of fluoridation more than half a century ago may have been premature.

On the whole, however, Americans seem to have grown accustomed to the fluoridated water that comes out of their taps and are more likely to get up in arms about other foreign substances in their water, such as the microbial contaminant *Cryptosporidium,* which caused diarrheal illness in some 400,000 residents of Milwaukee, Wis., in 1993—and may have contributed to as many as 100 deaths.

—*Jeff Wallenfeldt*

New Drugs Approved by the Food and Drug Administration, January 1996–July 1997

Priority approvals[1]			
Generic name (brand name)	**Manufacturer**	**Use**	**Selected side effects**
albendazole (Albenza)	SmithKline Beecham	cystic disease caused by pork tapeworm larvae and dog tapeworm larvae	changes in liver enzymes; abdominal pain; nausea; vomiting; headache
amlexanox (Aphthasol)	Block Drug	ulcers of oral mucous membrane	transient local pain, stinging, and/or burning
anagrelide (Agrylin)	Roberts	thrombocythemia (elevated blood platelet count)	headache; diarrhea; edema (accumulation of fluid in the tissues); palpitation; abdominal pain; muscle weakness; dizziness; shortness of breath
atorvastatin (Lipitor)	Warner-Lambert; Pfizer	high cholesterol levels	constipation; flatulence; indigestion; abdominal pain
bentoquatam (IvyBlock)	EnviroDerm	skin protection against poison ivy, oak, and sumac	[none of significance]
betaine (Cystadane)	Orphan Medical	elevated homocysteine levels resulting from homocystinuria (a metabolic disorder)	nausea; gastrointestinal distress; diarrhea
corticorelin ovine triflutate (Acthrel)	Ferring	diagnostic aid for determining cause of Cushing's syndrome	flushing of face, neck, and upper chest; rapid heartbeat; low blood pressure; difficulty breathing; chest tightness
delavirdine (Rescriptor)	Pharmacia & Upjohn	HIV infection	rash; nausea; headache; fatigue; changes in liver enzymes
docetaxel (Taxotere)	Rhône-Poulenc Rorer	breast cancer in patients who have not responded to standard therapies	low white blood cell count; anemia; low platelet count; fluid retention; rash; hair loss; nausea; vomiting; diarrhea; low blood pressure; inflammation of the mouth; changes in liver enzymes
donepezil (Aricept)	Eisai; Pfizer	Alzheimer's disease symptoms	nausea; diarrhea; insomnia; vomiting; muscle cramps; fatigue; loss of appetite
gemcitabine (Gemzar)	Lilly	pancreatic cancer	low white blood cell count; nausea; vomiting; fever; edema (accumulation of fluid in the tissues); rash; flulike symptoms; hair loss
indinavir (Crixivan)	Merck	HIV infection	kidney stones; elevated levels of the pigment bilirubin (a sign of impaired liver function); abdominal pain; weakness; nausea; diarrhea; vomiting; headache; taste disturbance
irinotecan (Camptosar)	Pharmacia & Upjohn	colorectal cancer in patients whose disease has relapsed or progressed on 5-fluorouracil therapy	diarrhea; low white blood cell count; nausea; vomiting; abdominal cramping
ivermectin (Stromectol)	Merck	strongyloidiasis and onchocerciasis (parasitic worm infestations)	dizziness; loss of strength; itching; diarrhea; fatigue; abdominal pain; loss of appetite; constipation; nausea; vomiting
latanoprost (Xalatan)	Pharmacia & Upjohn	relief of intraocular pressure in open-angle glaucoma	increased brown coloring of the iris of the eye; blurred vision; ocular stinging and/or itching
midodrine (ProAmatine)	Roberts	orthostatic, or postural, hypotension (reduction in blood pressure when assuming upright position)	high blood pressure; scalp itching; goosebumps; chills; urinary urge, frequency, and/or retention
nelfinavir (Viracept)	Agouron	HIV infection	diarrhea; nausea; flatulence; rash
nevirapine (Viramune)	Boehringer Ingelheim; Roxane	HIV infection (in combination with other drugs)	severe rash; changes in liver enzymes
ritonavir (Norvir)	Abbott	HIV infection	nausea; diarrhea; vomiting

New Drugs Approved by the Food and Drug Administration, January 1996–July 1997

Generic name (brand name)	Manufacturer	Use	Selected side effects
Priority approvals[1]			
sodium phenylbutyrate (Buphenyl)	Ucyclyd	urea cycle disorders (a group of congenital metabolic diseases)	absence of menstrual periods; body odor; taste aversion; decreased appetite
topotecan (Hycamtin)	SmithKline Beecham	ovarian cancer	low white blood cell count; nausea; vomiting; diarrhea; constipation; abdominal pain; hair loss; fatigue; fever
troglitazone (Rezulin)	Parke-Davis	Type II diabetes	infection; headache; pain
urea C-14 (Pytest)	Tri-Med	breath test for detection of *Helicobacter pylori*	[none of significance]
Standard approvals[2]			
adapalene (Differin)	Galderma	acne	skin redness and/or scaling, dryness, itching, burning, stinging, tingling
ardeparin (Normiflo)	Wyeth-Ayerst	prevention of deep-vein thrombosis following knee replacement	bleeding; blood-containing swelling at injection site (hematoma); low platelet count; fever; anemia; constipation; rash
azelastine (Astelin)	Carter-Wallace	seasonal nasal allergies	bitter taste; drowsiness; weight gain; muscle pain
brimonidine (Alphagan)	Allergan	open-angle glaucoma and elevated ocular pressure	oral dryness; ocular itching, burning, stinging, and/or congestion; blurred vision; headache; sensation of foreign body in eye; development of follicles (cavities) in mucous membrane of eye; ocular allergic reactions; drowsiness
butenafine (Mentax)	Penederm	athlete's foot	burning; stinging; itching
cabergoline (Dostinex)	Pharmacia & Upjohn	hyperprolactinemic disorders (a group of endocrine conditions)	nausea; headache; dizziness; constipation; fatigue; postural hypotension (drop in blood pressure when assuming upright position)
cefipime (Maxipime)	Bristol-Myers Squibb	urinary tract infections, skin infections, pneumonia	rash; vein inflammation; pain
cerivastatin (Baycol)	Bayer	high cholesterol levels	inflammation of nasal lining; inflammation of sinuses; joint pain; indigestion; muscle pain; peripheral edema (accumulation of fluid in tissues); insomnia
cidofovir (Vistide)	Gilead	cytomegalovirus infection of the retina	protein in the urine; nausea; vomiting; loss of strength; neutropenia (decrease in the white blood cells known as neutrophils); rash; headache; diarrhea; hair loss; chills; loss of appetite; anemia; increased blood-creatinine levels (a sign of kidney dysfunction); fever; infection; shortness of breath; abdominal pain
danaparoid (Orgaran)	Organon	prevention of deep-vein thrombosis in elective hip surgery	pain; fever; nausea; urinary tract infection; constipation; rash
ferumoxides (Feridex)	Advanced Magnetics	medical imaging for diagnosis of liver lesions	back pain; dilation of blood vessels; pain; low blood pressure
ferumoxsil (GastroMARK)	Advanced Magnetics	medical imaging for diagnosis of intestinal disorders	nausea; vomiting; diarrhea; abdominal cramping; upset stomach; flatulence; tingling sensation in the mouth
fexofenadine (Allegra)	Hoechst Marion Roussel	seasonal allergy symptoms (*e.g.*, nasal inflammation, itchy eyes)	nausea; drowsiness; upset stomach
fosfomycin tromethamine (Monurol)	Forest; Zambon	uncomplicated urinary tract infection	diarrhea; vaginitis; nausea; headache; dizziness
fosphenytoin (Cerebyx)	Warner-Lambert	epileptic and neurosurgical seizures; short-term substitution for oral phenytoin	burning; itching; tingling sensations

New Drugs Approved by the Food and Drug Administration, January 1996–July 1997

Standard approvals[2]			
Generic name (brand name)	Manufacturer	Use	Selected side effects
glatiramer acetate (Copaxone)	Teva	relapsing-remitting multiple sclerosis	injection site reaction; vasodilation; chest pain; loss of strength; infection; nausea; joint pain; anxiety; increased muscle tension
imiquimod (Aldara)	3M Pharmaceuticals	genital and perianal warts	skin redness, erosion, flaking, ulceration, hardening, and/or scabbing; swelling
iodixanol (Visipaque)	Nycomed	diagnostic imaging of blood vessels	chest pain; nausea; headache and/or migraine; vertigo; rash; taste disturbance
lispro insulin (Humalog)	Lilly	diabetes	allergic reactions; itching; low blood sugar
meropenem (Merrem)	Zeneca	complicated intra-abdominal infections; pediatric bacterial meningitis	diarrhea; nausea; headache; rash
mibefradil (Posicor)	Roche	high blood pressure; chronic stable angina	headache; runny nose
miglitol (Glyset)	Bayer	Type II diabetes	abdominal pain; diarrhea; flatulence
mirtazapine (Remeron)	Organon	depression	low white blood cell count; drowsiness; nausea; weight gain
nilutamide (Nilandron)	Hoechst Marion Roussel	adjunct to castration surgery for metastatic prostate cancer	nausea; hot flushes; constipation; abnormal vision; impaired adaptation to darkness; pain; impotence; breast enlargement
olanzapine (Zyprexa)	Lilly	psychotic disorders	postural hypotension (drop in blood pressure when assuming upright posture); weight gain; drowsiness; dizziness; personality disorder; increased muscle tension; inflammation of nasal lining
olopatadine (Patanol)	Alcon	itching associated with allergic conjunctivitis	headache; ocular burning and/or stinging
penciclovir (Denavir)	SmithKline Beecham	recurrent oral herpesvirus infection	headache
pentosan (Elmiron)	Baker Norton; Alza	bladder pain or discomfort associated with interstitial cystitis	abdominal pain; diarrhea; hair loss; nausea; headache; rash; upset stomach
pramipexole (Mirapex)	Pharmacia & Upjohn; Boehringer Ingelheim	Parkinson's disease symptoms	hallucinations; impaired movement; drowsiness; dry mouth
remifentanil (Ultiva)	Glaxo Wellcome	general anesthesia	respiratory depression; slowed heartbeat; low blood pressure; skeletal muscle rigidity; nausea; vomiting
ropivacaine (Naropin)	Astra	local anesthesia	low blood pressure; slowed heartbeat; slowed fetal heartbeat in childbirth; nausea; vomiting; tingling sensations; back pain
samarium (Quadramet)	Cytogen	relief of pain in bone cancer	low white blood cell count; decreased hemoglobin; bleeding; irregular heartbeat
sparfloxacin (Zagam)	Rhône-Poulenc Rorer	community-acquired pneumonia; acute bacterial infection in chronic bronchitis	sunlight sensitivity; diarrhea; nausea; headache; upset stomach; dizziness
tamsulosin (Flomax)	Boehringer Ingelheim	benign enlargement of prostate gland	dizziness; abnormal ejaculation; inflammation of nasal lining; drowsiness; infection; loss of strength; back pain
tazorotene (Tazorac)	Allergan	psoriasis; acne	skin dryness, redness, scaling, discoloration, burning, fissuring, and/or itching; localized swelling
technetium Tc 99m tetrofosmin (Myoview)	Medi-Physics	diagnostic imaging of heart muscle	high blood pressure; torsades de pointes (a type of irregular heart rhythm); vomiting; abdominal discomfort; skin allergy; low blood pressure; dizziness; elevated white blood cell count

New Drugs Approved by the Food and Drug Administration, January 1996–July 1997

Generic name (brand name)	Manufacturer	Use	Selected side effects
Standard approvals[2]			
tiludronate (Skelid)	Sanofi Winthrop	Paget's disease	nausea; diarrhea; upset stomach
tizanidine (Zanaflex)	Athena Neurosciences	muscle spasticity	changes in liver enzymes; dry mouth; drowsiness; loss of strength; dizziness
topiramate (Topamax)	Ortho-McNeil	seizures	drowsiness; incoordination; dizziness; slowed movement; speech disorder; abnormal movement of eyeballs (nystagmus); tingling sensations; fatigue; difficulty concentrating; confusion; depression; anxiety
toremifene citrate (Fareston)	Schering-Plough; Orion	metastatic breast cancer in postmenopausal women with estrogen receptor-positive or receptor-unknown tumors	hot flushes; sweating; nausea; vaginal discharge; dizziness; pain; vomiting
trandolapril (Mavik)	Knoll	high blood pressure	cough; dizziness; diarrhea
urea C-13 (UBT Breath Test)	Meretek	diagnosis of *Helicobacter pylori*-associated ulcers	[none of significance]
valsartan (Diovan)	Novartis	high blood pressure	viral infection; fatigue; abdominal pain; headache; dizziness
zafirlukast (Accolate)	Zeneca	asthma	headache; nausea; diarrhea
zileuton (Zyflo)	Abbott	asthma	nausea; upset stomach; pain; abdominal pain; loss of strength
Biologics or vaccines[3]			
arcitumomab (CEA-Scan)	Immunomedics	medical imaging for diagnosis of colorectal cancer	possible allergic reactions
capromab pendetide (ProstaScint)	Cytogen	medical imaging for diagnosis of prostate cancer	elevated levels of the pigment bilirubin (a sign of impaired liver function); high blood pressure; low blood pressure
diphtheria and tetanus toxoids and acellular pertussis vaccine adsorbed (Infanrix)	SmithKline Beecham	immunization against diphtheria, tetanus, and pertussis	redness and/or swelling at injection site; drowsiness; poor appetite; vomiting
hepatitis A vaccine (Vaqta)	Merck	prevention of hepatitis A infection	fever; sore throat; abdominal pain
imciromab pentetate (MyoScint)	Centocor	medical imaging for diagnosis of damage to heart muscle	dry mouth; injection-site pain; fever
interferon-beta-1a (Avonex)	Biogen	relapsing forms of multiple sclerosis	fever; chills; muscle aches; fatigue; weakness
nofetumomab (Verluma)	Boehringer Ingelheim	medical imaging for diagnosis of lung cancer	fever; rash and/or hives; allergic reaction
respiratory syncytial virus immune globulin (RespiGam)	MedImmune	prevention of respiratory syncytial virus infection	fever
reteplase (Retavase)	Boehringer Mannheim	dissolution of blood clot in acute heart attack	bleeding; nausea; low blood pressure; fever
New indications, formulations, or combinations			
acitretin (Soriatane)	Roche	severe psoriasis (new form of an existing drug)	lip inflammation; hair loss; skin peeling; changes in liver enzymes; risk of birth defects
albuterol sulfate CFC-free metered aerosol (Proventil-HFA)	3M Pharmaceuticals; Schering Plough	asthma (chlorofluorocarbon-propellant-free formulation)	palpitations; chest pain; rapid heart rate; tremors or nervousness
alendronate (Fosamax)	Merck; Wyeth-Ayerst	prevention of osteoporosis in postmenopausal women (previously approved only for osteoporosis treatment)	abdominal pain; muscle pain; constipation; diarrhea; flatulence; headache

New Drugs Approved by the Food and Drug Administration, January 1996–July 1997

New indications, formulations, or combinations			
Generic name (brand name)	Manufacturer	Use	Selected side effects
allopurinol injection (Zyloprim)	Glaxo Wellcome	uric acid elevation in chemotherapy patients (injectable formulation; previously available as tablet)	rash; elevated white blood cell count; injection-site reaction
alprostadil injection (Edex)	Schwarz Pharma	erectile dysfunction	penile pain; prolonged erection; bleeding; bruising
alprostadil transurethral (Muse)	Vivus	erectile dysfunction	penile pain; prolonged erection; urethral burning and bleeding; low blood pressure; dizziness; vaginal burning in partner
alteplase (t-PA; Activase)	Genentech	acute ischemic stroke (previously approved for heart attack)	intracranial bleeding
amphotericin B cholesteryl sulfate complex (Amphotec)	Sequus	aspergillosis infection in patients unresponsive to or unable to tolerate conventional amphotericin B therapy (active ingredient previously approved for fungal infections in nonliposomal form)	chills; fever; low blood pressure; rapid heartbeat; increased blood-creatinine levels (a sign of kidney dysfunction); nausea
amphotericin B lipid complex (Abelcet)	The Liposome Co.	invasive fungal infections in patients unresponsive to or unable to tolerate amphotericin B (previously approved for aspergillosis in patients unresponsive to or unable to tolerate amphotericin B)	chills; fever; increased blood-creatinine levels (a sign of kidney dysfunction); gastrointestinal bleeding; respiratory failure; multiple organ failure; sepsis
azithromycin (Zithromax)	Pfizer	AIDS-related *Mycobacterium avium* complex infection; urinary and genital infections in males; pediatric community-acquired pneumonia (previously approved for other respiratory, skin, and urinary tract infections)	diarrhea; nausea; abdominal pain
bismuth subsalicylate/ tetracycline/metronidazole (Helidac)	Proctor & Gamble	duodenal ulcer associated with *Helicobacter pylori* infection (separate ingredients previously approved for other uses)	nausea; diarrhea; abdominal pain; dark-colored stools
bleomycin (Blenoxane)	Bristol-Myers Squibb	malignant pleural effusions (exudation of fluid into the pleural membranes as a complication of lung cancer; previously approved for squamous cell carcinoma, lymphoma, and testicular carcinoma)	local pain; lung inflammation; development of fibrous tissue in the lungs; low blood pressure; skin redness; rash; hair loss
brompheniramine maleate (Efidac 24)	Alza	over-the-counter antihistamine/decongestant (formerly prescription-only)	[not available]
budesonide (Pulmicort Turbuhaler)	Astra	asthma (oral-inhalation form; previously available as nasal spray)	respiratory infection; headache; pain; oral fungal infection; voice alteration
buproprion hydrochloride sustained-release (Wellbutrin SR)	Glaxo Wellcome	depression (previously approved but withdrawn from market)	headache; dry mouth; insomnia; nausea; dizziness; agitation; sore throat
buproprion hydrochloride sustained-release (Zyban)	Glaxo Wellcome	smoking cessation (previously approved for depression)	headache; dry mouth; insomnia; nausea; dizziness; agitation; sore throat
calcipotriene cream (Dovenex)	Bristol-Myers Squibb	psoriasis (cream form; previously available as ointment)	rash; itching; dermatitis
cefuroxime axetil (Ceftin)	Glaxo Wellcome	early Lyme disease (previously approved for other infections)	diarrhea; Jarisch-Herxheimer's reaction (increase in symptoms of syphilis); vaginitis
clarithromycin (Biaxin)	Abbott	*Helicobacter pylori*-associated duodenal ulcers (in combination with omeprazole); community-acquired pneumonia in children (previously indicated for prevention and treatment of AIDS-related *Mycobacterium avium* complex and other infections)	diarrhea; nausea; taste disturbance; upset stomach; abdominal pain; headache

New Drugs Approved by the Food and Drug Administration, January 1996–July 1997			
New indications, formulations, or combinations			
Generic name (brand name)	Manufacturer	Use	Selected side effects
cromolyn sodium (Gastrocrom)	Rhône-Poulenc Rorer	mastocytosis (an immunologic disorder; previously approved for nasal allergies)	headache; diarrhea; itching; nausea; muscle pain
cyclosporine microemulsion (Neoral)	Novartis	rheumatoid arthritis unresponsive to methotrexate; severe recalcitrant psoriasis (previously approved for organ rejection)	high blood pressure; kidney dysfunction; headache; gastrointestinal disturbances; excessive hair growth
daunorubicin liposomal formulation (DaunoXome)	NeXstar	AIDS-related Kaposi's sarcoma (liposomal formulation; formerly available in nonliposomal formulation for leukemia)	blood cell suppression; back pain; flushing; chest tightness; cardiac symptoms
dexfenfluramine (Redux)*	Interneuron; Wyeth-Ayerst	obesity (new formulation of the drug fenfluramine)	diarrhea; dry mouth; drowsiness; risk of primary pulmonary hypertension (increased resistance to blood flow in the arteries that supply the lungs)
divalproex (Depakote)	Abbott	prevention of chronic migraine headache; complex partial seizures (previously approved for treatment of epilepsy and manic phase of bipolar disorder)	nausea; upset stomach; diarrhea; vomiting; weakness; fatigue; drowsiness; dizziness; risk of liver failure
estradiol controlled-release film (Alora)	TheraTech; Proctor & Gamble	flushing associated with menopause; vulvar and vaginal atrophy; low estrogen levels due to removal or failure of ovaries (new form of estradiol)	[not available]
estradiol controlled-release patch (Fempatch)	Warner-Lambert	estrogen replacement therapy in menopausal women and those with low estrogen levels due to removal or failure of ovaries; abnormal uterine bleeding due to hormonal imbalance (new form of estradiol)	bloating; dizziness; depression; breast pain
estradiol vaginal ring (Estring)	Pharmacia & Upjohn	local treatment for vaginal and urogenital postmenopausal atrophy (vaginal insert formulation)	vaginal discomfort and/or discharge; abdominal pain; nausea; back pain; headache
ethinyl estradiol and norethindrone acetate (Estrostep)	Warner-Lambert	contraception (new form of estradiol and norethindrone)	nausea; breast tenderness; headache; bloating; weight gain
etoposide phosphate (Etopophos)	Bristol-Myers Squibb	small-cell lung cancer, testicular tumors (new formulation of etoposide)	low blood cell count; nausea; vomiting; chills; fever; rapid heart rate; shortness of breath; low blood pressure
fluoxetine (Prozac)	Lilly	bulimia (previously approved for depression and obsessive-compulsive disorder)	loss of strength; flu syndrome; nausea; upset stomach; insomnia; anxiety; sleepiness; tremor
fluticasone propionate (Flovent)	Glaxo Wellcome	asthma (oral inhalation form; formerly available as nasal spray for nasal inflammation)	sore throat; nasal congestion; respiratory infection; flu; headache; oral candidiasis (fungal infection of mouth); hoarseness
fluvoxamine maleate (Luvox)	Solvay; Pharmacia & Upjohn	obsessive-compulsive disorder (OCD) in children and adolescents (previously approved for OCD in adults)	nausea; headache; loss of strength; diarrhea; constipation; indigestion; agitation; hyperactivity; depression; painful menstruation; flatulence; rash
ganciclovir intraocular implant (Vitrasert)	Chiron; Roche	AIDS-related cytomegalovirus infection of the retina (implantable formulation)	temporary decrease in visual acuity; eye infection; retinal detachment; cataracts
ganciclovir oral formulation (Cytovene)	Roche	AIDS-related cytomegalovirus infection of the retina (oral formulation)	fever; abdominal pain; diarrhea; nausea; low white blood cell count
interferon alpha (Roferon-A)	Roche	chronic hepatitis C (previously approved for chronic myelogenous leukemia, hairy cell leukemia, and Kaposi's sarcoma)	anemia; low white blood cell count; low platelet count; fever; chills; muscle pain; loss of appetite; nausea; headache
ipratropium bromide/albuterol sulfate (Combivent)	Boehringer Ingelheim	chronic obstructive pulmonary disease (COPD; combination of ingredients previously approved separately for COPD and asthma)	headache; bronchitis; difficulty breathing; coughing; respiratory infection

New Drugs Approved by the Food and Drug Administration, January 1996–July 1997

New indications, formulations, or combinations			
Generic name (brand name)	Manufacturer	Use	Selected side effects
itraconazole (Sporanox)	Janssen	onychomycosis (fungal infection of toenails and fingernails) and fungal infections of skin (previously approved for other fungal infections)	changes in liver enzymes; gastrointestinal disorders; rash; high blood pressure; low blood pressure; headache; muscle pain; vertigo
lansoprazole (Prevacid)	TAP Holdings	eradication of *Helicobacter pylori* (with clarithromycin and/or amoxicillin) in duodenal ulcer disease; maintenance of healing in erosive esophagitis (previously approved for treatment of duodenal ulcer, erosive esophagitis, and hypersecretion of stomach acid)	abdominal pain; diarrhea; nausea
levofloxacin (Levaquin)	Ortho-McNeil	acute maxillary sinusitis; acute bacterial exacerbation of chronic bronchitis; community-acquired pneumonia; uncomplicated skin and skin-structure infections; complicated urinary tract infection; acute kidney infection (new form of ofloxacin)	nausea; diarrhea; vaginitis; flatulence; itching; dizziness; insomnia
levonorgestrel two-rod implant [no brand name]	Wyeth-Ayerst	contraception (previously available in six rods as Norplant)	heavy menstrual bleeding; painful menstruation; spotting; absence of menstrual periods; acne; breast pain; headache; nausea; nervousness; vaginal infection and itching; weight gain
miconazole (Monistat 3)	Johnson & Johnson Advanced Care Products	over-the-counter three-day treatment for vaginal yeast infection (formerly prescription-only)	vaginal itching and burning; abdominal cramping; headache; rash
minoxidil (Rogaine)	Pharmacia & Upjohn	over-the-counter hair-growth treatment for male and female hair loss (formerly prescription-only)	skin irritation; eczema
nicotine gum (Nicorette)	SmithKline Beecham	over-the-counter smoking-cessation therapy (formerly prescription-only)	oral tingling; bleeding of gums; diarrhea; upset stomach; nausea; hiccups; tooth disorders
nicotine inhaler (Nicotrol)	McNeil	smoking cessation aid (oral inhalation form; previously available as skin patch)	mouth and/or throat irritation; upset stomach; nausea; diarrhea; hiccups; headache
nicotine nasal spray (Nicotrol NS)	McNeil; Pharmacia & Upjohn	smoking cessation aid (nasal-spray form; previously available as skin patch)	nasal and throat irritation; runny nose; watering eyes; sneezing; coughing
nicotine patch (Nicotrol)	McNeil	over-the-counter smoking-cessation aid (formerly prescription-only)	rash; increased heart rate
nizatidine (Axid AR)	Whitehall Robins	over-the-counter heartburn treatment (formerly prescription-only)	anemia; rash
norgestimate/ethinyl estradiol (Ortho Tri-Cyclen)	Ortho	acne in women seeking contraception (previously approved only for contraception)	nausea; vomiting; abdominal cramping and bloating; breakthrough bleeding
ofloxacin ophthalmic solution (Ocuflox)	Allergan	corneal ulcers (previously approved for bacterial conjunctivitis)	ocular burning, stinging, redness, dryness, and/or light sensitivity; blurred vision
ofloxacin tablets (Floxin)	Johnson & Johnson	pelvic inflammatory disease (previously approved for other infections)	nausea; headache; insomnia; vaginal itching; dizziness; diarrhea; vomiting; rash
omeprazole (Prilosec)	Astra and Merck	*Helicobacter pylori*-induced duodenal ulcers (in combination with clarithromycin); gastric ulcers; symptomatic gastroesophageal reflux disease (previously approved for duodenal ulcers, erosive esophagitis, and gastrointestinal reflux disease)	dizziness; rash; constipation; cough; back pain

New Drugs Approved by the Food and Drug Administration, January 1996–July 1997

New indications, formulations, or combinations

Generic name (brand name)	Manufacturer	Use	Selected side effects
paroxetine (Paxil)	SmithKline Beecham	obsessive compulsive disorder, panic disorder (previously approved for depression)	weakness; sweating; nausea; decreased appetite; drowsiness; dizziness; insomnia; tremor; nervousness; ejaculatory disturbance
polifeprosan/carmustine implant (Gliadel)	Guilford; Rhône-Poulenc Rorer	recurrence of central nervous system tumor glioblastoma multiforme (previously available in different formulation)	fever; pain; abnormal healing; fluid accumulation in brain; confusion; sleepiness
pravastatin (Pravachol)	Bristol-Myers Squibb	reduction of heart attack risk and slowing of progression of coronary atherosclerosis (previously approved for cholesterol lowering)	rash; heartburn; fatigue; headache; dizziness
progesterone bioadhesive vaginal gel (Crinone)	Columbia Labs; Wyeth-Ayerst	infertility due to progesterone deficiency (new form of progesterone)	breast enlargement; sleepiness; constipation; nausea; perineal pain; headache; abdominal pain; nervousness; excessive nighttime urination; depression; decreased libido
ranitidine bismuth citrate (Tritec)	Glaxo Wellcome	duodenal ulcer associated with *Helicobacter pylori* (in combination with clarithromycin; previously approved as separate active ingredients for different uses)	diarrhea
sertraline (Zoloft)	Pfizer	obsessive-compulsive disorder (previously approved for depression)	headache; nausea; diarrhea; dizziness; mouth dryness; fatigue; indigestion; tremor; sweating
somatropin (Humatrope)	Lilly	short stature in Turner's syndrome (a chromosomal anomaly), somatotropin deficiency in adults (previously approved for growth failure in children due to inadequate hormone secretion)	injection-site pain
somatropin (Nutropin)	Genentech	short stature in Turner's syndrome (previously approved for growth failure in children due to inadequate hormone secretion)	injection-site pain
somatropin (Saizen)	Serono	growth failure in children due to inadequate hormone secretion (active ingredient previously available)	injection-site reaction; thyroid deficiency; low blood sugar
somatropin (Serostim)	Serono	physical wasting and malnutrition in AIDS (active ingredient previously available)	musculoskeletal discomfort; swelling of hands and feet
sumatriptan (Imitrex)	Glaxo Wellcome	cluster headache (previously approved for migraine headache)	tingling; weakness; warm/hot sensation; feeling of heaviness or tightness
terbinafine tablets (Lamisil)	Sandoz	onychomycosis (fungal infection of toenails and fingernails; formerly available in cream form for athlete's foot, jock itch, and ringworm)	diarrhea; rash; upset stomach; changes in liver enzymes; itching; taste disturbance; nausea; abdominal pain
tretinoin cream (Avita)	Penederm	acne (active ingredient previously available)	skin swelling, crusting, and/or blistering; sensitivity to sunlight
valacyclovir (Valtrex)	Glaxo Wellcome	initial episode of genital herpesvirus infection (previously approved for herpes zoster [shingles] and recurrent genital herpes)	nausea; headache; diarrhea; dizziness

[1]New compounds (*i.e.*, new molecular entities) to treat serious illnesses for which no adequate alternative therapy exists.
[2]New compounds that provide some, little, or no therapeutic gain over products already available.
[3]Products such as serums, toxins, blood components, etc., used to prevent, treat, or cure disease.
*Withdrawn from market in September 1997.

—*prepared by Danielle Foullon*

Safety Issues: The Paradox of Effective Vaccines

Vaccine safety as a media topic reached new heights in 1997. The popular press charged that the international pharmaceutical industry was vested in selling existing vaccines, which generate annual revenues ranging in the billions of dollars; scientific papers explored the complexities of developing new vaccines; and national policy makers wrestled with fundamental matters of vaccine safety. It may seem surprising that so much attention is being given to such a well-established preventive health measure. The concerns surrounding vaccines are evidence of the power of anecdotes, the limitations of science, the rise of consumerism (*i.e.,* the questioning of "establishment" dictums), and the inherent uncertainty that arises whenever technology advances.

To understand the vaccine safety issues, it is helpful to appreciate that "safety" is more than one thing. First, in legal terms, it is the "relative freedom from harmful effect" that is afforded when a product is prudently administered. Second, in practical terms, vaccine safety is the result of a massive effort spanning research, development, laboratory and clinical testing, production in stringently regulated facilities, and careful evaluation of all data accumulated prior to licensure, as well as postlicensure vigilance to ensure proper, safe, and effective use. Finally, in media terms, the focus is rarely on safety per se when vaccines are successful but rather on their perceived shortcomings.

In the United States responsibility for vaccine safety rests with the federal government. While the Food and Drug Administration (FDA) has official regulatory authority over vaccines, safety is ultimately achieved through the concerted efforts of scientists, doctors, nurses, parents, and manufacturers. But history is replete with examples of ways the public's perception of risk has become the driving force behind changes in the manner in which vaccines are used by entire countries.

In the 1970s concerns over pertussis (whooping cough) vaccine safety resulted in a decline in consumer confidence, plummeting immunization rates, and national epidemics of the disease in Great Britain and Sweden. In the early 1980s similar concerns in the U.S. threatened the vaccine supply as hundreds of lawsuits forced companies to cease production. Nearly 20 years later those concerns have not vanished. The U.S. Public Health Service Task Force on Safer Childhood Vaccines affirmed recently that the stability of the national immunization program continues to depend on public confidence in vaccines. After examining all aspects of vaccine safety, the task force issued recommendations to ensure safety at every step of the pathway (from basic science through production and use) and to strengthen the systems to monitor vaccine reactions.

Polio: a case in point

The news media have clearly documented what has become the paradox of immunization. Simply stated, although vaccines must be as safe as possible in order to be licensed for use to prevent disease in healthy children, adolescents, and adults, no pharmaceutical product is ever 100% safe. In the aftermath of the summertime polio epidemics that raged through communities in the 1940s and early '50s—paralyzing children, filling iron-lung wards of hospitals, and leaving vast misery in their wake—the first polio vaccine, which became available in 1955, was perceived to be a precious gift from science. The first clinical trial of Jonas Salk's killed, or inactivated, poliovirus vaccine (IPV) involved more than one million U.S. schoolchildren in the first, second, and third grades. The day after the field testing concluded, the vaccine was licensed, and shortly thereafter parents lined up their children in droves for injections. By 1960 vast numbers of U.S. children and adults had received polio shots, and the annual incidence of paralytic polio had dropped to less than 2 per 100,000. In that same year Albert Sabin's preparation of live attenuated (weakened) oral poliovirus vaccine (OPV) was approved, and it soon became the predominant vaccine used in the U.S. and most other countries.

Alan Mothner—Associated Press

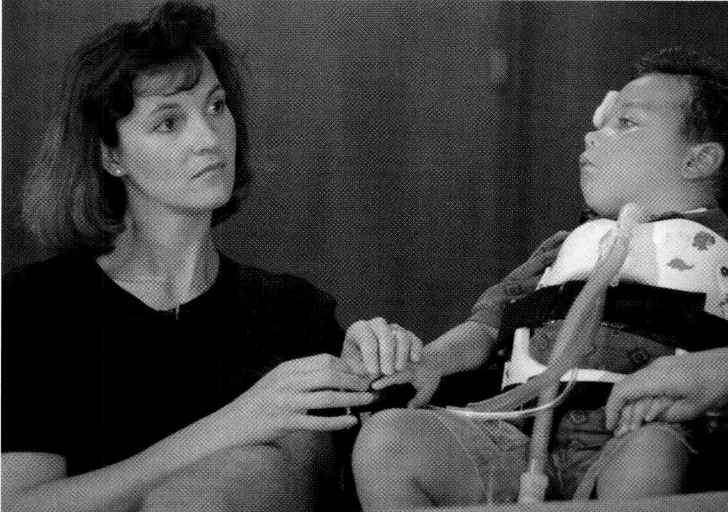

Routine immunization of infants with oral polio vaccine results in about eight cases of paralytic disease in the U.S. each year. Gordon Pierson—one of the unlucky ones—appeared with his mother, Susan (left), before an advisory committee on immunization practices on June 19, 1996.

By 1997 polio was no longer a familiar or feared disease in the U.S. There had been no infection due to the naturally occurring virus for more than 15 years. There had, however, been about eight cases of disease reported annually that were due to the vaccine itself. This phenomenon, called vaccine-associated paralytic poliomyelitis (VAPP), occurs when the weakened oral vaccine reverts to an aggressive virus that once again can cause disease. The risk may be perceived to be quite rare—affecting about one person per million recipients of oral polio vaccine and their susceptible contacts. But today, because polio has been eliminated from the entire Western Hemisphere and because an alternative vaccine exists, even that low level of risk is unacceptable to many. After intense public debates, both the American Academy of Pediatrics (AAP) and the Advisory Committee on Immunization Practices of the Centers for Disease Control and Prevention (CDC) recently recommended a transition to increasingly greater use of the safer IPV—especially for the first two (of four) childhood doses, when the risk of neurological virulence from OPV appears to be the greatest.

The performance of the polio vaccine has not changed over the past 40 years; rather, it is the public's perception of the balance

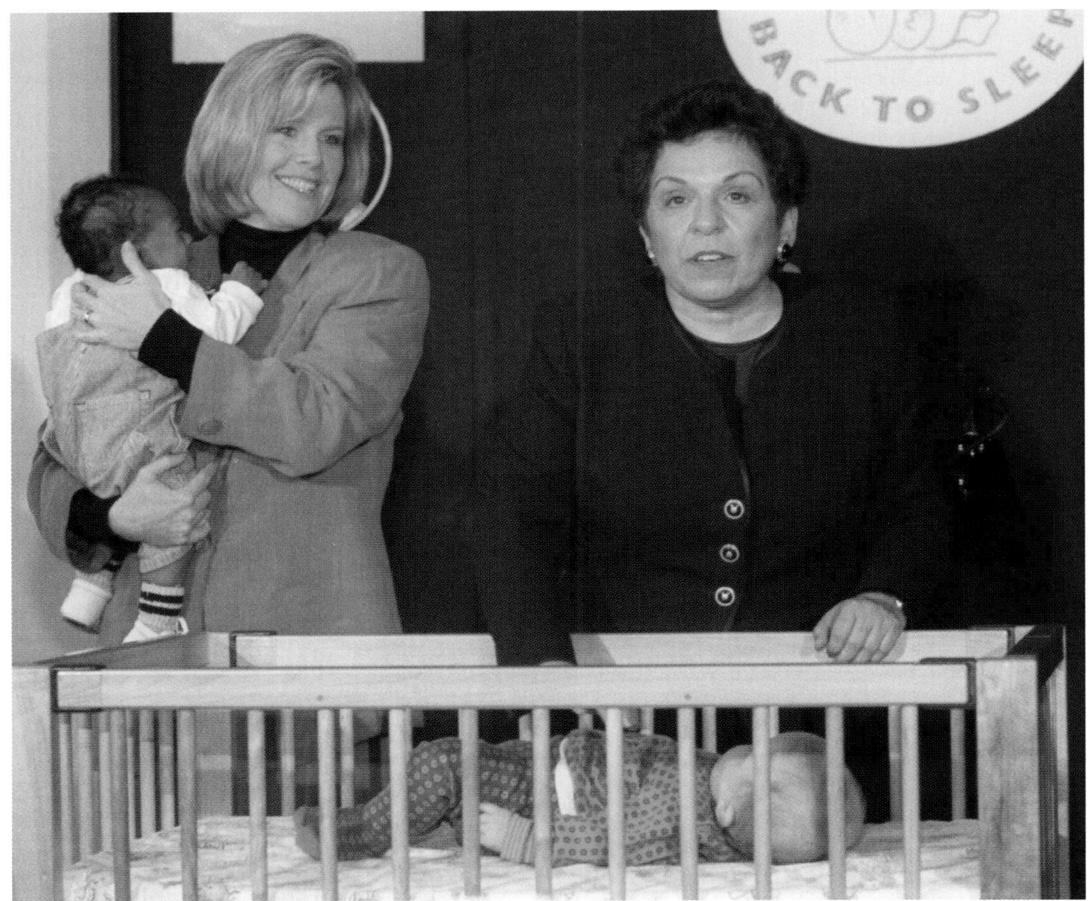

Ken Cedeno—Associated Press

Tipper Gore (left), wife of U.S. Vice Pres. Al Gore, and Secretary of Health and Human Services Donna Shalala have championed a campaign to put infants to sleep on their backs (or sides). That campaign has led to a sharp decline in the incidence of sudden infant death syndrome and helped quell many parents' concerns that vaccines might be a cause of SIDS.

of risks versus benefits that has altered. The debates about polio vaccine safety center on several questions: How should potential benefits to individuals versus those to society be balanced, especially when they could be in conflict? How much is society willing to pay for the safer vaccine in order to prevent the rare occurrence of VAPP? How should the potential benefits of the new AAP and CDC recommendations for the U.S. population as a whole be measured against the potential effects that they might have on the global polio-eradication program—especially when too early a shift from OPV to IPV on an international scale could slow eradication progress in less-developed countries? Can the existing public and private systems for the delivery of vaccines handle the more complex immunization schedule required for IPV when the long-relied-upon OPV is so easily administered? Even if systems were equipped for the change, could it be accomplished without risking decreased immunization rates and outbreaks due to other vaccine-preventable diseases? For many reasons the recent polio policy decision represents and illuminates the broader vaccine safety debate.

Safety's many subtleties

How much risk is associated with various vaccines? That question was intensively studied by a panel of experts convened by the Institute of Medicine of the National Research Council. Two in-depth reviews of all available information on the safety of childhood vaccines—case reports, papers, and reported safety problems—were published in 1991 and 1994. The IOM reports documented that extremely rare adverse events due to vaccination do, in fact, occur. The reviewers found that the existing data were sufficient to establish a causal relationship between measles vaccine and low blood platelet counts (creating a risk of bleeding), between OPV and VAPP, and between measles vaccine and death from measles infection, but the evidence was against any link between vaccines and infantile spasms or sudden infant death syndrome (SIDS).

There were many more conditions, however, for which the data were not clear-cut. It is this grey area that is especially troubling for some parents, who, on the one hand, want to protect their children as much as they can but, on the other hand, are fearful of the risks. Here, while sound science cannot *prove* that a risk does not exist, large and carefully conducted studies can provide the reassurance that if a risk does exist, it is extremely rare—perhaps so rare as to be immeasurable. Determining actual risk becomes even more difficult with extremely rare conditions that are known to have other infectious or metabolic causes, such as encephalopathy (involving widespread destruction or degeneration of brain tissue); when the lag time between the inciting event (vaccination) is years distant from the condition it is presumed to cause (*e.g.,* learning disabilities); or when comparative studies are difficult to conduct because the vaccine is highly effective and very few individuals have not been immunized.

Alleged risks

A broad array of adverse reactions (most notably allergic, autoimmune, and neurological conditions) have been alleged to occur as a consequence of vaccination. Testing the validity of those allegations would require epidemiological and microbiological data, which often are not available. Dispelling fears about potential adverse reactions, therefore, is difficult.

For many years it was thought that SIDS might be a sequela, or aftereffect, of vaccination. Carefully conducted studies in large populations, however, failed to find such an association. Infants are the target group for immunizations because they are at the highest risk for the infections that vaccines prevent. It so happens that infants receive vaccines at about the same age that developmental delays and other neurological symptoms are most commonly diagnosed and that SIDS tends to claim infants' lives. Not surprisingly, this "coincidence" may be difficult to untangle—and for parents of affected children, it may be difficult to believe. Fortunately, in the past several years a hard-hitting and apparently quite effective public education campaign, "Back to Sleep," recommending putting infants to sleep on their backs rather than on their stomachs, clearly lowered the SIDS mortality rate and thereby offered reasonable assurance to parents that vaccination was not a likely cause of SIDS.

There are other ongoing vaccine-safety controversies that have yet to be resolved. For example, in the early 1960s a cancer-causing virus of monkeys called SV40 was found to have contaminated some lots of OPV grown in monkey kidney cells. Before this was realized, millions of children had received the potentially contaminated products. Tracking and follow-up of vaccine recipients in the U.S. and Sweden for more than 40 years, however, failed to find an increased incidence of cancer in these populations. Moreover, such a risk is minimized today because there are now sophisticated technologies, such as polymerase chain reaction (PCR), available to detect minute quantities of an adventitious (foreign) agent in the vaccine supply.

NEWS CAP

Inhaler Users Holding Their Breath

Many of the estimated 24 million people in the United States who suffer from asthma and other respiratory diseases rely on devices known as metered-dose inhalers (MDIs), which use small quantities of chlorofluorocarbons (CFCs) to propel medication into the lungs. Because studies have shown quite clearly that CFCs contribute to the depletion of the ozone layer, efforts are presently under way around the world to eliminate all CFC production. In March 1997 the Food and Drug Administration (FDA) announced plans to begin replacing MDIs with inhalers that are CFC-free. Those plans caused considerable alarm among patients.

A survey of 20,000 asthma sufferers conducted by a patient advocacy group, the Allergy and Asthma Network/Mothers of Asthmatics, Inc., indicated that most supported the elimination of the environmentally hazardous CFCs and the development of new inhalers. What they feared, however, was that the FDA would phase out existing MDIs without first ensuring that the new ones worked as well.

"People shouldn't panic," said John Jenkins, director of the FDA's division of pulmonary drug products. "It's frightening for patients when they can't breathe, and they come to rely on medications. And when they hear the government is going to take away their medication, people get scared. But there will be time. We're not proposing to eliminate CFCs until new products adequately serve patients' needs."

According to the FDA's transition strategy, the phase-out of CFC-containing inhalers will not take place until reliable replacements that have proved acceptable to users have been on the market for at least one year. Moreover, sufficient supplies of the new varieties of MDIs will have to be made widely available to all who need them. One reassuring sign to those who suffer from respiratory illnesses is that medical groups such as the American Lung Association and the American Academy of Allergy, Asthma and Immunology have expressed their support for the FDA plans.

Science Source/Photo Researchers

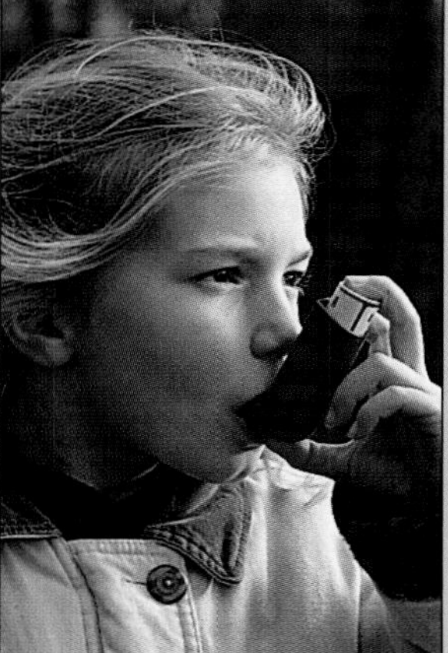

New chlorofluorocarbon-free metered-dose inhalers must eventually replace those that millions of asthma sufferers in the U.S. now depend upon.

Although FDA officials would not speculate on a completion date for the transition to CFC-free inhalers, it seems likely that the process will take years.

So far, only one new inhaler-delivered drug, albuterol, a bronchodilator marketed under the name Proventil HFA, which uses hydrofluoroalkane gas as a substitute for CFCs, has received FDA approval. Made available to the public in January, Proventil took seven years and $100 million to develop. Other products are currently under review. One trade group, the Washington, D.C.-based International Pharmaceutical Aerosol Consortium, estimated that at least 11—and perhaps as many as 30—CFC-free MDIs would be approved by the turn of the century.

—*Sherman Hollar*

Safety questions have also been raised about the diphtheria-pertussis-tetanus (DPT) vaccine. Rare but quite serious neurological illnesses had been blamed on the DPT vaccine. Efforts to reassure the public were only partially successful because a unified surveillance system was lacking; furthermore, experts did not always agree on what symptoms were vaccine-related. DPT is made from killed, inactivated preparations of the whole cell of the pertussis toxin, which includes dozens of cellular components that are thought to be associated with side effects, (*e.g.,* redness and pain at the injection site, prolonged crying, and—rarely—seizures or coma). A 15-year effort involving the scientific and public health communities, parents, and the pharmaceuticals industry led to the production of new *acellular* pertussis (aP and DTaP) vaccines, made from one or more inactivated, purified, or recombinant (genetically engineered) antigens, which cause fewer reactions. Whether acellular pertussis is entirely safe will be learned only with increased use and ongoing surveillance over many years.

Liability

In an atmosphere of urgency and compromise, medical, legal, and consumer groups worked with Congress to enact into law the National Childhood Vaccine Injury Act of 1986. As a result, the federal government instituted mandates for office record keeping, scientific studies of vaccine reactions, distribution of vaccine information for families and patients, and a national surveillance system to monitor adverse events. Liability was addressed by the creation of the National Vaccine Injury Compensation Program, a no-fault approach to compensation for injury, which relies on an established table of compensable injuries. Litigation shifted to this relatively simplified and straightforward system, which ascribed an untoward reaction to a vaccine if (1) it occurred within a certain time frame, (2) another cause of illness was not present, and (3) certain legal requirements were met.

Operational since 1988, the program, financed by an excise tax on every dose sold, covers routinely given vaccines. As of July 1997, more than 1,250 awards had been made to families or individuals. By streamlining adjudication, the program avoids the long, burdensome civil process, which in the 1980s sometimes resulted in inconsistent jury awards. While cash payments cannot adequately compensate for injury suffered, they remove the financial burden for families in the unfortunate instances where an unanticipated reaction occurs.

By most standards the federal system has achieved its goals of compensating individuals, stabilizing the supply and price of vaccines, and reducing health care provider and manufacturer liability. Only a small number of lawsuits are filed annually against vaccine manufacturers, and there is little evidence that plaintiffs whose cases are rejected by the federal system or who choose not to accept payment from the national program seek compensation elsewhere. The IOM studies suggested that most injuries and deaths that follow vaccination are non-vaccine-related. Rather, they are most often the consequence of prenatal, metabolic, or other kinds of developmental conditions. If anything, close analysis of the available data affirms that the high standards of safety and efficacy that society expects of pharmaceutical products (such as vaccines) that are routinely given to healthy children and adults are being met.

A proper perspective

While more is known today than ever before about the inherent safety of vaccines, the uncertainties of the past are never far away. One example is the confusion surrounding the hearing loss of Heather Whitestone, Miss America of 1995. Initially, her deafness was reported in the *New York Times* and other media sources as having been vaccine-caused, but it was later confirmed to be the result of complications from meningitis caused by an infection with *Haemophilus influenzae* type b (Hib), a once-prevalent pediatric condition that has been virtually eliminated by Hib vaccines that became available in the late 1980s. Indeed, had a vaccine been available when Whitestone was a child, she and many in her generation would not be deaf today. The confusion and furor that arose about that mistaken initial report serve as a reminder of the enormous power of the media and the potential for widespread dissemination of misinformation.

Properly communicating the advantages of immunization presents an ongoing challenge. Because vaccines prevent disease in healthy individuals beginning as early as the newborn period, the tragedies that would have occurred had they not been available are never seen and thus may be hard to appreciate. Furthermore, though vaccines are given to individuals, they convey an immeasurable benefit to the community as well. Thus, society has a vested interest in preventing infectious illness, which, in the U.S.,

A baby in the Philippines is vaccinated against paralytic poliomyelitis—a disease that may well have seen its day by the end of the current century, thanks to the mass-immunization programs that are being waged in every country that is still affected by the crippling infectious disease.

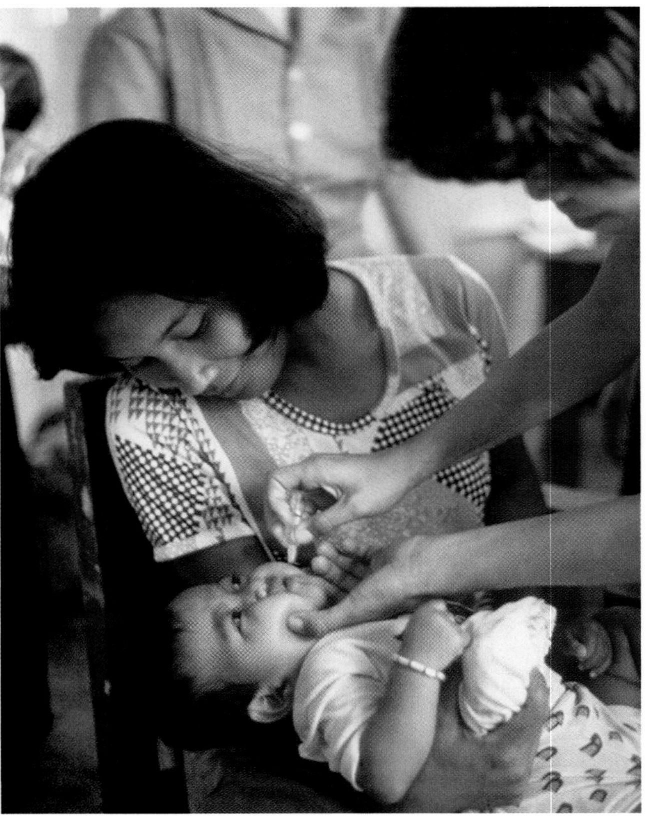

EPI/WHO

translates into laws that require children to be immunized before they are allowed to enter school.

The benefit-risk ratio of vaccines is never static. On one hand, the diminished incidence of preventable disease is welcome. On the other hand, the absence of disease that vaccination brings about often leads to a decreased familiarity with the devastating effects of the diseases vaccines prevent. In the absence of illness, concerns shift toward matters of safety and whether, in fact, vaccines are needed. Not giving vaccines, however, would result in lost opportunities to eradicate disease (*e.g.,* smallpox and polio), and society could once again see epidemics of major proportions.

Fortunately, the science of communicating risk continues to advance. The goals are to learn what factors influence individual perception of risk and what types of communication do the best job of informing the public and/or changing behavior. The educational level, experiences, beliefs, attitudes, and values of every potential recipient need to be considered. Other considerations in risk-benefit communication are the individual's ability or inability to control risks and the reasons that a person judges one type of risk to be more or less significant than another.

The concerns about vaccine safety need to be placed in context. There is far more good news than bad. The past generation has witnessed unprecedented immunization advances. About 10,000 cases of meningitis a year that were previously caused by the *H. influenzae* type b organism have simply disappeared, thanks to widespread use of the Hib vaccine (the first dose of which is given at two months of age). The absence of meningitis represents a quiet victory in the war against infectious diseases. Immunization rates in U.S. children are now the highest they have ever been, and the infectious diseases they prevent have reached new lows. In July 1997 Pres. Bill Clinton, who had made raising national immunization rates a high priority of his administration, announced that the child-immunization goal for 1996—90% of two-

NEWS CAP MHA 98

Grapefruit's Powerful Punch

The potency of a number of commonly prescribed drugs, including several used to treat allergies and high blood pressure, is dramatically increased if they are taken with even a single glass of grapefruit juice. In fact, some patients have inadvertently overdosed when they chose grapefruit juice to wash down their medication.

That may sound like pulp fiction to some, but in reality the so-called grapefruit juice effect is a well-documented phenomenon. Since 1989, when the effect was first reported in the medical literature, numerous studies have shown that grapefruit juice greatly enhances the body's ability to absorb certain drugs. Among the symptoms that have been attributed to the grapefruit juice effect are dizziness, facial flushing, accelerated heartbeat, headache, and drowsiness.

Until recently, medical experts were at a loss to explain why drinking grapefruit juice helps to boost the absorption of drugs into the body. A study, led by Kenneth S. Lown of the University of Michigan Medical School, Ann Arbor, and published in *The Journal of Clinical Investigation* (May 15, 1997) confirmed what a few researchers had suspected. It found that components in grapefruit juice inhibit the ability of an enzyme, known as CYP3A4, to break down drugs in the liver and small intestine. This allows drugs to accumulate and linger longer in the bloodstream, which thereby increases their potency and their potential to cause adverse effects.

The 12-day study involved 10 healthy male volunteers who were admitted to the University of Michigan General Clinical Research Center and put on diets entirely devoid of fruits and vegetables. Beginning on day 6, the men were served an 8-oz (235-ml) glass of grapefruit juice with breakfast, lunch, and dinner. On days 4, 6, and 11, each man took a 10-mg tablet of felodipine (Plendil), a drug used to treat hypertension. After the first glass of juice on day 6, concentrations of the drug in each man's bloodstream had more than tripled since day 4, when the felodipine tablets had been taken only with water. By day 11 the felodipine concentrations had quadrupled. In addition, each of the volunteers exhibited low concentrations of the CYP3A4 enzyme.

Although felodipine was the only drug that was employed in the study, other drugs may trigger the grapefruit juice effect. After the study appeared in print, the American Heart Association strongly urged patients not to take any of the following drugs with grapefruit juice:

- nimodipine (Nimotop), nifedipine (Adalat, Procardia), and verapamil (Calan, Isoptin, Verelan)—drugs widely prescribed for the treatment of high blood pressure and congestive heart failure
- cyclosporine (Sandimmune, NeOral), which helps prevent rejection in transplant recipients
- terfenadine (Seldane), for treating allergic disorders

At least one earlier study had indicated that drinking grapefruit juice even 24 hours before taking medication may have the same effect as drinking the juice with medication. Thus, patients who take the drugs mentioned above may want to avoid drinking grapefruit juice altogether.

Investigation of the grapefruit juice effect will likely continue. The specific substance in grapefruit juice responsible for inhibiting the CYP3A4 enzyme has yet to be identified. Some pharmacologists speculate that once this substance has been isolated, adding it to drugs could lower the dosage needed.

—Sherman Hollar

UPI

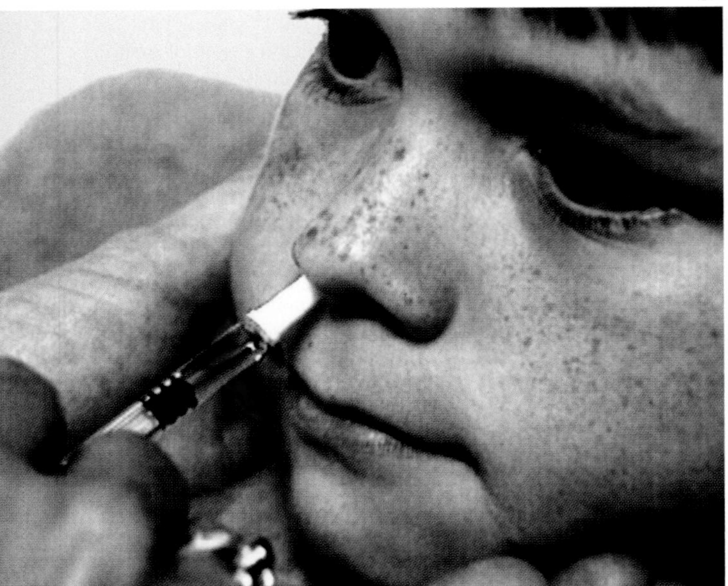

A California youngster participates in a nationwide trial of a new vaccine aimed at preventing influenza in healthy children. Whereas 18% of those who received a placebo succumbed to flu's miseries during the 1996–97 season, all but 1% receiving the experimental vaccine were protected.

year-olds having received three critical doses of vaccines—had been achieved. (In 1992 the overall immunization level was only 55%.)

Thanks to the World Health Organization's Expanded Programme on Immunization, children in every corner of the world are being fully immunized. Mass-polio-immunization campaigns are being waged in every country that is still affected by paralytic polio; eradication of the crippling disease is predicted for early in the 21st century.

Over the past year, there have been exciting advances in vaccine science. Among them is a promising vaccine against Lyme disease. Another is the development of technology for producing "edible" vaccines, in which genetically engineered potatoes or bananas could be used as the vehicles for delivering antigens that protect against infant diarrhea; production of such crop-based vaccines would be feasible and potentially cost-effective in less-developed countries.

Further, a recently concluded trial of a nasal-spray flu vaccine for children showed that two tiny squirts (in one or two doses) were remarkably effective; only 1% of the more than 1,000 children treated with the vaccine contracted flu during the 1996–97 winter. Pending FDA approval, a nasal-spray influenza vaccine may be available as early as 1999.

Because nothing can replace the trust the public places in physicians and health care providers, today's health care professionals must stay current with the science of vaccines and be prepared to address questions and concerns that discerning consumers are likely to have. Not all patients will accept reassurance and choose to be immunized or have their children immunized. Ultimately, it is trust—a fragile resource—that will continue to provide vaccine safety assurance.

—N. Regina Rabinovich, M.D., M.P.H., and Geoffrey Evans, M.D.

Stress and the Blood-Brain Barrier

About a century ago the German scientist Paul Ehrlich introduced the concept of a "blood-brain barrier" when he demonstrated that dye intravenously injected into the body stained most organs but not the brain. That barrier, a tight sheath of cells surrounding the capillaries of the brain, has long been viewed as a kind of physiological Checkpoint Charlie. Normally, it lets only small, vital molecules such as water, oxygen, and carbon dioxide into brain cells while keeping out larger, potentially poisonous molecules (*e.g.,* antibiotics). But if a group of researchers in Israel is correct, then an inadvertent "mega-experiment" involving Israeli soldiers in the Persian Gulf War may have shown that when people are under acute stress, the blood-brain barrier temporarily becomes permeable—as if normally well-armed guards at a strategic crossing point had fallen asleep on the job.

Inadvertent drug experiment

Israeli soldiers who took the drug pyridostigmine to protect themselves against possible nerve-gas attacks may have absorbed some of the drug into their brains and suffered unanticipated adverse consequences as a result. Neurosurgeon Alon Friedman and coinvestigators at the Life Sciences Institute of the Hebrew University, Jerusalem, and the Sackler School of Medicine, Tel Aviv University, suspected that stress had something to do with the soldiers' symptoms; the researchers were able to mimic the human reactions in laboratory mice. Their findings, published in *Nature Medicine* (December 1996), not only may revise conventional scientific thinking about the impermeability of the blood-brain barrier but could alter the way doctors and pharmacists advise patients to take standard medications.

The story behind this accidental insight starts in the synapses (sites where nerve impulses are passed from one nerve cell, or neuron, to another) in the peripheral nervous system (PNS). The PNS comprises all the nerves (except the optic nerve) outside the central nervous system (CNS). Normally, firing neurons of the parasympathetic nervous system (the part of the autonomic nervous system that increases secretions, enhances the tone and contractility of smooth muscles, slows the heart, and stimulates digestion) release the neurotransmitter acetylcholine, which opens channels in the membranes of adjoining PNS neurons for the transmission of an electrochemical nerve impulse. A crucial enzyme, acetylcholinesterase, breaks down acetylcholine after passage of the impulse and thereby prevents a buildup of the neurotransmitter in the PNS; the enzyme has the same effect in the CNS. Thus, if and when an acetylcholinesterase inhibitor penetrates into the brain, it will cause a buildup of acetylcholine in the brain, as it does in the periphery, and could trigger convulsions. Poisonous organophosphate nerve gases (such as soman) will inactivate acetylcholinesterase, leading to an acetylcholine overload and thus to convulsions and other symptoms associated with CNS activation—but only when the soman has had an opportunity to penetrate into the brain.

Pyridostigmine, another cholinesterase inhibitor, is a large molecule and one that will not permeate the blood-brain barrier under normal conditions. Instead, it binds with acetylcholinesterase in the PNS only and would not normally have any central effects. For this reason, the drug is commonly given to combatants who

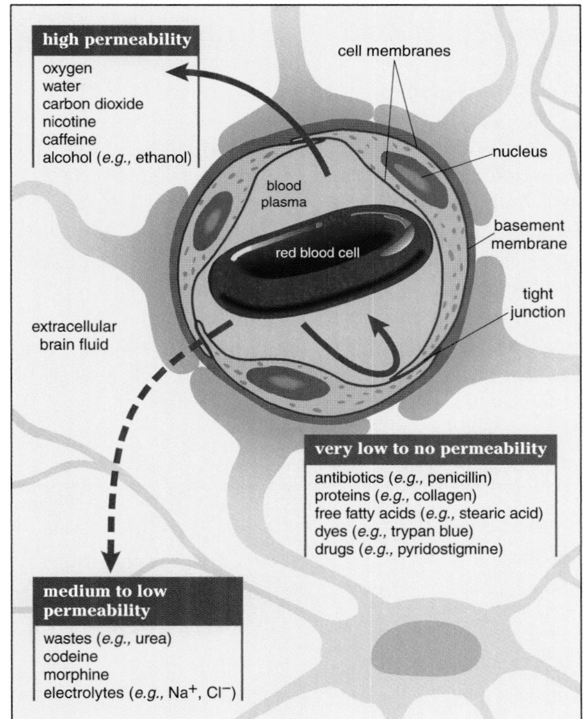

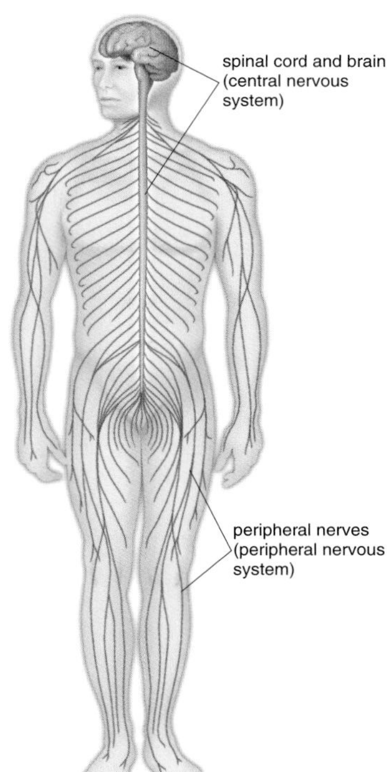

(Far right) Modified from an original illustration by Harwin Studios

The permeability of the blood-brain barrier to various substances depends on factors such as the molecular size, electrical charge, and relative solubility of the agent in question. An "inadvertent" experiment involving Israeli soldiers in the Persian Gulf War suggests that another important factor may be stress. The anti-nerve-gas drug pyridostigmine, which normally acts in the peripheral nervous system, may have "leaked" across the blood-brain barrier in the combatants to whom it was given, causing untoward central-nervous-system effects.

face the threat of chemical warfare; no other pharmaceutical is known to offer this protection.

Under conditions of stress, however, the blood-brain barrier will become "leaky," and some pyridostigmine would then be able to enter the CNS. Once there, it would act on nerve cells, releasing acetylcholine in a manner similar to that which occurs in the PNS. This effect of pyridostigmine in the brain would result in a central accumulation of acetylcholine and hence toxicity of central origin (producing drowsiness, insomnia, headache, etc.).

An earlier study of soldiers pretreated with pyridostigmine during the days of Iraqi missile attacks on Israel showed that many had experienced side effects that seemed to involve the CNS—*e.g.,* drowsiness, insomnia, headaches, nervousness, and difficulties in focusing attention. Friedman, who was a medical corps physician in the Israeli defense forces during the Gulf War, knew from much previous research that stress raises the concentrations of epinephrine and other stress-related hormones in the blood; moreover, a study reported in 1991 found that the same hormones can loosen the tight junctions between the cells that make up the blood-brain barrier. Putting those pieces of information together, Friedman and his team speculated that wartime anxiety had weakened the soldiers' blood-brain barriers, which allowed pyridostigmine to penetrate into brain cells, where it produced the CNS symptoms.

In mice and men, in war and peace

To test this hypothesis, the Israeli researchers performed an experiment in which they subjected a group of mice to a "forced swim protocol." The test involved placing a mouse in the middle of a deep pool so that it had to swim for a specific time period, with no option for rest—a stressful situation that may be loosely analogous to fighting in a war. The researchers stressed some mice (putting them through two consecutive four-minute forced swims) but not others. They injected the mice in both groups with varying doses of pyridostigmine or a similar drug, physostigmine, and 10 minutes later sacrificed the mice and measured acetylcholinesterase activity in their brain cells. This indicated how much of the enzyme had been bound up and inhibited by the drug and thus was an indirect measure of the amount of pyridostigmine or physostigmine that had penetrated the blood-brain barrier.

What they found was that the pyridostigmine dose required for reducing acetylcholinesterase activity by 50% in the brains of the stressed mice was only 1/100 of the dose required for doing the same in nonstressed mice—an indication that the blood-brain barriers of the stressed animals had been severely weakened. Pharmacologist Israel Hanin at the Chicago Stritch School of Medicine, Loyola University, Maywood, Ill., commented in the same issue of *Nature Medicine* that the "classical textbook view" teaches that the blood-brain barrier is highly effective at keeping "undesirable molecules" out of the brain. "This may certainly be the case under normal conditions," said Hanin, "but during stress, this premise appears to fall apart."

Such a finding raises important concerns about other pharmaceuticals. Penicillin, for example, which is meant to act outside the brain, can cause convulsions if it enters the CNS. If stressful situations can directly weaken the blood-brain barrier, it may not take a war to evoke the necessary level of stress that could compromise the brain's defenses to drugs; marital troubles, tension on the job, or even overdoing an exercise routine might be adequate. Hanin concluded that scientists need to gain a better understanding of this phenomenon so that appropriate new drugs can be designed "for use during war and peace."

—*Wade Roush, Ph.D.*

Adolescent and Adult Immunization

Childhood immunization programs in the United States and around the world have been so successful that many children will grow up without any knowledge of the diseases that modern vaccines have prevented. Smallpox has been eradicated from the globe. There is no evidence that polio has been transmitted within North America in nearly 20 years. The wide application of measles vaccine now offers the hope that this potentially serious viral infection too will be eliminated. And in just the past decade, the nearly universal use of the *Haemophilus influenzae* type b (Hib) vaccine in the U.S. has reduced the incidence of childhood meningitis and pneumonia, both devastating diseases, from 20,000 to fewer than 300 cases per year. In fact, historic low rates of infection have been achieved for all 10 of the vaccine-preventable diseases for which children are routinely immunized.

Most vaccines given in childhood appear to provide lifelong protection, with a few notable exceptions. Booster immunizations with tetanus toxoid have traditionally been recommended at 10-year intervals throughout life, and outbreaks of measles among adolescents, some of whom had been immunized as children, prompted public health officials to recommend a second dose of measles vaccine for children between the ages of either 4 and 6 years or 11 and 12 years and for certain adults who are considered to be in high-risk groups, such as health care workers, students entering postsecondary school, and international travelers.

In addition, vaccines are available to prevent three diseases that are of substantial public health impact among adults: influenza, pneumococcal disease (infection of the bloodstream and cerebrospinal fluid), and hepatitis B. Influenza and pneumococcal disease are responsible for some 50,000–60,000 deaths among adults in the United States each year, more than the number of deaths

NEWS CAP MHA 98

Diabetes Redefined

In June 1997 an international panel of experts convened by the American Diabetes Association (ADA) issued new guidelines for diagnosing and classifying diabetes mellitus—the fourth leading cause of death in the United States and a major cause of morbidity and mortality worldwide. The threshold for a diagnosis of diabetes has been lowered from 140 mg/dl (milligrams of glucose per deciliter of blood)—a level that had been established in 1979—to 126 mg/dl. The committee also strongly recommended that all adults aged 45 years and older undergo screening for diabetes and begin early treatment if the findings indicate a high blood sugar level. If the results are normal, retesting every three years is advised. Individuals at high risk should be tested at an earlier age and more frequently. These guidelines, issued after the panel conducted a two-year review of more than 15 years of published scientific literature, received almost immediate endorsements from the American Medical Association, the National Institute of Diabetes and Digestive and Kidney Diseases, and the Centers for Disease Control and Prevention, as well as the World Health Organization, which is expected to adopt similar guidelines.

In essence, diabetes has been redefined. Research has shown that the onset of serious diabetes-related problems such as blood vessel damage can occur when the concentration of sugar in a person's bloodstream is as low as 126 mg/dl. Such damage may result in blindness, kidney failure, heart disease, and stroke, and severe diabetic nerve damage often leads to the amputation of feet or legs. In addition to lowering the diagnostic cutoff point from 140 to 126, the new definition includes an "impaired" blood glucose status (levels between 110 and 125 mg/dl). A reading within this range is considered a risk factor for future diabetes and its complications. A major clinical trial is under way to test the assumption that patients in the impaired category who begin treatment as soon as possible can avoid or delay the development of diabetes. (Those who have already been diagnosed as having diabetes and are being treated will not be affected by the new numbers.)

Other diabetes risk factors include obesity, high blood pressure, a high-density lipoprotein level of 35 mg/dl or lower and/or a triglyceride level of 250 mg/dl or higher, having a first-degree relative with diabetes, and having delivered a baby weighing over 4.1 kg (9 lb) or had a previous diagnosis of gestational diabetes. Population groups that are at greater-than-average risk are Native Americans, African-Americans, Latinos, and Asians.

By promoting widespread testing in adults over age 45, physicians may be able to identify up to 2 million of the estimated 8 million cases of undiagnosed diabetes in the U.S.—about 16 million Americans have diabetes, but only half are diagnosed. Diabetes is called a silent killer because in the early stages the absence of symptoms allows the disease to do hidden damage to the body; often patients have the disorder for seven years or more before they are diagnosed and may become aware that they have diabetes only after one of its life-threatening complications has developed.

According to the new recommendations, in order for a diagnosis to be made, the initial test result must be confirmed by a second test on a different day. The new cutoff figures are based on the results of a fasting plasma glucose (FPG), a simple blood test done after a fast of at least eight hours. The FPG is the preferred test—and the one that the committee recommended for universal use because it is convenient (usu-

caused by motor vehicle crashes or AIDS. People chronically infected with hepatitis B virus are at high risk of developing chronic liver disease and, potentially, liver cancer. The estimated annual cost to society of caring for patients with these preventable infections is over $10 billion. Consequently, influenza, pneumococcal, and hepatitis B vaccines are routinely recommended for adults who are at risk of contracting the diseases or suffering from their complications. In marked contrast to childhood vaccines, however, the use of these "adult" vaccines is far from universal (*see* Table, page 332).

Shots: not just for tots

The wide promotion of childhood immunization has given the impression that vaccines are only for children. Adult immunization is not routine for a number of reasons. Whereas preventive care is a cornerstone of pediatric medicine, this is less the case with the health care services that the majority of adults receive. Adolescent and adult visits to doctors do not revolve around regularly scheduled immunizations (as they do for children), and, in contrast to the legal requirement that children be fully immunized before entering school, few workplaces require immunizations for employees (with the exception of certain laboratories and health care facilities). Furthermore, adult vaccines are often not as effective as childhood vaccines. Because advancing age tends to be accompanied by a decline in immune function, vaccines that are given in adulthood may have diminished effectiveness. Despite this fact, pneumococcal vaccine prevents serious pneumococcal disease in 60% of adults, including the elderly. Influenza vaccine prevents complications from flu in 70% of adults immunized, and 90% of healthy older adults will mount a protective immune response to the three-dose series of hepatitis B vaccine.

ally done in the morning after an overnight fast), easy to administer, and relatively inexpensive. Two other tests that may be used for diagnostic purposes are the casual plasma glucose (taken at any time of day without regard to food intake) and the less-convenient, more expensive oral glucose tolerance test (requiring a 10–16-hour fast and blood glucose measurement before and at several time intervals after drinking a glucose-containing liquid). When either of the latter tests is done, the diabetes diagnosis level is 200 mg/dl. Finger-prick tests, often available at health fairs, and urine tests are not considered reliable diagnostic tools.

The ADA committee also recommended a change in nomenclature. The old terms, *insulin-dependent diabetes mellitus (IDDM)* and *non-insulin-dependent diabetes mellitus (NIDDM),* have been replaced by type 1 and type 2 diabetes, respectively. A relatively small proportion (about 5% to 10%) of the total number of people who have the disease have type 1 diabetes. Type 1, which largely affects children and young adults who tend to be slim, is an autoimmune disease in which the body destroys the cells in the pancreas that produce insulin. People with type 1 generally fail to produce any insulin and must take insulin shots daily in order to survive. The much more common type 2 diabetes occurs mostly in people who are over 40 and overweight. In type 2 diabetes the body continues to produce insulin but is unable to use it properly or does not make enough. Treatment depends on the stage at which a diagnosis is made. While it almost always requires lifestyle changes such as losing weight, exercising, and stopping smoking, it may also involve taking insulin or oral antidiabetic drugs (thus, the previous distinction between insulin and non-insulin dependency is not accurate). Although less severe than type 1 diabetes, type 2 is a greater cause for concern because it is approaching epidemic proportions, and its prevalence is expected to escalate as the population ages.

"We feel passionately that people need to take diabetes more seriously," said James R. Gavin III of the Howard Hughes Medical Institute, Chevy Chase, Md., and chair of the Expert Committee on the Diagnosis and Classification of Diabetes Mellitus. In the U.S. more than 178,000 will die this year from the disease or related complications. Diabetes is also the leading cause of new cases of blindness, as well as the most frequent cause of nontraumatic lower-limb amputations. People with diabetes are two to four times more likely to develop heart disease or to suffer a stroke than are those without the disease. Although these facts are grim, Gavin stressed that the new definition should have a major impact on public health: "The earlier we pick up the disease and the more aggressive we are in treating it, the greater the likelihood we'll be able to avoid these kinds of complications."

—*Afrodite Mantzavrakos*

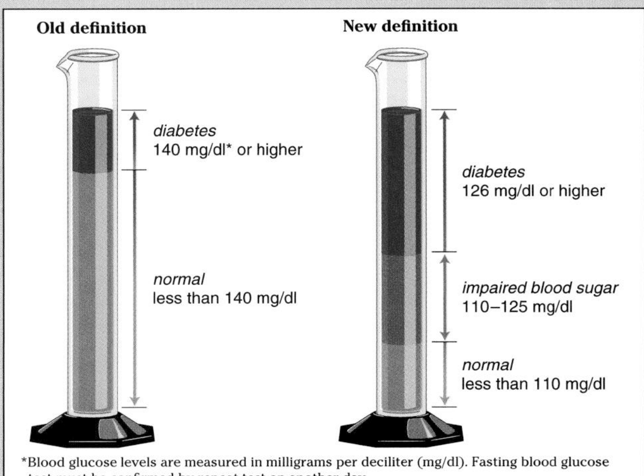

*Blood glucose levels are measured in milligrams per deciliter (mg/dl). Fasting blood glucose test must be confirmed by repeat test on another day.

Adult Vaccines: Current Use and Impact

Disease	Estimated annual deaths (number)	Estimated vaccine efficacy in healthy adults (percentage)	Current vaccine utilization[1] (percentage)	Additional preventable deaths per year[2] (number)
Influenza	20,000	70	55	6,300
Pneumococcal infection	20,000–40,000	60	30	8,400–16,800
Hepatitis B	6,000	90	10	4,860
Tetanus-diphtheria	<25	99	40	<15
Measles, mumps, and rubella	<30	95	variable	<30
Travelers' diseases (cholera, typhoid, Japanese encephalitis, yellow fever, poliomyelitis, and rabies)	<10	variable	unknown	<10

[1]The percentage of targeted groups who have been immunized according to current recommendations. Rates vary among different targeted groups. Data for influenza and pneumococcal vaccines apply to persons aged 65 and older.

[2]Calculated as: (potential additional vaccine utilization) × (estimated vaccine efficacy) × (estimated annual deaths).

Sources: Centers for Disease Control and Prevention, unpublished data; 1994 National Health Interview Study; *Adult Immunization: A Report by the National Vaccine Advisory Committee, 1994.*

Although some vaccines are contraindicated in people with severe allergies to components such as egg protein (some vaccines are grown in fertile eggs), misconceptions about who should *not* have adult vaccines abound. Adults can safely be vaccinated with most vaccines *even if* they:

- have had a reaction to a previous vaccine consisting of mild-to-moderate local tenderness, redness, swelling, or fever under 40.5° C (105° F)
- have a mild acute illness or a low-grade fever at the time of receiving a vaccine
- are receiving antimicrobial therapy for a current infection or are in the process of convalescing from a recent illness
- live in the same household as a pregnant woman
- have had recent exposure to an infectious disease
- are currently breast-feeding
- have a history of allergies, including allergy to penicillin or other antibiotics (excluding anaphylactic reactions to neomycin or streptomycin)
- have a family history of adverse reactions to vaccination, seizures, or allergies to medications

Adult protection: stepped-up efforts

Recognizing the unacceptably low rates of adult immunization, the U.S. Department of Health and Human Services in 1997 launched the Adult Immunization Initiative, a broad program involving many federal agencies as well as the broader community of research scientists, vaccine and biotechnology companies, managed-care organizations, health insurance providers, state and local immunization programs, and public and private health care professionals. The goals of this multifaceted initiative are to:

- increase the demand for adult vaccinations by improving public awareness of them
- increase the capacity of the health care system to deliver vaccines to adults
- support and expand financing mechanisms to ensure the efficient delivery of vaccines to adults
- increase support for research on all aspects of vaccine-preventable diseases of adults

As the initiative moves into full gear, its success will be measured by the widespread use of existing vaccines in those at greatest risk and the development of safe and effective new vaccines for this population. Given the vaccine tools that are currently available, adult immunization has typically focused on the administration of influenza and pneumococcal vaccines to prevent these infections mainly in the elderly but also in some adults at high risk of suffering severe infections.

Most adults who develop serious pneumococcal disease have been hospitalized within the previous five years for some medical problem. Hospitalization, then, is one important notable opportunity to immunize the segment of the population that is most at risk for pneumococcal disease. Strategies for the reduction of vaccine-preventable diseases in adults include targeting a number of situations where those at risk of developing severe infections are already in contact with health care providers. Computer reminder systems are a particularly useful means of encouraging health care providers to take advantage of existing opportunities to immunize adult patients. Increasingly, immunization campaigns are reaching large groups of adults by offering vaccines in such convenient places as shopping malls, workplaces, churches, and retirement centers.

To minimize missed opportunities, public health officials are now recommending that an initial assessment of immunization status be made for all adults beginning at age 50. The rapid growth of medical services delivered in managed-care settings may help to solidify and realize this objective, as "age-appropriate" immunization is expected to become one of the standard measures of the quality of care that managed-care organizations deliver. As there are a growing number of vaccines in development that are specifically aimed at preventing infections that occur most frequently among adolescents and young adults, an adolescent-immunization assessment is also likely to become a routine part of physician visits.

Recommendations: adolescents and young adults

Ten vaccines are routinely recommended for all children, and five of these are recommended for adolescents and adults to boost their immunity to tetanus, diphtheria, measles, mumps, and rubella (German measles). The immunization schedule during the preteen and teenage years currently focuses on completing the immunizations initiated in childhood. A routine health care visit at age 11–12 serves as an opportunity to complete the childhood immunization series and to address other preventive health issues for the adolescent.

Epidemics of measles in the United States during 1989–91 demonstrated the need for a second dose of measles vaccine to protect those who remain susceptible to measles despite the single shot received early in life. Thus, those who did not receive two doses during childhood should receive a second dose as adolescents. Unless there are specific contraindications, the formulation that should be used for the second dose is the MMR (combined measles, mumps, and rubella) vaccine.

Tetanus and diphtheria boosters are usually recommended every 10 years; an alternative strategy, however, recommended by the American College of Physicians, is a single adulthood booster at age 50 for those who have received their childhood series.

Although adults constitute fewer than 5% of all chicken pox (varicella) cases, more than 50% of the deaths that result from this infection occur in adults. Therefore, *all persons* 13 years of age and older who do not have a reliable history of having had chicken pox and have no evidence of antibodies to the virus are considered to be susceptible and should be vaccinated. Early in 1995 the long-awaited varicella vaccine was licensed in the U.S. Because of the severity and complications of the disease when it occurs in young adults, the Advisory Committee on Immunization Practices of the U.S. Public Health Service recommends two doses of the vaccine for those aged 13 and over.

Recommendations: older adults and the elderly

Immunization with pneumococcal and influenza vaccines is recommended for all adults aged 65 and over. (In the U.S. both vaccines are covered by Medicare.) Younger persons who are at high risk for these infections and their complications should also receive the two vaccines. While influenza vaccine must be given annually to provide protection against new influenza virus strains that circulate each year, protection conferred by pneumococcal vaccine is long-lasting, and most adults at risk for the disease require only one dose. Persons at highest risk for disease (such as those without functioning spleens or those with compromised immune function), however, should receive a second dose of the pneumococcal vaccine five or more years following the first dose.

Vaccines for special groups and situations

There are certain people in certain situations for whom vaccination recommendations differ from the above routines. These include:

- susceptible individuals who have had intimate contact with a person infected with a vaccine-preventable disease
- pregnant women
- immunocompromised adults (*e.g.,* organ transplant recipients, persons on long-term steroid and/or immunosuppressive medication, and people with HIV/AIDS, cancer, diabetes, alcoholism, cirrhosis of the liver, or kidney failure)
- international travelers headed for certain destinations
- individuals such as health care workers, microbiology laboratory personnel, and the military who are exposed or at risk of exposure to infectious agents

Specific recommendations for these special cases have been made by the Advisory Committee on Immunization Practices and are published in special supplements to *Morbidity and Mortality Weekly Report* of the Centers for Disease Control and Prevention (CDC).

Flu vaccine 1996–97

The influenza virus has the capacity to regularly change its characteristics. This capacity gives it the potential to evade even the immune system of a person who has previously had influenza or who was immunized with a vaccine prepared for a previous year. Because the influenza viruses in circulation are different from one year to the next, vaccines must be tailor-made each year. Owing to this high variability, the Food and Drug Administration (FDA), the agency charged with the licensing and regulating of vaccines, and the World Health Organization convene meetings in January and February that are attended by leading virologists, influenza experts, vaccine manufacturers, and public health officials. These groups carefully review the global influenza situation. Data from laboratories around the world are analyzed in an effort to determine the most suitable components of the forthcoming year's influenza vaccine. Pharmaceutical manufacturers then return to their laboratories and vaccine-production facilities to begin the labor-intensive process of growing influenza virus in eggs in order to produce, test, prepare, bottle, and distribute millions of doses of vaccine in time for the usual late-fall-through-winter flu outbreaks. There is always a potential, of course, for flu predictions to be wrong, and occasionally the vaccines are not as

Before selecting his produce, this Minnesota shopper gets a flu shot. Influenza vaccine, recommended annually for all adults aged 65 and older, prevents serious flu complications in 70% of those who receive it.

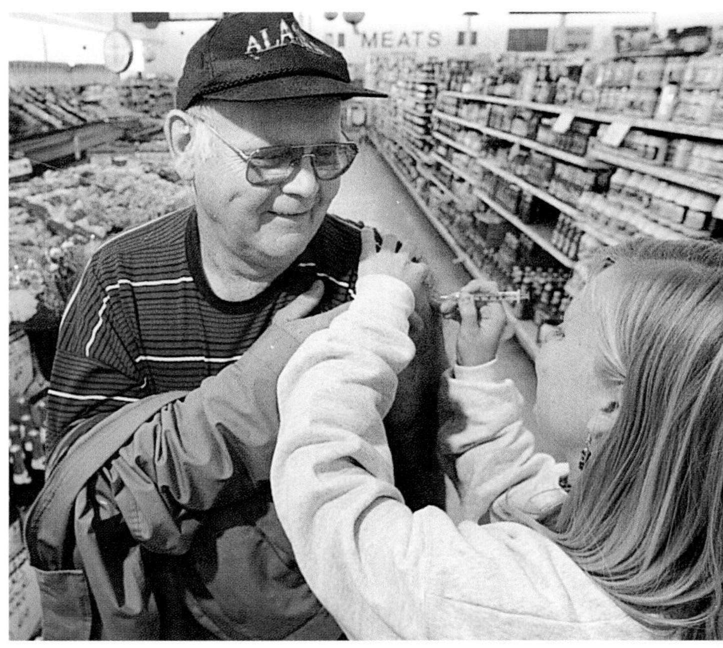

Buzz Magnuson—Saint Paul Pioneer Press

protective as they need to be. Unfortunately, by the time either of these circumstances occurs, it is usually too late for a manufacturer to start again and produce sufficient lots of vaccine that can be used for that year's flu season. Probably as a result of the diligent collection and review of data, however, this has not been a problem.

During the 1996–97 influenza season, routine testing determined that one manufacturer's influenza vaccine had a shorter shelf life than anticipated and lost some of its potency from the time it was produced to the time that it was in clinics around the country ready to be administered. Since it could not be ensured that the use of these vaccine lots would provide adequate protection, especially for individuals at high risk of suffering flu complications (in particular, those with serious chronic underlying medical conditions), many batches were recalled. The CDC and the FDA recommended revaccination with a vaccine from a lot of known potency only for those who had received the recalled vaccine *and* were at high risk for flu complications. The biological

NEWS CAP MHA 98

Disease Eradication: Progress Report

The past year (1996–97) saw substantial progress toward the goal of global eradication of two terrible diseases: poliomyelitis and guinea worm disease (dracunculiasis). Only one other scourge of humankind, smallpox, has been officially eradicated from the world. *Eradication,* which differs from *control* or *elimination,* means that zero incidence of a disease is achieved globally, such that further control measures are not necessary.

The World Health Organization (WHO) initially selected guinea worm disease as a candidate for eradication in 1986. Though the original target eradication date of 1995 was not met, major progress has been made; only 34,000 cases were reported outside of The Sudan in 1996 (in contrast to an estimated 3 million cases worldwide at the start of the eradication campaign in 1986), and 6 of the 18 countries that are still affected (Cameroon, India, Senegal, Yemen, Chad, and Kenya) are on the verge of achieving eradication. The Sudan, which reported almost 120,000 cases—78% of the 1996 global total—is the exception; its program to protect people from the parasitic disease continues to be hampered by civil war. The progress of the campaign to eradicate guinea worm disease was additionally marked in early 1997 when WHO officially certified Pakistan, Iran, and 19 other countries as being "free of dracunculiasis transmission."

Dracunculiasis is transmitted by contaminated drinking water from stagnant ponds or open wells that harbor a tiny water flea (*Cyclops*) containing the embryonic guinea worm parasite. The fleas release worm larvae, which grow and reproduce inside the human body. Female worms migrate within the body to the lower legs and sometimes to various other parts of the body, such as breasts or scrotum, and then emerge through the skin as slender worms that can be up to 90 cm (one yard) long. When the infected person enters a body of water, larvae from the emerging worm are released and are eaten by *Cyclops,* and the vicious circle continues. Victims suffer painful blisters, incapacitation (sometimes for months), and, in the worst cases, permanent crippling and/or secondary infections. Unlike polio or smallpox, the disease is not vaccine-preventable. The dracunculiasis-eradication strategy involves (1) installing wells that supply pumped water to replace open ponds or step wells that require people to enter the water, (2) routinely filtering (or boiling) all drinking water to remove or kill the fleas, (3) teaching people not to contaminate their drinking water, and (4) treating the contaminated water source with a chemical insecticide (temephos [Abate]) that kills *Cyclops.*

Polio, which has been targeted for eradication by the year 2000, has been reduced from about 35,000 *reported* cases in 1988 (though about 300,000 cases are believed to have actually occurred that year) to fewer than 4,000 cases reported worldwide in 1996. Most remaining cases of polio are in Africa and the Indian subcontinent. No cases of polio attributed to wild (naturally occurring) virus have been reported in the Americas since 1991.

The poliovirus attacks certain cells of the brain stem

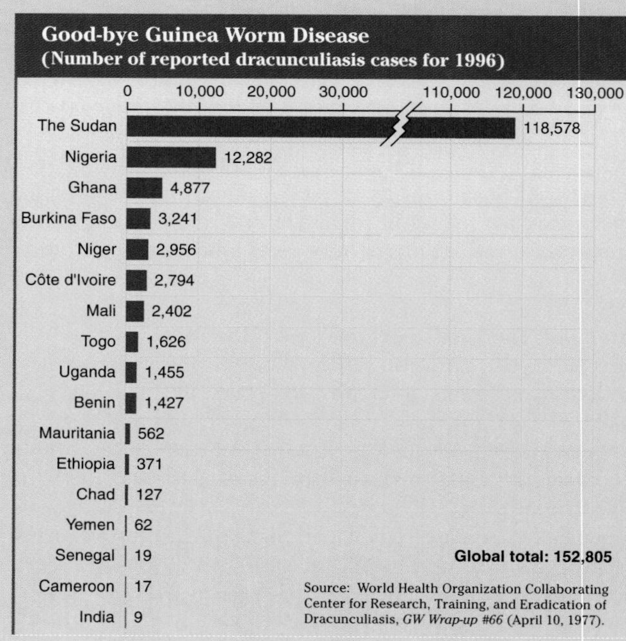

Good-bye Guinea Worm Disease (Number of reported dracunculiasis cases for 1996)

Source: World Health Organization Collaborating Center for Research, Training, and Eradication of Dracunculiasis, *GW Wrap-up #66* (April 10, 1977).

basis for the decline in potency is unknown; fortunately, this was a highly unusual circumstance. Moreover, the efficient recall demonstrated that there is a system in place to respond when something goes wrong.

New vaccines on the horizon

With the growing demand for cost-effective preventive health care strategies, it will be important to increase investment in molecular biology and immunology, as these are the scientific disciplines that will provide the necessary tools and approaches for vaccine development. At the same time, however, efforts are being made to improve the delivery of the vaccines that are now available to adults. Both improvement in the performance of existing vaccines and the creation of new vaccines are likely to enhance the acceptance of immunization as a safe, effective preventive strategy by adult patients in the public at large and by health care providers.

and spinal cord. Though not every infected person has symptoms, everyone who contracts the virus can infect others. Eradication strategies include: (1) achieving and maintaining high vaccination coverage of children under one year of age with at least three doses (preferably four) of oral vaccine, (2) establishing effective epidemiological and laboratory surveillance systems to track and evaluate all suspected cases, and (3) providing supplemental vaccination to interrupt wild poliovirus transmission. The ultimate goal is to track and eliminate every last microscopic bit of wild virus remaining in the world.

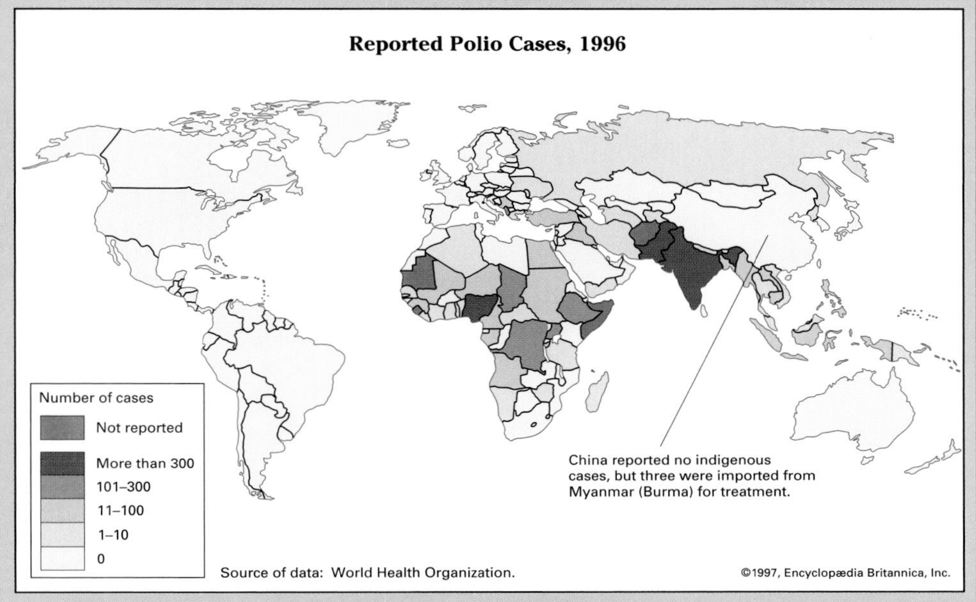

The impending victories against dracunculiasis and polio have spawned new campaigns to wipe out two other infectious diseases: measles and lymphatic filariasis. In May 1997 WHO adopted a resolution calling for the elimination of lymphatic filariasis, a mosquito-transmitted parasitic disease that affects some 120 million persons in tropical Asia, Africa, and the Americas, often causing grotesquely swollen limbs or genitals ("elephantiasis"). The methods to rid the world of this malady are to reduce the opportunity for mosquitoes to bite humans and to treat infected persons with safe and effective drugs.

The Pan American Health Organization, which aims to eliminate measles from the Americas by 2000, reported roughly 2,000 confirmed cases of that disease in the Western Hemisphere in 1996, compared with about 150,000 cases reported annually in the same area in the 1980s. Measles will likely be officially slated by WHO for global eradication as soon as polio eradication has been completed.

Meanwhile, in March 1997 the Free University of Berlin convened 40 infectious disease specialists from around the world for a weeklong workshop. Among other items on its agenda were the review of key biological, economic, and sociopolitical criteria that make eradication of an infectious disease feasible. Workshop attendees also examined specific ways that eradication programs can be used to strengthen ongoing health services, as well as how the latter can support the former, and they considered potential alternatives for initiating and coordinating eradication campaigns. The proceedings of the Berlin workshop will be published in an expanded book form, entitled *The Eradication of Infectious Diseases,* in 1998.

A much larger conference on global disease elimination and eradication as critical future public health strategies will be held in Atlanta, Ga., in February 1998 under the auspices of more than 17 international health organizations. That conference is likely to move beyond the exciting discussions begun in Berlin and will actually identify the specific diseases with the greatest potential for elimination or eradication at that time.

—Donald R. Hopkins, M.D., M.P.H.

Among the most promising new vaccine products intended for adolescents, adults, and the elderly that are currently in the development pipeline and expected to be available in the near future are:

- flu vaccines that will be administered in the form of nose drops or sprays rather than shots
- pneumococcal vaccines with enhanced potency over those in current use
- varicella vaccine to prevent herpes zoster (shingles), a common and painful nerve infection in adults caused by the same virus that causes chicken pox
- an acellular pertussis (whooping cough) vaccine for adults (in the past few years, such vaccines have been developed for children; compared with vaccines made from whole-cell pertussis, the acellular products cause many fewer adverse reactions yet have a high degree of efficacy)
- a vaccine against the bacterium *Helicobacter pylori,* which is responsible for gastric ulcer disease and has been linked to the development of gastric cancer
- vaccines against the sexually transmitted diseases herpes simplex virus infection, gonorrhea, and chlamydia
- a vaccine to prevent Lyme disease, an increasingly prevalent acute inflammatory tickborne disease caused by the spirochete *Borrelia burgdorferi*

NEWS CAP MHA 98

Hazards on the Highway

In 1997 researchers at the University of Toronto released the results of a study they conducted to find out what impact the use of cellular telephones by drivers has on their driving performance. The study, published in the February 13 issue of *The New England Journal of Medicine*, confirmed what many people had suspected—that the chance of being involved in a collision increases when a driver is simultaneously making a phone call or carrying on a telephone conversation.

Jeff Zaruba—AllStock/PNI

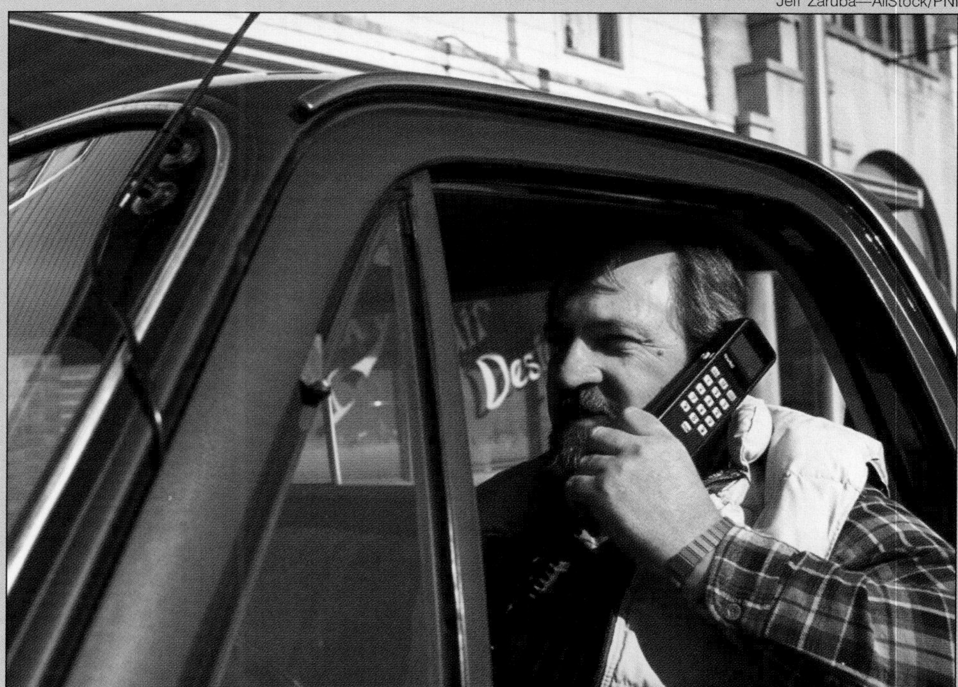

Talking on the phone while navigating through traffic may be as dangerous as driving after having had too much to drink. Several countries have taken the step of outlawing the use of cellular phones by drivers.

After analyzing the cellular telephone records of 699 drivers who had been involved in traffic mishaps, the researchers, Donald A. Redelmeier, a professor of medicine, and Robert J. Tibshirani, a statistician, concluded that drivers using cellular phones are more than four times as likely to be involved in a crash as those minding only the road. That risk is about the same as that of a driver with a blood alcohol level of 0.1%. Ironically, there seemed to be one advantage to having a car phone: 39% of the drivers used their cellular telephones to call for help after a crash had occurred. Perhaps the study's most surprising finding, however, was that the use of hands-free speakerphones offered no safety advantage over the use of handheld cellular phones. The danger, according to the Canadian researchers, was not that the manual dexterity of the drivers was limited but rather that people talking on cellular phones could not—or did not—give their full attention to driving. Brazil, Israel, and Switzerland are among the countries that have banned the use of cellular phones by those behind the wheel.

Another potential driving hazard fueled heated discussion in 1997. Airbags, which have been credited with saving hundreds of lives, especially in head-on collisions, have been *responsible* for the deaths of at least 38 children in the United States since 1993. It had become generally accepted, even by those who defended the use of the devices, that small adults—

While substantial barriers currently block the development of vaccines that protect against the mycobacterial disease tuberculosis, the human immunodeficiency virus (HIV), responsible for AIDS, and the mosquito-transmitted parasitic disease malaria, active research on all of these is currently in progress in laboratories around the world. The ability to prevent these diseases would indeed have a profound public health impact.

No scientific advance of the present century has had as important an effect on public health as immunization. Yet as society approaches the 21st century, medical science has only begun to scratch the surface of the potential to prevent human suffering caused by infectious illnesses and their common complications. New technologies will undoubtedly change the way a variety of once-dreaded diseases are viewed; thanks to the protection that immunizations will offer, maladies that are incurable or that require expensive, complicated, and presently only partially effective therapies will no longer occur.

Scientists already possess a great many of the tools that are needed to proceed full speed ahead with new vaccine development; most of them, however, have not yet been fully exploited. Many other tools, technologies, and novel vaccines are on the horizon—or should soon be visible in the distance.

—Bruce G. Gellin, M.D., M.P.H., and Robert F. Breiman, M.D.

especially small women—were also at risk for serious and even fatal injury from the deployment of airbags during collisions. Hoping to put the brakes on injuries and deaths due to airbags, the National Highway Traffic Safety Administration (NHTSA) enacted legislation in 1997 permitting automobile manufacturers to reduce by 20–35% the force with which airbags deploy.

The NHTSA also recommended that in certain types of vehicles (*e.g.,* those without backseats), manufacturers install switches by which passenger-side airbags may be turned off and that car dealers be given the authority to deactivate bags in any vehicle when so requested by the owner. Another proposal was the implementation of "smart" airbags that deploy according to the size of the occupant and the force of the crash. It was agreed, however, that it would take several years to complete the development and testing of smart bags.

Because most severe injuries and deaths from airbags occur when children and adults are riding unrestrained or without proper restraints, the NHTSA and other safety groups offered the following tips for the public:

- Children should be placed in a safety device appropriate to their age and size. Infants up to one year of age and weighing up to 9 kg (20 lb) should be placed in a rear-facing safety seat; children over one year, weighing up to 18 kg (40 lb) and measuring up to 100 cm (40 in) in height, in a forward-facing seat; and children over 18 kg and 100 cm in height, in a booster seat until regular lap and shoulder belts fit them properly. Parents should read the instructions that come with safety seats and follow them exactly.
- Infants in rear-facing safety seats should be placed in the backseat of the automobile. A rear-facing safety seat should never be used in the front seat of an automobile equipped with a passenger-side airbag.
- Children under age 12 should ride in the backseat. (This is required by law in six European countries and Australia.) If this is not possible, the seat should be moved all the way back.
- All occupants of a motor vehicle should use lap and shoulder belts properly.

Experts in the field of traffic safety agree that if these guidelines are followed, the risk of airbag-associated injuries is significantly lowered.

—Robert Rauch

Although airbags are credited with having saved hundreds of lives, children and small adults are at risk for serious and even fatal injury from the deployment of airbags during collisions.

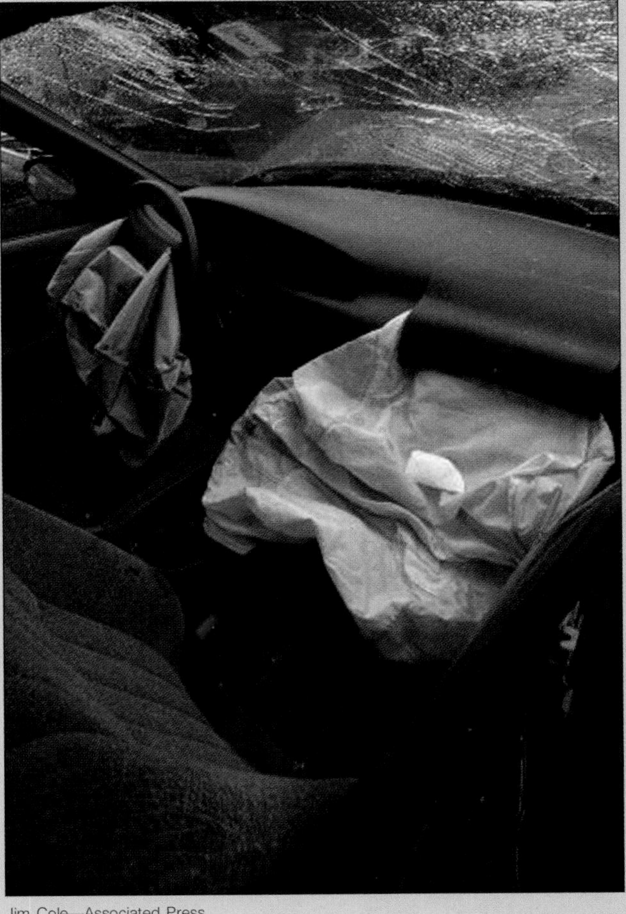

Jim Cole—Associated Press

NEWS CAP MHA 98

Pedestrians in Peril

Mean Streets, a report jointly compiled by the Surface Transportation Policy Project (STPP) and the Environmental Working Group (EWG) and issued in April 1997, revealed that the most basic form of transportation, walking, is an increasingly dangerous activity. In the United States approximately 6,000 pedestrians per year die after being hit by automobiles. In addition, some 110,000 pedestrians are injured in traffic accidents each year.

Why so many injuries and deaths? Surprisingly, perhaps, the reason is not the failure of walkers to perform the age-old safety measure—looking both ways before crossing any thoroughfare. Rather, the STPP and the EWG concluded that pedestrian safety is suffering because it is a low priority of the U.S. government and highway engineers, whereas vehicle safety and traffic flow management are high priorities. The *Highway Capacity Manual,* a widely used guide in the roadway engineering industry, in fact, defines *pedestrians* as "traffic flow interruptions!"

The report also indicated that only 1% of federal highway safety funds is spent on improving roads for "pavement pounders" and bicyclists, despite the fact that pedestrians (about a quarter of whom are senior citizens who find it difficult to cross a street before traffic signals change) account for 14% of all motor-vehicle-related deaths. Furthermore, 55% of total pedestrian fatalities occur in growing residential communities, not major metropolitan areas. Many large cities, however, are also unsafe for walking.

Randy Wells—Tony Stone Images

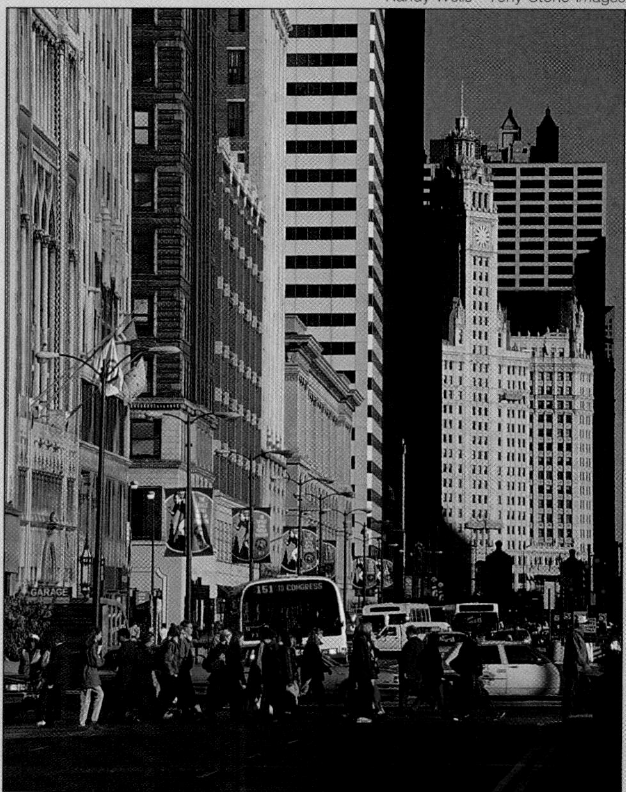

Walkers cross Michigan Avenue during rush hour in Chicago, where pedestrians account for 23% of all automobile-related fatalities. In the U.S., 110,000 pedestrians are injured in traffic accidents each year.

In their report the STPP and the EWG ranked the following five U.S. metropolitan areas as having the meanest streets:

- Fort Lauderdale, Fla.
- Miami, Fla.
- Atlanta, Ga.
- Tampa–St. Petersburg–Clearwater, Fla.
- Dallas, Texas

On the other hand, the following have the most walker-friendly streets:

- Pittsburgh, Pa.
- Milwaukee, Wis.
- Boston
- Rochester, N.Y.
- New York City

Contending that citizens have been forced to yield to motor vehicles for too long, pedestrian-safety advocates are now pushing for legislation at the federal level. Their first step toward achieving pedestrian-friendly streets was to lobby for a more proportionate allocation of federal highway-safety funds. Specific improvements suggested include building more sidewalks, providing bicycle and pedestrian paths, and erecting speed bumps and traffic circles to discourage speeding. As part of an effort to call attention to pedestrian-safety concerns, the Campaign to Make America Walkable also identified 12 top pedestrian complaints (dubbed by the campaign the walkers' "dirty dozen"): sidewalks with missing sections, poor sidewalk surfaces, obstructed sidewalks, bad sidewalk maintenance, narrow sidewalks, missing curb ramps, poorly designed street crossings, the failure of motorists to stop at crosswalks, barriers on walking routes, high traffic levels, motorists shortcutting through neighborhoods, and locations with documented histories of traffic accidents.

In 1997 Pres. Bill Clinton submitted to Congress a reauthorization package for the 1991 Intermodal Surface Transportation Efficiency Act, at the same time proposing an increase in funding for an "Enhancements" program that currently provides funds for pedestrian and bicycle projects. With any luck, as a result of these efforts, pedestrian safety and the clean air that walking promotes may at long last get a green light.

—*Jackie Orihill*

Rheumatic and Musculoskeletal Disorders Update

Arthritic, other rheumatic, and musculoskeletal conditions are so common that most people sooner or later will consult their physician for such a problem. Collectively, they account for the overwhelming majority of acute and chronic pain syndromes and may involve the joints, bones, cartilage, muscles, tendons, ligaments, or the lubricating sacs between any of these structures, called bursas.

One chronic nonarticular musculoskeletal ailment (one that does not involve the joints), low-back pain, is estimated to affect up to 100 million people in the United States alone at any one time. According to the Arthritis Foundation, 2.1 million Americans suffer from rheumatoid arthritis, a progressive, often crippling autoimmune inflammatory disease of the membrane lining the joints (the synovial membrane), which results in bone and cartilage damage throughout the body and for which there is—as yet—no cure. Osteoarthritis, which destroys the cartilage that normally cushions the bones (articular cartilage), is a noninflammatory wear-and-tear disorder and a main cause of disability among older people. Autoimmune and inflammatory disorders such as systemic lupus erythematosus (lupus, or SLE) and the tickborne infection Lyme disease, caused by the spirochete *Borrelia burgdorferi,* are also rheumatic conditions.

Each of these in its own way can be devastating to the joints or organs they affect; sometimes they can be fatal. Equally great numbers of people are affected by such nonarticular conditions as bursitis, tendinitis, fibromyalgia, and certain primary diseases of bone. In just the past few years, the advances in the understanding, diagnosis, prevention, and treatment of many of these rheumatic and musculoskeletal conditions have been impressive; indeed, some would call them revolutionary. Osteoporosis (the loss of bone density potentially leading to fractures), which eventually affects most women, is in the midst of its own revolution; thanks to the attention that has been given to this serious and prevalent problem, its development is now readily prevented or else recognized and effectively managed.

In addition to these leaps forward, there are also vexing ethical-legal questions surrounding certain rheumatic conditions and their treatment. Increasingly, some of the thornier issues—*e.g.,* those concerning on-the-job injuries, untoward reactions to medications, and questionable reimbursement decisions by insurance companies—are being adjudicated in courtrooms.

Focus on fibromyalgia

Pain is the body's way of warning people that something is wrong. Pain is usually defined as an unpleasant sensation in response to a stimulus that causes organ or tissue damage or perceived bodily injury. Yet during any given month, most adults have occasional discomfort for which there may be no significant or identifiable stimulus. A smaller but not insignificant population complains of constant or recurrent widespread musculoskeletal pain on a near-daily basis. The latter group may have fibromyalgia, a prevalent, albeit poorly understood syndrome fraught with controversy. Among the reasons that fibromyalgia is considered controversial are that some patients have a history of psychiatric illness, which suggests they are more likely to have a mental, not physical, illness and, at best, there are few corroborating physical findings. In contrast to many other rheumatic diseases, there are no definitive laboratory or imaging studies for diagnosing fibromyalgia. Thus, many physicians tell their patients that the "pain is in your head."

Fibromyalgia, which was first described nearly 200 years ago, has also been called variously *fibrositis, myofasciitis, myofascial pain syndrome,* and *musculoskeletal rheumatism.* An estimated three million to six million people in the United States have fibromyalgia; women sufferers outnumber men 10 to one.

Clues to a cause. The cause of fibromyalgia is not known. Because most patients have flulike symptoms when they first seek a physician's care, viruses have been suspected, but the few studies to date that have investigated the role of infectious diseases were unable to find either a viral, a bacterial, or a fungal cause. Symptoms of fibromyalgia are remarkably similar to those of so-called chronic fatigue syndrome. While both conditions are notable for their symptoms of pain and fatigue, more patients with chronic fatigue syndrome than fibromyalgia also complain of fever, sore throat, and rash.

Typically, patients with fibromyalgia find that major stress, such as the death of a loved one or on-the-job pressure, precipitates or aggravates the disease. Stress, however, is also known to worsen other diseases. Furthermore, otherwise-healthy individuals may complain of sore muscles after tense or unpleasant interactions with another person (hence the expression "you give me a pain in the neck").

Many investigators suspect that sleep deprivation may induce fibromyalgia. Most patients with fibromyalgia have poor sleep patterns; they awaken frequently during the night—sometimes because of pain, other times free of pain—and even in the absence of pain, they generally feel unrefreshed upon rising in the morning. Studies performed in Canada revealed that patients with fibromyalgia have a disturbance of non-rapid eye movement (non-REM) sleep. The studies showed that when normal volunteers were awakened frequently during non-REM sleep, they often developed fibromyalgic symptoms. As most people know, inadequate sleep commonly results in daytime fatigue, heightened sensitivity to pain, and moodiness.

Neurotransmitters, such as serotonin and endorphins, are normally produced by the brain and other nervous system tissues in response to a painful stimulus. Researchers postulate that such neurotransmitters affect sleep and mood. Furthermore, neurotransmitters play a part in helping maintain the blood supply to the muscles. If these chemical substances are deficient, there may not be enough oxygen carried by the blood to the muscles to maintain their vitality and proper function. Whenever body tissues need more oxygen, lactic acid accumulates, causing variable degrees of pain.

There are intriguing connections here. Is there a link between specific neurotransmitters, sleep, mood, and muscle pain that eventually will explain fibromyalgic symptoms? It seems possible, but at present no one knows for sure.

Sites of pain. Symptoms of fibromyalgia are primarily musculoskeletal pain and stiffness. Pain tends to occur in predictable sites in the neck, upper back, shoulders, lower back, thighs, and knees. Dampness and cold tend to aggravate these complaints, whereas heat gives relief. Other symptoms include tingling in the extremities, headaches, cold sensitivity, and irritable bowel syndrome. The ligaments, tendons, and muscles surrounding joints are usually discretely sensitive to touch (tender points), yet no characteristic pathological changes have ever been detected. Often, upon physical examination, muscle spasms are evident; otherwise, there are few concrete physical findings.

Fibromyalgia is diagnosed on the basis of a careful physical examination, since specific tests are not available. The American College of Rheumatology has published diagnostic guidelines based on the presence of chronic pain and a number of distinct tender points; these guidelines, however, are intended mainly for research. Although the mere existence of this disorder has been questioned by some physicians, to suffering patients it is quite real. Recognizing fibromyalgia as an entity means that patients are more likely to receive helpful, targeted treatment.

Enlightened treatment. For most patients the best way to manage fibromyalgia and other chronic pain syndromes is with a comprehensive approach. Certain principles are paramount in the management of fibromyalgia or any chronic pain syndrome. The physician must have respect for the patient's pain and conduct a careful search for underlying or precipitating causes. While there is no single predictable treatment for fibromyalgia, most patients can achieve partial or complete relief.

An advanced aquatic exercise program helps women with fibromyalgia and other painful rheumatic conditions alleviate debilitating symptoms by strengthening and conditioning large major muscle groups.

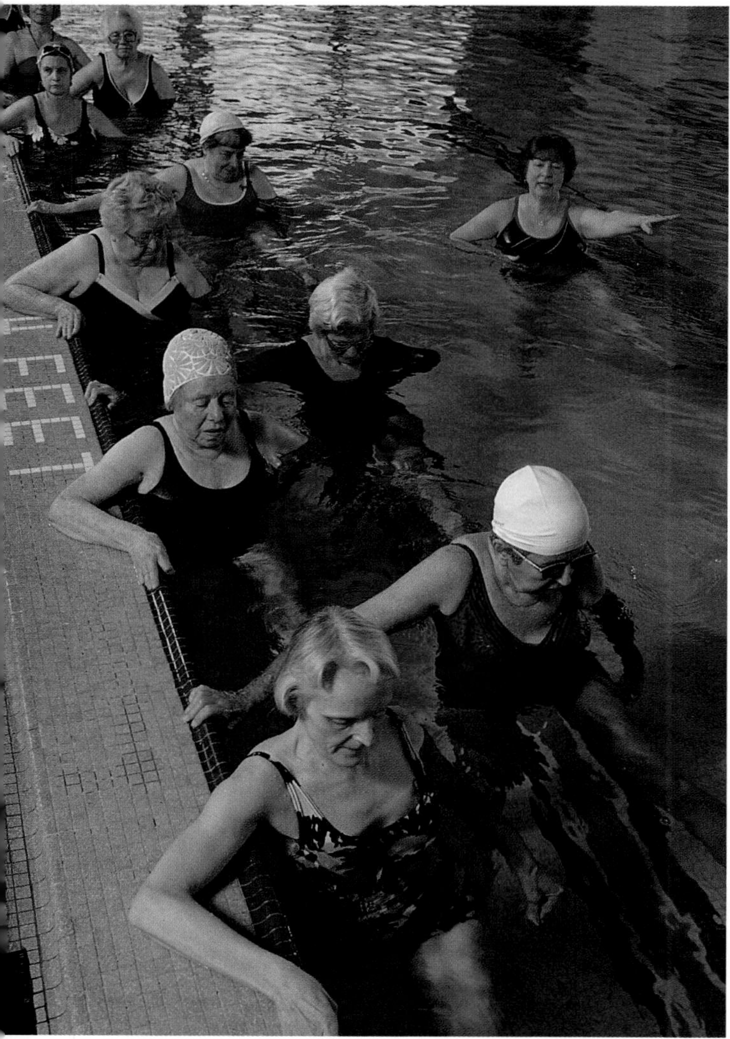

Arthritis Foundation

An important component of treatment is an adjustment in attitude on the part of patients and physicians. Unfortunately, many physicians have dismissed their patients as complaining neurotics. The first step is for a physician to reassure patients that their symptoms are real and that they are not "crazy," as others may have suggested to them. A physician, of course, cannot guarantee patients with fibromyalgia that their disease will be completely cured. Those who have experience in treating the condition, however, can assure them honestly that others with similar conditions are now well. Having hope is important; patients who embrace this hopeful outlook often become their own best source of support. Fear, on the other hand, intensifies pain.

Some patients who have encountered dismissal by health professionals are enraged and frustrated at not being able to get answers from otherwise qualified and respected health professionals. Understandably, they may turn to unproven remedies and quackery. Some of these are dangerous and costly. Others might actually be benign, inexpensive, and helpful.

Because "deconditioning" of muscles may be a cause or an effect of fibromyalgia, graduated exercise-based conditioning is essential. Aerobic exercise that utilizes large muscle groups, such as walking, biking, or swimming, is an excellent conditioner, as it serves to increase the supply of oxygen and nutrients to the muscles. The fibromyalgia patient may at first have a low tolerance for exercise, yet most patients using the "slow as you go" technique can gradually build up to a level required for conditioning. Most patients also get a much-needed psychological boost from exercising on a regular basis.

Flexibility exercises with assistance (passive) or without (active) help stretch underused, contracted muscles. Many physicians recommend warm pool therapy for patients with fibromyalgia. Exercising in warm water conditions and strengthens muscles and builds endurance; the buoyancy of the water and the resistance it provides are ideal for those who have pain and stiffness. Some fibromyalgia sufferers have found relief from other physical modalities, including simple hot or cold packs, massage therapy, acupuncture, chiropractic manipulation, and relaxation techniques.

A balance of rest and activity is critical to the recovery process. The proper activity threshold will vary from patient to patient. "Overdoing it" exacerbates stress, and stress is a key provoker of symptoms in patients with fibromyalgia. Therefore, patients should be counseled about pacing their activity. Recognizing stress's warning signs, learning how to avoid stress, and finding useful strategies for handling it when it is unavoidable are all integral to a successful fibromyalgia management program.

Medications play an important role in the treatment of fibromyalgia, but independent of the treatment components described above, drug therapy will most likely fail. Medication regimens must be tailored to the individual. No two patients will respond to the same drugs the same way. There are numerous options, including analgesics, nonsteroidal anti-inflammatory drugs (NSAIDs), muscle relaxants, hypnotics (sleeping pills), and antidepressants.

Because fibromyalgia is a pain-amplification syndrome, analgesics (pain relievers) are usually beneficial. These run the gamut from simple aspirin to narcotics such as codeine, although physicians prescribe the latter variety of analgesics only as a last resort because of their addicting properties. Acetaminophen often relieves pain when patients take it, but compliance may be poor because over-the-counter medications are viewed by some patients as unimportant. Ibuprofen and other NSAIDs help somewhat, but to date there have been few reported studies of their effectiveness. Many such investigations, however, are currently under way. Some NSAIDs have notable gastrointestinal tract side effects. A safe alternative to NSAIDs and narcotics is the prescription drug tramadol, a pure analgesic that works in part like a narcotic but without having the addictive properties of narcotics. Tramadol also works as a selective serotonin reuptake inhibitor, which means that it positively influences neurotransmitters that might play a causative role in fibromyalgia.

Because sleep is so important to the daytime well-being of patients with fibromyalgia, several newer hypnotics such as zolpidem, which help normalize non-REM sleep without the "hangover" of most sleeping pills, are useful in treating fibromyalgia. First, however, patients should alter their "sleep hygiene," making adjustments in such elements as bed comfort, ambient temperature, noise level, and prebedtime eating and exercise.

Physicians frequently prescribe antidepressant drugs even in the absence of overt clinical depression. The doses required for pain relief and a sense of well-being are less than those used to treat depression. Traditionally, tricyclic antidepressants like amitriptyline enable patients with fibromyalgia to feel better. In recent years selective serotonin reuptake inhibiting agents like fluoxetine (Prozac) have been widely prescribed; they may work in part by raising the patient's pain threshold and in part by alleviating the sleep disturbance. Muscle relaxants such as cyclobenzaprine play a similar role by improving sleep and relieving pain.

Soaring rates of repetitive strain injuries

In November 1996 California became the first U.S. state to regulate occupational practices that often lead to repetitive strain injury (RSI)—the fastest-growing category of workplace injury. Currently, mandatory federal guidelines aimed at preventing such injury in workplaces nationwide are being developed. RSIs are defined as a musculoskeletal syndrome provoked by personal, household, occupational, or sports activities that are repetitious. The onset is often insidious and without a history of specific trauma. Rather, the repetition of many small traumas (microtraumas) may cause the problem.

Meatpackers to data processors. Muscle strain in the forearm, tendinitis (painful and inflamed tendons) of the wrist or hand, and nerve impingement may all be forms of RSI. Occasionally, blood vessels are involved; overuse of muscles may exceed the available blood supply, which diminishes or compromises

A waitress with carpal tunnel syndrome (CTS) struggles with her task at hand—getting the table cleared for the next customer. CTS is an occupationally induced repetitive strain injury that affects ever-increasing numbers of people in the workforce. Treatments, including wrist splints, exercises, cortisone shots, and surgery, may help temporarily, but long-term relief often depends on ceasing or modifying the provoking activity.

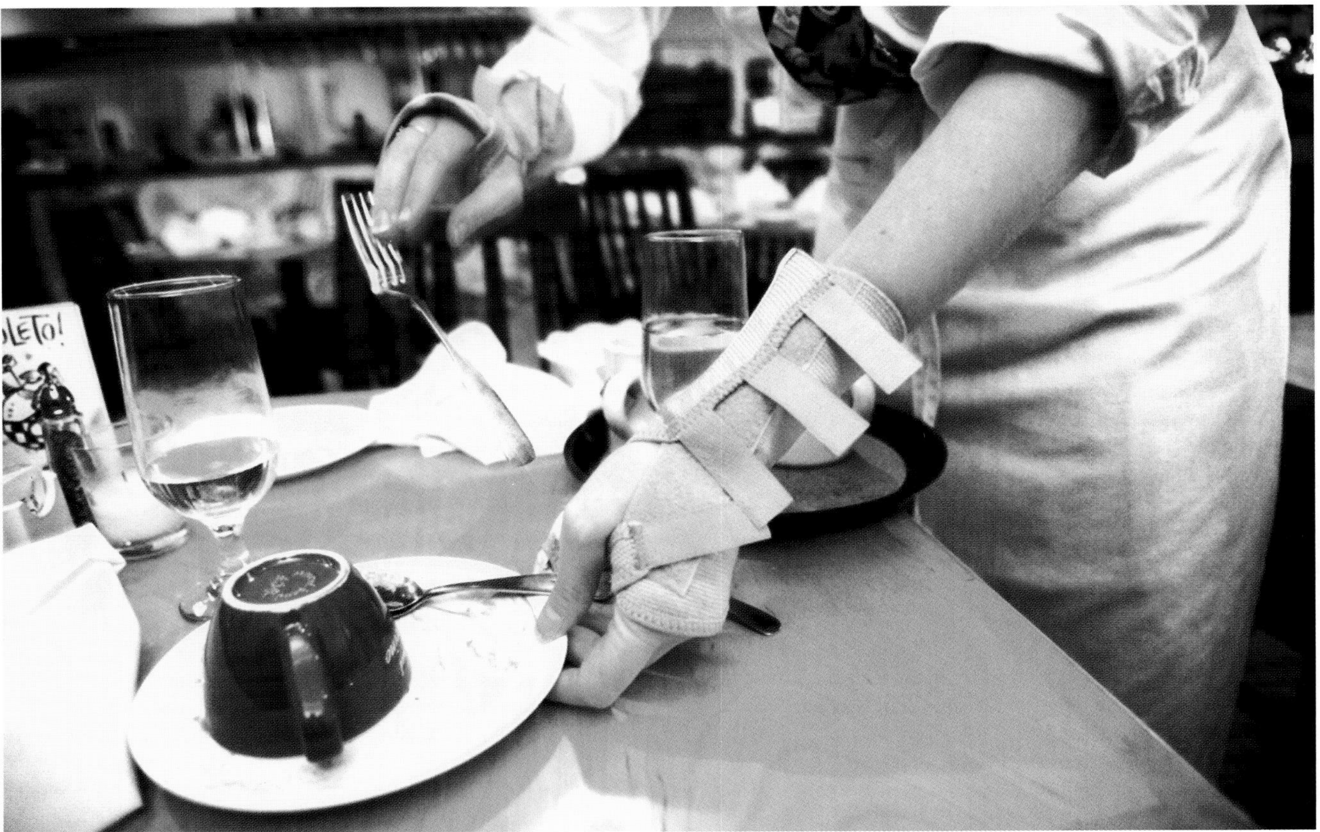

Paul Shoul—Impact Visuals/PNI

Hank Morgan—Science Source/Photo Researchers

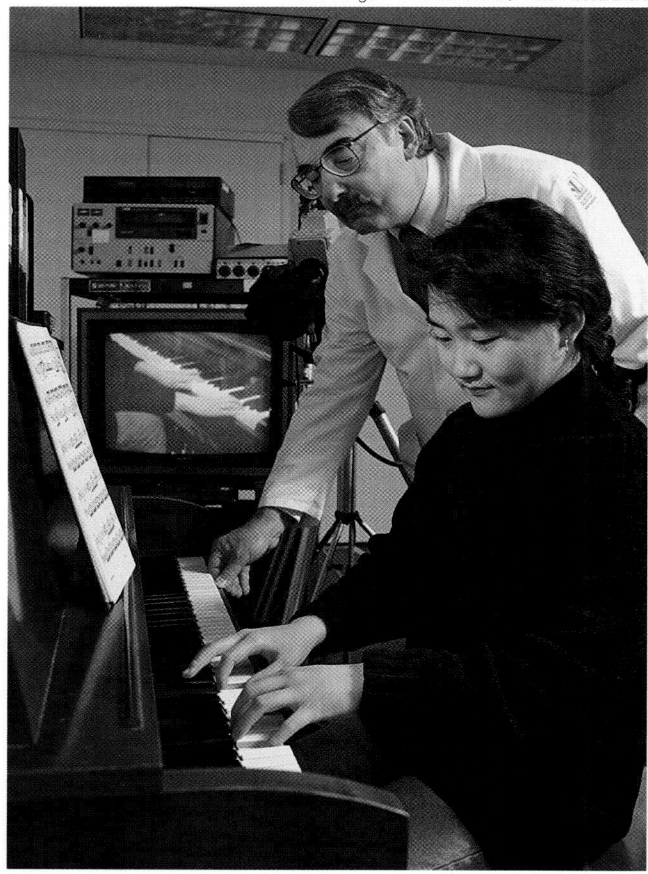

The playing style of a piano student with repetitive strain hand injuries and tendinitis in her right forearm is being videotaped; this will enable her to see the flaws in her technique that contribute to her debilitation.

blood flow to the extremities and results in pain. Carpal tunnel syndrome (CTS) is the most commonly recognized type of nerve-compression RSI. In this condition tendons, ligaments, and blood vessels compress the median nerve, which extends along the forearm and hand and passes through a narrow bony canal in the wrist (carpal tunnel). Tendinitis, diabetes mellitus, arthritis, wrist fracture, underactive thyroid gland, and pregnancy are some fairly common conditions that may lead to CTS. Excessive typing, hammering, chopping, knitting, keypunching, and playing a musical instrument are examples of activities that may promote tendinitis and CTS. Thus, secretaries, carpenters, pianists, meat-packers, data processors, and many more are at risk.

Getting to the root of the problem—and relieving it. The patient's history and a careful physical examination provide the principal clues that enable a correct diagnosis of RSI. Nerve conduction testing, which measures the speed of the electrical signals that run along the median nerve as it passes through the carpal tunnel, is an electrodiagnostic study that helps establish the presence of CTS and other nerve-impingement syndromes. Occasionally, specialized studies such as magnetic resonance imaging are done to pinpoint a specific cause of an RSI.

Treatment depends upon the specific cause. CTS, for example, may respond to splinting, local injections of corticosteroids into the wrist, or surgical release of the carpal tunnel by cutting an overlying protective ligament. Yoga-based exercises may reduce some patients' pain by increasing local circulation. To ensure long-term relief, most patients with RSI must make changes in the technique and often in the equipment they use to perform the activity that provoked the problem in the first place.

In 1997 the U.S. government began to review the best workplace practices with the intention of publishing a manual so that the successes of companies that have eased the burden of RSIs can be made known to other companies. Federally sponsored research is also under way seeking cause-and-effect links between specific kinds of work and specific injuries.

Tricky nature of cause and effect

Trauma plays a key role in fractures, sprains, RSIs, torn cartilage (meniscus) of the knee, reflex sympathetic dystrophy (an excruciating sympathetic nervous system pain syndrome), and certain cases of osteoarthritis. Although trauma has been associated with the onset of fibromyalgia, gout, rheumatoid arthritis, and other connective tissue diseases, there is considerable controversy as to whether trauma is a relevant specific cause or just a coincidental event.

Even experts cannot always prove a cause-and-effect relationship between a specific rheumatic disease and the traumatic event that preceded it (the proximate cause). An in-line skater who crashes into a parked automobile may sustain a fracture to the wrist; if that blunt-trauma injury is immediately followed by swelling or bleeding into the injured wrist and forearm tissues, there is fairly irrefutable evidence that a traumatic life event (the skater's impact with the car) and the symptoms (bleeding, pain, and swelling) are connected. If the wrist never heals properly, however, chronic wrist discomfort, sometimes aggravated by overuse, may develop. Wrist-related disability experienced years after the skating injury may not have such a clear explanation. In fact, in most cases of chronic rheumatic disease, the precise mechanism may be unclear.

Some specialists suspect that certain rheumatic disorders such as osteoarthritis result from trauma that causes cracking of cartilage or a minimal tearing of the soft tissues that support joints. Others hypothesize that emotional or physical stress so alters the immune system that susceptibility to systemic disorders such as rheumatoid arthritis (a long-term destructive connective tissue disease that results from the body's attacking healthy joint tissue) increases; some scientific evidence supports this contention.

Attempts to establish a link between a traumatic event and the development of rheumatic symptoms can easily get into murky medicolegal waters. Patients, no matter how badly injured, are often suspected of malingering (feigning illness for the purpose of gaining some desired end). Insurance companies usually reimburse for proximate injuries such as fractures and sprains but often balk at compensating patients who subsequently develop osteoarthritis, fibromyalgia, reflex sympathetic dystrophy, or rheumatoid arthritis—conditions often associated with lifelong suffering and disability. One recent study showed that fibromyalgia was common after neck injuries. Another indicated that 77% of patients litigating because of trauma-related fibromyalgia continued to receive treatments after they settled their legal cases in or out of court. These findings suggest strongly that these patients were not malingering. This situation becomes more important and

(Left) Mehau Kulyk—Science Source/Photo Researchers;
(right) Dorothy Littell Greco—Stock, Boston

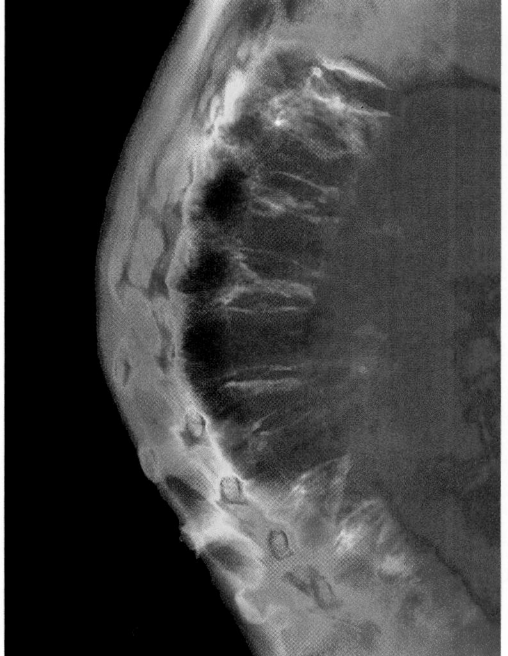

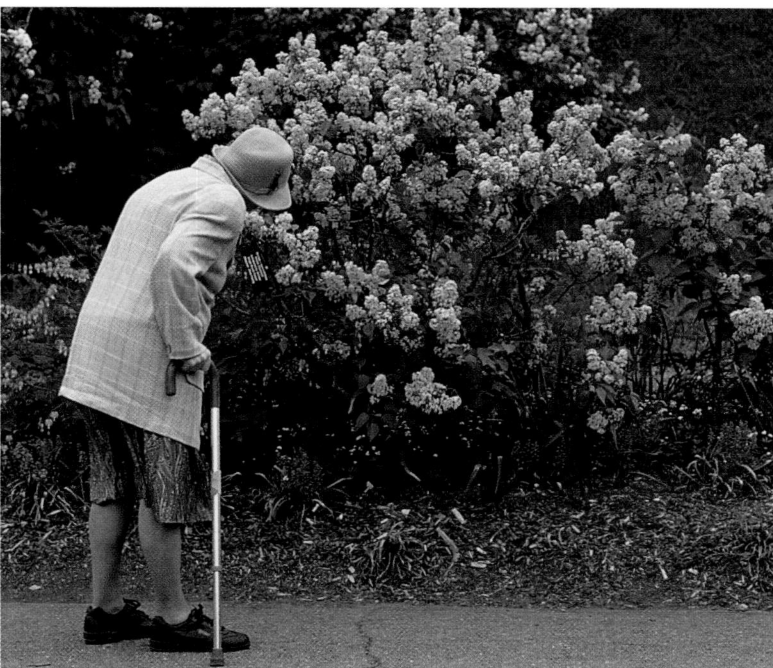

(Left) A color-enhanced X-ray of the curved thoracic spine of a patient with advanced osteoporosis shows how vertebrae have become compressed. Pain and loss of height are common effects of the condition. Fortunately, state-of-the-art diagnostic equipment and enlightened means of preventing loss of bone-mineral density are brightening the outlook for future generations of elderly females.

indeed more vexing as more people live long enough to develop conditions such as osteoarthritis. For example, late in life many former athletes develop osteoarthritis in joints that were frequently subjected to trauma. Increasingly, the association between trauma and arthritis is being decided by lawyers, judges, and juries in the courtroom rather than by physicians and other medical scientists in the clinic or the laboratory.

The challenge of osteoporosis

Osteoporosis is a thinning of the bones secondary to progressive loss of calcium and deterioration of the skeletal supporting structures. Some bone loss is a natural consequence of aging, but it is accelerated in osteoporosis. It is not a new disease; however, during the past few years interest in its detection and treatment has exploded. Osteoporosis affects more than 25 million people in the United States. Untreated, it leads to 1.5 million painful, disabling fractures annually. Hip fractures may be fatal; up to 20% of those who experience them die within the first year of the injury. Hip fractures in postmenopausal women result in long-term care in a nursing home in about 20% of cases.

Osteoporosis affects most women and some men. Both sexes begin losing calcium from their bones during their 20s and 30s. Women lose it faster than men, particularly after menopause, when levels of estrogen, the female hormone that helps to maintain the integrity of bone, diminish. Most cases of osteoporosis are menopause-related; during the 5–15 years following menopause, women typically lose 15% of their bone mass. Certain endocrine or metabolic diseases such as those affecting the gonads (sex glands), thyroid gland, parathyroid glands, and adrenal glands may also lead to osteoporosis. Regardless of specific cause, certain people are more inclined than others to develop the disease. Those at greatest risk are Caucasians and Asians, people of short or thin stature, those with a family history of the disease, smokers, those who consume alcohol in excess, women who reach menopause before age 45 (either naturally or after hysterectomy), and men with hypogonadism (functional incompetence of the testes). Osteoporosis should be suspected in patients with a history of many fractures, particularly after minimal trauma.

Silent but complicated. Osteoporosis is a silent disease because most patients are without symptoms until they develop the conspicuous complications—*e.g.,* painful fractures, a measurable loss of height, or spinal deformity. A prominent protuberance at the back of the neck ("dowager's hump") or a markedly bent-over posture characterizes the spinal deformity. These complications may take many years to develop after the onset of the osteoporotic process; without appropriate diagnostic testing, however, there can be no certainty about when and whether osteoporosis has begun.

The disease is suspected when risk factors become apparent during the susceptible years, but it takes a knowledgeable patient or health care provider to ask the right questions. Several imaging methods, from traditional X-rays to computed tomography (CT) scans to special radiographic techniques such as dual photon absorptiometry, have been used to diagnose the condition. These procedures, however, either lack diagnostic specificity, take an inordinately long time to perform, have high costs, or expose the patient to excessive radiation. Over the past decade a procedure known as dual-energy X-ray absorptiometry (DEXA) has become the diagnostic method of choice. With DEXA the patient's radiation exposure is minimal; moreover, the test is easily performed at relatively low cost and takes a maximum of 20–30 minutes.

Nevertheless, the cost is high enough to prohibit mass screening of patients without apparent risk factors. Fortunately, less-expensive, more portable apparatuses that depend largely on ultrasonic sources of energy are expected to come onto the market soon. They will make it possible to screen large numbers of patients; those for whom a preliminary diagnosis of osteoporosis is made then will be selected to undergo DEXA testing.

Treatment options. The optimal management of osteoporosis, like that of so many musculoskeletal disorders, is based on a comprehensive therapeutic protocol that involves appropriate patient education, medications, mineral supplements, diet, and exercise. The purposes of treating osteoporosis are to: (1) increase bone mass, which thereby reduces fracture risk, (2) stop or reverse bone loss by inhibiting bone resorption, (3) maximize physical functioning, and (4) prevent falls, because even a minor tumble can cause painful fractures in a patient with poor bone mass.

Estrogen is essential to the maintenance of proper bone mineralization; a lack of it results in loss of bone density. This important female hormone is therefore the medication of choice in treating postmenopausal osteoporosis. Seven to 10 years of estrogen therapy, started immediately after menopause, reduces the incidence of vertebral and hip fractures by 50%. Estrogen is also effective in older women who are many years past menopause. Estrogen is almost always given in conjunction with the hormone progesterone to prevent endometrial (uterine) cancer. For a variety of reasons, however—breast tenderness, bloating, postmenopausal vaginal bleeding, weight gain, and concerns about estrogen-induced breast cancer among them—only 29% of postmenopausal women are compliant with long-term hormone replacement therapy.

Calcitonin, another hormone, has been available as a treatment for 30 years; it partially reverses osteoporosis by slowing bone resorption, but because it must be self-administered via an intramuscular injection, chronic adherence to this regimen is poor. Moreover, it is not especially well tolerated. Within the past few years, the Food and Drug Administration (FDA) has approved a nasal-spray form of calcitonin, which has local rather than systemic side effects. Intranasal calcitonin reverses calcium loss from bone, but to date there are no published data indicating that it can prevent osteoporotic fractures.

Alendronate is the newest and most effective of a class of drugs known as bisphosphonates. According to several reported studies, alendronate administered in oral form once daily can help increase bone density and prevent fractures, deformity, and loss of height. It reduces the rate of fractures by nearly 48%. Alendronate must be taken exactly as prescribed in order to maximize its absorption through the gastrointestinal tract and minimize heartburn. All drugs used for the treatment of osteoporosis have the potential to cause side effects, which, of course, physician and patient together should weigh against the benefits. A diet rich in calcium, mainly in the form of dairy products, along with calcium and vitamin supplements, is an essential part of almost any preventive or therapeutic program.

Moderate weight-bearing aerobic exercise helps maintain calcium balance and optimal bone mineralization. Walking is especially beneficial. A supervised medical exercise program may be required for severely affected patients. Falls are the most common cause of fractures. Thus, exercises that increase strength and endurance and special environmental accommodations, such as unobstructed pathways, proper lighting, and carpeting, are important means of preventing falls and protecting against their effects. These measures are an integral aspect of the total treatment program, especially among the elderly.

Fortunately, accurate state-of-the-art diagnosis, along with some combination of carefully selected medications, diet, and exercise, is now preventing the pain, suffering, and deformity that were so often associated with undetected and untreated osteoporosis in the past. The availability of these preventive and therapeutic measures becomes ever more important as the population worldwide ages. Though the cost of treatment can be high, the health care expenditures for *untreated* osteoporosis in years to come would be substantially greater.

Corticosteroids: the ecstasy and the agony

Ever since the late 1940s, when Philip S. Hench and his colleagues at the Mayo Clinic in Rochester, Minn., discovered that a "miraculous" substance isolated from the cortex of the adrenal gland (initially called *compound E* and later named *cortisone*) had a dramatic effect on patients with rheumatoid arthritis, this drug has been the subject of much debate. Cortisone is a steroid hormone that is naturally released from the adrenal glands in response to stress.

That the synthetic form of cortisone is a potent anti-inflammatory drug capable of relieving the pain and suffering of most inflammatory forms of arthritis is unquestioned. When analgesics and NSAIDs fail to relieve the pain and inflammation in rheumatoid arthritis, cortisone and similar corticosteroid drugs (*e.g.,* prednisone, hydrocortisone) usually succeed—not only in lessening the pain, reducing the inflammation, and improving joint function but also in giving the patient an initial sense of well-being. Patients with certain conditions such as polymyalgia rheumatica, a disorder of the elderly characterized by muscular pain and stiffness in the shoulders, neck, and pelvic area, respond so dramatically within 24 hours of receiving even a modest dose of the drug that cortisone is used for diagnostic purposes; a rapid therapeutic response is an indicator of the condition. Cortisone has saved the lives of many patients with arthritis-related connective tissue disorders such as lupus, which can involve the brain, kidneys, heart, and blood vessels. It is also effective in treating numerous other rheumatic and nonrheumatic conditions; these include disease of the adrenal glands, severe allergic conditions, asthma, and ulcerative colitis, to name a few. Patients who have had organ transplants may need to take corticosteroids for the rest of their life to prevent graft rejection.

The downside of corticosteroid administration lies in its predictable side effects. These include weight gain, fluid retention, high blood pressure, muscle weakness, and skin fragility. The potential to develop a puffy moon-shaped face, flushed cheeks, fullness in the neck ("buffalo hump"), and growth of hair in undesirable places (*e.g.,* on the face in women) after a few years may be of great concern to some patients, even when the drug is needed for survival. Cortisone may also place the patient at risk for certain disorders such as diabetes, infections, psychosis, and avascular necrosis (a deterioration of bone related to a loss of blood circulation to one or many joints). Patients who take the drug for a long time may need total joint replacements to alleviate pain and restore lost musculoskeletal function. Virtually all patients taking the drug in high-enough doses over a long-enough period of time will develop unwanted reactions.

Corticosteroid drugs can also cause osteoporosis when taken over a period of time. Because so many patients are on long-term corticosteroid treatment and so many patients develop osteoporosis as a result, the American College of Rheumatology recently issued the first guidelines for the management of steroid-induced osteoporosis. The organization recommends that patients have baseline bone mineral densitometry testing at the initiation of treatment and at subsequent intervals. Postmenopausal women should be on hormone replacement therapy unless it is otherwise contraindicated. Patients are advised to consume 1,500 mg of calcium daily (dietary and/or supplemental) along with at least 800 international units of vitamin D to increase absorption of calcium. Daily weight-bearing exercise is recommended, as are smoking cessation, very moderate alcohol intake, and a prudent diet. Physicians should also be aware of the patients' muscle strength, balance, gait, and visual acuity to assess their risk of falling and should inquire about any home-environment factors that may increase the risk of falls.

The devastating side effects of cortisone in some patients may quickly overshadow its benefits and sometimes even its lifesaving outcome. Even patients who clearly would not have survived without cortisone may have second thoughts about taking the medication and question their physicians' judgment in prescribing the drug. Under such circumstances some patients have sought legal recourse, even though there may not have been a suitable medical alternative and even though they were warned of the consequences. When a health care provider offers cortisone as a therapeutic option, patients should ask lots of questions about benefits and risks. If there is any doubt in either the patient's or the physician's mind about such a choice, it is always wise to seek a second opinion.

—*Warren A. Katz, M.D.*

NEWS CAP MHA 98

Osteoarthritis: No Easy Answers

Can a dietary supplement cure osteoarthritis, the most common type of arthritis that eventually affects most people? The cause of osteoarthritis is complex, but wear and tear of cartilage is probably largely responsible. Cartilage is composed of collagen—a strong, tightly woven protein—and other substances, chondroitin sulfate and its derivative, glucosamine sulfate. These chemicals are the building blocks for extremely large molecules that mesh with one another, trapping water and thus creating a cushioning sponge. This biophysical phenomenon allows cartilage to act as a shock absorber—for example, when people walk. When the cartilaginous interwoven arcade breaks down, as in osteoarthritis, chondroitin sulfate and glucosamine sulfate, being smaller molecules, leak out. It is no wonder then that patients with osteoarthritis of the knee have pain when they bear weight. Conventional wisdom holds that replacing chondroitin sulfate and glucosamine sulfate would restore destroyed cartilage. Studies in the early 1980s did suggest that glucosamine could slow cartilage breakdown in animals, perhaps by stimulating its growth.

Now, 15 years later, popular magazines, best-selling books, including one called *The Arthritis Cure,* the *New York Times,* national television shows, and health food stores have been promoting chondroitin sulfate and glucosamine sulfate as nutritional supplements for the treatment of arthritis. The theoretical argument for their use is intriguing because both are essential for the maintenance and repair of cartilage. Individual testimony about their effectiveness in relieving arthritis pain is rampant, but testimony is not science! Although several small, short-term controlled studies in humans do attest to a modest decrease in joint symptoms, there is no clear-cut evidence that these agents prevent or reverse cartilage destruction in osteoarthritis. Furthermore, although the substances are widely available in stores that sell nutritional supplements, the Food and Drug Administration has not approved them.

Pending further investigation, even if patients choose to use glucosamine and chondroitin, they should also follow more conventional guidelines. The American College of Rheumatology recommends analgesic and anti-inflammatory medications, exercise, physical therapy, joint protection, self-help aids, and total joint replacement if necessary.

—*Warren A. Katz, M.D.*

Widely advertised nutritional supplements sold as osteoarthritis "cures" have not been shown to do what their promoters claim: reverse cartilage destruction. Nor are they cheap! These two bottles cost $68.

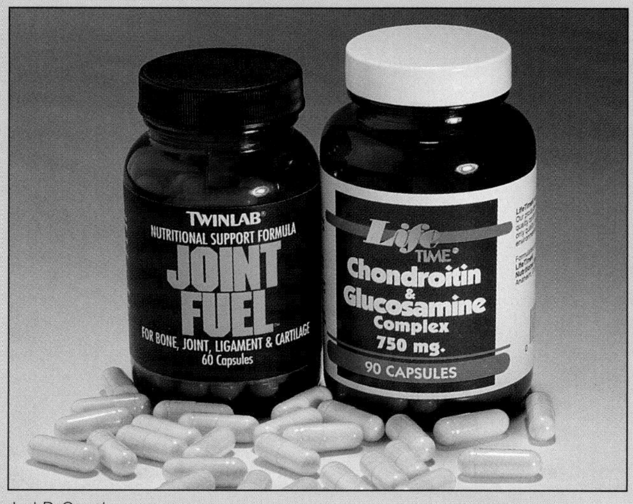

Joel DeGrand

College Crisis: Booze Before Books

It is a Thursday night; Linda, a 19-year-old sophomore, heads for the bar around the corner from her dorm. She easily slips past the bouncer with her fake ID and finds her boyfriend and his friends at the end of the bar. She begins drinking, and though she knows it will mean another Friday of missed classes, she continues into the wee hours. The next morning, she wakes with her face buried in the bathmat, her head throbbing. Her roommate passes the bathroom door and asks, "Good time last night?" Linda does not respond. In fact, Linda does not remember last night.

According to a recent survey conducted by the Carnegie Foundation, college presidents across the United States cite alcohol abuse as the number one problem on campus. Yet alcohol remains readily available to nearly every student on nearly every campus. The U.S. is not alone. There is probably not a Western industrialized country in which students attending institutions of higher learning do not abuse alcohol. While alumni of virtually any college anywhere in the world may amuse themselves recalling their fondest drinking exploits, recent public health research suggests that the effects of heavy drinking on the student drinker and those around him or her are devastatingly destructive. Yet they are widely overlooked.

Campus complacence

Drinking—legal and underage—is the most widely and passively accepted social activity on U.S. college campuses. The question shouted across the dining hall on Friday nights is not "What are you doing tonight?" but "Where are you gonna get trashed [or pissed or loaded] tonight?" Some students find getting drunk a refuge from what they consider overwhelming pressures; others claim that they simply lack other things to do. Whatever the reason, students binge drink at very high rates and thereby jeopardize all aspects of their student lives: social, academic, and personal.

Excessive drinking is not a new phenomenon on campus. In colonial days Harvard University's annual graduation processions were led by a county sheriff—not for ceremonial reasons but rather to ensure that student rowdiness was kept under control. The tradition at Harvard has continued, and so has the problem of inebriated collegians that spawned it. But should heavy drinking still be seen as an acceptable and necessary part of the Harvard—or any college—experience? Those who have taken a close look at college drinking and its effects think not.

A few years ago, researchers at the Harvard School of Public Health conducted a nationwide survey of more than 17,000 students attending 140 four-year U.S. colleges in 40 states. Their goal was to determine the extent of binge drinking by college students and look at the ensuing health and behavioral problems that binge drinkers create for themselves and others. Results showed that most (84%) college students drink during the school year, and almost half (44%) binge drink. "Binge drinking" is defined as five drinks in a row for men, four for women, one or more times in a two-week period. Half of those who binge drink are frequent bingers, which means they have drunk in such a manner three or more times in a two-week period. A drink is defined as a 360-ml (12-oz) can or bottle of beer, a 120-ml (4-oz) glass of wine, a 360-ml can or bottle of wine cooler, or a shot (37 ml [1.25 oz]) of liquor, straight or in a mixed drink. That eye-opening study, published in the *Journal of the American Medical Association* (Dec. 7, 1994), provided the clearest picture to date of the seriousness of the problem. Two more recent studies also found binge-drinking rates on U.S. campuses to be high: two of every five students drink excessively on a regular basis.

Harvard researchers have continued to study the campus binge-drinking problem. Their findings have helped determine when "social" drinking becomes distinctly "antisocial," suggested which students are most likely to become binge drinkers and suffer the consequences, and pinpointed steps that college administrators, parents, and students can take to begin to solve the serious campus problem.

Statistics compiled by the Center on Addiction and Substance Abuse at Columbia University, New York City, indicate that white male college students drink more then white females and more than black and Latino students of both sexes, that students spend $5.5 billion on alcohol annually (which is more than they spend on nonalcoholic beverages and books combined!), and that students in the northeastern U.S., which has the greatest concentration of colleges, drink more than students in the South or the West.

One thing is consistent: the more a student drinks, the more likely that student is to suffer alcohol-related problems—in the present and in the future. Frequent bingers are 7–10 times more likely than nonbinge drinkers to engage in such dangerous activities as having unprotected sex, getting into trouble with the police, and driving while drunk. The Harvard survey results revealed that among frequent binge drinkers, 62% of men and 49% of women drove after drinking some amount of alcohol and that 40% of men and 21% of women reported that they drove after having five or more drinks. For many people, drinking heavily in college sets a pattern of lifelong alcohol abuse. One study followed college-age alcohol abusers into adulthood and discovered that at age 60, 59% were still abusers.

Secondhand consequences

A group of junior-year university students are gathered in one of their dorm rooms watching a video movie during midterm-exam season. They are all tired and engrossed in the suspense-filled film. When a few loud shouts are heard outside, they simply turn up the volume. But the noise outside swells, and violent words are exchanged. A brawl has broken out between groups of obviously drunken students. Nothing can be seen from the window, so one junior steps outside to see what is going on. Just as his eyes adjust to the dark, a beer bottle strikes the side of his face, slashing his cheek from eye socket to chin.

Binge drinkers not only hurt themselves; they hurt those in their environment—friends and strangers alike. Their drunken actions run from annoying to life-threatening. A majority of college students at some time experience adverse consequences from other students' drinking. At the least severe, they find that their studies and their own social lives are regularly disrupted because drunken friends need someone to escort them home, foot the bar bill or taxi fare, hold the bucket, clean up the vomit, bandage a wound, apply ice to a nasty shiner, or nurse them through the next day's hangover.

While some might dismiss being awakened in the middle of the night by a group of drunken students as just part of the college "experience," most cannot deny the more lasting consequences of being pushed, hit, assaulted, insulted, or humiliated by a binge drinker. The most severe and damaging consequences are associated with explicitly antisocial and violent actions on the part of the drinker, including unwanted sexual advances, blatant sexual assault, and so-called date rape.

Secondhand effects of binge drinking are felt by almost everyone. Not surprisingly, on campuses with very high binge-drinking rates, nonbinging students are likely to suffer secondhand effects. But even on campuses with relatively few binge drinkers, a majority of students living on campus are likely to experience some adverse consequences of others' intoxication at some time. On an individual level, the more a particular student drinks, the more likely he or she is to associate with binge drinkers and become the victim of secondhand binge effects. While all students can become the targets of secondhand binge effects, binge drinkers themselves are more likely than their nonbinging counterparts to be victims of their peers' drunken actions.

The binge-drinking risk

A freshman fraternity pledge is found dead of pulmonary edema (abnormal accumulation of fluid in the lungs) on the floor of his dorm room. Although the medical examiner would not say whether alcohol was the cause of his death, the facts are clear: that night, along with a handful of other pledges, he was locked in a closet with a keg of beer and not allowed out until they had consumed the entire 61 liters (16 gal). Arriving home, he passed out and choked on his own vomit.

The drinking rates of different types of students at different schools vary greatly. The single best predictor of binge drinking in college is living in or belonging to a fraternity. More than half of fraternity-house residents and nearly half of sorority-house residents are frequent binge drinkers. In early 1997 a handful of national fraternities announced their intention to go "dry" and prohibit drinking in their houses. Among members of Greek societies, there is a long-standing culture of frequent and deliberate heavy drinking that does not seem likely to end soon. Through hazing rituals and wild parties, frequent indulgence begets even more frequent indulgence. Fraternity members (both those who live in a fraternity house and nonresident members) who did not binge in high school often succumb to heavy drinking once they arrive on campus.

Surveys indicate that fraternity and sorority residents are the students who are most likely to consider heavy drinking a campus problem; despite that concern, their parties and antics rage on. Every year local newspapers carry "horror stories" about some of the doings inside the houses. Worst cases may involve racist and misogynistic practices, rituals in which pledges are forced to perform disgusting or self-abasing acts, and brutal clashes between fraternity and nonfraternity students that may result in hospitalization or even death. They all have one thing in common: regular, heavy use of alcohol.

Robert E. Daemmrich—Tony Stone Images

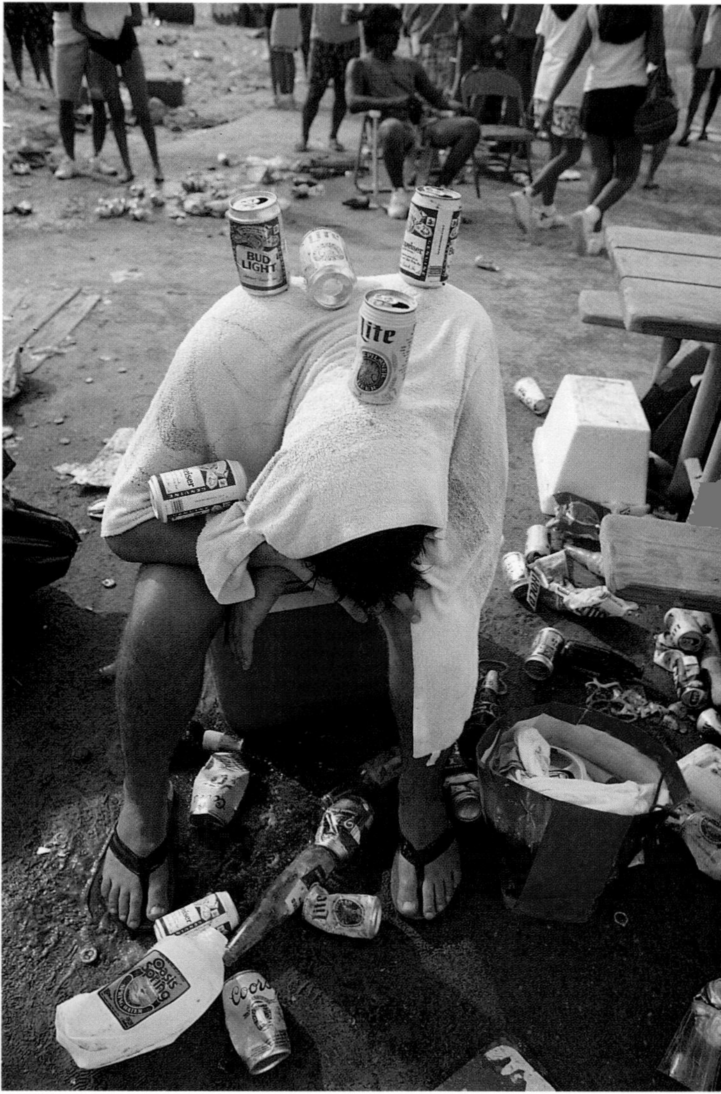

The rather unsavory aftermath of a spring-break bash. Is this what college memories are made of? For too many students the answer may be "yes." Alcohol abusers create problems for themselves and problems for others; most students on today's campuses at one time or another experience the adverse consequences of other students' alcohol binges.

Sports involvement also seems to predict binge drinking. The more involved a student is in sports, the more likely that student is to binge drink. Nearly two-thirds of male students who are seriously involved in competitive college athletics binge drink, whereas fewer than half of male students who are not on an athletic team abuse alcohol. These statistics suggest that even among those whose top concern should be their physical condition, the message—that there are serious health-related consequences of excessive alcohol consumption—apparently has not motivated a change in behavior.

There are two other special groups whose drinking patterns suggest that they are at high risk of becoming full-fledged binge drinkers: women and freshmen. Women are particularly at risk when it comes to college drinking, both as drinkers and as victims of others' drunken behavior. According to recent research, women metabolize ethanol (alcohol) at a slower rate than men and therefore begin experiencing alcohol's effects after fewer drinks. (Those studies took into account lower weights and leaner body masses in women.) When the Harvard survey on binge drinking was done, female students reported having experienced alcohol-related problems (*e.g.,* being hungover, missing a class, getting into an argument, having unplanned or unsafe sex) after fewer drinks than men. This led the authors of the study to modify their definition of binge drinking to be gender specific (four drinks in a row for women, as opposed to five in a row for men); all previous studies had used the same amounts of ethanol consumed for both sexes. With this adjustment, the proportion of females in the Harvard study who met the definition of binge drinker approached but did not equal the proportion of males in that category.

Women's heightened susceptibility to alcohol-induced effects puts them in particular danger. Unaware of the gender differences, women often attempt to drink as much as their male friends—and wind up in some fairly uncomfortable circumstances as a result. Sorority members appear to be at highest risk of all college students (including members of fraternities) for alcohol-related health and behavior problems. Sorority women are less likely than their male counterparts to have been heavy drinkers in high school but are just as likely to begin binge drinking during their first year of college.

Because there is a direct correlation between binge drinking and experiencing secondhand binge effects, women drinkers, again, seem to be at considerable risk. Women students are the most frequent victims of unwanted sexual advances, sexual assault, and date rape. In addition, female students tend to be less willing than male students to recognize their own problem drinking and therefore are probably less likely to seek help when it is truly needed.

The U.S. minimum-drinking-age law, which took effect in 1985, does not seem to deter students under age 21 from consuming alcohol. The best evidence for this is the drinking levels of college freshmen. Eager to fit in, first-year students are often influenced by what they perceive to be the binge-drinking norms of the campus. Typically, there is simply not enough time for freshmen to find their social niche before the beer starts flowing—so they assimilate quickly to the dominant lifestyle. At schools that have high binge-drinking rates, two out of three freshmen binge during their first semester at school, and more than half of them do so within their first week! Why do they start binge drinking even before they have bought their first textbook? Most freshmen students acknowledge that they drank more in their first months away from home than they ever expected to. When asked why, most claim it is "because more drinking goes on here than in high school."

Sober-minded questions

Drinking is a complex behavior that is influenced by many factors. Although not all of these can be pinpointed or controlled, research has helped uncover some factors that can be targeted for change through a combination of policy, education, and consumer choice. Parents have a particularly important role to play. Although the focus here is on the problems associated with college-age drinking, long before the college application process begins, youngsters need to be educated about the adverse effects of alcohol. Parents and teachers should insist on quality programs that begin in the primary grades and continue through high school. Although many become first-time binge drinkers as college freshmen, those who start early—whether in junior high or high school—usually do not give it up once they get to college.

Jon Riley—Tony Stone Images

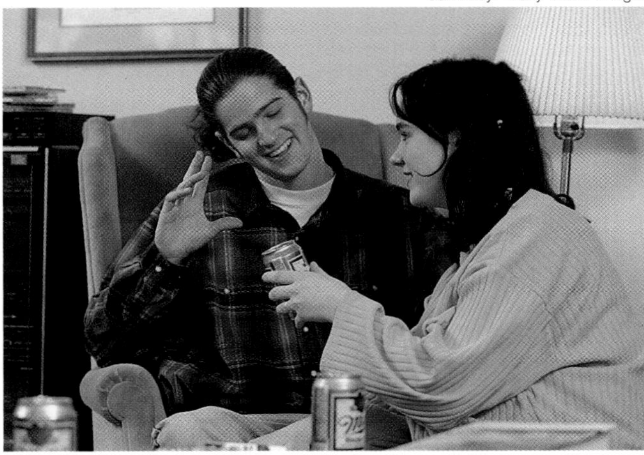

He says, "I'll pass." She says, "Oh, come on." Drinking is a complex behavior influenced by a great many factors. There are clear gender differences in the ability to tolerate alcohol; unfortunately, only after they have paid the consequences do some college women realize that they cannot consume as much alcohol as their male counterparts.

Parents can also play an active role when it comes to choosing the right college. Visiting a college is the best way to learn about the social atmosphere and student life on campus. Some questions that parents and prospective students may want to ascertain the answers to are as follows:

- What kinds of activities are scheduled for weekends?
- Do organized academic programs and extracurricular activities accommodate a diversity of student interests?
- Is alcohol consumption a routine part of weekend activity?
- Are there many abstainers on campus?
- Is alcohol that is sold in the environs cheap? Are $2 pitchers easy to come by? Are kegs allowed on campus?
- How prominent is sorority-fraternity life? Is it supported by the university? How many students are *not* members of sororities and fraternities?
- Who lives in dorms? Underclassmen only? Or do upperclassmen stay on campus, too?
- Is the library open evenings and weekends?
- Does the school spend money on controlling drinking or preventing irresponsible drinking? Does it sponsor liquor-free events?

Confronting campus consumption: a 12-step start

Campus drinking rates vary greatly from one school to another. At some schools as few as 1% of students binge drink, while at others 70% do. Heavy drinking clearly creates a self-perpetuating culture; campuses known for their high drinking rates attract students who were binge drinkers in high school and remain so in college. Unless comprehensive steps are taken involving everyone on campus, including the top administrators, the vicious circle will continue.

It is important for administrators to start prevention programs early—focusing on first-year students. The structure and content of these educational efforts need to be carefully considered and tailored to the individual campus. There are some pertinent questions that must be asked. If participation in substance-abuse-prevention programs is elective, will those at highest risk be reached? Is there much encouragement of students to be *responsible* drinkers? Do programs convey that the university regards binge drinking as a serious problem?

The following 12-step program was designed for campuses with a drinking problem. Though it is aimed at college presidents, deans, and administrators, prospective students and parents can use it to determine the extent to which a college is committed to dealing with its alcohol problems.

1. *Assess the ways in which alcohol is affecting your college.* It is easy to deny alcohol's impact on campus life. Spending time on campus over the weekend is a good way to learn about extracurricular activities. Talk to security guards, or drive around with them to see what they see.
2. *Admit that your college, like most other colleges, has a problem.* The prevalence of binge drinking on most campuses is no secret, and denial is counterproductive.
3. *Show your commitment to substance-abuse prevention.* Meaningful prevention strategies for ensuring students' safety must be reflected in budgets, not just in speeches.
4. *Do not cut corners or think binge drinking can be conquered in a day.* Alcohol abuse has been present on college campuses for centuries; programs to prevent such abuse must be ongoing.
5. *Involve everyone in the solution.* The school's health and security services, obviously, must take part in alcohol-abuse-prevention efforts; coaches, athletic department staff, and other faculty members also need to get involved.
6. *Involve the local community.* Local merchants often supply alcohol to underage students and offer large volumes of alcohol for cut-rate prices. In turn, student drunkenness often disrupts and damages the local community.
7. *Establish the rights of nonbinge-drinking students.* Administrators should support nonbinge drinkers in their activities as actively as they discourage or condemn binge drinkers.
8. Target disruptive behavior for disciplinary action. In concert with students, develop and enforce a code of conduct.

Partying, hazing, and other alcohol-associated antics have long been staples of fraternity (and sorority) life. That distinction of Greek societies, however, may be starting to fade; in 1997 several fraternities across the U.S. announced their intention to go dry. (Below) Industrious and civic-minded sorority sisters and fraternity brothers have taken on a decidedly constructive project: rehabbing a home in a low-income area.

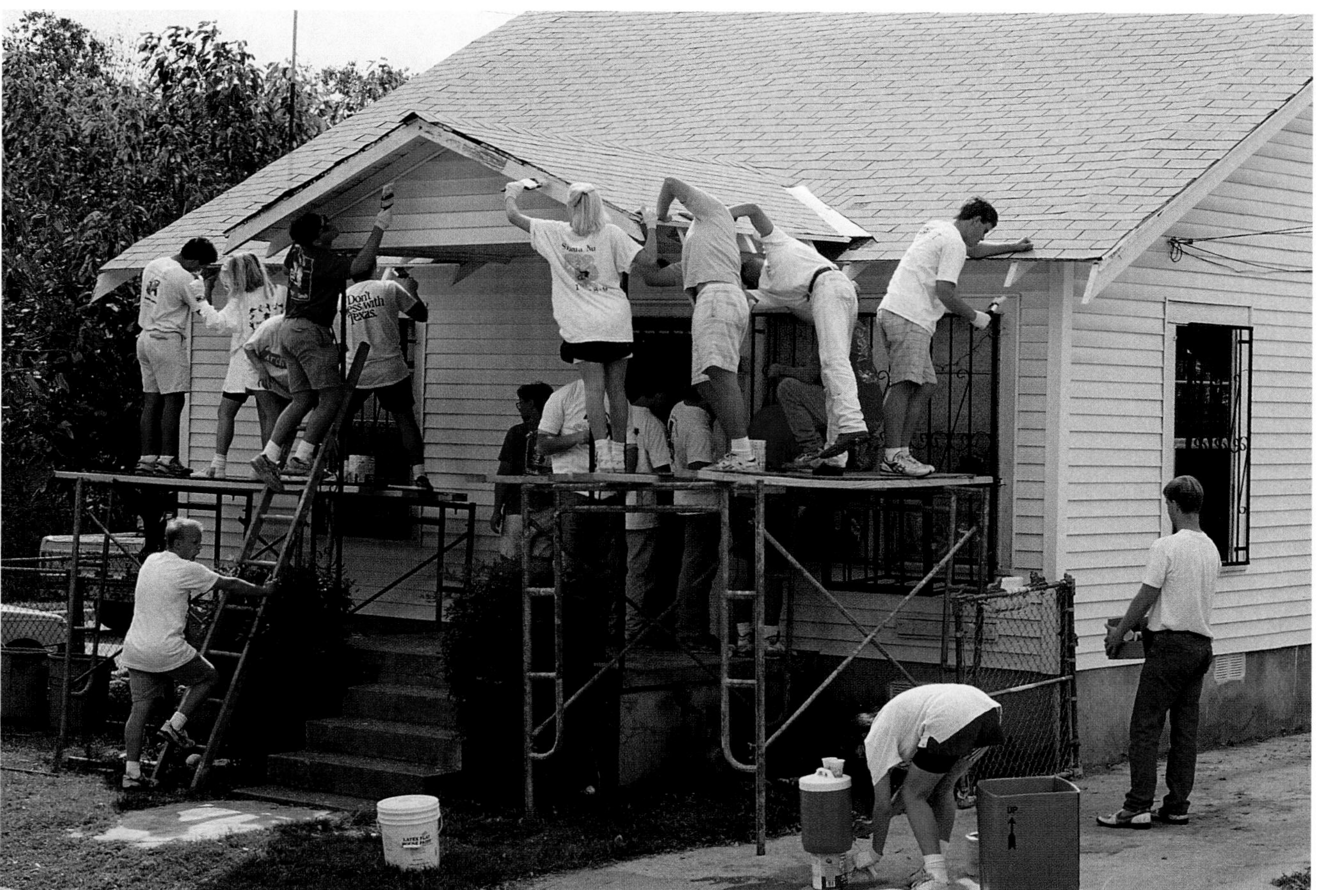

Robert E. Daemmrich—Tony Stone Images

9. *Address the problem-drinking that occurs among fraternities and sororities.* These organizations must be held accountable for serving underage students in their houses and for providing an environment in which frequent binge drinking is not only considered socially acceptable but condoned.
10. *Provide a full-time education for a full-time tuition.* Hold classes on Friday and require attendance. Schedule Friday exams. A college should not act as an enabler for students who choose to binge drink from Thursday through Sunday.
11. *Encourage problem drinkers to seek help or treatment.* Campus health services should be familiar with treatment resources and readily refer students to them.
12. *Start freshman orientation long before other students arrive on campus.* The data show that very few freshmen anticipated getting drunk at all during their freshmen year, but half reported having been drunk in the most recent month. Catch them early! Freshmen will respond positively to initiatives they might later spurn, particularly if the initiatives represent an opportunity to meet their classmates under sober conditions.

Colleges cannot advance their core mission—to provide a safe and stimulating learning and living environment—if they disregard a problem as pervasive as binge drinking. Like other difficult and deeply entrenched social problems, this one will not be solved overnight or with a magic bullet.

—Henry Wechsler, Ph.D., and Charles Deutsch, Sc.D.

Acupuncture in Addiction Treatment

A journalist who was writing a feature article on alternative medicine interviewed the head of an acupuncture clinic, who then suggested he have a demonstration treatment. Two days later the writer returned to the clinic, saying the acupuncturist must have "pushed the wrong button." He elaborated by explaining that he usually enjoyed a few drinks after work, but since his treatment, he had lost interest in drinking. Acupuncture, he claimed, had "ruined his social life."

Acupuncture, a major component of the ancient tradition of Chinese medicine, is currently used in approximately 700 substance-abuse programs in the U.S., Europe, and locations as diverse as Trinidad, Saudi Arabia, and Nepal. Clinical evidence supports this use; acupuncture has been shown to reduce the impact of withdrawal symptoms from alcohol, opiate drugs such as morphine and heroin, and cocaine. It also diminishes the craving associated with some of the most commonly abused substances, including nicotine.

In addiction treatment, acupuncture is a nonverbal, nonthreatening first-step intervention that has an immediate calming effect on clients. As an initial form of substance-abuse therapy, it has been shown to improve patients' overall treatment response.

Acupuncture needles are thin stainless steel shafts inserted under the surface of the skin. Addiction treatment uses locations on the external ear; thus, the needles are inserted very shallowly. Patients may notice a local warmth and tingling in the area around the needles. There may also be an electrical sensation or heaviness felt in other parts of the body. Some patients feel sleepy after initial treatments—a reaction that is normal in the addiction recovery process and generally does not last very long. A few patients develop a brief headache at the end of a treatment session. In rare cases a "needling reaction" occurs, in which the patient feels dizzy and light-headed and may actually faint during treatment or upon getting up afterward—a reaction that is also seen in many medical and dental settings.

Substance-abuse programs use sterile, disposable needles that are discarded in a special container as soon as they are removed. The insertion of acupuncture needles never causes bleeding. About 10% of the time, however, ear treatment sites will bleed *after* the needles are removed. Therefore, standard precautions are taken to ensure that others are not exposed to the client's blood.

"Pointed" action

Acupuncture's demonstrated effectiveness in veterinary medicine is usually cited as proof that it produces more than just a placebo effect. More than a hundred individual acupuncture points have been identified on the human ear alone. These specified points are physiologically distinct—*e.g.,* they are measurably warmer than surrounding tissue by a fraction of a degree. A standard acupuncture textbook summarizes the functions of five main ear points as follows:

- **sympathetic point**—commonly used in the treatment of conditions that involve disruption of the sympathetic and/or parasympathetic nervous systems; its stimulation relieves pain, promotes relaxation of internal organs, and dilates (widens) blood vessels
- ***Shen-men* ("spirit gate") point**—commonly used for treatment of neuropsychiatric disorders; has both sedating and antiallergenic effects
- **lung point**—used for pain relief, control of excess sweating, and treatment of various respiratory conditions
- **liver point**—used in the treatment of hepatitis, anemia, pain syndromes (neuralgia), muscle spasms, and eye diseases
- **kidney point**—aids in the relief of neurasthenia (nervous exhaustion), lassitude, headache, and urogenital problems

A pet cat, suffering from nerve damage after having fallen from a window, is treated with acupuncture. The widely demonstrated effectiveness of acupuncture in veterinary medicine is often cited as evidence that it produces more than simply a placebo effect.

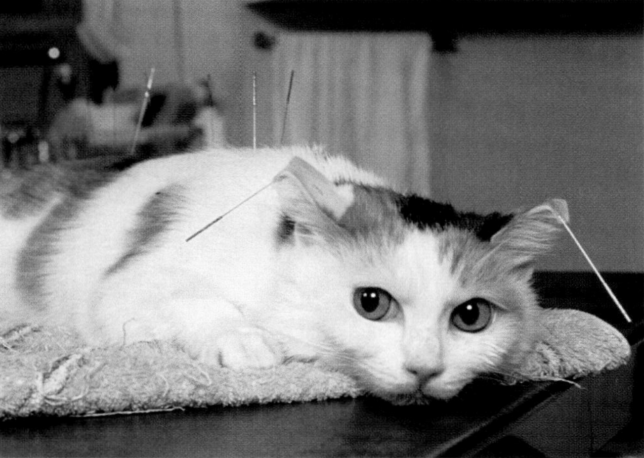

Kaku Kurita—Gamma Liaison

Traditional Chinese theory associates each of the 2,000 identified acupuncture points on the human body with particular external structures, internal organs, and body functions, including emotions. Western medical studies have linked acupuncture to the release of various nervous system chemicals such as endorphins (natural morphinelike substances, or painkillers); ACTH, or adrenocorticotropic hormone (an anti-inflammatory agent); and neurotransmitters like serotonin and norepinephrine that are involved in pain and affect sleep, mood, and appetite.

These theoretical correlations, however, are complex and variable; no single chemical mechanism has been established to explain acupuncture's unique effectiveness. Rather, it appears that acupuncture enhances the integrity of the autonomic nervous system, which activates muscle and glandular tissues and governs the body's involuntary actions. By supporting basic functions such as circulation, wound healing, and various immune and neurological functions, acupuncture promotes homeostasis, the balanced functioning of the "whole person."

In 1973 a Chinese doctor was the first to report successful treatment of addiction withdrawal symptoms with acupuncture. H.L. Wen, a neurosurgeon in Hong Kong, observed that opium addicts who had undergone surgery and received acupuncture for postoperative pain relief experienced few withdrawal symptoms. The patients had been given electroacupuncture (needles connected to a low-voltage alternating current) to the lung point on the external ear. Subsequently, Wen conducted clinical studies that established acupuncture as a valuable treatment for other forms of addiction.

South Bronx protocol

Acupuncture treatment for drug and alcohol problems was primarily developed at Lincoln Hospital (now the Lincoln Medical and Mental Health Center), a New York City-run public facility in the impoverished South Bronx. The substance-abuse division at Lincoln is a state-licensed treatment program that has provided more than 500,000 acupuncture treatments in the past 20 years. Initially, in 1974, the Lincoln Clinic detoxification program used Wen's method, applying a weak electrical stimulation through a fine needle to the lung point on the ear. Patients reported being more relaxed, having fewer opiate withdrawal symptoms, and being able to participate in longer periods of therapy.

It was only accidentally discovered that electrical stimulation was not necessary to produce symptomatic relief. In fact, simple manual needling produced a more prolonged effect. Patients were able to receive acupuncture just once a day and experience suppression of their withdrawal symptoms throughout the day. Such manual needling also was found to reduce craving, especially for alcohol and heroin—an effect that had never been described previously.

Over a period of years, this author and colleagues at the Lincoln Clinic developed the so-called five-point formula, utilizing some combination of the five external ear acupuncture points cited above to treat most substance-abuse disorders. From the traditional Chinese perspective, it makes sense to use such a single basic formula for this broad group of patients, who tend to be both emotionally and physically depleted.

Chinese medicine describes the absence of inner calm that typifies this state of depletion as "empty fire" (*xu huo*), in which the "heat of aggressiveness" is said to burn out of control. It is easy to be confused by the aggressiveness that many addicts exhibit and conclude that the goal of treatment should be to "put out the fire" pharmacologically. In fact, addicts themselves often take this approach when they use highly sedating drugs. The "empty fire" condition, however, represents an illusion of power, an illusion that leads to more desperate chemical abuse and senseless violence. Acupuncture helps to restore patients' inner calm and control.

Lincoln Medical and Mental Health Center; photograph, Mary Linda Morales

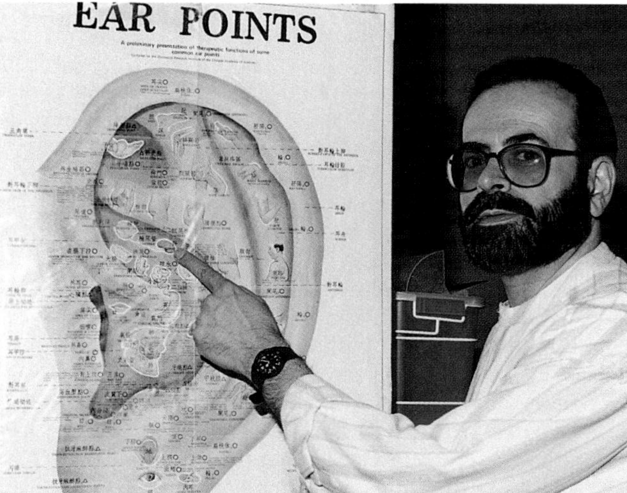

Over 100 distinct acupuncture points have been identified on the human ear. The Lincoln Clinic in New York City has developed a protocol for treating drug addiction that uses needles placed in three to five external ear locations, which Carlos Alvarez, of Lincoln's staff, indicates above.

An example from the Lincoln Clinic program illustrates the treatment of "empty fire." B.K. is a single mother with a long history of impulsive child abuse and drug addiction. She had given birth to four children before the age of 18, never having had a chance to grow and mature herself. When she entered the program, B.K. was extremely jittery and hostile toward her counselor. In the first interview, she talked incessantly about pressures and problems at home. But after just one acupuncture treatment, she reported she was "like a changed person." In her second interview she told her counselor, "My kids said I didn't act the same at all." That interview proved to be much more constructive and detailed than the first. B.K. has continued in treatment, and the Lincoln program staff are very enthusiastic about her new calm and constructive outlook.

Treatment is provided in a large group setting for a duration of about 45 minutes, with each client having needles placed in three to five points per ear. The group setting not only enables many patients to be treated at once; it also enhances acupuncture's effectiveness. Experience has demonstrated that participants in groups of more than six experience greater relaxation and relief from withdrawal symptoms. By contrast, those treated individually or in groups of fewer than six tend to be self-conscious and easily distracted.

The location of ear points and the technique of insertion can be taught effectively in a 70-hour apprenticeship-based program. Typically, clinicians involved in many aspects of substance-abuse treatment learn to administer acupuncture under the general supervision of licensed or certified acupuncturists; this arrangement allows for acupuncture to be integrated with existing medical and psychosocial services in a convenient, flexible, and cost-effective way. Since 1990 more than 2,000 clinicians have been trained to provide acupuncture through the substance-abuse program at the Lincoln Clinic, which works in conjunction with the National Acupuncture Detoxification Association (NADA). One of NADA's missions is to promote the use of the Lincoln model nationwide, as well as to ensure that acupuncture detoxification programs and facilities maintain rigorous standards.

Calm and confident without chemicals

Clients often describe acupuncture as a unique kind of balancing experience: "I was relaxed but alert"; "I was able to relax without losing control." Those who are depressed or tired say that they feel more energetic. Patients respond best when acupuncture treatment is administered quickly, without a lot of discussion, examination, and other preliminaries. The lack of verbal communication and interpersonal action during the administration of acupuncture is especially valuable at a time when the client may be experiencing acute physical withdrawal symptoms (such as aching, headache, nausea, sweating, muscle cramping, and cravings), as well as intense anxiety and/or depression. In conjunction with acupuncture, the Lincoln program uses an herbal formula known as "sleep mix." The formula, drunk as a tea, consists of inexpensive herbs, including peppermint, chamomile, yarrow, skullcap, hops, and catnip, all of which are commonly used in Europe and are said to have calming effects upon the nervous system. This herb mix also stimulates blood circulation and promotes the elimination of waste products and toxins.

One of the striking characteristics of the group acupuncture treatment setting is that each patient seems comfortable in his or her own space; the quiet 45-minute period is conducive to personal reflection and self-assessment. As one patient put it, "I sat and thought about things in a slow way like I did when I was 10 years old." Acupuncture treatment promotes awareness of various relaxing bodily processes. Patients gradually gain confidence that their minds and bodies can function in a more balanced and autonomous manner. After just a few treatments, most substance abusers who receive acupuncture treatment come to realize that the technique works largely by revealing their own internal capabilities—capabilities that they can realize without adding external chemicals.

Consider J.J., a woman who was six months pregnant and addicted to crack cocaine. She showed up one day anxious and nervous at a NADA-run clinic. "I can't tell you much about myself," she told the staff, "because my husband is out in the street with a baseball bat, and he'll hit me in the knees if I say too much." The program provided an emergency acupuncture treatment and conducted a simplified admissions interview. Two weeks later the patient brought her husband in and said, "This is my husband; he doesn't have a drug problem, but he is nervous. Can you help him?" Both of them received acupuncture that day. The woman needed a protective environment in which she was not vulnerable to her husband's physical abuse; he needed a treatment setting in which he did not feel threatened and was not subjected to verbal questioning or challenges. In fact, the whole process was so supportive and calming that the husband was able to begin trusting his wife and encouraging her detoxification.

James Marshall

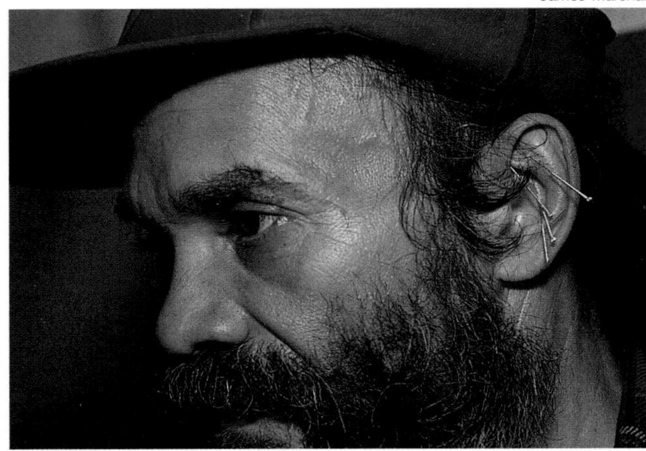

Acupuncture is a nonverbal, nonthreatening first step in substance-abuse treatment. It has an immediate calming effect and has been shown to improve the overall treatment response of most clients. Stainless steel needles are inserted shallowly; the client may notice a local warmth or slight tingling in the general insertion area.

Acupuncture is most often used in conjunction with group rehabilitation programs such as Alcoholics Anonymous and Narcotics Anonymous and provides an excellent foundation for both well-established 12-step recovery programs. Acupuncture and 12-step programs have much in common. Participation in both is independent of diagnosis and level of recovery. Both have a "one-day-at-a-time" philosophy. In both components of treatment, participants draw on the collective strength of the group and gain comfort and inspiration from others who are managing their recovery well. Both approaches are simple, reinforcing, nurturing, and convenient, and both emphasize self-responsibility in the recovery process.

Clinical outcomes

A number of controlled studies have been conducted on human subjects, using various modified versions of the Lincoln Clinic protocol. In 1987 a placebo-controlled study by Milton Bullock and colleagues in Minneapolis, Minn., assessed the value of acupuncture as a treatment for alcoholism. Fifty-four chronic alcohol abusers were randomly assigned to receive acupuncture either at points specifically related to addiction or at nearby locations not specifically related to addiction (placebo sites). Subjects were treated in an inpatient setting but were free to leave the program each day. The study showed that those in the former group had higher rates of attendance of counseling and other psychosocial elements of treatment, less self-reported need for alcohol, diminished desire to drink, and fewer actual drinking episodes. Two years later the same group of investigators replicated their study, using a larger sample (80 subjects) over a longer follow-up period (six months). Of 40 alcohol abusers in the treatment group (receiving acupuncture to specific ear sites), 21 completed the treatment, whereas only one of 40 controls stayed enrolled during the full protocol.

The investigators concluded: "We believe that our results are encouraging enough for other research groups to validate the efficacy of acupuncture in the treatment of various subsets of the alcoholic population." Acupuncture intervention can reduce craving for alcohol in poorly motivated individuals and, as the previously mentioned example of the journalist suggests, even in those who may not be motivated to give up the substance at all.

Acupuncture has been recognized as a particularly important innovation in the treatment of addictions to cocaine and crack cocaine, for which there are presently no effective pharmaceutical therapies. The Lincoln Clinic acupuncture-based program is the largest outpatient program for crack cocaine patients in the world, with some 400 patients attending the program on a regular basis. About 60% of new crack-dependent patients give a series of clean urine tests within several weeks of entering treatment; more than 65% complete the first three months of treatment.

Amphetamine abusers experience similar dramatic improvement. A detoxification facility in Portland, Ore., reported that prior to the incorporation of acupuncture into its treatment protocol, only 5% of amphetamine users continued in treatment, whereas 90% stayed on in the program after acupuncture was introduced.

Marijuana abuse has also been curbed with acupuncture treatment. Primary marijuana abusers experience a prompt reduction in their craving for pot; they also report improved mental well-being.

Heroin-withdrawal symptoms are reduced by acupuncture. Treatments may be given up to three times a day to inpatients or once daily to outpatients, during which time they taper their use of drugs. Acupuncture is often used with pharmaceutical agents such as methadone for this purpose.

Lincoln Medical and Mental Health Center; photograph, Mary Linda Morales

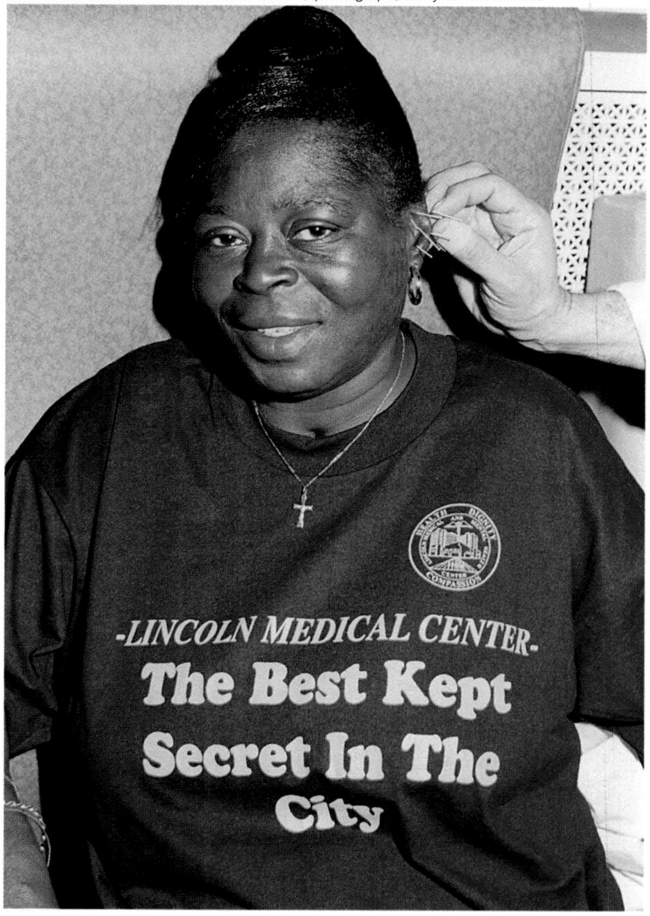

About 250 substance abusers a day are treated in the Lincoln Clinic's acupuncture detox program. Clients report relief from withdrawal symptoms, less craving, clearer thinking, and decreased anxiety. A special program addresses the needs of addicted women and mothers.

Methadone-maintenance patients receive acupuncture in various settings. Methadone is a potent synthetic narcotic that is effective for treating addiction to heroin and other narcotics. It suppresses withdrawal symptoms, causes no euphoria, and enables recovering addicts to lead relatively normal, productive lives. But it is also an addictive drug. Acupuncture seems to reduce secondary symptoms of methadone use (*e.g.,* sweating, constipation, and sleep problems) and is especially valuable during the progression from methadone to abstinence.

The Lincoln Clinic has established the Maternal Substance Abuse Acupuncture Services for pregnant women who are crack-cocaine-dependent or addicted to other drugs. These women need a drug-free form of treatment, as well as one that addresses their other prenatal needs. Notably, 90% of women in the Lincoln program are drug-free at the time of delivery. Moreover, those women who abstain from drugs for most of their pregnancy deliver babies of average weights. By contrast, women who abuse drugs throughout gestation are at high risk of having low-birth-weight babies, who generally begin life with many developmental difficulties and health risks.

Female patients are often trapped in destructive and exploitative relationships; the Lincoln program encourages them to become drug-free not solely for the sake of the baby. This emphasis on recognizing their own self-worth is vital to the program's success and is well aided by the reflective daily group acupuncture sessions.

Nicotine addiction

In office-based practices and many other outpatient settings, acupuncture is frequently used to treat nicotine addiction. Usually a "press needle" is placed in the lung point on both ears. Press needles are shaped like a thumb tack so that patients can manipulate them gently three minutes at a time, three times a day. The needles are left in place for a week or two, and treatment continues over a period of one to two months.

Treatment of heavy smokers often produces dramatic results. The effect is not immediate, however, so patients will continue to smoke after the insertion of the needles. At the beginning of treatment, their skepticism is usually quite evident; about 4–10 hours after the insertion of the needles, however, clients experience a sudden aversion to smoking. Typically, they will put out a cigarette just after lighting it. At this time they have no withdrawal symptoms; they simply feel no desire to smoke—an effect lasting as long as the needles are in place. Whether they can continue their abstinence after the treatment period ends depends on their motivation and willpower. The primary advantage of acupuncture in quitting smoking is that it encourages a rapid reduction in nicotine use, which most habituated smokers can easily tolerate in the early stage of treatment and which in turn often enhances the course of the entire treatment process.

"Street sobriety"

One of the most serious problems affecting society today is substance abuse. Substance abuse is linked to many other societal ills. High rates of addiction are directly or indirectly associated with high crime rates and high rates of illness and injury. In many communities today drug abuse is so rampant that it threatens to overwhelm the limited resources that are available to deal with it. Acupuncture, in this light, offers a compassionate, convenient, and cost-effective foundation for psychosocial rehabilitation.

NEWS CAP MHA 98

Ashes to Ashes: Tobacco and Health Update

Two major developments in 1997 signaled what may be the beginning of the end for the U.S. tobacco industry. On April 25, more than three decades after the first surgeon general's report on the lethal effects of smoking, a federal judge in Greensboro, N.C., ruled that the Food and Drug Administration (FDA) had the authority to regulate the conditions of sale and the labeling of cigarettes. Although the rights of tobacco companies to advertise their products were protected, most opponents of tobacco applauded the ruling.

More controversial was the agreement reached in June between several tobacco giants—RJR Nabisco, Philip Morris, Brown & Williamson, and Lorillard—and their legal opponents in dozens of liability lawsuits. In exchange for an annual $5 billion cap on payments for past wrongdoing and immunity from future class-action suits against them, the companies agreed, among other concessions, to pay $368.5 billion in damages to claimants over the next 25 years and to scrap ads featuring such recognizable characters as Joe Camel and the Marlboro Man. Many health experts, however, among them former surgeon general C. Everett Koop and former FDA commissioner David A. Kessler, felt that the penalties against the companies were not severe enough and urged Congress to develop a national policy to fight tobacco addiction.

Overshadowed somewhat by the controversy surrounding the tobacco industry were a number of published studies that accumulated new evidence of the medical dangers of smoking. These studies either found or confirmed that:

- For nonsmokers, regular exposure to the cigarette smoke of others nearly doubles the risk of heart disease. As many as 50,000 people in the U.S. die of heart attacks every year as a result of secondhand smoke.
- Women who smoke during pregnancy give birth to babies with nicotine levels in their bodies as high as those seen in adult smokers. These newborns most likely spend their first few days of life suffering nicotine withdrawal.
- Lung development in teenage smokers is impaired even if tobacco consumption is as low as five cigarettes per day. Adolescent girls, who are now taking up smoking at a faster rate than boys, are at a greater risk than boys for lung damage from smoking. Each day an estimated 3,000 teens in the U.S. begin to smoke.
- The risk of age-related macular degeneration, the leading cause of severe visual impairment among elderly Americans, is more than doubled by the use of tobacco. Macular degeneration (the deterioration of the center of the retina), a condition for which medical treatment is effective in only a small percentage of patients, joins a growing list of serious smoking-related diseases.
- Each year thousands of young children suffer nicotine poisoning after swallowing cigarettes or cigarette butts. Such ingestions often result in vomiting, nausea, convulsions, slowed respiration, and abnormal heart rhythms.
- Although the health risks from smoking cigars are less than those from smoking cigarettes, cigar smokers are at a much higher risk than nonsmokers of developing lung, mouth, and throat cancers. Cigar sales nevertheless have risen dramatically in recent years as the fad for stogie smoking has caught fire in the U.S. Because it is not customary for cigar smokers to inhale, many of them erroneously believe that cigars are not addictive. Nicotine from cigars is, in fact, easily absorbed through the mucous membranes of the mouth.

Innovative approaches to publicizing the medical dangers of tobacco use and promoting a smoke-free environment were undertaken by several organizations in 1997. The American Medical Association (AMA) launched an ad campaign featuring a Superman-like cartoon hero—the Extinguisher—who appeared on television shows and in person at Discovery Zone stores to educate children about the dangers of smoking. One humor magazine, *The Annals of Improbable Research,* awarded an "Ig-Nobel Prize" for medicine to five tobacco company scientists—one posthumously—who had concluded that "nicotine is not addictive." Among other groups, the American Cancer Society ran satiric ads attacking the glamorous image of cigar smoking.

Outside the U.S. there were also numerous efforts to light into the problem of lighting up. The Geneva-based World Health Organi-

Once this foundation has been established and the drug abuser's fears are reduced, the focus of treatment can shift away from relieving unpleasant withdrawal symptoms to overcoming dependence on chemical substances and taking steps toward long-term social and emotional recovery. The ultimate aim of any addiction treatment is for participants to achieve "street sobriety." That means that those who were once hooked on harmful substances are able to adopt a healthy, productive, *drug-free* lifestyle—despite the continuing presence of drugs in their environment.

—Michael O. Smith, M.D.

zation sponsored a "World No-Tobacco Day" on May 31, issuing press releases, fact sheets, a poster, and an advisory kit on measures to reduce tobacco use. The Goethe Endowment for Nonsmoking, established by a German physician, presented the Goethe Challenge Trophy to the AMA for its hard-hitting antismoking efforts; the trophy commemorates the German poet Johann Wolfgang von Goethe (1749–1832), who was among the first to describe the health risks associated with second-hand smoke. In an improbable development during the Peruvian hostage crisis (Dec. 17, 1996–April 22, 1997), nonsmoking hostages insisted on establishing smoke-free areas in the Japanese ambassador's residence in Lima, where they were being held captive by leftist Túpac Amaru guerrillas. In Israel government officials initiated a $5.7 billion lawsuit against cigarette manufacturers, making Israel the only country other than the U.S. to have sued tobacco companies.

Whether health warnings about smoking or the backlash against the tobacco industry will be able to significantly decrease the numbers of smokers worldwide remains to be seen. Demand for cigarettes continues to run high in countries such as France, China, and Vietnam.

Sadly and ironically, shortly before the death on January 15 of Oscar Auerbach, the pathologist who first linked smoking to cancer, experts projected that more than five million people in the U.S. now under 18 will die prematurely from smoking-related diseases.

—Katherine I. Gordon

Jack Higgins—Chicago Sun-Times

OBITUARIES

Joe Camel, 45; Cigarett

Joseph S. "Smokin' Joe" Camel died yesterday. He was 45 (9 human years). Only recently doctors discovered the two lumps on his back were malignant and inoperable.

In effect, walking a mile, for this camel, was no longer possible.

He leaves no Known survivors.

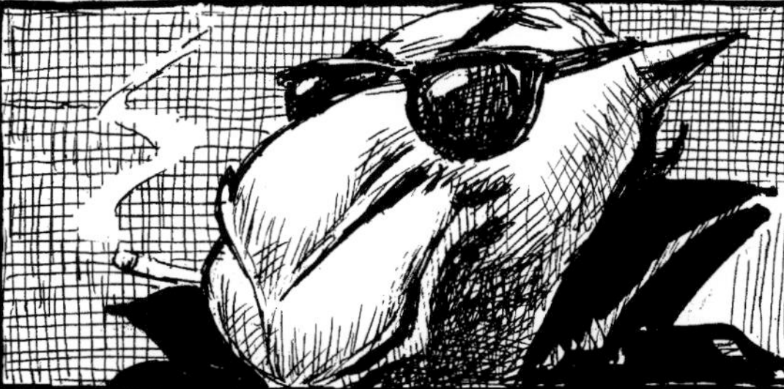

Cigarette "Smokesman."

In lieu of flowers, contributions to the American Cancer Society (No cigarette coupons please). His ashes will be scattered at a nearby playlot.

Cutting-Edge Heart Surgeries

Recent advances in technology have enabled heart surgeons to develop revolutionary new procedures and greatly improve existing ones. Using a laser, surgeons can pierce tiny holes in the heart muscle, a technique called transmyocardial laser revascularization, which relieves chest pain due to inadequate blood flow through the coronary arteries (the vessels that supply blood to the heart muscle). Minimally invasive techniques for bypassing blocked coronary arteries and replacing defective heart valves are being tested and refined, with the hope that they may eventually replace conventional techniques that not only are more costly but also require a longer convalescence and carry higher risks of complications. This report reviews five innovative surgical procedures that have evolved in the past few years. Although the results to date appear promising, it should be noted that the data are still preliminary. More experience will be needed before surgeons can develop specific guidelines for the use of these new procedures and determine which patients are likely to benefit most.

Bypass versus angioplasty: continuing debate

The introduction of the heart-lung machine in the 1950s revolutionized the field of cardiac surgery. By rechanneling blood flow and allowing oxygenation to occur outside the body (rather than, as normally, in the lungs), the heart-lung machine made it possible for surgeons to work in a "bloodless" field. With the heart stopped and blood flow diverted, they could perform procedures such as coronary artery bypass graft, or CABG (a common treatment for patients with narrowing of the coronary arteries), with much greater accuracy than was possible when they worked on an organ in constant motion.

Conventional CABG (surgeons generally pronounce the acronym "cabbage") surgery requires that the surgeon open the patient's chest with a 30-cm (12-in)-long incision and, using a saw, divide the sternum (breastbone) in two to gain access to the heart. The cutting of the sternum is one of the most traumatic aspects of open-heart surgery; it is a source of postoperative pain, may entail a lengthy recuperation, and can be associated with other complications, including infection. Even use of the heart-lung machine has disadvantages, including the possibility of an allergic reaction to the tubing used to rechannel the blood and the risk of postoperative complications such as arrhythmia (disordered heart rhythm) and lung and neurological problems. Because of these drawbacks and because of the high costs of bypass surgery, medical scientists have long sought alternative methods for opening blocked arteries.

One such technique, developed in the 1970s, is a nonsurgical procedure called percutaneous transluminal coronary angioplasty, or balloon angioplasty (or, simply, angioplasty). The procedure involves widening the lumen (the interior hollow portion) of the artery at one or more points. This is accomplished by introducing a catheter, or tube, into the artery and guiding it to the site where a fatty deposit in the arterial wall is interfering with blood flow. Once the tube is in place, a balloonlike device at its tip is inflated, compressing the fatty material, reopening the lumen of the artery, and reestablishing patency of the artery (*i.e.,* its capacity for normal blood flow).

The relative merits of balloon angioplasty and CABG have been debated for several years. Angioplasty's proponents cite the procedure's lower cost and shorter recuperation period compared with bypass surgery. Supporters of CABG note the higher rate of repeat blockage associated with angioplasty and the more frequent need for additional angioplasties within the first three months after the procedure. A surgical procedure that would combine the better long-term results of CABG with the advantageous decrease in both recovery time and hospital stay of angioplasty would be ideal. For selected patients this compromise may be found in so-called mini-CABG surgery.

"Mini-CABG": way of the future?

In the mini-CABG procedure, the surgeon gains access to the heart through a relatively small (4–12-cm [about 1½–4½-in]) incision. The sternum need not be divided, and the heart-lung machine is not used. Mini-CABG was first described in 1967. Today it is in limited use in carefully selected patients. Although eliminating the use of the heart-lung machine avoids some postoperative complications, the mini-CABG procedure too has its drawbacks. The smaller incision is more technically demanding, and it takes some time for the surgical team to learn and master the procedure. Fewer patients are eligible, and the results are less consistent than those of conventional bypass surgery.

Patients with narrowing of only one of the coronary vessels currently represent the largest group of candidates for mini-CABG surgery, particularly patients whose disease is limited to the left coronary artery. (The left and right coronary arteries arise from the aorta; the left coronary artery immediately divides into two main branches. Smaller subsidiary arteries branch from these three large vessels.) Typical candidates fall into two groups. One consists of patients with coronary artery disease involving the left coronary artery system but whose right coronary arteries either are undiseased or, despite being narrowed, are not amenable to surgical treatment. The second category includes patients who have narrowing or complete obstruction of the right coronary artery that cannot be treated by angioplasty. Another good candidate would be a patient who has coexisting health problems that would contraindicate use of the heart-lung machine. Patients are generally not considered eligible for mini-CABG if it appears that they will eventually require surgery with the heart-lung machine because of additional heart disease or if more than three of their coronary arteries are diseased.

In the mini-CABG procedure, the incision is made over the left fifth rib. The left internal mammary artery, which receives its blood supply from the aorta, is the vessel most commonly used in single-vessel coronary artery bypass. To locate this artery, some surgeons use a small fiber-optic camera inserted between the fifth and sixth ribs and directed toward the underside of the sternum. The heart is exposed through an incision in the pericardium, the membranous sac that surrounds it. The internal mammary artery is removed from the interior of the chest wall and connected to the coronary artery beyond the point of narrowing. The incisions are then closed after the surgeon has confirmed the final position of the graft. When the target lesion (*i.e.,* the fatty deposit) is in the right coronary artery, the incision is made on the right side of the chest, and the same steps are followed. Some surgeons have reported using a T-shaped graft for lesions in two vessels, pro-

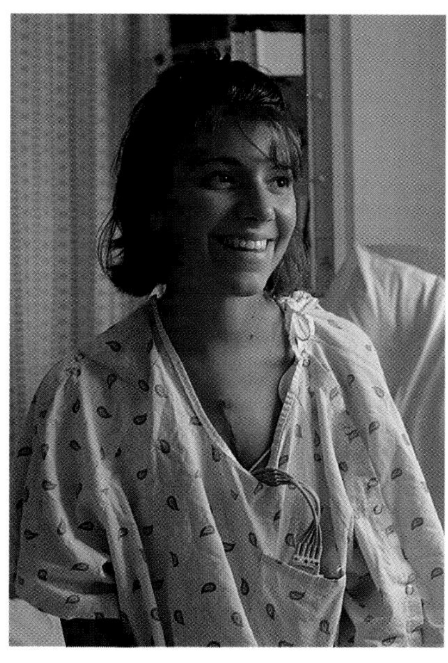

Larry Hamel-Lambert for U.S. News & World Report

Three days after minimally invasive surgery to repair a defective mitral valve, this recent Ohio State University graduate does not even need a bandage to cover the 7.6-cm (3-in)-long incision in her chest.

viding both can easily be reached through the limited chest incision. In this procedure the internal mammary artery is further connected to a simultaneously removed segment of an artery from either the arm or the stomach.

The results from initial trials of mini-CABG surgery in selected patients with single coronary artery disease have been promising. The percentage of grafts remaining open during the first several months after surgery is comparable to that of conventional CABG surgery in similar groups of patients. At present, mini-CABG surgery is limited to patients who have certain characteristics of coronary anatomy and certain types of artery narrowing. Clearly, a full-scale evaluation of mini-CABG surgery comparing it with conventional CABG is required before guidelines for its use can be developed. As experience with mini-CABG surgery grows, it will undoubtedly be applied to patients with a wider variety of coronary problems.

Mini-CABG procedures cost an average of 30% less than conventional CABG surgery. As noted above, however, the new procedure requires extensive training and much practice. As Stephen Westaby, at the Oxford Heart Centre, John Radcliffe Hospital, wryly observed in a 1995 editorial in the *British Heart Journal,* "A certain degree of surgical skill is needed to suture a 1.5 mm mammary artery to a moving target of 2 mm in diameter."

Port-access surgery

To avoid the problem of the "moving target," some investigators have been experimenting with valvular and bypass surgery using minimally invasive techniques similar to those of the mini-CABG but using the heart-lung machine. Surgeons at Stanford University and New York University have described a minimally invasive technique for both establishing heart-lung bypass and preserving the heart muscle while the heart is stopped. Heart-lung bypass is established via the femoral artery and vein in the thigh. A balloon-tipped catheter is then used to block the flow of blood out of the heart, and a preservation solution is infused into the heart via the coronary vessels. This method was shown to preserve heart function comparably to conventional approaches, in which access to the arterial system is obtained via the aorta and access to the venous system via the right-sided chambers of the heart. Infusion of preservation solution in this method requires that a clamp be used to compress (and occlude) the aorta.

Mario Pompili and his colleagues at Stanford have combined these techniques with a small "window" incision, or port, enabling them to gain access to the heart in a fashion similar to the mini-CABG procedure described above. Using custom-made instruments and a fiber-optic video camera to help them see inside the chest cavity, they replaced the mitral valve in 15 healthy dogs. (The mitral valve is a unidirectional heart valve that controls blood flow from the left atrium to the ventricle.) All of the animals survived with no impairment in overall heart function.

To date, approximately 240 people worldwide have had heart surgery using the port-access system. Results at this point must be viewed as preliminary. The procedure may not be appropriate for some patients, such as those with hardening of the aorta and extensive atherosclerosis (accumulation of fatty deposits in the arteries), in whom the manipulation of the balloon-tipped catheter could be dangerous. Likewise, surgeons must currently rule out patients whose femoral artery is too small or diseased to allow use of a femoral catheter (which is needed to transport oxygenated

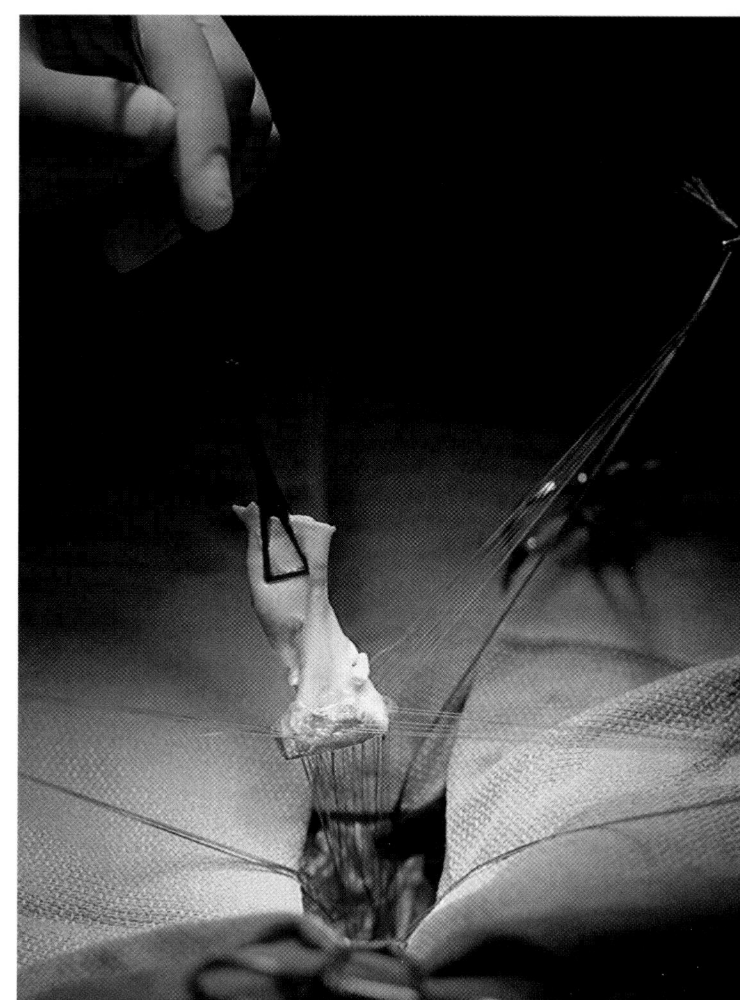

A replacement heart valve is sutured into place in a port-access procedure. During the operation the patient's blood circulation is maintained by the heart-lung machine, with access through the femoral vessels in the thigh.

Jeffrey Macmillan for U.S. News & World Report

blood from the heart-lung machine). The results of clinical trials, expected to be published in 1998, will be influential in establishing criteria for the selection of candidates for port-access surgery.

Transmyocardial laser revascularization

Patients with chest pain may be treated with various conventional therapies, either medical or surgical. In some cases, however, the coronary vessels are so narrowed by disease that surgical bypass procedures are not feasible. Such patients may have severe, intractable chest pain due to restricted blood supply to the heart muscle and may be unable to get relief from medication. Transmyocardial laser revascularization (TMR or, sometimes, TMLR) is a new procedure under investigation for treating patients with chest pain that cannot be alleviated by conventional therapies.

In TMR the surgeon uses a laser to bore numerous small channels in the heart muscle. In theory, this allows increased blood flow to these areas. While these channels were initially thought to mimic the blood circulation of reptilian hearts (in which such channels exist naturally), the true mechanism by which TMR ameliorates intractable chest pain remains unclear. Since its initial evaluation nearly 35 years ago, the procedure—as well as the normal physiology of the reptilian heart—has been the subject of substantial research. Artificial channels have been created in the hearts of experimental animals by the insertion of acupuncture needles, the implantation of tubes, and the insertion of segments of vein.

Current studies suggest that destruction of tissue by the laser may stimulate the growth of new blood vessels, which provides increased blood supply to the heart muscle and thus relieves chest pain. Another theory is that pain relief results from the destruction by the laser of pain nerve fibers in the heart muscle.

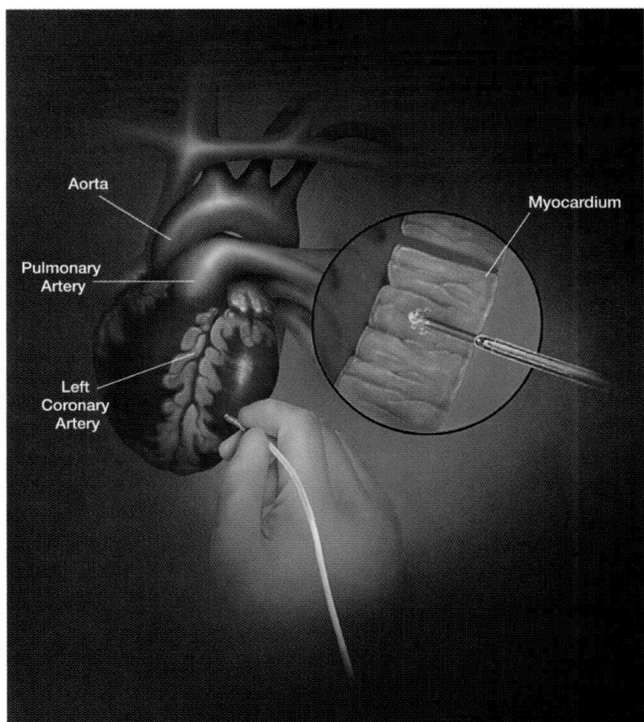

Early TMR procedures used a carbon dioxide laser and approached the heart from the exterior. Recently, at many institutions, a different type of laser, the holmium:YAG laser, has been used, penetrating the heart tissue from the outside or inserted into the heart to create channels from the inside out. The laser energy from the holmium:YAG laser allows for slow healing and delayed scar formation, which help to keep the channels open. The carbon dioxide laser, however, may produce less heat and thus cause less overall tissue injury.

TMR has had varying results in experimental animals. Some investigators have observed increased blood flow and improved heart muscle function after TMR. Others have reported a relatively high rate of reclosure of the channels. Early clinical experience with humans has been promising, however; a substantial number of patients have experienced reduced chest pain and overall improvement in heart blood flow.

In a recent national multicenter trial involving 200 patients, TMR produced a reduction in chest pain, improvement in cardiac blood flow, and a decrease in the number of postprocedure hospital admissions. These initial findings are encouraging. It remains to be demonstrated, however, whether this therapy will be effective in patients who have had a prior heart attack affecting the front wall of the heart (the most critical area) and in those with severe congestive heart failure. As with other recent surgical advances, the patient population for whom this procedure is most effective has yet to be fully established.

Assistance for the failing heart

Cardiac transplantation has been remarkably successful as a therapy for congestive heart failure. Nearly 85% of patients are alive one year after transplantation, and nearly 65% survive for five years. When compared with the two-year survival rate of 20–30% for patients managed medically (*i.e.,* treated with medication) for severely debilitating heart failure, transplantation clearly represents the best therapy for end-stage heart disease. Because of the current shortage of donor organs, however, cardiac transplantation provides effective therapy for only about 2,000 U.S. patients per year. As a consequence, 20–30% of all those awaiting heart transplants die before they can receive a suitable donor organ. Increasing demand has prompted an effort to develop alternatives to transplantation. One of the most successful of these has been the left ventricular assist device (LVAD).

LVADs are pumping devices that are connected to the patient's left ventricle (providing inflow of blood) and aorta (outflow). By augmenting the flow of blood through the left side of the heart, LVADs support the circulation and increase blood flow to the other vital organs of the body. The LVAD is implanted in a "pocket" created under the skin of the abdomen and is powered by either a small electric generator (the size of a "fanny" pack) or a pneumatic air-driven pump (the size of a small shopping cart). The LVAD can be adjusted to beat either in or out of synchrony with the patient's normal heartbeat. LVADs are currently indicated for patients with profound congestive heart failure

In the procedure known as transmyocardial laser revascularization, the surgeon uses a laser to bore numerous small channels in the heart muscle. The technique shows promise for relieving chest pain and improving blood flow to the heart muscle.

Courtesy of CardioGenesis Corporation, Sunnyvale, Calif.

who are also candidates for LVAD therapy as an intermediate step, or "bridge," to transplantation and (1) whose heart conditions may be worsening in the intensive care unit despite maximal medical therapy, or (2) who are unable to be weaned from the heart-lung machine following open-heart surgery.

Recipients of these devices have shown measurable improvement in heart function and ability to carry out their normal daily activities—both of which translate into overall improvement in the functioning of other vital organs. As a result of being generally in better physical condition than patients without LVADs, recipients are better candidates for heart transplants. Paradoxically, the availability of LVADs has prolonged the waiting time to transplantation for patients who are not LVAD recipients by saving some percentage of those who otherwise would have died while awaiting a suitable organ.

Now, however, trials are under way using LVADs as a so-called destination therapy rather than as a "bridge" to transplantation. The fact that short-term LVAD support has been shown to improve overall physiological functioning suggests that long-term LVAD use may slow the progression of congestive heart failure. On the basis of these promising results, the Randomized Evaluation of Mechanical Assistance Therapy as an Alternative in Congestive Heart Failure, or REMATCH, trial began in 1996 to compare medical therapy with LVAD support. To be eligible to participate in REMATCH, patients must be ineligible for cardiac transplantation. Most of those in the study are over 65, which automatically eliminates them from consideration as transplant recipients. The early success with LVADs has already led to wider use, and it seems certain that these devices will become increasingly common worldwide during the next decade.

The "Batista" procedure

The ventricular remodeling technique called the Batista procedure—after its developer, Brazilian surgeon Randas J.V. Batista—is an operation for the treatment of some kinds of end-stage heart failure. Championed for more than 15 years by its originator, the operation has only recently begun to receive serious consideration.

The Batista procedure contradicts conventional medical wisdom in that it consists of removing living tissue from the heart. Candidates for the procedure are people whose hearts have become so enlarged that they are distended (stretched out) and have lost the ability to pump effectively. The operation consists of the removal of a piece of tissue from the left ventricle (*see* diagram). The opening is then eliminated by suturing the two edges together. The net result is that the size of the heart is reduced, which has the effect of restoring some of the lost contractile function. Patients with this particular kind of end-stage heart failure often have poorly functioning mitral valves as well. Surgeons performing the Batista procedure can surgically strengthen the mitral valve at the same time.

Since 1994 Batista has operated on more than 300 patients in southern Brazil. The surgery, often performed in only rudimentary medical facilities, has been relatively successful. Scientific evaluation of the results is somewhat difficult, however, owing to the lack of data regarding the stage of disease of each patient and his or her postoperative course. Batista has reported a relatively high mortality rate, which some critics attribute to poor patient selection and others to the inherent risks of the procedure itself.

Another Brazilian surgical team reported their experience with 13 patients in whom force of contraction of the left ventricle was improved and ventricular diameter reduced. They also reported a 60-day survival rate of 83%. Their report of four patients who developed postoperative arrhythmia prompted U.S. surgeons to add antiarrhythmia medications to the routine postoperative care of such patients.

Surgeons in Japan have reported performing the Batista procedure in 24 patients; their results showed an improvement in the pumping function of the left ventricle throughout the reported 4½-month follow-up period. Patrick McCarthy and colleagues at the Cleveland (Ohio) Clinic Foundation have reported the outcomes in 53 patients who underwent the Batista procedure. Approximately 98% of the patients were still alive six months after surgery. Like the surgical teams mentioned above, they too reported an overall improvement in ventricular function and reduction in ventricular size. Ninety-one percent of their patients were able to be removed from the transplantation waiting list. Ultimately, however, 12 patients required relisting for transplantation; 9 developed worsening heart failure after the surgery and required implantation of an LVAD; and 3 experienced relapsing heart failure early after surgery.

Because of the substantial percentage of patients who require LVAD insertion or transplantation following the Batista operation, the Society of Thoracic Surgeons in the U.S. has recently suggested that only medical centers with LVAD implantation and heart transplantation capabilities be allowed to perform the operation in its current form. There is general consensus worldwide

The Batista Procedure

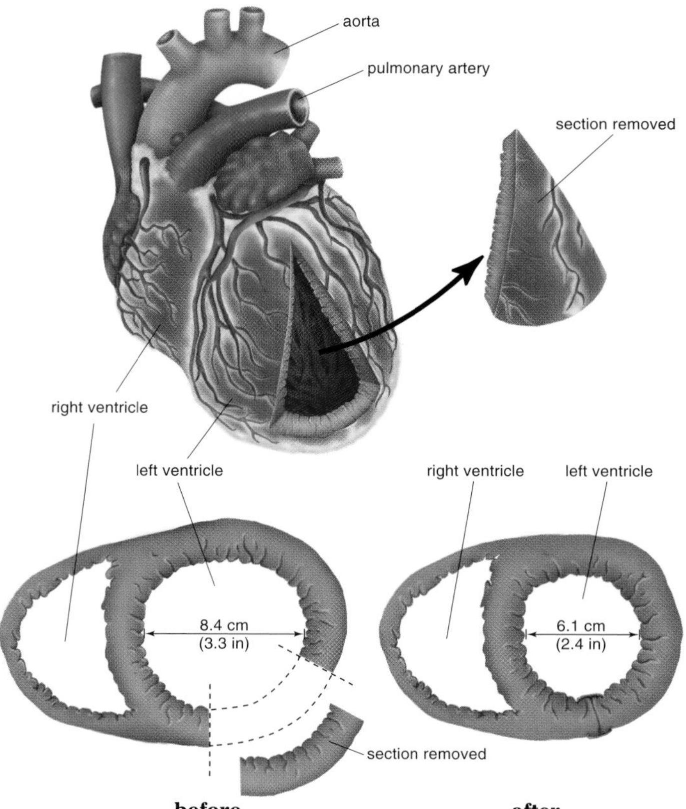

A diagram shows the ventricular remodeling technique known as the Batista procedure, in which removal of a piece of tissue from the left ventricle effectively reduces the size of the distended failing heart.

Adapted from information obtained from Patrick McCarthy, Cleveland Clinic Foundation that a registry should be created of patients undergoing the Batista operation to expedite evaluation of this intriguing—and incompletely understood—new surgery.

At the frontier

The five innovative procedures described above represent the "cutting edge" of cardiac surgery. Their recent successes in clinical trials approved by the U.S. Food and Drug Administration follow many years of animal research. While a number of potential complications have been anticipated, it is impossible for medical scientists to predict all the risks related to these procedures. Thus, the long-term success of these exciting new techniques depends on increased sophistication preoperatively (careful patient selection), intraoperatively (improved surgical techniques and increased experience with the procedures), and postoperatively (development of excellent methods of medical management).

—Robert E. Michler, M.D., and Jonathan M. Chen, M.D.

NEWS CAP MHA 98

Glimmer of Hope for Old Eyes

On Jan. 29, 1997, a team of doctors from the University of Chicago Medical Center transplanted fetal retinal pigment epithelial cells into the left eye of an 80-year-old volunteer, Pearl Van Vliet, who was suffering from age-related macular degeneration, a common and debilitating eye disease. The six-person surgical team, led by ophthalmologist J. Terry Ernest and retinal surgeon Samir Patel, inserted a one-millimeter (0.039-in) microsphere containing about 250,000 cells under the patient's retina during a novel two-hour operation. The researchers chose fetal cells because they grow rapidly and are less likely than mature cells to provoke an immune response. The fetal cells, collected after a medically necessary second-trimester abortion, were grown and formed into tiny microspheres in the laboratory.

During extensive studies in animals, this approach led to vigorous growth of fetal cells both in test tubes and after their insertion under the retinas of living animals. Because there is no animal model for macular degeneration, the only true way to assess the procedure's clinical value was to conduct human trials. The surgery on Van Vliet was the first in the U.S.; four more patients were scheduled to undergo the same operation by the same Chicago team. Doctors in Sweden had tried a similar procedure on a small series of patients, whose eyesight did not improve as a result.

The Chicago results, although preliminary, are extremely encouraging. Six months after their insertion, the cells continued to grow steadily, as had been hoped. Moreover, the cells had not triggered any inflammatory response or rejection, which had been one of the physicians' greatest concerns. Although the patient reported slightly better vision in her treated eye, the researchers could not detect improvement (she remained legally blind) and did not expect a change, at least for several additional months. "We don't really expect to reverse the damage," explained Ernest, "but we hope to be able to halt the relentless progression of the disease. That would make us very happy."

More than three million people in the U.S. alone suffer from macular degeneration; 20% to 35% of all people over 75 have various stages of the disease, and autopsy studies indicate that most people over 70 already have some evidence of it. There are 200,000 new cases each year, which makes it as common as breast cancer. That number is expected to double by 2030 as the population ages. The disease causes gradual loss of central vision by damaging the cells in the macula, the region of the retina at the center of the field of vision that is responsible for seeing fine detail. Patients first lose the ability to see details and are soon unable to read. Although laser treatment can sometimes slow the spread of some forms of the disorder, there is no proven effective treatment for the advanced stages of macular degeneration.

The cell-transplant procedure, though extremely delicate, is similar to what retinal surgeons do routinely. Using a microscope to view the precise area, the surgeon cuts three tiny holes in the eye to admit miniature instruments and a fiber-optic light source. The novelty in this case—and the difficulty—lay in creating the tiny retinal opening and inserting the microsphere without damaging either the patient's retina or the transplanted cells.

Approximately a dozen spheres for transplantation can be obtained from a single fetal eye; the availability of appropriate fetal cells, however, is quite limited, and the physicians continue to search for an alternative source of cells. Only about 5% of all abortions are performed during the second trimester; at most hospitals they are offered only when termination of the pregnancy is required for medical reasons or the fetus has a severe chromosomal abnormality. Rigorous ethical guidelines established prior to clinical testing prohibit surgeons from mentioning the potential use of fetal cells to a pregnant woman until after she has decided to have an abortion. Only then is she asked if she will donate the cells—which would otherwise be discarded—for transplantation.

—John Easton

Hormone Replacement Therapy in Perspective

With the average life expectancy of women in the U.S. and all other industrialized countries now more than 70 years and in some cases over 80, many women will be postmenopausal for at least one-third of their lives. (Menopause is the cessation of menstruation.) As a consequence, the management of menopause and the role of hormone replacement therapy have become an area of considerable interest to women and their physicians—and a source of controversy as well.

Many women and a substantial number of physicians insist that menopause is a natural event and should not be "medicalized." On the other side of the issue are those who feel that the years of postmenopausal life that women have gained as a result of medical advances can be made healthier and more productive by means of appropriate intervention. The debate hinges on the wisdom and necessity of replacing the natural female hormone estrogen, which is produced by the body during the reproductive years but declines with age and falls to extremely low levels after menopause.

In the U.S. between one-sixth and one-quarter of postmenopausal women currently take some form of estrogen. Indeed, Premarin, the most commonly used form of the hormone, is the most frequently prescribed brand-name medication in the U.S. Studies of international pharmaceutical sales suggest that estrogen use by women aged 45–70 varies considerably around the world. American women are the most likely to take estrogen, followed by those in the United Kingdom and Scandinavia; women in other Western European countries rank a distant third.

Estrogen supplementation was first introduced in the 1940s. Originally, it was directed solely at the relief of menopausal symptoms such as hot flashes. Although the hormone is highly effective for this purpose, many women discontinued the therapy almost immediately because of troublesome side effects, which ranged from vaginal bleeding to nonspecific symptoms such as irritability, swelling, nausea, bloating, and breast tenderness. In any case, estrogen alone was usually given, and most women took the hormone only for relatively short periods of time—a few months to a year. This regimen was known as estrogen replacement therapy, or ERT.

In the 1970s a number of studies demonstrated that ERT increased the risk of uterine cancer in women who had not undergone hysterectomy (surgical removal of the uterus). To reduce this risk, a regimen of estrogen plus a progestin—called hormone replacement therapy, or HRT—was substituted. (The progestins are a group of natural and synthetic hormones with effects like those of the female hormone progesterone.) Today this combination treatment is the standard therapy for women with a uterus, while ERT is used by women who have undergone a hysterectomy.

Studies of the effects of HRT revealed not only that it was safe—*i.e.,* did not cause uterine cancer—but that it apparently had certain unexpected health benefits. Compared with women who did not use hormones, for example, women taking HRT appeared to have some degree of protection against the development of heart disease and osteoporosis, conditions responsible for a large proportion of deaths and disability among aging women. In recent years these potential benefits of HRT have been widely investigated, and other positive effects have been suggested by this research, among them protection against colon cancer and, perhaps, Alzheimer's disease.

Heart health

Cardiovascular disease is the most common cause of death in women in the developed world. Indeed, in the U.S. alone, coronary heart disease (*i.e.,* disease of the coronary arteries, which supply blood to the heart muscle) is responsible for the death of approximately 230,000 women every year. More than 30 epidemiological studies have shown that postmenopausal women who use estrogen are at lower risk for heart disease than those who do not. This effect has been attributed partly to estrogen's favorable impact on cholesterol levels and partly to its capacity to improve blood flow via direct effects on the smooth muscle of the arteries. While most of the data on estrogen's cardiovascular effects come from studies of the use of estrogen alone, recent data suggest that these benefits are not diminished by the concomitant use of a progestin.

The question of the effects of estrogen alone versus estrogen plus a progestin was addressed in a 1995 report from the Postmenopausal Estrogen/Progestin Interventions (PEPI) trial. PEPI was a three-year study of 875 healthy postmenopausal women between the ages of 45 and 64 who were randomly assigned to take either a placebo, estrogen alone, or one of three estrogen-progestin combinations. Both estrogen alone and the estrogen-progestin combinations were found to increase high-density lipoprotein cholesterol (HDL, the "good" cholesterol) and reduce low-density lipoprotein cholesterol (LDL, the "bad" form, which has been linked to heart disease). Blood pressure and insulin levels, two other important risk factors for heart disease, were not adversely affected by the hormone replacement regimens. The PEPI trial was too short and too small, however, to provide a basis for drawing firm conclusions about heart disease risk.

In 1996 investigators from the Nurses' Health Study published data confirming the beneficial effects of postmenopausal HRT on the incidence of cardiovascular disease. This study has monitored the health status and lifestyles of more than 200,000 female nurses over a period of more than 20 years and has provided a vast amount of data on questions pertaining to women's health. Of the more than 59,000 postmenopausal study participants between 1976 and 1992, 770 had heart attacks or died from heart disease and 572 had strokes. Women who were on estrogen alone had a 40% decrease in the risk of heart disease compared with those who were not using hormones; those taking estrogen plus a progestin had a 60% reduction in heart disease risk below that of nonusers. The benefits were limited to women currently using hormones or those who had discontinued hormone therapy within the past three years. Doses of 0.3 or 0.625 mg/day of estrogen were equally effective. The researchers found little association between the risk of stroke and current or past use of estrogen, either with or without a progestin. These data support but do not prove the cardiac benefits of estrogen alone or in combination with a progestin.

A critical feature of all major studies of HRT and cardiac risk to date is their inability to prove cause and effect. That is, the data show an association between hormone use and reduced incidence of heart disease, but they do not show that hormone use

Sharon J. Wohlmuth—KRT

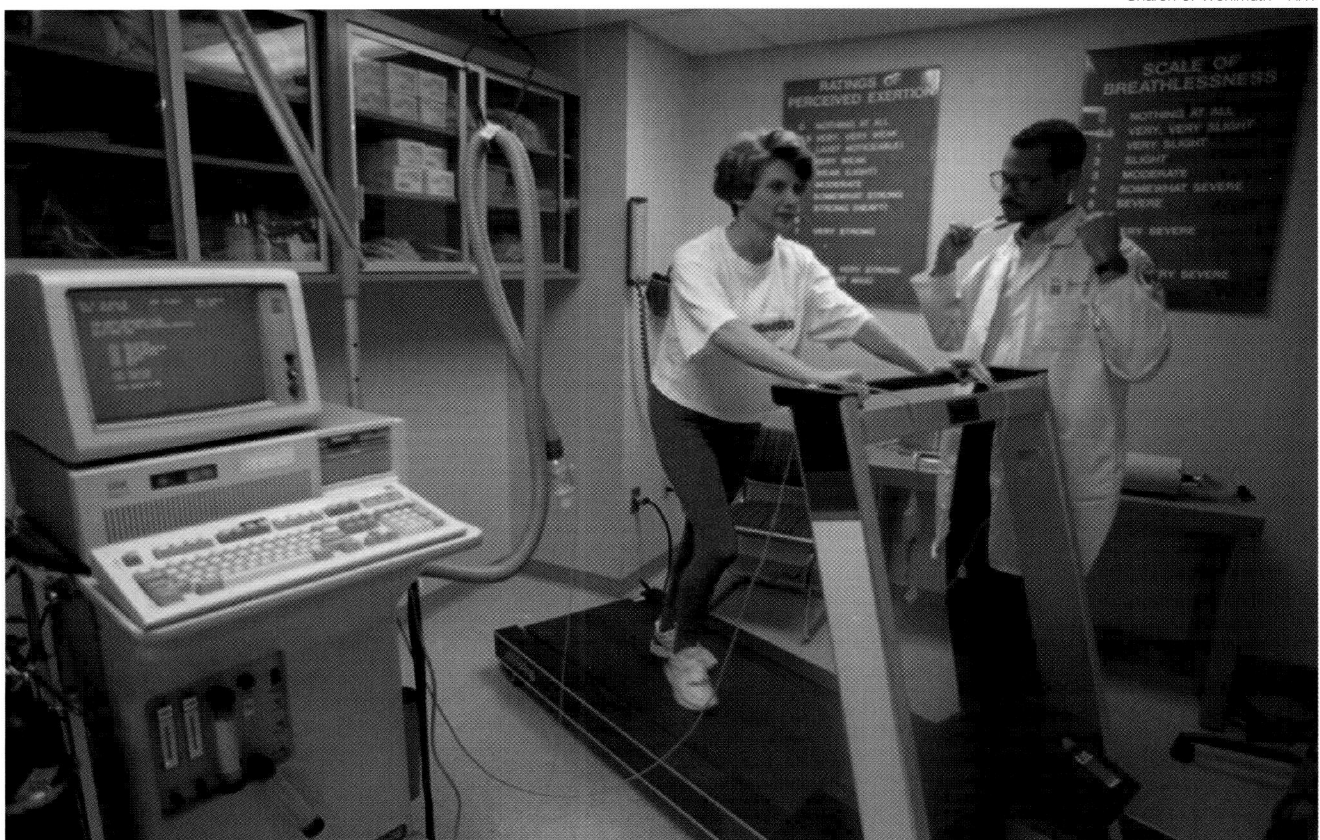

At Temple University Hospital in Philadelphia, a woman who takes hormone replacement therapy works out on a treadmill. More than 30 epidemiological studies have found that postmenopausal hormone replacement reduces a woman's risk of cardiovascular disease.

is the reason for the reduction. It is possible that women who take hormones are healthier to begin with and more likely to receive regular medical care than those who do not. Only a randomized trial (in which participants are assigned to treatment and control groups on a random basis) can address this possibility. Such a trial is, in fact, taking place in the U.S. under the direction of the Women's Health Initiative. In this investigation (which is now in the process of recruiting volunteers and is expected to enroll some 160,000 participants), 25,000 postmenopausal women will be randomly assigned to take hormones (estrogen alone if they have had a hysterectomy or estrogen and a progestin if they have not) or a placebo. This procedure should eliminate the possibility that observed differences in outcome between the groups are due to bias in the selection of their members. The risk of a variety of health problems, including heart disease and osteoporosis, will be evaluated over time.

Because of the documented association between oral contraceptive use and increased risk of blood clots, scientists have been concerned that estrogen use might promote the formation of blood clots in veins of the legs (a condition called thrombophlebitis) or lungs (pulmonary embolism). Three large studies have shown that current but not past use of HRT is associated with a small risk of such events. Research conducted at the University of Oxford found that the risk was 300% higher for current users and was highest during the first three years of use. A similar study from the state of Washington also showed a 300% increase in the risk of clot formation, with the rate of risk being related to the dose of estrogen prescribed. Finally, an analysis of data from the Nurses' Health Study found that the risk of pulmonary embolism was doubled in current users of HRT compared with nonusers. Still, the average increased risk reported in these studies translates into only one additional case of blood-clot development per 5,000 estrogen users per year, which makes it a low-probability event indeed.

It should be noted that despite evidence of the cardiovascular benefits of postmenopausal estrogen, Premarin is currently approved by the U.S. Food and Drug Administration (FDA) only for use in relief of hot flashes and genitourinary symptoms of menopause and prevention of osteoporosis. Prevention of heart disease is not listed in the FDA's indications for the drug at this time.

Benefits for bone

Bone fractures are a major cause of injury, disability, and death among the elderly, as well as being a major source of health care expenditures. Annually, in the U.S. alone, nearly 65,000 women die from complications following hip fracture. A large number of observational studies (those like the Nurses' Health Study, in which the health status of a population is monitored over time) and a smaller number of randomized trials have documented the beneficial effects of HRT on bone density. Estrogen apparently slows the natural process of bone resorption, with the result that bone mass is increased. It also influences bone density by increasing the level of vitamin D in the blood and promoting the absorption of calcium. Improved bone density, in turn, appears to translate into a decreased incidence of fractures.

Studies of hip fracture in postmenopausal women show that those taking HRT have significantly fewer fractures—anywhere from 25% to 40% fewer, depending on the study. Importantly, research also shows that bone loss invariably resumes when HRT is stopped, paralleling the natural skeletal changes seen after menopause. Thus, continuous hormone therapy—to the end of life—presumably would be required for maintaining bone density.

While scientists know that estrogen has a positive effect on bone density, the effects of combination regimens have been a matter of question. This issue was addressed in a recent report from the PEPI trial. After three years the women assigned to the placebo group had lost an average of 1.8% of bone density in the spine and 1.7% in the hip, while those assigned to any of the four hormone regimens had gained bone density at both sites. The trial did not last long enough to measure effects of HRT on fracture rates, but the Women's Health Initiative will further investigate this issue.

Marnie Crawford Samuelson—KRT

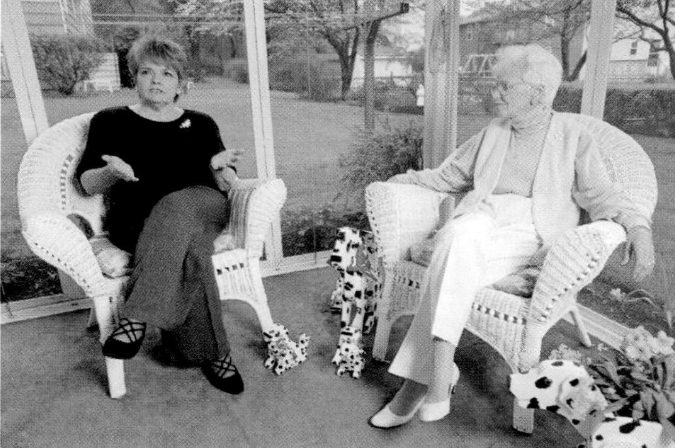

A Providence, R.I., woman and her daughter-in-law are among the some 160,000 participants in the Women's Health Initiative, the largest U.S. study ever to focus solely on the health problems of women.

Colon cancer prevention

Recently several studies have suggested that the use of HRT may reduce the incidence of and deaths from colon cancer, the third most common cancer (and the third most common cause of cancer deaths) in U.S. women. Scientists speculate that this effect could be related to estrogen's ability to reduce the concentration of bile acids in the colon. The largest study done to date looked at the medical records of 897 women who had died of colon cancer; these subjects were drawn from a group of more than 400,000 postmenopausal women followed as part of a study begun by the American Cancer Society in 1982. This investigation found that women currently using HRT were 50% less likely than nonusers to die of colon cancer, while former users had a 30% reduction in fatal colon cancers.

These results were echoed by several smaller studies. Investigators in Wisconsin studying 694 postmenopausal women with colon cancer and 1,622 healthy controls found that recent users of estrogen (with or without a progestin) had a 50% lower chance of developing colon cancer, although there was no difference between users and nonusers in incidence of rectal cancer. A smaller study from the University of Washington, which compared 193 women with colon cancer and 194 similar subjects with no history of the disease, showed that HRT reduced the risk of colon cancer by about 40%. Like the work on the connection between HRT and breast cancer, none of these studies can be considered definitive because of their design. Thus, the Women's Health Initiative findings on colon cancer risk will also be eagerly awaited.

An anti-Alzheimer's drug?

Laboratory studies of the effects of estrogen on neurons (nerve cells) suggest that the hormone may enhance the survival of these cells and limit the accumulation of beta-amyloid, a protein whose deposition in the brain is associated with Alzheimer's disease. The possibility that estrogen might prevent or forestall the development of Alzheimer's disease has aroused much enthusiasm. So far, however, studies examining the relationship between HRT and dementia have had mixed results.

One of the most promising studies was reported in 1996. The study population consisted of some 1,100 elderly New York City women participating in a long-term investigation of aging and health. The women were free of Alzheimer's disease and Parkinson's disease at the time they entered the study, and none had experienced a stroke. Over time, the annual rate of Alzheimer's disease was 2.7% among women who took estrogen, compared with 8.4% among those who did not. Similar beneficial effects of estrogen were seen in women followed as part of the Baltimore (Md.) Longitudinal Study on Aging, sponsored by the National Institutes of Health. These data, published in June 1997, showed that the risk of developing Alzheimer's disease was reduced by 50% in the women who took estrogen.

In contrast, another large study that focused on younger postmenopausal women failed to show any difference in a variety of tests of cognitive function between those who took estrogen and those who did not. Again, examination of the possible relationship between estrogen replacement and mental function will be an integral part of the Women's Health Initiative.

The negatives

If all of the evidence about HRT were positive, or even merely suggestive of benefits, deciding whether to take it would be an easy matter. Unfortunately, this is not the case.

Effects on the uterus. An undisputed side effect of ERT is increased risk of cancer of the uterus or the uterine lining (endometrium). As noted above, the major preventive strategy has been administration of a progestin either continuously or cyclically. Adding a progestin to the regimen has also been shown to decrease the likelihood that abnormal cells will develop in the uterus, a condition that can set the stage for cancer. In addition to having their blood lipids and bone density regularly evaluated, women in the PEPI trial underwent a uterine biopsy annually or

(continued on page 365)

NEWS CAP MHA 98

Making Sense of the Mammography Muddle

While there is strong agreement that mammograms help reduce the rate of death from breast cancer among women aged 50 and older, controversy continues about the value of mammography screening for younger women. Recently, women in their 40s received conflicting—and confusing—advice.

In January 1997 a consensus conference convened by the U.S. National Institutes of Health (NIH) concluded that the scientific evidence to date was not strong enough to warrant a universal recommendation that all women in their 40s get screening mammograms. The group declined to issue a guideline but instead left it to women in this age-group to make the decision individually after weighing the risks and benefits.

The NIH's failure to take a stand was sharply criticized by many medical and women's groups, which immediately launched a campaign that led even the U.S. Congress to become involved, unanimously passing a nonbinding resolution in favor of breast cancer screening for women aged 40–49. The American Cancer Society, the leading voluntary cancer organization, called the public debate confusing and in March 1997 issued a simple new guideline for all women 40 and older: get a mammogram once a year.

Less than a week later, the advisory board of the National Cancer Institute (NCI) also issued a recommendation endorsing regular mammograms for women in their 40s. The NCI board suggested screening every one to two years for women in this age-group who are at average risk; those who are at a high risk for breast cancer were advised to get medical advice about when and how often to get mammograms. The guidelines also emphasized that women should have a regular breast examination by a physician, since mammography is far from foolproof.

Mammograms are low-dose X-rays used to visualize breast tumors. They are intended to help detect these growths at the earliest stages, when they are small and believed to be most treatable. Most authorities agree that the procedure is more reliable in older women, whose breast tissue is less dense, than in women who are premenopausal. Also limiting the usefulness of mammography in younger women is the fact that tumors are sometimes more aggressive in this age-group and may grow more rapidly during the intervals between screening.

The NIH's reevaluation of mammography for women in their 40s was prompted by newly available data from long-term trials conducted during the 1960s and '70s in several different countries; data from Sweden were particularly notable. The overall evidence showed that within 7 to 10 years after screening, breast cancer mortality was not significantly lower in women who underwent mammography in their 40s than in similar women who did not. The consensus conference report noted, however, that 7–10 years may not be sufficient for a decline in mortality to become apparent. It also observed that current mammography technology may be better than that used in the past, so the survival benefits may be underestimated by the available research.

Will and Deni McIntyre—Science Source/Photo Researchers

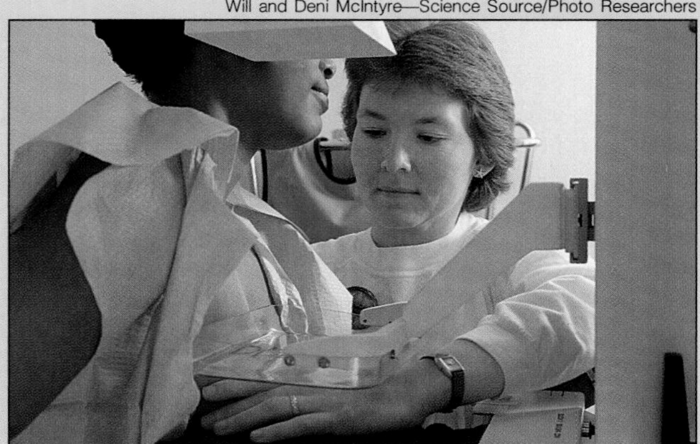

Regular mammographic screening has been shown to lower breast cancer mortality in women 50 and over. The impact on the death rates of younger women is less clear, however, and has stirred heated debate.

The decision not to recommend routine mammograms for younger women was initially reported as unanimous, but some who participated in the consensus conference had second thoughts, which led to one resignation and the unusual step by two others of filing a "minority report" endorsing mammography screening in the 40–49 age-group. NCI director Richard Klausner, who had been critical of the conference report, accepted the NCI advisory board's recommendation. Pres. Bill Clinton, in turn, urged that insurance plans cover the costs of screening for women in the younger age-group.

Some scientists and women's advocacy groups were disappointed with this turn of events. They contended that the benefits of screening for women under 50 have yet to be proved and suggested that the government's decision had been largely political—in other words, because mammography is one of the few tools for early diagnosis of breast cancer, equivocal support for screening might be interpreted by some as insensitivity to an important women's health issue.

—Cristine Russell

(continued from page 363)
whenever medically indicated (*e.g.,* in case of unusual bleeding). Of the women taking estrogen in the form of conjugated equine estrogens (Premarin and similar preparations, in which the hormone is derived from the urine of pregnant mares), 60% had abnormal uterine biopsies at some point in the trial. As a result, more than half of the women assigned to take estrogen alone discontinued the drug sometime during the three years of study. In contrast, fewer than 3% of women taking a placebo or one of the estrogen-progestin combinations had abnormal uterine biopsies, and 80% of women in these groups stayed on their assigned regimen throughout the duration of the trial. Although this investigation was neither large enough nor long enough to assess the participants' risk of uterine cancer, it is noteworthy that the single case of uterine cancer was seen in a woman in the placebo group.

Breast cancer. Fear of breast cancer is one of most frequently cited reasons for avoiding or ending HRT. About 180,000 cases of breast cancer are diagnosed in the U.S. each year, which makes it the most common nonskin cancer in American women. It is second only to lung cancer as a cause of cancer deaths in women, taking about 45,000 lives annually. Despite years of research, the relationship between HRT and breast cancer risk remains unclear. This uncertainty was reflected in three reports published in 1995.

First, investigators from the Nurses' Health Study addressed the risk of breast cancer in postmenopausal women taking estrogen alone or estrogen plus a progestin. They found that while the type of hormone regimen did not have a significant effect on breast cancer risk, the woman's age and duration of hormone use did. In particular, women who took hormones for five years or less showed no increased risk, whereas among those who took HRT for longer periods, breast cancer incidence increased by about 40%. Increased risk was limited to those women taking hormones at the time and seemed to disappear two years after HRT was stopped.

In contrast, the other two studies published around the same time failed to show any increased risk for breast cancer among women taking HRT. In one of these, conducted at the University of Washington, investigators interviewed 537 breast cancer patients aged 50 to 64 and 492 randomly selected women in the same age-group with no history of breast cancer. Data analysis showed no connection between HRT use and breast cancer risk. A larger study of similar design gave the same result. Information about 3,130 breast cancer patients and 3,698 similar women without breast cancer living in four states was reviewed for any link between HRT and breast cancer risk. No increased risk was observed, even with long durations of therapy. Results did not vary according to family history of breast cancer, personal history of benign breast disease, alcohol intake, or type of HRT.

As with the investigations of HRT and heart disease, none of these studies is considered definitive. The women in these trials who used HRT may have had different risk factors for breast cancer (*e.g.,* age at onset of menstruation, age at first pregnancy) than those who did not. In addition, medical care (*e.g.,* frequency of mammography) of the two groups may have varied. Again, a definite conclusion can come only from a randomized controlled trial. It is hoped that this kind of information will come out of the Women's Health Initiative. In the meantime, many authorities consider the findings from the Nurses' Health Study to be the most persuasive of the three because of the large number of participants and the long duration of the study. Moreover, the Nurses' Health Study is prospective in design (*i.e.,* all participants were initially healthy), and its findings are therefore considered more reliable than those of the other two investigations, both of which were retrospective.

It should be emphasized, however, that a diagnosis of breast cancer does not inevitably translate into death from breast cancer. Indeed, a somewhat surprising finding from a number of small studies is that HRT users who are found to have breast cancer have a better prognosis than women who are not taking HRT at the time of their diagnosis. Many breast cancer survivors and their physicians are even beginning to question the long-held assumption that postmenopausal women with a history of the disease must never take estrogen. So far, however, very few objective data exist on this subject.

A secondary but nonetheless significant issue is the effect of HRT on mammography. Postmenopausal women who take hormones have denser breasts than those who forgo HRT, and the density of breast tissue may affect the reliability of the mammographic image. Indeed, the researchers from the University of Washington suggested that the current use of HRT is associated with lower specificity and sensitivity of screening mammography. If hormone use does indeed reduce the accuracy of mammography, it could decrease the effectiveness of the technique as a screening method and delay the diagnosis of breast cancer until the disease has reached a more advanced stage.

Today's HRT—and tomorrow's

In the U.S. estrogen is most commonly given in the form of conjugated equine estrogens, which are administered orally. Women who have not had a hysterectomy usually take a progestin in addition. Depending on the formulation of the drug, the progestin may be supplied concurrently with estrogen or intermittently. Concurrent administration suppresses proliferation of the endometrial tissue, which thus reduces the possibility that abnormal cells will develop. When a progestin is given intermittently, its periodic withdrawal from the woman's system causes shedding of the endometrial lining (*i.e.,* bleeding). Both strategies are designed to prevent the development of uterine or endometrial cancer. Not surprisingly, many women prefer the concurrent regimen and are more likely to continue hormone therapy when it does not involve the inconvenience of monthly bleeding.

A variety of hormone preparations have recently been tested to see if they have benefits over the widely used regimen of estrogen plus medroxyprogesterone. One of the experimental therapies involved a combination of ethinyl estradiol (a synthetic estrogen and the most common estrogen component of many oral contraceptives) with the progestin norethindrone acetate. Overall, studies showed that women who followed this regimen had good relief from hot flashes, experienced no withdrawal bleeding, and showed improved bone mineral density and favorable changes in HDL/LDL ratios. Further, they were well protected against proliferation of endometrial tissue. The dose of estrogen used was lower than that in many oral contraceptive preparations. It is too early to tell what impact this therapy will have on breast and colon cancer risk. Other areas of ongoing research include the development of innovative agents, such as raloxifene (an estrogen-like compound that acts selectively on the body's estrogen-sensitive tissues), and exploration of a possible role for natural estrogens derived from plant sources (phytoestrogens).

Risk versus benefit: a delicate balance

A frustrating problem for women and their doctors alike is the fragmented nature of the current information about HRT. Recently, researchers have begun to try to integrate the effects of HRT on multiple diseases rather than focusing studies on a single condition. At the same time, they have begun to address the question of the net health benefits of HRT. One study following this approach used data on 41,000 postmenopausal women who had participated in the Iowa Women's Health Study. The investigators found that the overall death rate of women who used HRT was 22% lower than that of nonusers. The HRT users had a 25% reduction in heart disease deaths, a 50% reduction in hip fractures, and a 30% reduction in colon cancer incidence. They also had a 25% increase in breast cancer incidence and a 400% increase in uterine cancer compared with those who did not take HRT.

A smaller study looked at a group of 232 postmenopausal women who began HRT within three years of menopause and used it for at least five years, compared with 222 age-matched postmenopausal women who did not use hormones. The average length of use was 17 years. All of the women in both groups belonged to a health maintenance organization and theoretically had access to similar medical care. The overall death rate was 50% lower in the women who took HRT. This reduction in mortality was due largely to a decrease in deaths from cardiovascular disease, the rate of which was reduced by more than 50%. There was no difference between the two groups in the death rate from cancer of all types, but those who took hormones had a 90% increase in breast cancer mortality.

A similar analysis of death rates and causes of death has also been carried out, using data from the Nurses' Health Study. A detailed examination showed that women who were taking hormones at the time had a 40% lower risk of death than those who had never taken hormones. The effect of HRT was particularly striking among women who had risk factors for heart disease; these women accounted for 70% of the study population, and their risk of death was decreased by 50% while they were on hormones. For the 13% of women who were at low risk for heart disease, there was much less benefit, about a 10% reduction. The survival benefits of hormone therapy were attenuated after 10 or more years of use, however, because the risk of death from breast cancer increased by 43% after 10 years of taking hormones, which thus partially counterbalanced the positive effects on cardiac risk.

Many women successfully manage the symptoms of menopause without hormone replacement. This 59-year-old Californian found all the relief she needed in yoga and a program of regular exercise.

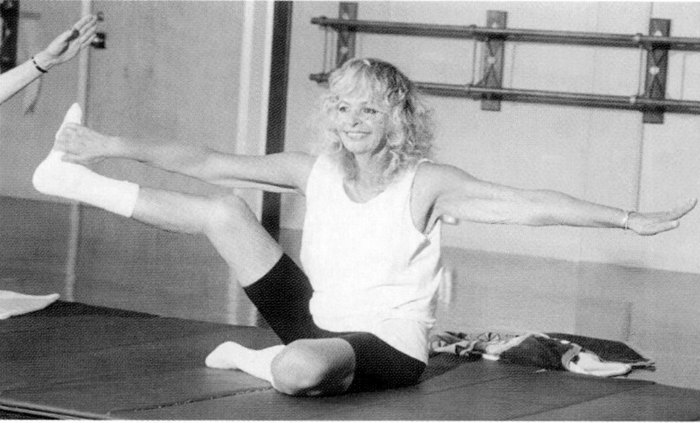

Ygnacio Nanetti—KRT

Although the results of these three studies are provocative, they must be regarded with the same reservations as the results of any other observational study. The Women's Health Initiative, with its randomized design, should provide more definitive results about the general and disease-specific effects of HRT.

But what to do now?

Results from the Women's Health Initiative will not be available until after the year 2000. In the meantime, many women and their physicians will have to make a decision about HRT. On the basis of the data currently available, a group of investigators from several Massachusetts medical centers have designed an algorithm, or decision pathway, to help women determine their own personal risk-benefit profile. The model uses as its major variables the factors that put women at risk for heart disease, osteoporosis, and breast cancer. Under the assumptions of this model, HRT should increase life expectancy for nearly all postmenopausal women, in some cases up to three years, depending on the woman's personal risk factors for heart disease and breast cancer. For women who have at least one of five risk factors for heart disease (diabetes, evidence of heart enlargement, hypertension, high cholesterol, or smoking), HRT is calculated to prolong life expectancy; this holds true even for women with first-degree relatives (mother or sister) with breast cancer. Only for women who have both a strong family history of breast cancer (defined as having two or more first-degree relatives with breast cancer) and no risk factors for heart disease or hip fracture does the risk of HRT-related breast cancer outweigh the potential benefits for heart and bone. This "decision tree" should be used by women in consultation with their doctors. While it cannot provide a definitive answer, it may be a useful aid in the decision-making process.

A key consideration for any woman who may be thinking about HRT is her personal reasons for taking hormones and the efficacy of alternative ways to meet these objectives. Certainly, the effectiveness of diet and exercise in reducing heart disease risk is well-documented, as is the importance of controlling diabetes, hypertension, and obesity. Estrogen should not be regarded simply as a substitute for these or any other health-promoting measures. Alendronate (Fosamax), a drug approved in 1995, has been shown to increase bone mass and thereby decrease fracture risk; promising new agents for the treatment of osteoporosis are under development. Decreasing dietary fat and increasing fiber are useful strategies for lowering colon cancer risk. None of these approaches carries the risk for uterine or breast cancer that has been associated with ERT. A woman who is intent on, say, preventing osteoporosis may be best advised to pursue a regimen specifically designed for that condition.

For many women, however, the accumulating evidence of estrogen's beneficial effects for a variety of conditions means that they must give serious consideration to the use of ERT or HRT. It is hoped that further research will provide answers and peace of mind for those faced with this difficult decision.

—Nancy E. Davidson, M.D.

The information presented here reflects the most recent published statistical figures that were available to the editors of *Medical and Health Annual* in mid-1997. Sources include principal intergovernmental organizations—*e.g.,* the World Health Organization (WHO; Geneva), the United Nations (New York City), and their regional offices and affiliated organizations; national statistical and health offices worldwide; principal U.S. authorities—the National Center for Health Statistics, the Centers for Disease Control and Prevention, and the Environmental Protection Agency; and on-line resources of the Internet.

Certain terms used in this section have specific meaning in a public health context:

incidence New cases of a disease or condition diagnosed during a specified period of time; may be reported as the "total number of cases," or as a "rate per [1,000, 10,000, or 100,000]," when referred to a specified population.

safe water Treated surface and untreated but uncontaminated ground waters that are accessible within 200 meters (urban) or that can be obtained without excessive expenditure of time (rural).

attended birth Birth attended by a physician, nurse, midwife, trained primary health care worker, or traditional birth attendant.

The application of other terms may differ according to their national contexts—availability of "health services within one hour's travel" means availability of *appropriate* services (different for the U.S. and, say, India) in one hour's travel (travel services differing as much as health services).

Most of the figures provided are "best estimates" and may conceal a considerable range of variation—geographic, economic, or demographic—within any single national value. Because the scope and priorities of national data-collection systems differ greatly, coverage of some subjects may be incomplete.

Symbols and abbreviations:

...	not available
<,>	less than/greater than
≤	equal to or less than
≥	equal to or greater than
AIDS	acquired immune deficiency syndrome
UNDP	United Nations Development Programme
UNICEF	United Nations Children's Fund

World/Regional Summary

Outbreaks: Emerging and Reemerging Infectious Diseases, 1996–97

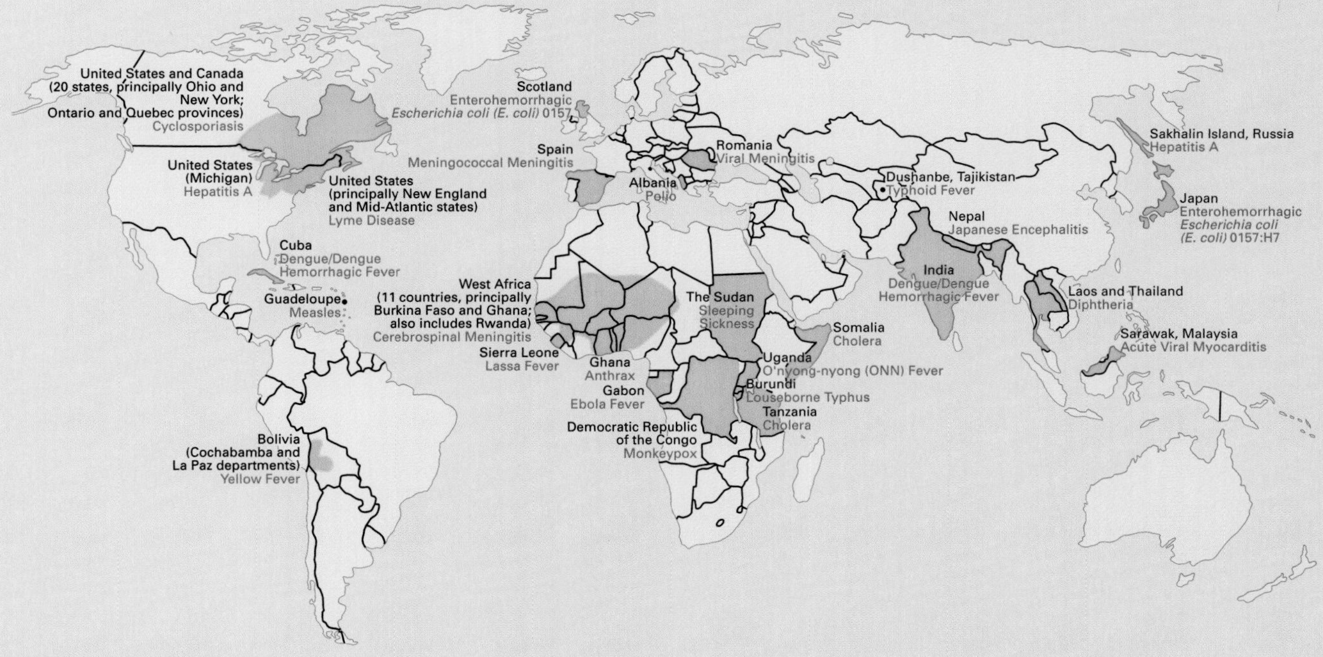

Health Indicators (World and Component Regions)

Continent/region/ bloc/country	Life expectancy		Other			
	Male (years)	Female (years)	Persons per doctor	Infant mortality per 1,000 births	Pop. having safe water (%)	Food (% FAO recommended minimum), 1992
WORLD	64.1	68.3	720	57.6	77	115
AFRICA	52.9	55.5	2,810	93.1	51	97
Central Africa	46.1	49.5	12,820	110.8	32	89
East Africa	47.5	49.5	12,330	107.1	42	81
North Africa	63.7	66.8	970	61.5	73	123
Southern Africa	61.8	66.9	1,680	53.2	69	109
West Africa	50.7	53.3	6,790	94.0	48	94
AMERICAS	68.4	74.7	520	32.5	88	126
Anglo-America[1]	72.4	79.2	390	7.8	100	139
Canada	74.7	81.7	460	6.2	100	116
United States	72.1	78.9	390	8.0	100	141
Latin America	66.0	71.9	650	41.7	80	116
Caribbean	66.6	70.9	490	52.6	74	106
Central America	64.6	70.1	1,190	44.3	66	107
Mexico	66.5	73.1	580	27.1	83	135
South America	66.0	71.8	670	46.0	81	113
Andean Group[2]	68.2	73.7	870	37.6	78	103
Brazil	63.8	70.4	680	57.2	87	118
Other South America	67.8	71.5	410	31.9	67	120
ASIA	64.5	67.5	980	54.8	74	113
Eastern Asia	69.7	73.6	620	24.0	71	117
China	69.1	72.4	630	26.0	67	116
Japan	76.6	83.0	550	4.2	100	124
South Korea	68.0	76.0	820	10.0	93	140
Other Eastern Asia	69.7	75.5	510	18.0	99	121
South Asia	58.7	59.8	2,360	78.8	80	104
India	58.7	59.8	2,170	73.0	81	108
Pakistan	62.0	64.0	2,060	79.0	79	100
Other South Asia	56.5	56.7	5,620	102.1	76	86
Southeast Asia	63.5	67.1	2,600	49.0	62	116
ASEAN[3]	64.6	68.3	2,550	42.2	66	116
Non-ASEAN	56.3	59.2	2,990	83.2	38	114
Southwest Asia	66.1	70.5	590	46.3	84	120
Central Asia	64.2	71.8	290	34.5	100	...
Gulf Cooperation Council[4]	68.1	71.3	640	26.5	93	115
Iran	65.8	68.2	1,600	54.6	84	119
Other Southwest Asia	66.5	70.9	680	50.4	76	122
EUROPE	68.7	77.1	290	10.9	100	133
Eastern Europe	63.3	73.9	280	16.4	100	123
Russia	58.0	72.0	240	18.0	100	...
Ukraine	65.3	74.7	230	14.0	100	...
Other Eastern Europe	67.9	75.5	380	16.0	100	123
Western Europe	73.4	80.0	300	6.1	100	135
European Union (EU)	73.3	80.0	300	6.1	100	136
France	72.9	81.1	360	6.1	100	144
Germany	72.5	79.0	310	5.6	100	126
Italy	73.8	80.4	190	6.6	100	141
Spain	73.2	81.1	250	6.0	100	151
United Kingdom	74.4	79.7	450	6.2	100	132
Other EU[5]	73.3	79.5	340	6.3	100	133
Non-EU	74.8	81.0	310	5.2	100	124
OCEANIA	71.6	76.7	520	24.2	88	122
Australia	75.4	81.1	450	5.7	100	120
Pacific Ocean islands	65.2	69.1	710	41.4	65	126

[1]Anglo-America includes Canada, the United States, Greenland, Bermuda, and St. Pierre and Miquelon.

[2]Bolivia, Colombia, Ecuador, Peru, Venezuela.

[3]Association of Southeast Asian Nations (Brunei, Indonesia, Malaysia, the Philippines, Singapore, Thailand, Vietnam).

[4]Bahrain, Kuwait, Oman, Qatar, Saudi Arabia, the United Arab Emirates.

[5]Finland, Greece, Ireland, Luxembourg, The Netherlands, Portugal, Sweden.

Household and Community Health Indicators (Selected Countries)[1]

	% persons in communities having:			% households having:	
	Health services (one hour's travel)	Safe water	Sanitary waste disposal	Inside toilet/ water closet	Refrigerator
AFRICA					
Algeria	98	78	91	68.9	...
Congo, Democratic Republic of the	26	42	18	...	...
Egypt	99	79	32	...	...
Ethiopia	46	25	19	55.2	...
Kenya	77	53	77	53.3	...
Morocco	70	55	41	50.2	...
Nigeria	51	51	58	7.0	...
South Africa	...	99	53	54.9	...
Sudan, The	70	60	22	...	...
Tanzania	42	38	86	...	...
NORTH AMERICA					
Canada	100	100	99	99.3	99.6
Mexico	93	83	72	45.0	23.0
United States	100	98	85	98.9	99.5
SOUTH AMERICA					
Argentina	71	71	68	95.1	...
Brazil	...	73	44	...	71.1
Colombia	81	85	85	77.9	...
Peru	44	72	57	35.7	70.3[2]
Venezuela	...	79	59	84.4	74.2
ASIA					
Bangladesh	45	97	48	12.5	...
China	88	67	24	25.2	25.0
India	85	81	29	23.7	6.9
Indonesia	93	62	51	51.5	...
Iran	88	90	81	43.6	...
Iraq	93	78	70	...	...
Japan	100	97	85[3]	74.7	98.9
Korea, North	80	...	74	...	...
Korea, South	100	93	100	51.3	93.1
Malaysia	88	78	94	...	...
Myanmar (Burma)	60	60	43	...	...
Nepal	...	63	18	6.1	...
Pakistan	55	74	47	25.1	...
Philippines	71	86	77	35.0	20.7
Saudi Arabia	97	95	86	...	...
Taiwan	...	86	69	94.2	99.1
Thailand	90	89	96	40.9	25.7
Turkey	100	80	83	70.6	83.1
Uzbekistan	...	62	22	...	...
Vietnam	90	43	22	...	...
EUROPE					
France	...	100	100	95.8	99.0
Germany	...	...	...	98.4	79.7
Italy	100	99	99	98.5	91.0
Poland	100	100	100	68.9	97.7[4]
Romania	100	100	49	...	...
Russia[5]	100	94	93	...	95.0
Spain	97	99	97	97.1	97.9
Sweden	100	100	100	98.0	...
Ukraine	100	97	49	49	...
United Kingdom	100	100	96	99.8	98.5
OCEANIA					
Australia	100	95	90	92.2	99.7
New Zealand	100	97	100[3]	97.1	76.5[6]

[1]Countries are selected on the basis of population.

[2]Metropolitan Lima.

[3]Urban households.

[4]Households of employed persons.

[5]Data refer to the former U.S.S.R.

[6]Combined refrigerator-freezers only.

Sources: UNICEF, *The State of the World's Children 1997*; *World Development Indicators 1997*; national statistical offices.

Maternal Health (Selected Countries)

	Percentage of deliveries				Deaths per 100,000 live births
	Prenatal care	Attended by trained personnel	Tetanus toxoid vaccine (pregnant women, 2 or more doses)	Babies of low birth weight (less than 2,500 g[1])	Maternal mortality
AFRICA					
Algeria	<40	77	52	9	160
Congo, Democratic Republic of the	...	...	33	15	870
Egypt	40–59	46	64	10	170
Ethiopia	40–59	14	22	16	1,400
Kenya	60–79	45	72	16	650
Morocco	<40	40	37	9	610
Nigeria	60–79	31	21	16	1,000
South Africa	≥90	82	26	...	230
Sudan, The	...	69	65	15	660
Tanzania	≥90	53	71	14	770
NORTH AMERICA					
Canada	≥90	99	...	6	6
Mexico	60–79	77	42	8	110
United States	≥90	99	...	7	12
SOUTH AMERICA					
Argentina	40–59	97	...	7	100
Brazil	60–79	81	70	11	220
Colombia	60–79	85	57	10	100
Peru	60–79	52	21	11	280
Venezuela	60–79	69	18	9	120
ASIA					
Bangladesh	<40	14	78	50	850
China	80–89	84	11	9	95
India	40–59	34	79	33	570
Indonesia	60–79	36	74	14	650
Iran	40–59	77	82	9	120
Iraq	40–59	54	72	15	310
Japan	≥90	100	...	7	18
Korea, North	≥90	100	95	...	70
Korea, South	80–89	98	...	9	130
Malaysia	60–79	94	79	8	80
Myanmar (Burma)	80–89	57	83	16	580
Nepal	<40	7	11	...	1,500
Pakistan	<40	19	36	25	340
Philippines	60–79	53	48	15	280
Saudi Arabia	80–89	82	62	7	130
Taiwan	...	...	...	...	8
Thailand	60–79	71	93	13	200
Turkey	40–59	76	38	8	180
Uzbekistan	...	...	...	...	55
Vietnam	≥90	95	82	17	160
EUROPE					
France	≥90	99	...	5	15
Germany	≥90	99	...	...	22
Italy	≥90	...	...	5	12
Poland	≥90	99	...	...	19
Romania	≥90	100	...	11	130
Russia	...		...	...	75
Spain	≥90	96	...	4	7
Sweden	≥90	100	...	5	7
Ukraine	...	100	...	...	50
United Kingdom	≥90	100	...	7	9
OCEANIA					
Australia	≥90	100	...	6	9
New Zealand	≥90	99	...	6	25

[1]Approximately 5½ lb.

Sources: WHO, *The World Health Report 1995;* UNICEF, *The State of the World's Children 1997.*

Infant/Child Health (Selected Countries)

	Deaths per 1,000 live births		Percentage of children immunized (age 12 months and under)			
	Infant mortality rate (deaths in first 12 months)	Child mortality rate (deaths in first 5 years)	Bacillus Calmette-Guérin (TB) vaccine	Diphtheria/ pertussis/ tetanus vaccine (3rd dose)	Oral polio vaccine (3rd dose)	Measles vaccine
AFRICA						
Algeria	51	61	93	83	83	77
Congo, Democratic Republic of the	119	185	46	26	27	39
Egypt	40	51	95	90	91	90
Ethiopia	114	195	63	51	48	43
Kenya	61	90	92	84	84	73
Morocco	61	75	93	90	90	88
Nigeria	114	191	57	27	27	40
South Africa	51	67	95	73	72	76
Sudan, The	69	115	88	76	77	74
Tanzania	100	160	92	88	86	82
NORTH AMERICA						
Canada	6	8	...	93	89	98
Mexico	27	32	98	92	92	90
United States	8	10	...	94	84	89
SOUTH AMERICA						
Argentina	24	27	96	66	70	76
Brazil	51	60	100	83	83	88
Colombia	30	36	99	93	95	84
Peru	41	55	96	95	93	98
Venezuela	20	24	91	68	85	67
ASIA						
Bangladesh	85	115	94	69	69	79
China	38	47	92	92	94	93
India	76	115	96	89	98	78
Indonesia	50	75	86	78	79	70
Iran	35	40	99	97	97	95
Iraq	57	71	99	91	91	95
Japan	6	4	91	85	91	68
Korea, North	23	30	99	96	99	98
Korea, South	8	9	93	93	93	92
Malaysia	11	13	97	90	90	81
Myanmar (Burma)	105	150	82	72	72	75
Nepal	81	114	61	63	62	57
Pakistan	95	137	75	35	37	53
Philippines	40	53	91	85	86	86
Saudi Arabia	34	29	93	97	97	94
Taiwan	5	6	...	...	...	...
Thailand	27	32	98	94	94	90
Turkey	44	50	42	51	51	42
Uzbekistan	50	62	95	89	99	81
Vietnam	34	45	96	93	94	95
EUROPE						
France	7	9	78	89	92	76
Germany	7	6	...	45	80	75
Italy	7	8	...	50	98	50
Poland	14	16	94	95	95	91
Romania	23	29	100	98	94	93
Russia	27	30	96	93	92	94
Spain	8	9	...	88	88	90
Sweden	4	5	...	99[1]	99	96
Ukraine	20	24	92	94	95	96
United Kingdom	6	7	...	92	94	92
OCEANIA						
Australia	7	8	...	95	72	86
New Zealand	7	9	20	84	84	87

[1]Diphtheria only.

Source: UNICEF, *The State of the World's Children 1997.*

Resources for Health Care (Selected Countries)

	Persons per doctor	Persons per dentist	Persons per nurse	Persons per pharmacist	Persons per midwife
AFRICA					
Algeria	1,030	3,470	…	10,200	…
Congo, Democratic Republic of the	15,580	913,070	1,360	634,510	…
Egypt	550	3,680	1,240	1,610	…
Ethiopia	30,200	…	12,810	123,080	…
Kenya	6,000	43,070	1,000	44,850	…
Morocco	2,940	22,730	1,930	10,520	295,770
Nigeria	4,690	77,430	1,640	15,840	1,610
South Africa	1,520	10,040	250	4,200	…
Sudan, The	10,000	…	…	…	…
Tanzania	22,568	…	…	…	…
NORTH AMERICA					
Canada	460	2,000	110	1,320	…
Mexico	580	18,260	610	…	…
United States	390	1,380	130	1,420	86,040
SOUTH AMERICA					
Argentina	380	1,520	1,854	44,490	…
Brazil	680	1,260	3,450	2,620	…
Colombia	910	2,420	720	…	…
Peru	940	2,790	1,480	3,740	6,300
Venezuela	630	2,570	390	3,640	…
ASIA					
Bangladesh	5,200	159,000	12,310	15,550	11,520
China	630	…	1,090	2,860	23,370
India	2,170	46,340	2,010	…	4,410
Indonesia	7,400	45,020	1,550[1]	52,340	…[1]
Iran	1,600	12,530	1,230[1]	…	…[1]
Iraq	2,180	11,570	1,450	12,280	…
Japan	550	1,560	140	790	5,480
Korea, North	380	…	…	…	…
Korea, South	820	3,440	390	1,060	5,380
Malaysia	2,300	11,910	540	15,630	…
Myanmar (Burma)	3,620	41,720	4,890	…	5,140
Nepal	12,550	…	6,750[1]	39,030	…[1]
Pakistan	1,910	48,740	5,890	31,940	6,770
Philippines	850	41,270	4,490	81,100	5,400
Saudi Arabia	520	8,330	340	9,050	…
Taiwan	770	2,980	370	1,110	25,260
Thailand	4,260	20,840	670	12,300	5,520
Turkey	970	5,360	1,093	3,550	1,640
Uzbekistan	290	5,200	90	13,160	1,110
Vietnam	2,490	…	1,310	10,820	5,860
EUROPE					
France	360	1,480	180	1,110	5,022
Germany	310	1,380	110[1]	1,860	…[1]
Italy	190	5,260	330	1,050	…
Poland	440	2,202	190	2,060	1,590
Romania[2]	560	3,600	…	3,540	…
Russia	240	3,150	150	20,320	1,270
Spain	250	3,190	230	990	6,290
Sweden	390	1,830	90[1]	1,520	…[1]
Ukraine	230	…	80[1]	…	…[1]
United Kingdom	670	3,230	200	1,540	2,350
OCEANIA					
Australia	450	3,660	124	1,590	…[1]
New Zealand	300	1,830	80[1]	1,010	…[1]

[1]Nurses includes midwives.

[2]Government-employed health personnel only.

Sources: International Monetary Fund, *Government Finance Statistics Yearbook* (1996); UNICEF, *The State of the World's Children 1997;* national statistical offices.

Institutional Resources

	% of central government expenditure on health	Hospitals			Access of population to essential drugs (%)
		Total number	Beds per 10,000 population	Occupancy rate	
AFRICA					
Algeria	…	181[1]	12	…	81–95
Congo, Democratic Republic of the	0.8	400	21	…	<50
Egypt	2.4	6,418	20	…	81–95
Ethiopia	5.1	86	3	…	50–80
Kenya	11.0	877	14	…	50–80
Morocco	2.9	201[2]	10[2]	63.8[2]	50–80
Nigeria	1.0	11,588	12	…	<50
South Africa	…	834[3]	39[3]	…	50–80
Sudan, The	…	…	8	…	<50
Tanzania	6.0	173	10	…	50–80
NORTH AMERICA					
Canada	4.9	1,079	50	…	>95
Mexico	2.2	1,539	10	64.7[1]	50–80
United States	23.4	6,580	46	64.6[4]	>95
SOUTH AMERICA					
Argentina	2.0	…	44	51.9[1]	81–95
Brazil	5.3	6,372	34	…	50–80
Colombia	5.4	947	14	57.2	50–80
Peru	6.0	427	17	…	50–80
Venezuela	10.0	610	26	69.7[1]	50–80
ASIA					
Bangladesh	5.0	903	3	…	50–80
China	0.3	67,857	26	69.0	50–80
India	1.7	15,067	7	…	50–80
Indonesia	3.3	971	6	…	50–80
Iran	8.9	653	15	…	81–95
Iraq	…	185	14	42.4	50–80
Japan	1.6	9,844	136	…	>95
Korea, North	…	…	135	…	50–80
Korea, South	0.5	…	32[5]	73.7[5]	>95
Malaysia	6.0	306	18	…	81–95
Myanmar (Burma)	4.0	717	6	…	<50
Nepal	5.0	114	3	…	<50
Pakistan	1.0	10,905	6	…	50–80
Philippines	3.0	1,723	11	62.1	50–80
Saudi Arabia	6.0	279	23	…	>95
Taiwan	…	828	49	…	50–80
Thailand	7.9	1,097	17	…	50–80
Turkey	2.6	962	22	…	>95
Uzbekistan	…	1,355	97	…	50–80
Vietnam	…	12,500	27	…	50–80
EUROPE					
France	21.7	3,810	118	75.1	>95
Germany	18.0	2,354	77	82.8	>95
Italy	11.3	1,912	67	72.5	>95
Poland	…	752	63	72.5	81–95
Romania	8.1	…	95	…	81–95
Russia	1.7	12,265	119	83.2	50–80
Spain	6.1	813	42	76.7	>95
Sweden	0.3	…	60	83.0	>95
Ukraine	…	3,900	130	…	81–95
United Kingdom	14.0	2,423	54	80.6	>95
OCEANIA					
Australia	13.4	1,071[6]	93[6]	…	>95
New Zealand	15.6	330	68	60.7[1]	>95

[1]Government hospitals only.

[2]Public sector only.

[3]Data exclude the former African independent states of Bophuthatswana, Ciskei, Transkei, and Venda.

[4]5,261 community hospitals only.

[5]General and specialized hospitals only.

[6]General hospitals only.

Sources: International Monetary Fund, *Government Finance Statistics Yearbook* (1996); UNICEF, *The State of the World's Children 1997;* national statistical offices.

Persons per Doctor
(World average: 720)

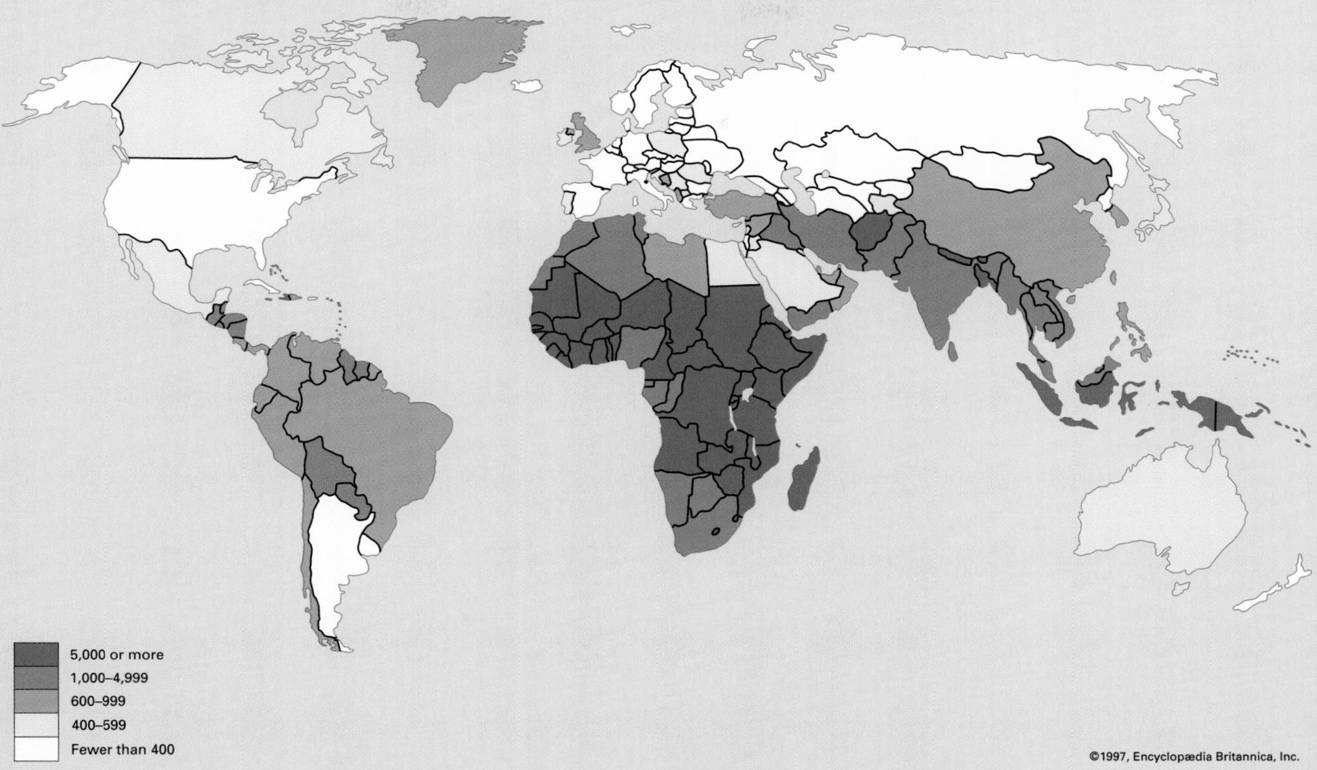

AIDS Cases Reported to WHO by Continent per Year Based on Reports Received Through Nov. 20, 1996

	New Cases						Cumulative Cases					
Year	Africa	Americas	Asia	Europe	Oceania	TOTALS	Africa	Americas	Asia	Europe	Oceania	TOTALS
1979	0	2	0	3	0	5	0	2	0	3	0	5
1980	0	185	1	7	0	193	0	187	1	10	0	198
1981	0	322	1	31	0	354	0	509	2	41	0	552
1982	2	1,156	1	90	91	1,340	2	1,665	3	131	91	1,892
1983	34	3,352	8	299	6	3,699	36	5,017	11	430	97	5,591
1984	199	6,680	8	732	76	7,695	235	11,697	19	1,162	173	13,286
1985	893	12,682	26	1,915	141	15,657	1,128	24,379	45	3,077	314	28,943
1986	5,038	21,322	85	3,897	251	30,593	6,166	45,701	130	6,974	565	59,536
1987	16,867	34,562	141	7,200	320	59,091	23,033	80,263	272	14,174	885	118,627
1988	28,234	47,697	158	10,852	598	87,539	51,267	127,960	430	25,026	1,483	206,166
1989	41,209	56,137	277	14,424	705	112,752	92,476	184,097	707	39,450	2,188	318,918
1990	54,448	65,051	540	17,436	779	138,254	146,924	249,148	1,247	56,886	2,967	457,172
1991	71,668	79,817	877	19,122	908	172,392	218,592	328,965	2,124	76,008	3,875	629,564
1992	71,946	101,969	2,117	20,990	871	197,893	290,538	430,934	4,241	96,998	4,746	827,457
1993	70,106	103,844	7,583	22,584	905	205,022	360,644	534,778	11,824	119,582	5,651	1,032,479
1994	68,025	92,957	14,665	25,117	1,006	201,770	428,669	627,735	26,489	144,699	6,657	1,234,249
1995	98,689	63,921	20,802	23,264	796	207,472	527,358	691,656	47,291	167,963	7,453	1,441,721
1996[1]	21,875	56,538	6,741	11,031	181	96,366	549,233	748,194	54,032	178,994	7,634	1,538,087
TOTALS	549,233	748,194	54,032	178,994	7,634	1,538,087	549,233	748,194	54,032	178,994	7,634	1,538,087

[1]Partial data.

Lifestyle-Related Mortality per 100,000 Population (Selected Countries)

	Cirrhosis of the liver		Diabetes mellitus		Atherosclerosis		Suicide		Motor vehicle accidents		Homicide	
	Males	Females	Males	Females	Males	Females	Males	Females	Males	Females	Males	Females
AFRICA												
Algeria	...	...	...	...	...	...	...	...	...	...	...	...
Congo, Democratic Republic of the	...	...	...	...	...	...	...	...	...	...	...	...
Egypt	–8.1–		–9.0–		...	...	–0.1–		–6.6–		–0.5–	
Ethiopia	...	...	...	...	...	...	...	...	...	...	...	...
Kenya	...	...	...	...	...	...	...	...	...	...	...	...
Morocco	...	...	...	...	...	...	...	...	...	...	...	...
Nigeria	...	...	...	...	...	...	...	...	...	...	...	...
South Africa[1]	8.5[2]	3.8[2]	15.5	26.1	...	...	8.4	2.2	32.5	11.3	36.2	7.4
Sudan, The	...	...	...	...	...	...	...	...	...	...	...	...
Tanzania	...	...	...	...	...	...	...	...	...	...	...	...
NORTH AMERICA												
Canada	10.2[2]	5.3[2]	16.3	18.4	5.5	8.1	21.0	5.4	16.1	7.6	2.5	1.2
Mexico	35.3[2]	10.3[2]	28.6	37.0	1.3	1.7	4.5	0.7	25.2	6.7	32.2	7.4
United States	12.9[2]	6.5[2]	20.4	24.6	5.0	7.7	19.8	4.4	22.7	10.6	13.8	3.8
SOUTH AMERICA												
Argentina	16.6[2]	5.2[2]	16.5	18.2	20.4	30.8	10.5	4.4	14.7	5.0	9.0	1.8
Brazil	–11.7–		–18.0–		...	...	7.4	2.1	31.2	8.9	130.6	9.0
Colombia[3]	6.0[2]	2.8[2]	9.9	16.2	4.2	5.6	7.4	2.1	31.2	8.9	130.6	9.0
Peru	–10.4–		–8.1–		...	...	–1.0–		–7.9–		–5.2–	
Venezuela	10.4[2]	3.7[2]	11.4	14.5	2.3	3.6	6.6	1.5	38.0	9.5	13.9	1.3
ASIA												
Bangladesh	...	...	...	...	...	...	...	...	...	...	...	...
China	21.1	11.6	4.6	6.0	...	...	23.7[4]	30.5[4]	16.5	7.0	5.2	3.7
India	24.5	10.6	11.2	13.3	...	...	...	...	28.3	12.2	7.5	5.5
Indonesia	...	...	...	...	...	...	...	...	...	...	...	...
Iran	...	...	...	...	...	...	...	...	...	...	...	...
Iraq	...	...	...	...	...	...	...	...	...	...	...	...
Japan	18.4[2]	8.3[2]	8.7	8.9	1.1	1.3	23.1	10.9	15.8	6.3	0.8	0.5
Korea, North	...	...	...	...	...	...	...	...	...	...	...	...
Korea, South	42.1[2]	9.6[2]	17.2	16.0	1.8	2.1	12.8	6.1	48.7	17.4	2.1	1.1
Malaysia	...	...	...	...	...	...	...	...	...	...	...	...
Myanmar (Burma)	...	...	...	...	...	...	...	...	...	...	...	...
Nepal	...	...	...	...	...	...	...	...	...	...	...	...
Pakistan	...	...	...	...	...	...	...	...	...	...	...	...
Philippines	7.5[2]	2.0[2]	5.5	6.3	2.9	3.3	0.9	0.4	6.6	2.9	0.3	0.4
Saudi Arabia	...	...	...	...	...	...	...	...	...	...	...	...
Taiwan	–21.0[2]–		–34.0–		...	...	...	...	...	...	...	...
Thailand	...	...	–6.2–		...	...	...	...	...	...	...	...
Turkey[5]	3.6	1.8	4.3	6.3	...	...	1.1	0.4	10.6	4.2	...	...
Uzbekistan	21.4	19.3	8.9	9.1	...	...	9.3	3.2	16.0	4.2	6.9	1.7
Vietnam	...	...	...	...	...	...	...	...	...	...	...	...
EUROPE												
France	22.6[2]	10.0[2]	9.5	13.2	2.3	2.4	31.6	11.5	22.4	8.1	1.4	0.8
Germany	32.7[2]	16.4[2]	18.8	35.8	14.9	30.6	22.9	8.6	17.3	5.9	1.5	0.9
Italy	33.1[2]	18.8[2]	24.5	40.7	15.7	23.8	12.1	4.1	26.6	7.6	3.9	0.6
Poland	16.7[2]	7.4[2]	10.4	17.5	168.0	234.9	24.7	4.5	29.9	7.6	4.5	1.6
Romania	50.1	28.6	9.4	10.9	83.0	106.0	18.5	4.9	23.5	6.8	7.5	2.5
Russia	16.9	10.9	5.6	11.6	45.7	82.0	65.9	12.9	49.9	13.4	49.3	13.5
Spain	27.4[2]	11.1[2]	15.7	27.9	15.4	26.4	11.0	3.4	26.7	7.9	1.3	0.5
Sweden	9.1[2]	4.0[2]	17.7	20.4	23.4	33.9	22.2	9.5	9.2	4.4	1.8	0.8
Ukraine	...	...	2.2	3.6	15.3	21.2	37.7	9.1	19.4	5.2	6.9	3.3
United Kingdom	7.9[2]	5.4[2]	10.5	11.7	3.1	6.4	11.9	3.3	9.1	3.8	1.4	0.6
OCEANIA												
Australia	8.3[2]	3.1[2]	14.6	14.5	3.4	6.2	18.7	4.5	15.8	6.3	2.4	1.3
New Zealand	4.6[2]	2.6[2]	13.3	13.2	2.3	3.4	20.5	5.4	25.1	10.2	1.9	0.8

[1]Estimates based on 60% of total deaths.
[2]Includes chronic liver disease.
[3]Estimates based on 75% of total deaths.
[4]Selected rural areas.
[5]Province and district capitals only.

Sources: WHO, *World Health Statistics 1995;* national statistical offices.

Environmental Pollution of the World

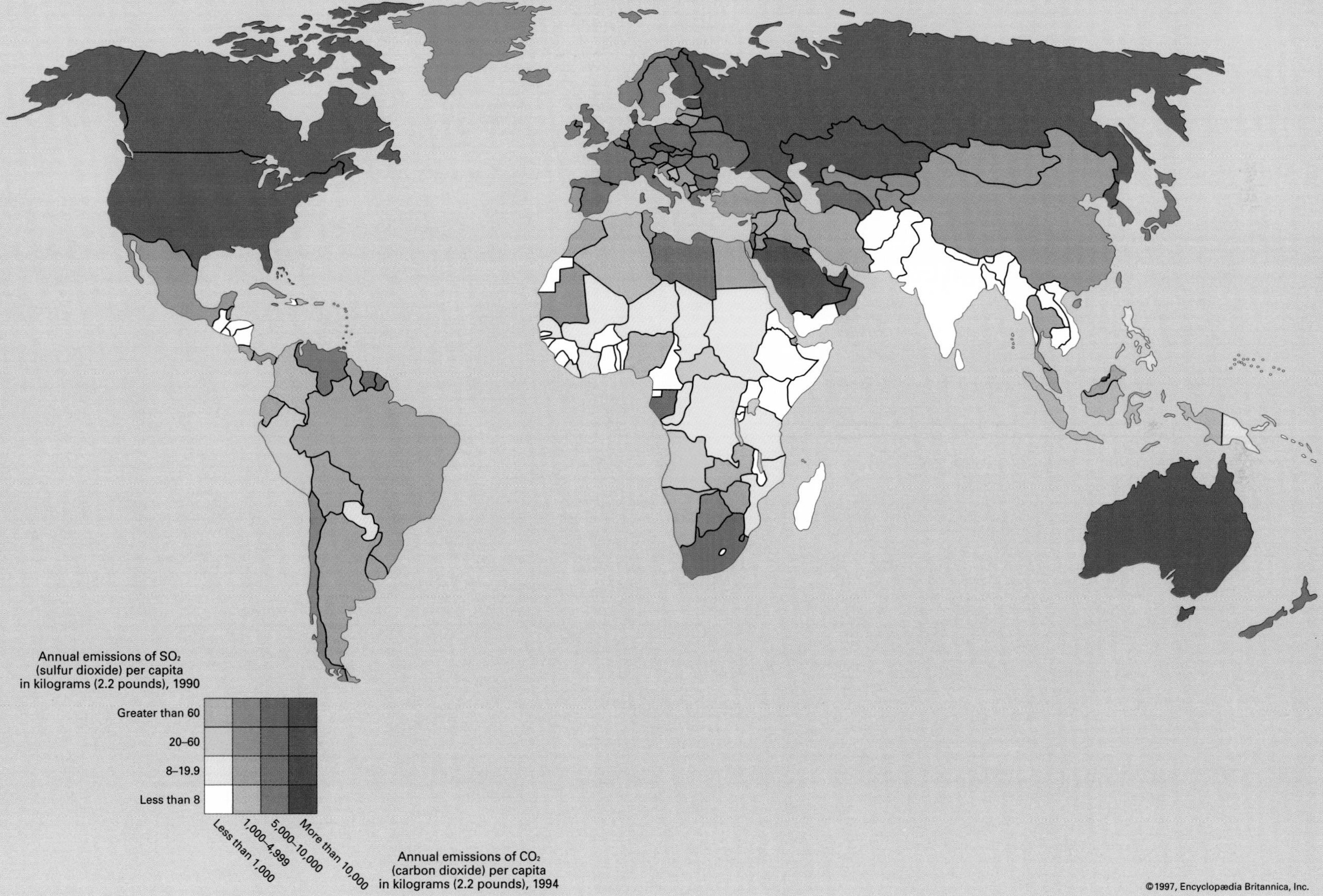

Annual emissions of SO_2 (sulfur dioxide) per capita in kilograms (2.2 pounds), 1990

Greater than 60
20–60
8–19.9
Less than 8

Less than 1,000
1,000–4,999
5,000–10,000
More than 10,000

Annual emissions of CO_2 (carbon dioxide) per capita in kilograms (2.2 pounds), 1994

United States, Deaths due to Injury, 1995
Selected causes by type of accident or manner of injury

TOTAL DEATHS DUE TO INJURIES	150,809
UNINTENTIONAL INJURIES/ACCIDENTS	91,437
Transport accidents	45,805
Railway	569
Highway	43,574
Water	762
Air and space	851
Poisoning and medical mishap	11,784
Drugs (licit and illicit), medications, and biologics	8,000
Gases and vapors	611
Complications of medical and surgical care	2,712
Falls	13,986
Fire	3,761
Lightning	87
Other accidents	17,612
Drowning	3,790
Inhalation and ingestion of food or other object	3,185
Firearm	1,225
Handgun	233
Other	992
Explosive material	170
Hot substance or object, corrosive material, and steam	97
Electric current	559
Adverse effects of drugs in therapeutic use	206
SUICIDE	31,284
HOMICIDE	22,552
Assault by firearm	15,551
Assault by cutting and piercing instrument	2,780
OTHER	5,536

Source: National Center for Health Statistics.

United States, National Health Care Expenditures by Kind, 1995

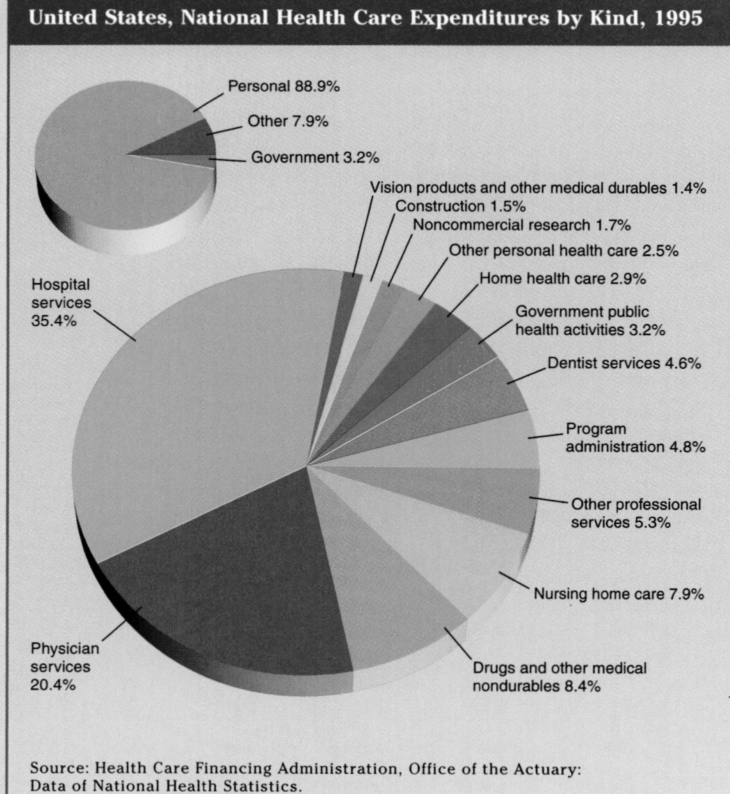

Source: Health Care Financing Administration, Office of the Actuary: Data of National Health Statistics.

United States,[1] Physicians by Specialty,[2] 1995

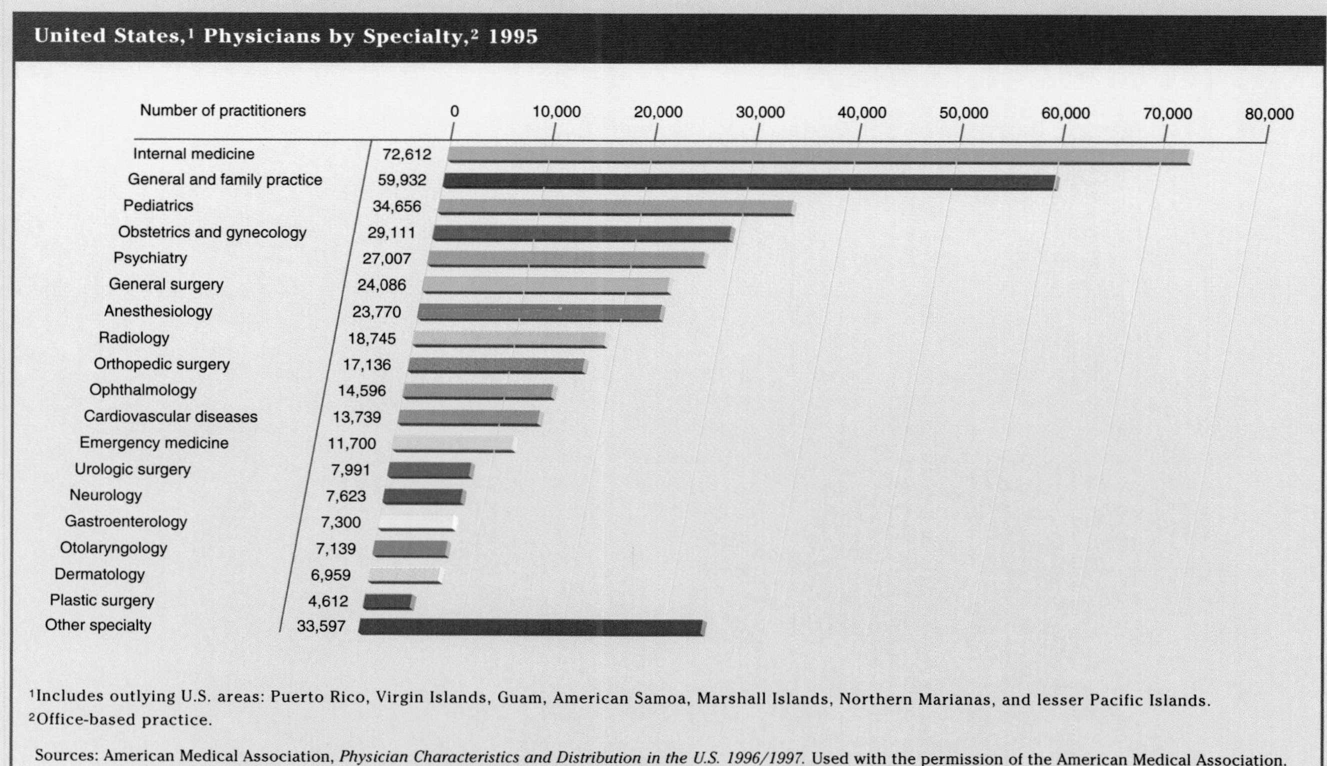

[1]Includes outlying U.S. areas: Puerto Rico, Virgin Islands, Guam, American Samoa, Marshall Islands, Northern Marianas, and lesser Pacific Islands.
[2]Office-based practice.

Sources: American Medical Association, *Physician Characteristics and Distribution in the U.S. 1996/1997.* Used with the permission of the American Medical Association.

Every Day in America

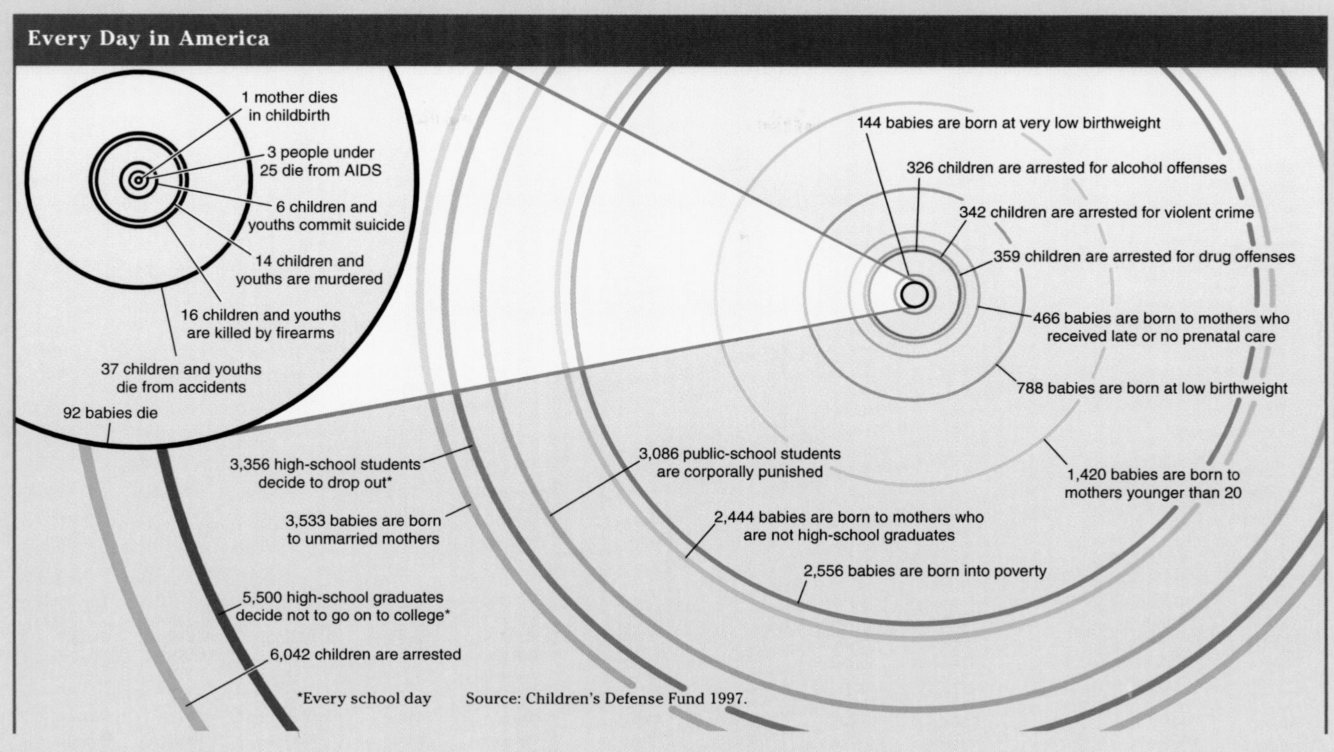
1 mother dies in childbirth
3 people under 25 die from AIDS
6 children and youths commit suicide
14 children and youths are murdered
16 children and youths are killed by firearms
37 children and youths die from accidents
92 babies die
144 babies are born at very low birthweight
326 children are arrested for alcohol offenses
342 children are arrested for violent crime
359 children are arrested for drug offenses
466 babies are born to mothers who received late or no prenatal care
788 babies are born at low birthweight
1,420 babies are born to mothers younger than 20
3,086 public-school students are corporally punished
2,444 babies are born to mothers who are not high-school graduates
2,556 babies are born into poverty
3,356 high-school students decide to drop out*
3,533 babies are born to unmarried mothers
5,500 high-school graduates decide not to go on to college*
6,042 children are arrested

*Every school day Source: Children's Defense Fund 1997.

Children Without Health Insurance in the U.S.

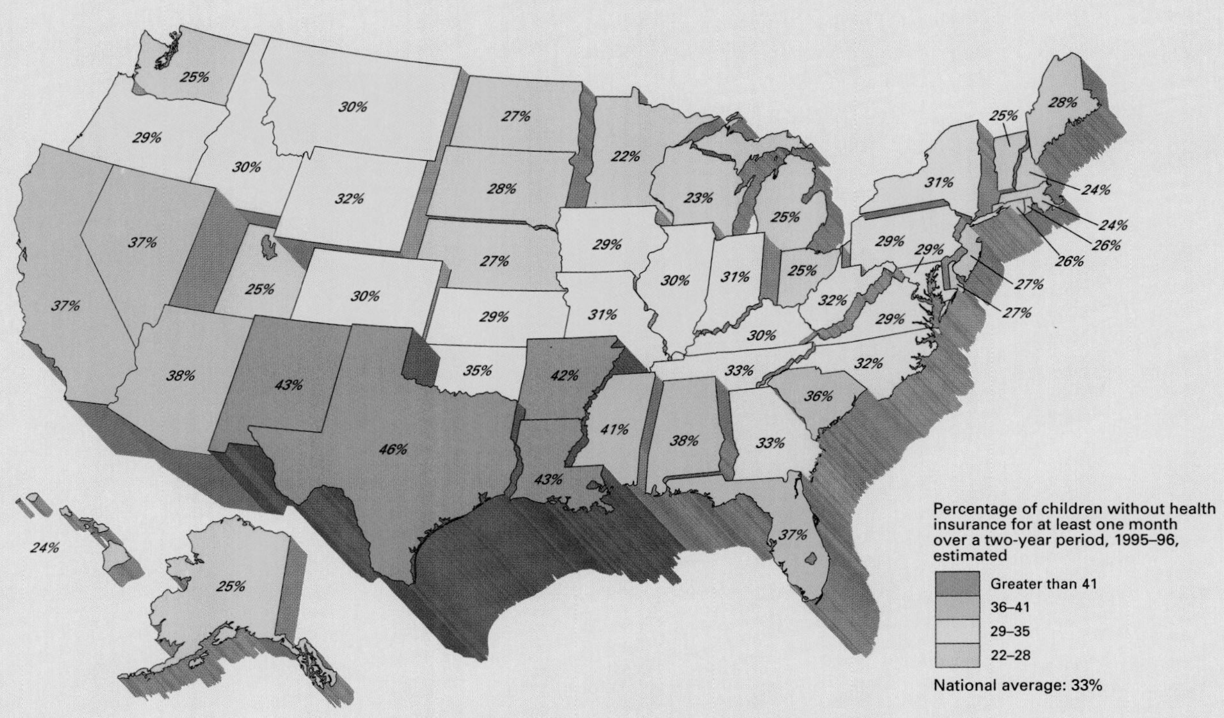
25%
29%
30%
30%
27%
32%
28%
22%
23%
25%
31%
28%
25%
24%
24%
26%
26%
37%
37%
25%
30%
27%
29%
29%
29%
30%
31%
25%
32%
29%
27%
27%
29%
31%
30%
33%
32%
38%
43%
35%
42%
36%
46%
41%
38%
33%
43%
37%
24%
25%
Percentage of children without health insurance for at least one month over a two-year period, 1995–96, estimated
Greater than 41
36–41
29–35
22–28
National average: 33%

Sports Participation in America

Number of Athletes (in millions) Seven Years of Age and Older Who Participated More than Once

SPORT	1996	1995	1994	1993	1992	1991	1990	1989	1988	1987	1986	1985
Exercise walking	73.3	70.3	70.8	64.4	67.8	69.6	71.4	66.6	62.3	58.1	53.5	41.5
Swimming	60.2	61.5	60.3	61.4	63.1	66.2	67.5	70.5	71.1	66.1	72.6	73.3
Bicycle riding	53.3	56.3	49.8	47.9	54.6	54.0	55.3	56.9	53.8	53.2	49.7	50.7
Exercising with equipment	47.8	44.3	43.8	34.9	39.4	39.2	35.3	31.5	28.9	34.8	32.0	32.1
Fishing	45.6	44.2	45.7	51.2	47.6	47.0	46.9	46.5	45.7	45.8	47.5	...
Camping	44.7	42.8	42.9	42.7	47.3	47.1	46.2	46.5	42.3	44.2	41.2	46.4
Bowling	42.9	41.9	37.4	41.3	42.5	40.4	40.1	40.8	37.9	40.1	34.2	35.7
Billiards/pool	34.5	31.1	34.0	29.4	29.3	29.6	28.1	29.6	32.4	29.3	...	23.0
Basketball	33.3	30.1	28.2	29.6	28.2	26.2	26.3	26.2	23.1	25.1	21.2	18.5
Boating (motor/power)	28.8	26.8	26.4	20.7	22.3	22.4	28.6	29.0	32.5	30.9	25.5	26.6
Hiking	26.5	25.0	25.3	19.5	21.6	22.7	22.0	23.5	19.9	17.4	17.0	21.1
Roller skating–in-line	25.5	23.9	19.5	12.4	9.7	7.3	3.6	...	...	...	...	...
Aerobic exercising	24.1	23.1	23.2	24.9	27.8	25.9	23.3	25.1	24.2	23.1	21.9	23.9
Golf	23.1	24.0	24.6	22.6	24.0	24.7	23.0	23.2	22.7	20.3	20.0	18.5
Running/jogging	22.2	20.6	20.6	20.3	21.9	22.5	23.8	24.8	22.9	24.8	23.1	26.3
Dart throwing	21.3	19.8	21.2	19.2	18.8	17.0	16.4	17.4	17.8	13.1	9.0	9.4
Softball	19.9	17.6	18.1	17.9	19.2	19.6	20.1	22.1	20.6	21.6	20.9	21.6
Hunting with firearms	19.3	17.4	16.4	18.5	17.8	17.1	18.5	17.7	...	...	...	...
Volleyball	18.5	18.0	17.4	20.5	22.1	22.6	23.2	25.1	22.0	23.6	20.7	20.1
Target shooting	15.7	13.9	12.2	12.8	12.3	11.5	12.8	...	...	...	...	...

Source: National Sporting Goods Association.

Environmental Pollution of the U.S.

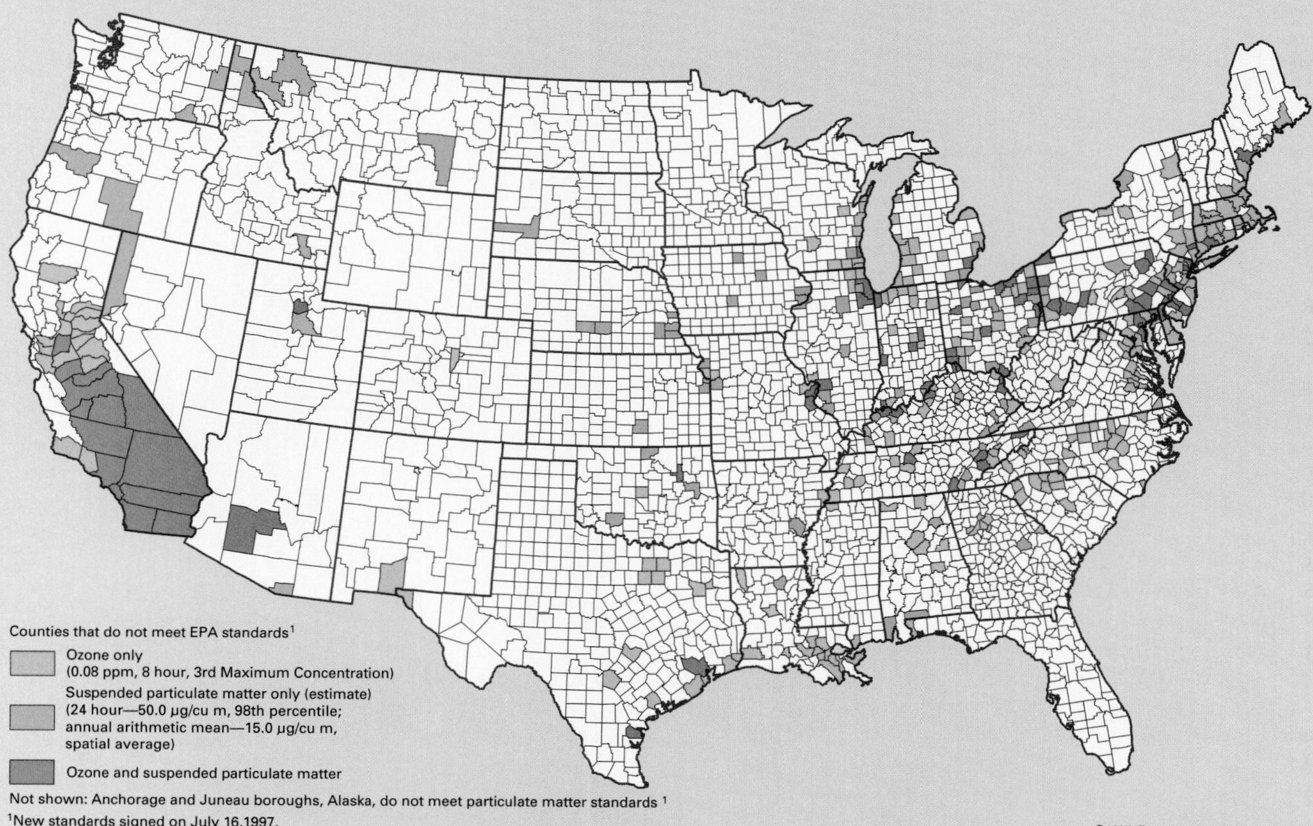

Not shown: Anchorage and Juneau boroughs, Alaska, do not meet particulate matter standards [1]

[1]New standards signed on July 16,1997.

Contributors to the World of Medicine

George J. Annas, J.D., M.P.H.
Assisted Suicide: No Constitutional Right
Edward R. Utley Professor of Health Law; Chair, Health Law Department; and Director, Law, Medicine, and Ethics Program, Boston University Schools of Medicine and Public Health

Lawrence J. Appel, M.D., M.P.H.
Getting to the Heart of Homocysteine (coauthor)
Associate Professor of Medicine, Epidemiology, and International Health, Johns Hopkins Medical Institutions, Baltimore, Md.

Richard L. Atkinson, M.D.
Body Weight: Biology, Not Behavior (coauthor)
Professor of Medicine and Nutritional Sciences and Director, Beers-Murphy Clinical Nutrition Center, University of Wisconsin at Madison Medical School

Laura D. Attardi, Ph.D.
P53: *Key to Many Cancers* (coauthor)
Postdoctoral Fellow, Center for Cancer Research, Massachusetts Institute of Technology, Cambridge

Henri Begleiter, M.D.
The Genetics of Alcoholism
Professor of Psychiatry and Neuroscience, State University of New York Health Science Center, Brooklyn, and Director, Collaborative Study on the Genetics of Alcoholism

Jeffrey D. Bernhard, M.D.
Itching
Professor of Medicine and Director, Division of Dermatology, University of Massachusetts Medical School, Worcester

Eric Block, Ph.D.
Is Everything Coming Up Roses for Garlic?
Professor of Chemistry, State University of New York at Albany

Lester E. Block, D.D.S., M.P.H.
Deconstructing Managed Care
Director, Graduate Studies in Public Health, School of Public Health, University of Minnesota, Minneapolis

Robert F. Breiman, M.D.
Adolescent and Adult Immunization (coauthor)
Director, National Vaccine Program Office, Centers for Disease Control and Prevention, Atlanta, Ga.

Malcolm K. Brenner, M.B., Ph.D.
Placental Blood Transplantation (coauthor)
Director, Cell and Gene Therapy Program, St. Jude Children's Research Hospital, Memphis, Tenn.

Francesco P. Cappuccio, M.D., M.Sc.
Salt: Shake the Habit? (coauthor)
Senior Lecturer in Medicine, St. George's Hospital Medical School, London

Jonathan M. Chen, M.D.
Cutting-Edge Heart Surgeries (coauthor)
Cardiothoracic Surgery Research Fellow, Department of Surgery, Division of Cardiothoracic Surgery, Columbia-Presbyterian Medical Center, New York City

James I. Cleeman, M.D.
Cholesterol Counts—More than Ever
Coordinator, National Cholesterol Education Program, National Heart, Lung, and Blood Institute, National Institutes of Health, Bethesda, Md. (article written in private capacity; no official support or endorsement by the National Heart, Lung, and Blood Institute or the National Institutes of Health is intended or should be inferred)

Marvin Cohen, D.D.S.
Help for Halitosis
Dentist in private practice; Chairman of the Board, Dental Science Corp.; President and Chief Executive Officer, A-H Clinic (sponsor of Antihalitosis Seminars); Past President and Chief Executive Officer, Ident Corp. of America; Past President, Neuromuscular Stress Management Consultants; and former faculty member, Washington University Dental School, St. Louis, Mo.

Ann C. Collier, M.D.
AIDS/HIV Update (coauthor)
Professor of Medicine, University of Washington School of Medicine, and Director, University of Washington AIDS Clinical Trials Unit, Seattle

Rick Curran
One Bold Plan for an AIDS Vaccine
Director of Communications, Albert B. Sabin Vaccine Foundation, New Canaan, Conn.

Nancy E. Davidson, M.D.
Hormone Replacement Therapy in Perspective
Breast Cancer Research Chair in Oncology, Johns Hopkins University School of Medicine, Baltimore, Md.

Peter Davies, Ph.D.
Alzheimer's Disease Update
Judith and Burton P. Resnick Professor of Alzheimer's Disease Research; Professor of Pathology and Neurosciences; and Director, Neurological Surgery Research, Albert Einstein College of Medicine of Yeshiva University, Bronx, N.Y.

Charles Deutsch, Sc.D.
College Crisis: Booze Before Books (coauthor)
Instructor in Health and Social Behavior, Harvard School of Public Health, Boston, and Director, National Committee on Higher Education and the Health of Youth

Nikhil V. Dhurandhar, Ph.D.
Body Weight: Biology, Not Behavior (coauthor)
Assistant Research Scientist, Department of Medicine, Clinical Nutrition Section, University of Wisconsin at Madison Medical School

John Easton
NewsCap: *Glimmer of Hope for Old Eyes*
Freelance writer and Director, Media Relations, University of Chicago Medical Center

Marc K. Effron, M.D.
Cardiovascular Disease Update
Director, Non-Invasive Cardiology, Scripps Memorial Hospital, and Clinical Assistant Professor, University of California, San Diego, School of Medicine, La Jolla

John W. Erdman, Jr., Ph.D.
Carotenoids: Can Carrots Prevent Cancer, Cataracts, and Coronaries? (coauthor)
Professor, Food Science and Human Nutrition, and Director, Division of Nutritional Sciences, University of Illinois at Urbana-Champaign

Kevin V. Ergil, M.A., M.S., L.Ac.
Acupuncture in the U.S.
Dean, Pacific Institute of Oriental Medicine, and acupuncturist and herbalist in private practice, New York City

Geoffrey Evans, M.D.
Safety Issues: The Paradox of Effective Vaccines (coauthor)
Chief Medical Officer, National Vaccine Injury Compensation Program, Health Resources and Services Administration, Rockville, Md.

Danielle Foullon
New Drugs Approved by the Food and Drug Administration, January 1996–July 1997
Assistant Managing Editor, *"The Pink Sheet"—Prescription Pharmaceuticals and Biotechnology,* FDC Reports, Chevy Chase, Md.

Floyd J. Fowler, Jr., Ph.D.
Taking the Pulse of the U.S. Population
Senior Research Fellow, Center for Survey Research, University of Massachusetts, Boston

Barry A. Franklin, Ph.D.
Sex and the Heart (coauthor)
Director, Cardiac Rehabilitation and Exercise Laboratories, William Beaumont Hospital, Royal Oak, Mich., and Professor of Physiology, Wayne State University School of Medicine, Detroit

M.J. Friedrich
Genetics Update
Associate Editor, Encyclopædia Britannica, Inc., Chicago

Bruce G. Gellin, M.D., M.P.H.
Adolescent and Adult Immunization (coauthor)
Medical Officer, Division of Microbiology and Infectious Diseases, National Institute of Allergy and Infectious Diseases, National Institutes of Health, Bethesda, Md.

Herman J. Gibb, Ph.D., M.P.H.
Arsenic-Tainted Drinking Water: Crisis in India and Bangladesh
Assistant Center Director, National Center for Environmental Assessment, U.S. Environmental Protection Agency, Washington, D.C.

John R. Gilbert, M.A.
Placental Blood Transplantation (coauthor)
Freelance biomedical editor-writer and Senior Consulting Editor, St. Jude Children's Research Hospital, Memphis, Tenn.

Katherine I. Gordon
NewsCap: *Ashes to Ashes: Tobacco and Health Update*
Editorial Coordinator, Encyclopædia Britannica, Inc., Chicago

Robert C. Hastings, M.D., Ph.D.
Leprosy at Century's End
Editor, *International Journal of Leprosy;* formerly Chief, Laboratory Research Branch, Gillis W. Long Hansen's Disease Center, Carville, La.

Sherman Hollar
NewsCaps: *Something to Wheeze About; Unforgettable Ewe: A Breakthrough in Cloning; Exercising Caution: Concussions and Athletes; Inhaler Users Holding Their Breath; Grapefruit's Powerful Punch*
Assistant Editor, Encyclopædia Britannica, Inc., Chicago

Donald R. Hopkins, M.D., M.P.H.
NewsCap: *Disease Eradication: Progress Report*
Associate Executive Director for Control and Eradication of Disease, The Carter Center, Atlanta, Ga.

Tyler Jacks, Ph.D.
P53: *Key to Many Cancers* (coauthor)
Associate Investigator, Howard Hughes Medical Institute, and Associate Professor of Biology, Center for Cancer Research, Massachusetts Institute of Technology, Cambridge

Dave Kajganish, W.F.R.
Medicine in the Middle of Nowhere
Lead Instructor for Hurricane Island Outward Bound School, Rockland, Me., and freelance writer

Warren A. Katz, M.D.
Rheumatic and Musculoskeletal Disorders Update
NewsCap: *Osteoarthritis: No Easy Answers*
Chief, Division of Rheumatology, Presbyterian Medical Center, University of Pennsylvania Health System; Clinical Professor of Medicine, University of Pennsylvania School of Medicine; and Director, The Philadelphia Osteoporosis Center

Steven J. Kittner, M.D., M.P.H.
Getting to the Heart of Homocysteine (coauthor)
Associate Professor of Neurology, Epidemiology, and Preventive Medicine, University of Maryland School of Medicine, Baltimore

Stephen Lock, M.D.
Britain's Health Service Pushes 50
Research Fellow, Wellcome Institute for the History of Medicine, London; and Medical Adviser, *Medical and Health Annual,* Encyclopædia Britannica, Inc.

Graham A. MacGregor, M.A.
Salt: Shake the Habit? (coauthor)
Professor of Cardiovascular Medicine, St. George's Hospital Medical School, London

Afrodite Mantzavrakos
UNICEF—50 Remarkable Years
NewsCaps: *A Tangled Web: Medical Advice in Cyberspace; Selling Kids on Poor Eating Habits; Diabetes Redefined; Zinc: Latest Weapon in the "Cold War"?*
Copy Editor, Encyclopædia Britannica, Inc., Chicago

Robert E. Michler, M.D.
Cutting-Edge Heart Surgeries (coauthor)
Director, Cardiac Transplantation Service, Division of Cardiothoracic Surgery, Columbia-Presbyterian Medical Center, and Associate Professor of Surgery and Director, Transplantation Research Laboratory, Columbia University College of Physicians and Surgeons, New York City

Amy C. Moore, B.S.
Carotenoids: Can Carrots Prevent Cancer, Cataracts, and Coronaries? (coauthor)
Graduate Research Assistant, Division of Nutritional Sciences, University of Illinois at Urbana-Champaign

Frances Munnings
Sex and the Heart (coauthor)
Freelance medical writer and editor, Minneapolis, Minn.

Gilbert S. Omenn, M.D., Ph.D.
Report Card on the Environment (coauthor)
Dean, School of Public Health and Community Medicine, University of Washington, Seattle, and Chair, Presidential/Congressional Commission on Risk Assessment and Risk Management

Jason M. Omenn
Report Card on the Environment (coauthor)
Researcher–Sales Representative, Environmental Home Center, Seattle, Wash.; formerly Research Associate, Northwest Pollution Prevention Resource Center

Jackie Orihill
NewsCaps: *Pedestrians in Peril; Puberty in U.S. Girls—New Norms; In-Line in the ER; Cardiac Emergencies: Nothing to Be Up in the Air About*
Index Editor, Encyclopædia Britannica, Inc., Chicago

Sandra Crouse Quinn, Ph.D.
Spreading the Gospel of AIDS Prevention (coauthor)
NewsCap: *Presidential Apology for the Study at Tuskegee* (coauthor)
Assistant Professor, Department of Health Behavior and Health Education, School of Public Health, University of North Carolina at Chapel Hill

N. Regina Rabinovich, M.D., M.P.H.
Safety Issues: The Paradox of Effective Vaccines (coauthor)
Chief, Clinical Studies Section, Division of Microbiology and Infectious Diseases, National Institute of Allergy and Infectious Diseases, National Institutes of Health, Bethesda, Md.

Alan M. Rapoport, M.D.
Making Headway Against Migraine
Director, The New England Center for Headache, Stamford, Conn.; Assistant Clinical Professor, Yale University School of Medicine, New Haven, Conn.; author, *Headache Relief,* and coauthor, *Headache Relief for Women: How You Can Manage and Prevent Pain* and *Headache Disorders: A Management Guide for Practitioners*

Robert Rauch
NewsCaps: *Hitting Stroke Below the Belt; Reality Bites; Hazards on the Highway*
Freelance editor and writer, Chicago

William Reed, M.D.
Sickle-Cell Disease Update (coauthor)
Fellow in Pediatric Hematology and Transfusion Medicine, Children's Hospital Medical Center, Oakland, Calif., and Irwin Memorial Blood Centers, San Francisco

Wade Roush, Ph.D.
Link...No Link; Stress and the Blood-Brain Barrier
Writer-reporter, *Science* magazine, Brookline, Mass.

Cristine Russell
NewsCaps: *Cancer Deaths: A Turning Point?; Selenium: A Supplement to Watch; Making Sense of the Mammography Muddle*
Freelance science writer, Darien, Conn., and Special Health Correspondent, *Washington Post*

Andrew A. Skolnick, M.S.
Traditional Chinese Medicine Under Scrutiny
Associate Editor, *Journal of the American Medical Association,* Chicago

Michael O. Smith, M.D.
Acupuncture in Addiction Treatment
Director, Substance Abuse Division, Lincoln Medical and Mental Health Center, Bronx, N.Y., and Assistant Professor of Psychiatry and Community Medicine, New York Medical College, Valhalla

David H. Spach, M.D.
AIDS/HIV Update (coauthor)
Associate Professor of Medicine, University of Washington School of Medicine, Seattle

Stephen B. Thomas, Ph.D.
Spreading the Gospel of AIDS Prevention (coauthor)
NewsCap: *Presidential Apology for the Study at Tuskegee* (coauthor)
Associate Professor, Department of Behavioral Sciences and Health Education, and Director, Institute for Minority Health Research, Rollins School of Public Health of Emory University, Atlanta, Ga.

Judith Anne Turow, M.D.
Pediatric Perspective on a "Lousy" Problem
Clinical Assistant Professor of Pediatrics, Jefferson Medical College, Philadelphia, and Fellow, American Academy of Pediatrics

Elliott P. Vichinsky, M.D.
Sickle-Cell Disease Update (coauthor)
Director, Department of Hematology/Oncology, Children's Hospital Medical Center, Oakland, Calif.

Jeff Wallenfeldt
NewsCaps: *Canadian Health Care: In Critical Condition?; Dr. Death's Very Still Lives; Furor over Fluoride in the U.K.*
Assistant Editor, Encyclopædia Britannica, Inc., Chicago

Henry Wechsler, Ph.D.
College Crisis: Booze Before Books (coauthor)
Director, College Alcohol Studies, Department of Health and Social Behavior, Harvard School of Public Health, Boston

Michael D. Yapko, Ph.D.
Spotlight on Brief Therapy
Clinical psychologist and marriage and family therapist in private practice, Solana Beach, Calif., and author of numerous books, including *When Living Hurts: Directives for Treating Depression, Hypnosis and the Treatment of Depressions,* and *Breaking the Patterns of Depression*

Glossary

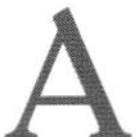

ACE inhibitor: any of a group of drugs (as captopril and enalapril) that are used to treat hypertension and heart failure and function by blocking the action of an enzyme (angiotensin converting enzyme) that affects blood vessel constriction—*also called* angiotensin converting enzyme inhibitor; *see also* hypertension

acetylcholine: a neurotransmitter that is released at the synapses of the autonomic nervous system and most neuromuscular junctions—*see also* autonomic nervous system; neurotransmitter

adrenaline: *see* epinephrine

allele: any of the different forms of a gene that can occur at a given locus, or site, on a chromosome

allogeneic: derived from or being individuals of the same species that are genetically dissimilar especially with respect to antigens; allogeneic transplants are typically recognized by the recipient's immune system as foreign and thus are rejected—*compare* syngeneic; *see also* antigen

amino acid: any of a group of over 100 organic compounds of which a subgroup of 20 are the building blocks of proteins, being joined by chemical peptide bonds to form long polypeptide chains that in turn combine with other amino acid chains; of these 20 amino acids, about half (nonessential amino acids) can be synthesized in the human body, while the remaining ones (essential amino acids) cannot be made in the body and must be obtained from the diet—*see also* peptide; protein

analgesic: any substance (as a nonsteroidal anti-inflammatory drug) that reduces sensitivity to pain without producing a loss of consciousness—*see also* nonsteroidal anti-inflammatory drug

anaphylactic: relating to, affected by, or causing a severe, sometimes fatal allergic reaction to a previously encountered substance or antigen (as penicillin or bee venom) to which the individual has become sensitized following initial contact; the reaction precipitates the release of histamine and related cellular substances into the body, which causes itching, hives, and, in more extreme cases, shortness of breath, a drop in blood pressure, and shock—*see also* antigen; histamine

androgen: any of a group of steroid hormones (as testosterone) that are produced mainly in the testes (paired male reproductive organs producing sperm) and also in minute quantities by the adrenal cortex (outer part of the adrenal glands) and ovaries (paired female reproductive organs producing eggs); induces the development of the male sex organs and male secondary sex characteristics (as facial and chest hair, deepening voice, and increase in muscle mass)—*see also* steroid; testosterone

anemia: a disorder in which the blood is deficient in red blood cells, hemoglobin, or total volume; symptoms include dizziness, fatigue, headache, difficulty in breathing during activity, and pale skin—*see also* hemoglobin; red blood cell

angina: chest pain usually due to decreased supply of oxygen to the heart muscle and generally associated with a blockage in one or both of the coronary arteries (pair of blood vessels supplying the heart)—*also called* angina pectoris

angina pectoris: *see* angina

angioplasty: a surgical procedure to widen the lumen (inner hollow portion) of a partly obstructed artery by introducing a catheter through the narrowed area, where a balloonlike attachment is inflated and then withdrawn—*also called* percutaneous transluminal angioplasty (PTA) or balloon angioplasty; *see also* catheter

angiotensin converting enzyme inhibitor: *see* ACE inhibitor

animal model: an animal similar to humans in its anatomy, physiology, or susceptibility to a pathogen and used in research to obtain results that can be applied in human medicine; also, a condition similar to a human condition or disease that occurs naturally in an animal or can be produced artificially

antibody: any of a large number of proteins that are produced by specialized cells (B cells) to attack an antigen in an immune response—*also called* immunoglobulin; *see also* antigen; protein

antigen: any substance (as a toxin, allergen, or enzyme) capable of stimulating an immune response

antioxidant: a substance (as beta-carotene) that inhibits reactions with or promoted by oxygen or peroxides and that protects the body from the effects of free radicals—*see also* beta-carotene; free radical

apoplexy: *see* stroke

apoptosis: the natural process of cell destruction that initiates an orderly breakdown and elimination of superfluous or defective cells—*also called* programmed cell death

atherosclerosis: a common condition of the arteries characterized by narrowing or obstruction due to deposits of cholesterol, fat, and other substances in the inner layer of the vessels; a major cause of angina (chest pain), heart attack, and stroke; often linked to high blood pressure, diabetes, and obesity—*see also* angina; cholesterol

autoimmune disease: a condition (as rheumatoid arthritis) caused by an immune response against the body's own tissues or cells

autologous: involving one individual as both donor and recipient (as of a tissue graft or blood transfusion)

autonomic nervous system: a part of the peripheral nervous system that activates muscular and glandular tissues (as of the stomach and heart) and governs involuntary actions (as digestion and heart rate); made up of the sympathetic and parasympathetic nervous systems—*compare* parasympathetic nervous system; peripheral nervous system; sympathetic nervous system

B

bacillus: any member of the genus *Bacillus,* a group of rod-shaped, spore-forming bacteria, some species of which cause disease in humans and animals; also, a rod-shaped bacterium of a genus other than *Bacillus*—*see also* bacterium

bacterium (plural **bacteria**): any of a group of one-celled microorganisms of different shapes (as round or spiral) that are found in soil, water, plants, and animals and may cause infection; the nature, severity, and outcome of the infection depend on the species of bacterium

balloon angioplasty: *see* angioplasty

benign: of a mild type or character, not threatening to health or life; also, not malignant—*compare* malignant

beta-adrenergic blocking agent: any of a class of drugs (as propranolol and atenolol) that block beta-receptor binding sites (as in the heart, lungs, and blood vessels) in order to inhibit the action of various substances (as epinephrine) that typically bind to and activate these receptors; used to treat and control various medical conditions, including cardiovascular disorders (as hypertension and irregular heartbeat), migraine headaches, and glaucoma—*also called* beta-blocker; *see also* beta-receptor; epinephrine; hypertension

beta-blocker: *see* beta-adrenergic blocking agent

beta-carotene: an antioxidant found in plants, mainly dark green and deep yellow vegetables and fruits (as sweet potatoes, spinach, carrots, pumpkin, and cantaloupe); converted in the body into vitamin A (retinol), an essential vitamin that aids in the prevention of night blindness and promotes healthy hair, teeth, gums, bones, skin, and mucous membranes—*see also* antioxidant

beta-receptor: any of a group of cellular sites in tissues that are supplied by the sympathetic nervous system and that bind to natural substances in the body (as epinephrine) or drugs, which results in an increase in the muscular contraction and beat of the heart and a relaxation of muscles in the bronchi (air passages leading to the lungs), intestines, and blood-vessel walls—*see also* epinephrine; sympathetic nervous system

blood-brain barrier: a physiological blockade created by the modification of capillaries (smallest blood vessels) that prevents many substances carried in the blood from crossing the capillary walls into the brain tissues

blood plasma: *see* plasma

bone marrow: a soft, vascular (supplied with blood vessels) connective tissue that occupies the cavities of most bones and occurs in two forms, one made up mostly of fat cells and whitish or yellowish in color and one containing little fat and producing red blood cells (reddish in color)—*see also* red blood cell

C

calcium: a silver-white element that is the most common mineral in the human body, found primarily in bones and teeth; critical in the prevention of certain bone diseases (as osteoporosis)

calcium channel blocker: any of a class of drugs that prevent calcium from entering smooth muscle cells (as of the heart) and thereby cause the tissue to relax; mainly used to treat cardiovascular conditions (as angina)—*see also* angina

cardiac arrest: the temporary or permanent cessation of heartbeat; often caused by myocardial infarction (heart attack)—*see also* myocardial infarction

cardiopulmonary resuscitation (CPR): an emergency medical procedure that is performed to restore normal breathing and circulation following cardiac arrest (cessation of heartbeat) and that involves clearing the airway to the lungs, mouth-to-mouth breathing, and external heart compression (depression of the victim's lower breastbone to constrict the heart and force blood into the circulatory system)—*see also* cardiac arrest

carotenoid: any of various pigments, usually of yellowish to reddish hue (as beta-carotene), that are found widely in plants and animals—*see also* beta-carotene

catheter: a tubular device for insertion into canals, vessels, or body cavities, usually to permit injection or withdrawal of fluids, to introduce and withdraw instruments, or to keep a passage open

central nervous system (CNS): the part of the nervous system that consists of the brain and spinal cord, to which sensory impulses are transmitted and from which motor impulses pass; functions as the body's main network of coordination and control—*compare* peripheral nervous system

cerebral cortex: the highly convoluted gray matter located on the outer surface of the cerebrum (the largest and most developed part of the brain) that controls higher intellectual activity and functions in the integration of sensory information and coordination of voluntary movement

cerebrovascular accident: *see* stroke

cholesterol: a fatty substance present in blood (transported in the form of lipoproteins) and body tissue that is manufactured primarily in the liver or is derived directly from certain foods (as butter or eggs) and functions as an important component of cell membranes and as a precursor of various biological substances (as steroid hormones); high levels of cholesterol in the blood are known to be associated with the development of atherosclerosis—*see also* atherosclerosis; lipoprotein; plasma; steroid

chondriosome: *see* mitochondrion

chronobiology: the study of biological rhythms; chronobiologists study the effect of time on living organisms and systems, especially in terms of cyclic or repetitive phenomena

circadian: characterized by or based on an approximately 24-hour period or cycle; circadian rhythms of living organisms are any of the repetitive biological activities or functions that occur at about the same time during every 24-hour period

clinical trial: a research activity that involves the administration of a test regimen (as a drug, vaccine, or procedure) to consenting humans to determine if the experimental treatment is safe and/or effective or to compare different regimens; typically, a specific set of criteria is used to determine the end point of the trial for each patient—*also called* therapeutic trial

CNS: *see* central nervous system

cognitive: of, relating to, or being conscious intellectual activity (as thinking, reasoning, perceiving, or remembering)

computed tomography (CT): an imaging technique involving X-rays that produces cross-sectional views of internal bodily structures—*also called* computerized tomography

concordance: the state of being similar with respect to one or more particular characteristics; used especially in reference to a pair of twins both of whom exhibit a given trait or disorder

contraindication: a condition or symptom that makes a particular treatment (as a drug) or procedure inadvisable

control group: subjects in a clinical trial or an experiment who are treated or followed as a comparison group and who typically do not receive any treatment during the investigation or who receive a standard treatment as opposed to the experimental one—*see also* clinical trial

corticosteroid: any of various steroid hormones (as cortisone) that are produced by the adrenal cortex (outer layer of the adrenal glands) and influence key biological functions in the body, including electrolyte and water balance and metabolism of carbohydrates, proteins, and lipids; the release of these hormones increases during stress, especially in anxiety and severe injury; natural and synthetic corticosteroids are used as replacement hormones in cases of deficiency caused by disease and as anti-inflammatory agents and immunosuppressants—*see also* cortisone; steroid

cortisone: a corticosteroid hormone that is produced naturally in small amounts and is used in a synthetic form (cortisone acetate) especially as a replacement hormone in cases of adrenal insufficiency and as an anti-inflammatory agent for various conditions (as rheumatoid arthritis)—*see also* corticosteroid

cowpox: a mild viral disease of cattle that is characterized by skin eruptions and that when transmitted to humans produces immunity to smallpox infection—*see also* smallpox

CPR: *see* cardiopulmonary resuscitation

CT: *see* computed tomography

cutaneous: of, relating to, or affecting the skin

D

defibrillate: to restore the normal heartbeat rhythm and rate to a heart in which the cardiac muscle of the atrium (upper heart chamber) or ventricle (lower heart chamber) is experiencing rapid and sometimes irregular contractions (as following a heart attack); a heart is defibrillated by means of a device (defibrillator) that delivers an electric shock to the heart either directly or through the chest wall

dementia: a condition of mental deterioration marked by lethargy, confusion, personality change, and a progressive decline in cognitive function, affecting memory, judgment, and reasoning

deoxyribonucleic acid: *see* DNA

diaphragm *1:* a dome-shaped sheet of muscle separating the thoracic (chest) and abdominal cavities; the diaphragm and intercostal rib muscles act together to control breathing; *2:* a flexible molded dome-shaped cap usually of thin rubber that is fitted over the uterine cervix to act as a contraceptive barrier

dioxin: any of several chemical compounds found in certain herbicides as toxic by-products formed during the manufacturing process; 2,4,5-T, an ingredient of Agent Orange (a defoliant formerly used in the U.S. and in the Vietnam War), contains an extremely toxic dioxin contaminant known as 2,3,7,8-TCDD, or 2,3,7,8-tetrachlorodibenzo-*p*-dioxin, which has been linked to serious side effects (as skin disease, muscular dysfunction, birth defects, nervous system disorders, and cancer)

diuretic: any of a class of substances that act on the kidneys to promote the formation and release of urine and are used to lessen the volume of fluid (as water) in the body

DNA (deoxyribonucleic acid): a large molecule that makes up the threadlike structures called chromosomes in the nucleus of a cell and contains the cell's genetic information

double-blind: related to or being an experimental procedure in which the identity of the test and control groups is known to neither the subjects nor the investigators during the course of the study—*see also* control group

E

endemic: restricted to or prevalent in a particular locality or region

endogenous: originating, arising, or produced within the body—*compare* exogenous

endometrium: the mucous membrane that lines the uterus and consists of three layers; thickens as the menstrual cycle progresses, and if an egg fails to implant, the two superficial layers are shed during menstruation, while the basal layer serves to regenerate the shed layers—*see also* uterus

endorphin: any of a group of proteins that occur naturally in the brain and possess potent analgesic (pain-blocking) properties

epidemic: an outbreak of disease affecting a large number of individuals within a population, community, or region at the same time—*compare* pandemic

epidemiology: a branch of medical science that deals with the incidence, distribution, and control of disease within a population

epinephrine: a colorless crystalline sympathetic-nervous-system-stimulating hormone that is secreted by the inner portion (medulla) of the adrenal glands and functions as the body's principal blood-pressure-raising hormone; used medically as a heart stimulant, vasoconstrictor (an agent that causes blood vessels to narrow), and muscle relaxant—*also called* adrenaline; *see also* sympathetic nervous system

erythrocyte: *see* red blood cell

estrogen: any of a group of steroid hormones that aid the development of female secondary sex traits (as breasts); drugs containing estrogen in natural or synthetic form are used to prevent pregnancy (as in oral contraceptives), to relieve symptoms associated with menopause (as hot flashes), and to prevent postmenopausal osteoporosis and heart disease—*compare* progestogen; progesterone; *see also* steroid

eugenics: a science concerned with the improvement of hereditary qualities of a breed or race (especially by influencing mating and reproduction)

euthanasia: the act or practice of killing hopelessly sick or injured individuals in a relatively painless way for reasons of mercy or allowing a hopelessly ill patient to die by taking less-than-complete measures to prolong life

exogenous: introduced from or produced outside the body—*compare* endogenous

F

fibrin: a white insoluble protein formed during the blood-clotting process

5-HT: *see* serotonin

folate: *see* folic acid

folic acid: a vitamin of the B-complex group that is required for normal production of red blood cells and synthesis of nucleoprotein (protein joined to nucleic acid); major food sources include green leafy vegetables, liver, dried beans, mushrooms, and whole-grain cereals—*also called* folate; *see also* red blood cell

free radical: an especially reactive atom or group of atoms possessing one or more unpaired electrons

G

gene: the physical unit of inheritance that consists of a segment of DNA and carries characteristics from parent to offspring; genes regulate the development, growth, and function of body cells and tissues—*see also* DNA

genome: the genetic material of a given individual or species

genotype: the genetic makeup of an organism as determined by the complex of genes inherited from both parents; also, the genetic constitution of one or more pairs of alleles (any of the different forms of a gene that can occur at a given locus or site on a chromosome)—*compare* phenotype; *see also* gene

graft: to surgically transplant living tissue (as skin, bone marrow, or an organ) from one part of the body to another or from one individual to another; also, the transplanted tissue itself

gram-negative: easily decolorized after treatment with an organic solvent (as alcohol or acetone) following staining with Gram's stain (a bacterial dye); gram-negative bacteria possess a thin cell wall surrounded by an outer membrane—*compare* gram-positive

gram-positive: resistant to decolorization after treatment with an organic solvent (as alcohol or acetone) following staining with Gram's stain (a bacterial dye); gram-positive bacteria possess a thick, rigid cell wall not surrounded by an outer membrane—*compare* gram-negative

H

HDL: *see* high-density lipoprotein

health maintenance organization (HMO): a public or private organization that provides comprehensive medical care to a group of voluntary subscribers on the basis of a prepaid contract and delivers those services for a fixed, prenegotiated fee

heart attack: *see* myocardial infarction

hematology: a branch of biology that deals with the blood and blood-forming organs

hematopoietic: relating to, involved in, or promoting the formation and development of blood cells in the living body

hemoglobin: the iron-containing pigment occurring in red blood cells that functions in the transport of oxygen from the lungs to tissues of the body and carbon dioxide from the tissues back to the lungs—*see also* anemia; red blood cell

hemolysis: the breakdown or destruction of red blood cells with the subsequent release of hemoglobin; may occur as a normal process affecting aged red blood cells or as an abnormal process (as in certain anemias or exposure to various chemicals and toxins)—*see also* anemia; hemoglobin; red blood cell

heterogeneity *1:* the quality or state of being heterogeneous; *2:* the production of a specific phenotype (observable trait) by more than one genetic mechanism—*see also* phenotype

heterogeneous: not uniform in structure, composition, or makeup (as a tumor or syndrome)

high blood pressure: *see* hypertension

high-density lipoprotein (HDL): a lipoprotein composed of a high proportion of protein and a low proportion of cholesterol; associated with a decreased probability of atherosclerosis and obstruction of blood vessels—*compare* low-density lipoprotein; *see also* cholesterol; lipoprotein; atherosclerosis

histamine: a substance found in body tissue that is formed by the breakdown of the amino acid histidine and is stored mainly in mast cells; released into the body in response to allergy, stress, or inflammation, causing dilation of capillaries (small blood vessels), contraction of smooth muscle (as of the lungs and uterus), and increased acid secretion in the stomach—*see also* amino acid; mast cell

hives: *see* urticaria

HMO: *see* health maintenance organization

homocysteine: an amino acid that is implicated as a factor in atherosclerosis and may function like cholesterol by contributing to the narrowing or obstruction of the arteries—*see also* amino acid; atherosclerosis; cholesterol

hypercholesterolemia: the presence of excess cholesterol in the blood; familial hypercholesterolemia is an inherited disorder marked by an increase of low-density lipoproteins in the blood plasma and their accumulation in body tissues—*see also* cholesterol; low-density lipoprotein; plasma

hypertension: a common, often asymptomatic condition in which the blood pressure (the force exerted by blood against the walls of the vessels) in either arteries or veins is abnormally high; may occur as a complication of a preexisting disorder (as of the kidneys or adrenal glands), pregnancy, or use of oral contraceptives but most often is of unknown cause; risk factors include obesity, cigarette smoking, high sodium intake, hereditary factors, and emotional or physical stress—*also called* high blood pressure

I

immunocompetent: possessing the capacity to mount a normal immune response—*compare* immunocompromised

immunocompromised: having an immune system that is impaired or weakened (as by drugs or illness)—*compare* immunocompetent

immunoglobulin: *see* antibody

incidence: the number of new instances of an illness occurring in a given time period—*compare* prevalence

inoculate: to introduce into the body, usually by means of injection, a small amount of a causative agent of disease (as a virus), an antibody, or an antigen in order to treat or prevent disease (as in vaccination); also, to introduce a microorganism into a laboratory culture in order to grow additional microorganisms for study, experimentation, or diagnostic purposes—*see also* antibody; antigen

L

LDL: *see* low-density lipoprotein

lesion: an abnormal change in the structure or function of a bodily organ or tissue due to injury or disease; may consist of gross anatomic changes visible to the unaided eye (as a cyst, nodule, or tumor), microscopic changes (as abnormally dividing cells), or biochemical changes (as abnormal antigens diagnostic of certain cancers)—*see also* antigen

leukocyte: *see* white blood cell

lipid: any of a diverse group of fats or fatlike organic compounds (as cholesterol and triglycerides) that are insoluble in water but soluble in organic solvents; lipids are stored in body tissues and serve as an energy reserve; lipids also play a role in the synthesis of important compounds in the body and are necessary for normal nervous system function; elevated lipid levels are sometimes characteristic of certain diseases (as atherosclerosis)—*see also* atherosclerosis; cholesterol; triglyceride

lipoprotein: any of a group of substances containing both lipid and protein that function in the transport of cholesterol in the blood—*see also* high-density lipoprotein; lipid; low-density lipoprotein; protein

low-density lipoprotein (LDL): a lipoprotein that is composed of a moderate proportion of protein and a high proportion of cholesterol; associated with an increased risk of atherosclerosis—*compare* high-density lipoprotein; *see also* atherosclerosis; cholesterol; lipoprotein

lycopene: the red pigment from which tomatoes and some berries and other fruits derive their characteristic color; functions as an antioxidant—*see also* antioxidant

lymphocyte: any of the white blood cells that originate from unspecialized stem cells and develop and mature in specialized lymphoid tissue (as of the bone marrow, spleen, or thymus) and are the cellular mediators of the immune system, recognizing and responding to foreign antigens; two principal types are B cells (or B lymphocytes), which secrete antibodies or serve as memory cells aiding in future recognition of antigens, and T cells (or T lymphocytes), which may assist in or suppress the production of antibodies in response to the antigen or may destroy antigen-bearing cells—*see also* antibody; antigen; stem cell; white blood cell

M

magnetic resonance imaging (MRI): a noninvasive diagnostic technique that relies on the response of individual atomic nuclei (particularly hydrogen nuclei) within an organism to powerful bursts of a magnetic field; resonant signals to a computer produce detailed images of soft body tissues that cannot be visualized by conventional X-rays or computed tomography (CT) scans

malignant: tending to produce death or deterioration by infiltration into tissue; having an unfavorable prognosis—*compare* benign

mast cell: a large cell found especially in connective tissue and containing granules that are storage sites for substances (as histamine) that mediate allergic reactions—*see also* histamine

melatonin: a hormone that is derived from serotonin and is secreted by the pineal gland, located deep within the brain; secreted especially in response to darkness and linked to the regulation of circadian rhythms—*see also* circadian; serotonin

meninges: the three membranes that cover and protect the brain and spinal cord and include the dura mater (tough fibrous outer layer), the arachnoid (delicate weblike middle layer), and the pia mater (thin inner layer supplied with blood vessels)

meta-analysis: a method of combining data from many experiments or studies to obtain statistical results that represent a synthesis of all data on a specific scientific question

metastasis: the process by which cancer cells spread to sites distant from that of the primary lesion and that results in the development of a similar lesion in a new location in the body—*see also* lesion

mitochondrion (plural **mitochondria**): a small threadlike structure that is the primary energy source of the cell—*also called* chondriosome

morbidity: a diseased state or abnormal condition; also, the rate of illness in a specific community or group

mortality: the condition of being subject to death; also, the rate of death in a specific community or group

MRI: *see* magnetic resonance imaging

myocardial infarction: damage to the heart muscle that occurs when one or more of the coronary arteries are blocked and the supply of blood to a portion of the heart muscle is interrupted; may be marked by sudden chest pain, shortness of breath, nausea, loss of consciousness, and sometimes death; risk factors include hypertension (high blood pressure), family history of cardiovascular disease, cigarette smoking, obesity, and high blood cholesterol—*also called* heart attack

N

neonatology: a branch of medicine concerned with the care, development, and diseases of newborn infants

nerve cell: *see* neuron

neuron: a nervous system cell that transmits and receives nerve impulses—*also called* nerve cell

neurotransmitter: a chemical substance (as serotonin) that transports nerve impulses across the synapses, or junctions, between neurons—*see also* serotonin; synapse

nonsteroidal anti-inflammatory drug (NSAID): a medication (as aspirin, ibuprofen, naproxen, or ketoprofen) used to relieve pain, stiffness, and inflammation, especially in conditions affecting the muscles, bones, and joints

NSAID: *see* nonsteroidal anti-inflammatory drug

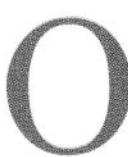

oncogene: a gene possessing the potential to cause a normal cell to become cancerous—*compare* proto-oncogene; *see also* gene

oxidation: the act or process of combining with oxygen

P

pandemic: the occurrence of a disease over a wide geographic area affecting an exceptionally high proportion of the population—*compare* epidemic

parasite: an organism living in, with, or on another organism

parasympathetic nervous system: a part of the autonomic nervous system that induces secretion, increases the tone and contractility of smooth muscle, slows the heart rate, and stimulates digestion; the neurotransmitter acetylcholine is the principal regulator of this system—*compare* autonomic nervous system; sympathetic nervous system; *see also* acetylcholine

pathogenesis: the origin and development of a disease or disease process

pathophysiology: the physical and biochemical processes underlying disturbances in a bodily function that accompany a particular syndrome or disease

PCR: *see* polymerase chain reaction

peptide: a compound that is composed of two or more amino acids joined by chemical bonds to adjacent amino acids and is usually derived from the partial breakdown of a protein—*see also* amino acid; protein

percutaneous transluminal angiography (PTA): *see* angioplasty

peripheral nervous system (PNS): the part of the nervous system external to the brain and spinal cord that carries sensory impulses to and motor impulses from the central nervous system and that comprises 12 pairs of cranial nerves arising from the brain and supplying mainly the head and neck and 31 pairs of spinal nerves arising from the spinal cord and dividing into many branches supplying mainly the trunk, arms, and legs—*compare* autonomic nervous system; central nervous system

PET: *see* positron-emission tomography

phenotype: the observable characteristics (as appearance or behavior) of an organism or group that are produced by interaction of the genotype (genetic constitution) with environmental influences—*compare* genotype

photosynthesis: the process by which green plants and certain microorganisms transform light energy into chemical energy; in green plants the light energy of the sun is absorbed by the pigment chlorophyll and used to produce carbohydrates (as glucose) from carbon dioxide and water, with oxygen being released as a by-product of the process

placebo: an inactive or innocuous substance used in controlled studies to test the effects of an active substance (as a drug) by serving as a basis of comparison; may be prescribed to patients when it is believed their condition is psychological rather than physical—*see also* placebo effect

placebo effect: a change in a patient's condition that is due not to the specific treatment given but to other factors (as the patient's belief in the treatment's effectiveness)

plaque *1:* a patch of fatty material deposited on the lining of an artery that can eventually narrow the vessel and obstruct blood flow; *2:* a sticky film on the teeth that harbors bacteria and is a cause of tooth decay; *3:* a brain lesion that is characteristic of Alzheimer's disease—*see also* lesion

plasma: the fluid part of a liquid (as blood, lymph, or milk), as distinguished from suspended material; blood plasma consists of water and its dissolved constituents (as salts, sugars, fats, proteins, and hormones)—*compare* serum

platelet: a small colorless disk-shaped component of the blood that assists in blood clotting by adhering to other platelets and to damaged tissue

pneumothorax: an abnormal condition characterized by the presence of air in the pleural cavity (the space between the membranous sac lining the lungs and chest wall) and that may result in lung collapse due to compression; causes include a penetrating chest wound or complication of lung disease; in the past the condition was sometimes artificially induced as a treatment for tuberculosis

PNS: *see* peripheral nervous system

polymerase chain reaction (PCR): a technique for rapidly synthesizing large quantities of a specific sequence of DNA; involves separating the paired strands of DNA and binding a primer molecule to the targeted DNA region on each strand in order to provide a reaction site for the enzyme DNA polymerase to begin its process of repeated copying of the given DNA sequence—*see also* DNA

positron-emission tomography (PET): a diagnostic imaging technique that detects evidence of collisions between electrons (negatively charged particles) and positrons (positively charged particles) emitted by radioisotopes (radioactive forms of elements) in the body; produces three-dimensional images that reflect and characterize the biochemical activity of tissues

potassium: an essential mineral found in foods (as bananas, meats, and bran) that facilitates contraction of muscles and transmission of nerve impulses, helps regulate fluid balance in cells, and promotes the release of energy from carbohydrates, proteins, and fats

prevalence: the proportion of individuals in a given population who are affected by a given disease—*compare* incidence

prion: an abnormal form of a normal protein, implicated as the cause of various infectious diseases of the nervous system (as bovine spongiform encephalopathy, also known as "mad cow" disease); derived from the term *proteinaceous infectious particle—see also* protein

proband: an individual who is the first family member identified as being affected with an inherited trait and from whom the pedigree (ancestral lineage) is traced in a genetic investigation to discover the trait's pattern of inheritance—*also called* propositus

progestagen: *see* progestogen

progesterone: a female steroid hormone that functions primarily to prepare the uterine lining for implantation of a fertilized egg and during pregnancy to ensure proper function of the placenta; used in synthetic forms as an oral contraceptive, to treat menstrual disorders, and to alleviate some cases of infertility in women—*compare* estrogen, progestogen; *see also* steroid

progestin: *see* progestogen

progestogen: any of a group of natural or synthetic hormones with progesterone-like effects—*also spelled* progestagen; *also called* progestin; *see also* progesterone

programmed cell death: *see* apoptosis

propositus: *see* proband

prospective study: a research protocol in which subjects who are healthy or untreated are followed from the present into the future and monitored for the development of a particular illness or the effects of a particular treatment—*compare* retrospective study; *see also* protocol

protease inhibitor: any of a group of compounds that slow or interfere with the chemical decomposition of proteins; includes several recently introduced drugs that, in combination with other agents, are effective in reducing the circulating levels of virus in many individuals who are infected with HIV (the virus that causes AIDS)

protein: any of numerous combinations of amino acids that occur naturally in the body and are among the most essential components of living cells and tissues; examples of proteins include enzymes, antibodies, hemoglobin, and some hormones; proteins found in foods (as poultry, milk, fish, eggs, cheese, dried beans, and nuts) are broken down during digestion into component amino acids, which are absorbed by the body and used by cells to form other proteins essential for normal body function—*see also* amino acid

protocol: a precise plan detailing the procedures to be followed for providing medical treatment or care or for conducting a medical or scientific experiment or study

proto-oncogene: a gene that has the potential to become (as by mutation) a cancer-causing gene, or oncogene—*compare* oncogene; *see also* gene

proximate cause: an event or factor that directly produces a usually foreseeable effect (as an injury) that otherwise would not have occurred

pruritus: a sensation that provokes the urge to scratch; also, localized or generalized itching or a condition marked by such itching

pulmonary embolism: a potentially fatal blockage of the pulmonary artery (the vessel supplying blood to the lungs) or one of its branches in a lung by foreign matter, most often a blood clot originating in a vein of the leg or pelvis; symptoms include labored breathing, chest pain, and shock

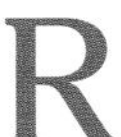

randomize: to select or assign in a chance way; in clinical trials, subjects are often randomized in test groups to minimize the effect of outside variables and reduce bias—*see also* clinical trial

receptor *1:* a protein molecule on or within a cell that selectively binds to various substances, including hormones, neurotransmitters, drugs, and viruses, and initiates specific cellular activity; *2:* any of the various sensory nerve endings in the skin, deep tissues, viscera, and sense organs (as the eyes or nose) that translate a stimulus into nerve impulses

red blood cell: any of the nonnucleated (lacking a nucleus) hemoglobin-containing cells of the human blood that transport oxygen to the tissues and are responsible for the red color of blood—*also called* erythrocyte; *compare* white blood cell; *see also* hemoglobin

retrospective study: a research protocol in which individuals who have a particular disorder are compared with unaffected individuals with respect to their previous exposure to a risk factor; also, research in which persons who have taken a particular drug or undergone a particular procedure in the past are compared with untreated individuals with respect to their present condition—*compare* prospective study; *see also* protocol

retrovirus: any of a group of viruses (as the AIDS-causing virus, HIV) that carry their genetic blueprint in the form of RNA and, by means of the enzyme reverse transcriptase, use RNA to synthesize DNA (a reversal of the process used by most other viruses and all cellular organisms); retroviruses include numerous tumor-causing viruses—*see also* DNA; RNA

ribonucleic acid: *see* RNA

risk factor: a characteristic (as an inherited trait) or circumstance (as an aspect of personal behavior or an environmental exposure) associated with an increased likelihood of developing a particular disease or condition

RNA (ribonucleic acid): a large molecule found in both the cell's nucleus and cytoplasm that plays a major role in the synthesis of protein; in the viruses known as retroviruses, RNA replaces DNA as the carrier of the genetic information—*see also* DNA

S

scourge: a cause of widespread or severe affliction; a destructive disease (as smallpox) that affects a large number of people over a broad geographic area

screening: testing of a population or group in order to detect a specific disease or calculate its prevalence—*see also* prevalence

serotonin: a natural chemical that constricts blood vessels, inhibits gastric secretion, stimulates smooth muscle, and serves as a neurotransmitter in the central nervous system; thought to be important in numerous neurological and psychiatric conditions—*also called* 5-HT; *see also* neurotransmitter

serum *1:* the clear watery fluid that moistens the surface of certain membranes (as the lining of the abdominal cavity) or is exuded when those membranes are inflamed; *2:* the clear yellowish fluid that separates from plasma when it clots—*compare* plasma

smallpox: a contagious, often fatal disease caused by a poxvirus (variola major) and typically characterized by sudden high fever, chills, and physical exhaustion followed by skin eruptions that progress from solid to fluid-filled to pus-containing lesions that scab and scar; a secondary strain of poxvirus (variola minor) causes a milder form of disease; no naturally acquired cases of smallpox have been reported since 1977

sodium: an element that functions within the body primarily to regulate fluid balance, transmit nerve impulses, and preserve the structural integrity and function of body cells; the most common sodium compound is sodium chloride (table salt)

spongiform encephalopathy: any of several degenerative disorders of the mammalian brain (as Creutzfeldt-Jakob disease in humans and "mad cow" disease in cattle) marked by the development of holes that give the brain tissue a porous, spongelike texture

stem cell: an unspecialized cell capable of giving rise to different types of cells

stenosis: a narrowing or constriction of a bodily passage or orifice (as a blood vessel or heart valve)

steroid: any of a large family of natural and synthetic substances comprising many hormones, vitamins, body constituents, and drugs (as cholesterol, corticosteroids, androgen, and estrogen) containing 17 carbon atoms arranged in four molecular rings and having various medical applications, including use as oral contraceptives, anti-inflammatory agents, and promoters of muscle growth and tissue regeneration—*see also* androgen; cholesterol; corticosteroid; estrogen

strain: a group of organisms (as subtypes of bacteria or laboratory mice) sharing or presumed to share similar structure or appearance but often having different physiology

stroke: a sudden neurological affliction usually caused by either rupture or obstruction of an artery that supplies blood to the brain; symptoms include dizziness, numbness, paralysis, impaired speech and vision, and confusion and may vary depending on the area of the brain that is damaged—*also called* cerebrovascular accident; *formerly called* apoplexy

sympathetic nervous system: the part of the autonomic nervous system that is concerned especially with preparing the body to react to situations of stress or emergency and that induces dilation of airways, sweating, increase in heart rate, relaxation of blood vessels in muscles, and inhibition of digestion; the neurotransmitters epinephrine and norepinephrine are the principal regulators of the system—*compare* autonomic nervous system; parasympathetic nervous system; central nervous system

synapse: the site where a nervous impulse is transmitted from one neuron to another by means of a chemical neurotransmitter—*see also* neurotransmitter

syngeneic: genetically identical especially with respect to antigens or immunologic reactions; identical twins are syngeneic—*compare* allogeneic; *see also* antigen

T

testosterone: a naturally occurring steroid hormone that is produced primarily in the testes (paired male reproductive organs producing sperm) and is the main androgen responsible for the development of the male sex organs and adult masculine characteristics—*see also* androgen; steroid

thalamus: the part of the brain that serves as a relay station to and from the cerebral cortex and functions especially in sensation and arousal.

therapeutic trial: *see* clinical trial

thrombolytic drug: an agent (as streptokinase or urokinase) that dissolves a thrombus (a blood clot formed in and attached to a blood vessel) and is used especially to treat myocardial infarction (heart attack), pulmonary embolism, and thrombosis of arteries (as those supplying the heart or brain) and deep-lying veins (as of the leg)—*see also* myocardial infarction; pulmonary embolism; thrombosis

thrombosis: the formation or presence of a clot within a blood vessel

tolerance: the ability to endure the effects of a drug or food or of a physiological insult without displaying the usual unfavorable effects; increased resistance to the usual effects of a drug due to continued use

trachea: a mucous-membrane-lined tube of fibrous and muscular tissue that is the airway, or main trunk of the respiratory system, by which air passes to and from the lungs; descends from the larynx and branches into the lungs' right and left bronchi—*also called* windpipe

transgenic: having chromosomes into which genes from another species have been incorporated either naturally or artificially

triglyceride: any of a group of lipids composed of one molecule of glycerol and three fatty acid molecules; triglycerides serve as energy reserves in fatty tissue and circulate in the blood in the form of lipoproteins—*see also* lipid; lipoprotein

U

ultrasound: a noninvasive and painless diagnostic technique that uses sound waves with frequencies above the audible range to produce a two-dimensional image; often used to examine and measure internal body structures and to detect bodily abnormalities; also used to reduce inflammation and accelerate healing in soft tissues (as muscles)

ultraviolet-A radiation (UVA): the long-wavelength radiation that is situated closest to the visible spectrum and that reaches the Earth's surface most often; responsible for tanning, sunburn, and other skin problems, including aging of the skin; not as damaging to the skin as ultraviolet-B radiation—*compare* ultraviolet-B radiation; *see also* ultraviolet radiation

ultraviolet-B radiation (UVB): the intermediate-wavelength radiation that reaches the Earth's surface only part of the time but when it does is the most damaging to the skin; responsible for sunburn and other skin damage, including cancer—*compare* ultraviolet-A radiation; *see also* ultraviolet radiation

ultraviolet light: *see* ultraviolet radiation

ultraviolet radiation: the radiation adjacent to the violet end of the visible spectrum that has a wavelength shorter than that of visible light and longer than that of X-rays; occurs naturally in sunlight—*also called* ultraviolet light; *see also* ultraviolet-A radiation; ultraviolet-B radiation

urticaria: an allergic reaction that is marked by transient itchy raised patches of skin that typically appear as white elevations surrounded by red inflammation and is most often triggered by food (as nuts and berries), drugs (as penicillin), or inhalants (as pollen) and less often by other factors, including exposure to heat, cold, or sunlight—*also called* hives

uterus: the muscular organ in female mammals that holds, protects, nourishes, and maintains the developing fetus—*also called* womb

UVA: *see* ultraviolet-A radiation

UVB: *see* ultraviolet-B radiation

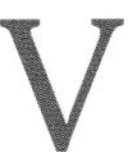

vaginal yeast infection: an infection of the female genital tract caused by the single-celled fungus *Candida albicans;* symptoms include a white vaginal discharge, inflammation, and irritation—*see also* yeast infection

vascular: supplied with or containing vessels and, especially, blood vessels

vasodilation: a widening of the interior hollow portion (lumen) of a blood vessel induced naturally by nerve impulses or artificially by drugs that relax smooth muscle

vector *1:* an organism (as a flea, mosquito, or mouse) that acts as a carrier, transmitting a disease-causing agent (as a parasite or virus) from an infected individual or source to an uninfected one; *2:* a sequence of genetic material into which foreign DNA is inserted for transport into a recipient host cell for the purpose of replicating additional foreign DNA; in the emerging field of human gene therapy, an inactivated retrovirus into which a therapeutic gene can be inserted for the possible cure of various diseases (as cystic fibrosis and some cancers)—*see also* parasite; retrovirus; virus

venous: made up of, carried on by, or occurring in the veins

ventricular fibrillation: rapid, irregular, and uncoordinated contraction of the heart's ventricles (lower chambers) that prevents the heart from pumping blood and results in fatal cessation of blood circulation; most commonly caused by myocardial infarction (heart attack)—*see also* myocardial infarction

ventricular tachycardia: abnormally rapid heartbeat that is generated by irregular electrical impulses originating within the heart's ventricles (lower chambers) and is usually caused by heart disease (as myocardial infarction or various abnormalities of the heart muscle)—*see also* myocardial infarction

viral load: the number of virus particles in a sample of blood plasma; used as a marker for disease progression in HIV (the virus that causes AIDS) infection

virus: a disease-causing agent that consists of genetic material (RNA or DNA) surrounded by a protein coat and, sometimes, an outer envelope composed of lipid and protein; capable of replicating only within a living host cell; more than 200 different viruses are known to cause disease in humans

visual acuity: the ability of the eye to resolve detail; a measure of the sharpness of vision

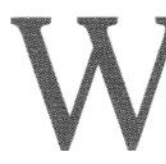

wasting: an unintended loss of weight and lean body tissue characteristic of many diseases, including cancer, tuberculosis, and AIDS

white blood cell: any of several kinds of white or colorless cells (as lymphocytes) of human blood that function in the immune defense system and tissue repair—*also called* leukocyte; *compare* red blood cell; *see also* lymphocyte

windpipe: *see* trachea

womb: *see* uterus

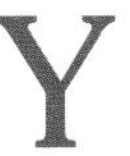

yeast infection: an infection caused by any of numerous single-celled fungi; can affect the skin, mouth, bloodstream, genitourinary tract, and virtually every organ system—*see also* vaginal yeast infection

yellow fever: a mosquito-borne viral infection, found primarily in tropical and subtropical regions, that is marked by rapid onset of headache, fever, nausea, vomiting, and bleeding: damage to the kidneys and liver may occur; in humans recovery is followed by lifetime immunity

Z

zeitgeber: an environmental factor (as sunlight or day length) that serves as a cue in regulating circadian rhythms—*see also* circadian

zoonosis (plural **zoonoses**): any disease that can be passed on to humans from a vertebrate animal host (as rabies, Lyme disease, and salmonellosis)

—prepared by Joan Narmontas, Associate Editor, Merriam-Webster, Incorporated

Index

This is a three-year cumulative index. Index entries to World of Medicine articles in this and previous editions of the *Medical and Health Annual* are set in boldface type, *e.g.,* **AIDS.** Entries to other subjects are set in lightface type, *e.g.,* alcohol. Additional information on any of these subjects is identified with a subheading and indented under the entry heading. The numbers following headings and subheadings indicate the year (boldface) of the edition and the page number (lightface) on which the information appears. The abbreviation *il.* indicates an illustration.

AIDS, *or* acquired immune deficiency syndrome **98**–146; **97**–164; **96**–268
  African-Americans **98**–150
  book reviews **97**–156
  emerging infectious diseases *map* **96**–247
  mortality and morbidity *table* **96**–250
  new FDA-approved drugs *table* **98**–315; **97**–330; **96**–409
alcohol
  aspirin interaction **97**–338
  bad breath cause **98**–311

All entry headings are alphabetized word by word. Hyphenated words and words separated by dashes or slashes are treated as two words. When one word differs from another only by the presence of additional characters at the end, the shorter precedes the longer. In inverted names, the words following the comma are considered only after the preceding part of the name has been alphabetized.
Examples:

Lake
Lake, Simon
Lake Charles
Lakeland

Names beginning with "Mc" and "Mac" are alphabetized as "Mac"; "St." is alphabetized as "Saint."

a

Dark-type numbers refer to the year of the edition, *e.g.*, **98–264** for the 1998 edition, page 264.

b

C

Dark-type numbers refer to the year of the edition, *e.g.*, **98**–264 for the 1998 edition, page 264.

d

Dark-type numbers refer to the year of the edition, *e.g.,* **98**–264 for the 1998 edition, page 264.

e

f

g

h

Dark-type numbers refer to the year of the edition, *e.g.,* **98**–264 for the 1998 edition, page 264.

i

j

k

Dark-type numbers refer to the year of the edition, *e.g.,* **98**–264 for the 1998 edition, page 264.

Dark-type numbers refer to the year of the edition, *e.g.*, **98**–264 for the 1998 edition, page 264.

O

Dark-type numbers refer to the year of the edition, *e.g.*, **98**–264 for the 1998 edition, page 264.

q

r

Dark-type numbers refer to the year of the edition, *e.g.*, **98**–264 for the 1998 edition, page 264.

Dark-type numbers refer to the year of the edition, *e.g.,* **98**–264 for the 1998 edition, page 264.

Dark-type numbers refer to the year of the edition, *e.g.*, **98**–264 for the 1998 edition, page 264.

t

u

Dark-type numbers refer to the year of the edition, *e.g.,* **98**–264 for the 1998 edition, page 264.

V

Dark-type numbers refer to the year of the edition, *e.g.*, **98**–264 for the 1998 edition, page 264.